Management of Temporomandibular Disorders and Occlusion

Sixth Edition

Jeffrey P. Okeson, DMD

Professor and Chair, Department of Oral Health Science
Director of the Orofacial Pain Center
College of Dentistry
University of Kentucky
Lexington, Kentucky

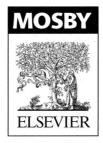

MOSBY

ELSEVIER

ELSEVIER
MOSBY

11830 Westline Industrial Drive
St. Louis, Missouri 63146

MANAGEMENT OF TEMPOROMANDIBULAR DISORDERS
AND OCCLUSION, EDITION 6

Notice

Knowledge and best practice in this field are constantly changing. As new research and experience broaden our knowledge, changes in practice, treatment, and drug therapy may become necessary or appropriate. Readers are advised to check the most current information provided (i) on procedures featured or (ii) by the manufacturer of each product to be administered, to verify the recommended dose or formula, the method and duration of administration, and contraindications. It is the responsibility of the practitioner, relying on his or her own experience and knowledge of the patient, to make diagnoses, to determine dosages and the best treatment for each individual patient, and to take all appropriate safety precautions. To the fullest extent of the law, neither the Publisher nor the Author assumes any liability for any injury and/or damage to persons or property arising out or related to any use of the material contained in this book.

The Publisher

Library of Congress Control Number: 2006940730

Senior Editor: John Dolan
Managing Editor: Jaime Pendill
Publishing Services Manager: Patricia Tannian
Senior Project Manager: Kristine Feeherty
Design Direction: Amy Buxton

Working together to grow libraries in developing countries

www.elsevier.com | www.bookaid.org | www.sabre.org

ELSEVIER   BOOK AID International   Sabre Foundation

Printed in the United States of America

Last digit is the print number: 9 8 7 6 5 4 3 2 1

This text is **personally** dedicated to my wife, Barbara,
for her continued unconditional love, support, and
understanding throughout my professional life,
and to my mother, Lois Okeson, and my father-in-law, Harold Boian,
for their many years of steadfast encouragement. I miss them greatly.

This text is **professionally** dedicated to all of our patients.
It is my hope that this text may in some
way help reduce their suffering.

About the Author
JEFFREY P. OKESON, DMD

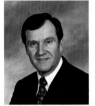

Dr. Okeson is a 1972 graduate of the University of Kentucky College of Dentistry. After graduation he completed two years with the Public Health Service in a rotating dental internship and direction of an out-patient clinic. He joined the faculty at the University of Kentucky in 1974. At present he is Professor, Chairman of the Department of Oral Health Science, and Director of the College's Orofacial Pain Center, which he established in 1977. The Center represents a multidisciplinary effort in the management of chronic orofacial pain problems. Dr. Okeson has developed several post-graduate training programs in the Center, including a Master of Science Degree in Orofacial Pain. Dr. Okeson has more than 200 professional publications in the areas of occlusion, temporomandibular disorders (TMDs), and orofacial pain in various national and international journals. Dr. Okeson's textbook, *Management of Temporomandibular Disorders and Occlusion*, is used in the majority of U.S. dental schools and has been translated into nine languages. In addition to this text, Dr. Okeson is also the author of *Bell's Orofacial Pains*. This text is also widely used in orofacial pain programs throughout the world.

Dr. Okeson is an active member of many TMD and orofacial pain organizations, holding many offices and serving on numerous commit-tees and boards. He is a past president and fellow of the American Academy of Orofacial Pain (AAOP). He is a founding diplomate and past president of the American Board of Orofacial Pain. He has been active in the AAOP, developing treatment and curriculum guidelines for TMDs and orofacial pain. He is the editor of the AAOP guidelines, titled *Orofacial Pain: Guidelines for Classification, Assessment, and Management*, Third Edition, which are used as treatment standards throughout the world. Dr. Okeson has presented more than 600 invited lectures on the subject of TMDs and orofacial pain in 48 states and 42 countries. At national and international meetings he is frequently referred to as "the world ambassador for orofacial pain." Dr. Okeson has received several teaching awards from his dental students, as well as the University of Kentucky Great Teacher Award. He is also the first-ever recipient of the Distinguished Alumni Award from the College of Dentistry.

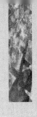

The study of occlusion and its relationship to function of the masticatory system has been a topic of interest in dentistry for many years. This relationship has proved to be quite complex. Tremendous interest in this area accompanied by lack of complete knowledge has stimulated numerous concepts, theories, and treatment methods. This, of course, has led to much confusion in an already complicated field of study. Although the level of knowledge today is greater than ever before, there is still much to learn. Some of today's techniques will prove to be our most effective treatments in the future. Other methods will be demonstrated as ineffective and will have to be discarded. Competent and caring practitioners must establish their treatment methods based on both their present knowledge and their constant evaluation of information received from the massive amount of ongoing research. This is an enormous task. I hope that this text will assist students, teachers, and practitioners in making these important treatment decisions for their patients.

I began my teaching career at the University of Kentucky in 1974 in the area of occlusion. At that time I believed there was a need for a teaching manual that presented the topics of occlusion and temporomandibular disorders (TMDs) in an organized, logical, and scientific manner. In 1975 I developed such a manual to assist in teaching my dental students. Soon, several other dental schools requested use of this manual for their teaching programs. In 1983 the CV Mosby Publishing Company approached me with the concept of developing this manual into a complete textbook. After two years of writing and editing, the first edition was published in 1985. I am very pleased and humbled to learn that this text is currently being used in most of the dental schools in the United States and has been translated into numerous foreign languages for use abroad. This is professionally very satisfying,

and it is my hope that the true benefit of this text is found in the improved quality of care we offer our patients.

It is a privilege to once again have the opportunity to update this text. I have tried to include the most significant scientific findings that have been revealed in the past 4 years. I believe the strength of a textbook lies not in the author's words but in the scientific references that are offered to support the ideas presented. Unreferenced ideas should be considered only opinions that require further scientific investigation to either verify or negate them. It is extremely difficult to keep a textbook updated, especially in a field in which so much is happening so quickly. Twenty-eight years ago, in the first edition of this text, I referenced approximately 450 articles to support the statements and ideas. The concepts in this edition are supported by nearly 2200 scientific references. This reflects the significant scientific growth of this field. It should be acknowledged that as future truths are uncovered, the professional has the obligation to appropriately respond with changes that best reflect the new information. These changes are sometimes difficult for the clinician because they may reflect the need to change clinical protocol. However, the best care for our patients rests in the most scientifically supported information.

The purpose of this text is to present a logical and practical approach to the study of occlusion and masticatory function. The text is divided into four main sections: The first part consists of six chapters that present the normal anatomic and physiologic features of the masticatory system. Understanding normal occlusal relationships and masticatory function is essential to understanding dysfunction. The second part consists of four chapters that present the etiology and identification of common functional disturbances of the masticatory system. Significant supportive documentation has been included in this edition. The third part consists of six chapters that present rational treatments for these disorders according to the significant etiologic factors. Recent studies have been added to support existing treatments, as well as for new considerations. The last part consists of four chapters that present specific considerations for permanent occlusal therapy.

The intent of this text is to develop an understanding of, and rational approach to, the study of masticatory function and occlusion. To assist the reader, certain techniques have been presented. It should be recognized that the purpose of a technique is to achieve certain treatment goals. Accomplishing these goals is the significant factor, not the technique itself. Any technique that achieves the treatment goals is acceptable as long as it does so in a reasonably conservative, cost-effective manner, with the best interests of the patient kept in mind.

ACKNOWLEDGMENTS

A text such as this is never accomplished by the work of one person, but rather represents the accumulation of many who have gone before. The efforts of these individuals have led to the present state of knowledge in the field. To acknowledge each of these would be an impossible task. The multiple listing of references at the end of each chapter begins to recognize the true work behind this text. There are, however, a few individuals whom I feel both obligated and pleased to acknowledge. First and foremost is Dr. Weldon E. Bell. Although we lost this giant in 1990, he remains my mentor to this day. He was the epitome of an outstanding thinker, information simulator, and teacher. Within the seven texts he wrote on TMD and orofacial pain lies enough information to keep a normal man thinking forever. He was a very special man, and I sorely miss him still.

I would like to thank Dr. Terry Tanaka of San Diego, California, for generously sharing his knowledge with me. Over the years I have come to value Terry's professional and personal friendship more and more. His anatomic dissections have contributed greatly to the profession's understanding of the functional anatomy of our complex masticatory system.

I would like to thank my colleague, Charles Carlson, PhD, for all that he has taught me regarding the psychology of pain. Charley and I have worked together for nearly 20 years in our Orofacial Pain Center, and I have seen him develop and successfully document his concepts of physical self-regulation. These techniques have helped many of our chronic pain patients. He has generously shared his ideas and concepts in Chapter 11.

I would also like to thank the following individuals for allowing me to use some of their professional materials and insights in this text: Dr. Per-Lennart Westesson, University of Rochester; the late Dr. Julio Turell, University of Montevideo, Uruguay; and Dr. Jay Mackman, Milwaukee, Wisconsin.

I need to also thank all of my residents at the University of Kentucky, both past and present, for keeping me alert, focused, and searching for the truth.

Last, but by no means least, I wish to express my gratitude to my family for their constant love, support, encouragement, and sacrifice during my writings. My mother and father inspired and encouraged me from the very beginning. My sons have understood the time commitment, and my wife has given up many evenings to my computer. I have been blessed with a wonderful, loving wife for 37 years, and her sacrifice has resulted in this textbook.

Jeffrey P. Okeson

Contents

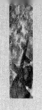

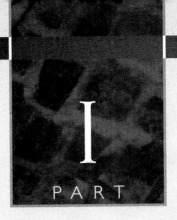

Functional Anatomy

The masticatory system is extremely complex. It is made up primarily of bones, muscles, ligaments, and teeth. Movement is regulated by an intricate neurologic control system composed of the brain, brainstem, and peripheral nervous system. Each movement is coordinated to maximize function while minimizing damage to any structure. Precise movement of the mandible by the musculature is required to move the teeth efficiently across each other during function. The mechanics and physiology of this movement are basic to the study of masticatory function. Part I consists of six chapters that discuss the normal anatomy, function, and mechanics of the masticatory system. Function must be understood before dysfunction can have meaning.

Functional Anatomy and Biomechanics of the Masticatory System

"Nothing is more fundamental to treating patients than knowing the anatomy."

—JPO

The masticatory system is the functional unit of the body primarily responsible for chewing, speaking, and swallowing. Components also play a major role in tasting and breathing. The system is made up of bones, joints, ligaments, teeth, and muscles. In addition, an intricate neurologic controlling system regulates and coordinates all these structural components.

The masticatory system is a complex and highly refined unit. A sound understanding of its functional anatomy and biomechanics is essential to the study of occlusion. This chapter describes the anatomic features that are basic to an understanding of masticatory function. A more detailed description can be found in the numerous texts devoted entirely to the anatomy of the head and neck.

FUNCTIONAL ANATOMY

The following anatomic components are discussed in this chapter: the dentition and supportive structures, the skeletal components, the temporomandibular joints (TMJs), the ligaments, and the muscles. After the anatomic features are described, the biomechanics of the TMJ are presented. In Chapter 2, the complex neurologic controlling system is described and the physiology of the masticatory system is presented.

DENTITION AND SUPPORTIVE STRUCTURES

The human dentition is made up of 32 permanent teeth (Fig. 1-1). Each tooth can be divided into two basic parts: the crown, which is visible above the gingival tissue, and the root, which is submerged in and surrounded by the alveolar bone. The root is attached to the alveolar bone by numerous fibers of connective tissue that span from the cementum surface of the root to the bone. Most of these fibers run obliquely from the cementum in a cervical direction to the bone (Fig. 1-2). These fibers are known collectively as the *periodontal ligament*. The periodontal ligament not only attaches the tooth firmly to its bony socket but also helps dissipate the forces applied to the bone during functional contact of the teeth. In this sense it can be thought of as a natural shock absorber.

The 32 permanent teeth are distributed equally in the alveolar bone of the maxillary and mandibular arches: 16 maxillary teeth are aligned in the alveolar process of the maxilla, which is fixed to the lower anterior portion of the skull; the remaining 16 teeth are aligned in the alveolar process of the mandible, which is the movable jaw. The maxillary arch is slightly larger than the mandibular arch, which usually causes the maxillary teeth to overlap the mandibular teeth both vertically and horizontally when in occlusion (Fig. 1-3). This size discrepancy results primarily from the fact that (1) the maxillary anterior teeth are much wider than the mandibular teeth, which creates a greater

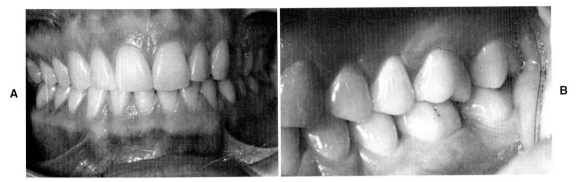

Fig. 1-1 Anterior **(A)** and lateral **(B)** views of the dentition.

arch width, and (2) the maxillary anterior teeth have a greater facial angulation than the mandibular anterior teeth, which creates a horizontal and vertical overlapping.

The permanent teeth can be grouped into four classifications as follows according to the morphology of the crowns.

The teeth located in the most anterior region of the arches are called *incisors*. They have a characteristic shovel shape, with an incisal edge. Four maxillary incisors and four mandibular incisors exist. The maxillary incisors are generally much larger than the mandibular incisors and, as previously mentioned, commonly overlap them. The function of the incisors is to incise or cut off food during mastication.

Posterior (distal) to the incisors are the *canines*. The canines are located at the corners of the arches and are generally the longest of the permanent teeth, with a single cusp and root (Fig. 1-4). These teeth are prominent in other animals such as dogs, and hence the name "canine." Two maxillary and two mandibular canines exist. In animals the primary function of the canines is to rip and tear food. In the human dentition, however, the canines usually function as incisors and are used only occasionally for ripping and tearing.

Still more posterior in the arch are the *premolars* (see Fig. 1-4). Four maxillary and four mandibular premolars exist. The premolars are also called *bicuspids* because they generally have two cusps. The presence of two cusps greatly increases the biting

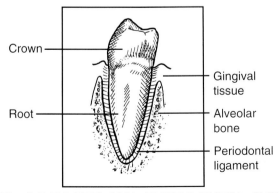

Crown —

Root —

Gingival tissue

Alveolar bone

Periodontal ligament

Fig. 1-2 TOOTH AND PERIODONTAL SUPPORTIVE STRUCTURES. The width of the periodontal ligament is greatly exaggerated for illustrative purposes.

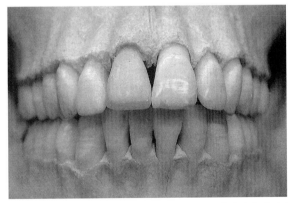

Fig. 1-3 The maxillary teeth are positioned slightly facial to the mandibular throughout the arch.

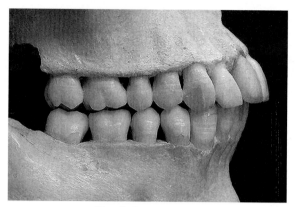

Fig. 1-4 Lateral view.

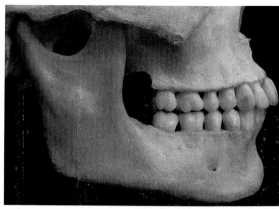

Fig. 1-5 Skeletal components that make up the masticatory system: maxilla, mandible, and temporal bone.

surfaces of these teeth. The maxillary and mandibular premolars occlude in such a manner that food can be caught and crushed between them. The main function of the premolars is to begin the effective breakdown of food substances into smaller particle sizes.

The last class of teeth, found posterior to the premolars, is the *molars* (see Fig. 1-4). Six maxillary molars and six mandibular molars exist. The crown of each molar has either four or five cusps. This provides a large, broad surface on which breaking and grinding of food can occur. Molars function primarily in the later stages of chewing, when food is broken down into particles small enough to be easily swallowed.

As discussed, each tooth is highly specialized according to its function. The exact interarch and intraarch relationships of the teeth are extremely important and greatly influence the health and function of the masticatory system. A detailed discussion of these relationships is presented in Chapter 3.

SKELETAL COMPONENTS

The masticatory system comprises three major skeletal components. Two support the teeth: the maxilla and mandible (Fig. 1-5). The third, the temporal bone, supports the mandible at its articulation with the cranium.

Maxilla

Developmentally, there are two maxillary bones, which are fused together at the midpalatal suture (Fig. 1-6). These bones make up the greater part of the upper facial skeleton. The border of the maxilla extends superiorly to form the floor of the nasal cavity, as well as the floor of each orbit. Inferiorly, the maxillary bones form the palate and the alveolar ridges, which support the teeth. Because the maxillary bones are intricately fused to the surrounding bony components of the skull, the maxillary teeth are considered to be a fixed part of the skull and therefore comprise the stationary component of the masticatory system.

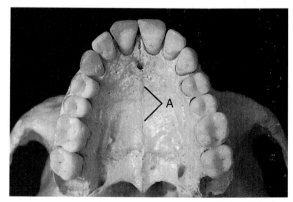

Fig. 1-6 The midpalatal suture *(A)* results from the fusion of the two maxillary bones during development.

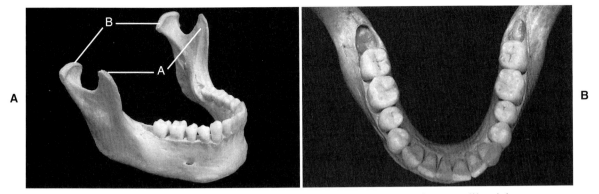

Fig. 1-7 A, The ascending ramus extends upward to form the coronoid process *(A)* and the condyle *(B)*. **B,** Occlusal view.

Mandible

The mandible is a U-shaped bone that supports the lower teeth and makes up the lower facial skeleton. It has no bony attachments to the skull. It is suspended below the maxilla by muscles, ligaments, and other soft tissues, which therefore provide the mobility necessary to function with the maxilla.

The superior aspect of the arch-shaped mandible consists of the alveolar process and the teeth (Fig. 1-7). The body of the mandible extends posteroinferiorly to form the mandibular angle and posterosuperiorly to form the ascending ramus. The ascending ramus of the mandible is formed by a vertical plate of bone that extends upward as two processes. The anterior of these is the coronoid process. The posterior is the condyle.

The condyle is the portion of the mandible that articulates with the cranium, around which movement occurs. From the anterior view it has medial and lateral projections, called *poles* (Fig. 1-8). The medial pole is generally more prominent than the lateral. From above, a line drawn through the centers of the poles of the condyle will usually extend medially and posteriorly toward the anterior border of the foramen magnum (Fig. 1-9). The total mediolateral length of the condyle is between 18 and 23 mm, and the anteroposterior width is between 8 and 10 mm. The actual articulating

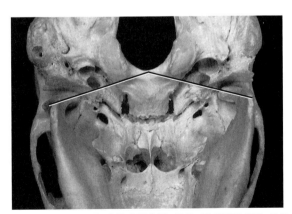

Fig. 1-9 INFERIOR VIEW OF SURFACE OF CRANIUM AND MANDIBLE. The condyles seem to be slightly rotated such that an imaginary line drawn through the lateral and medial poles would extend medially and posteriorly toward the anterior border of the foramen magnum.

Fig. 1-8 CONDYLE (ANTERIOR VIEW). The medial pole *(MP)* is more prominent than the lateral pole *(LP)*.

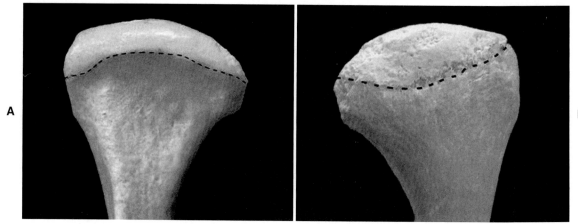

Fig. 1-10 CONDYLE. A, Anterior view. **B,** Posterior view. A dotted line marks the border of the articular surface. The articular surface on the posterior aspect of the condyle is greater than on the anterior aspect.

surface of the condyle extends both anteriorly and posteriorly to the most superior aspect of the condyle (Fig. 1-10). The posterior articulating surface is greater than the anterior surface. The articulating surface of the condyle is quite convex anteroposteriorly and only slightly convex mediolaterally.

Temporal Bone

The mandibular condyle articulates at the base of the cranium with the squamous portion of the temporal bone. This portion of the temporal bone is made up of a concave mandibular fossa, in which the condyle is situated (Fig. 1-11) and which has also

been called the *articular* or *glenoid fossa.* Posterior to the mandibular fossa is the squamotympanic fissure, which extends mediolaterally. As this fissure extends medially, it divides into the petrosquamous fissure anteriorly and the petrotympanic fissure posteriorly. Immediately anterior to the fossa is a convex bony prominence called the *articular eminence.* The degree of convexity of the articular eminence is highly variable but important because the steepness of this surface dictates the pathway of the condyle when the mandible is positioned anteriorly. The posterior roof of the mandibula fossa is quite thin, indicating that this area of the temporal bone is not designed to

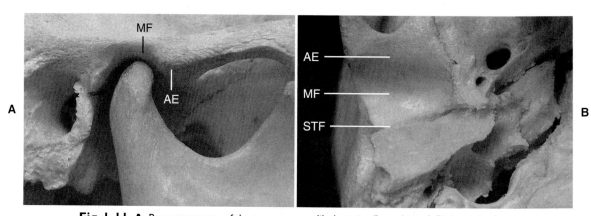

Fig. 1-11 A, Bony structures of the temporomandibular joint (lateral view). **B,** Articular fossa (inferior view). *AE,* Articular eminence; *MF,* mandibular fossa; *STF,* squamotympanic fissure.

sustain heavy forces. The articular eminence, however, consists of thick dense bone and is more likely to tolerate such forces.)

TEMPOROMANDIBULAR JOINT

The area where the mandible articulates with the cranium, the TMJ, is one of the most complex joints in the body. It provides for hinging movement in one plane and therefore can be considered a ginglymoid joint. However, at the same time it also provides for gliding movements, which classifies it as an arthrodial joint. Thus it has been technically considered a *ginglymoarthrodial joint*.

The TMJ is formed by the mandibular condyle fitting into the mandibular fossa of the temporal bone. Separating these two bones from direct articulation is the articular disc. The TMJ is classified as a compound joint. By definition, a compound joint requires the presence of at least three bones, yet the TMJ is made up of only two bones. Functionally, the articular disc serves as a nonossified bone that permits the complex movements of the joint. Because the articular disc functions as a third bone, the craniomandibular articulation is considered a compound joint. The function of the articular disc as a nonossified bone is described in detail in the section on the biomechanics of the TMJ later in this chapter.

The articular disc is composed of dense fibrous connective tissue, for the most part devoid of any blood vessels or nerve fibers. The extreme periphery of the disc, however, is slightly innervated.[1,2] In the sagittal plane it can be divided into three regions according to thickness (Fig. 1-12). The central area is the thinnest and is called the *intermediate zone*. The disc becomes considerably thicker both anterior and posterior to the intermediate zone. The posterior border is generally slightly thicker than the anterior border. In the normal joint the articular surface of the condyle is located on the intermediate zone of the disc, bordered by the thicker anterior and posterior regions.

From an anterior view, the disc is generally thicker medially than laterally, which corresponds to the increased space between the condyle and the articular fossa toward the medial of the joint (Fig. 1-13). The precise shape of the disc is

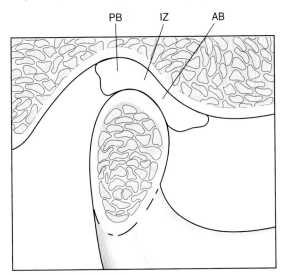

Fig. 1-12 ARTICULAR DISC, FOSSA, AND CONDYLE (LATERAL VIEW). The condyle is normally situated on the thinner intermediate zone *(IZ)* of the disc. The anterior border of the disc *(AB)* is considerably thicker than the intermediate zone, and the posterior border *(PB)* is even thicker.

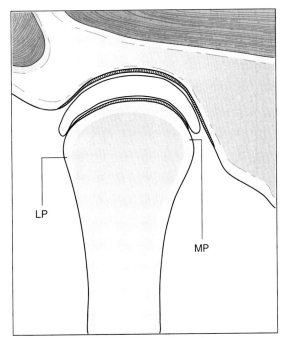

Fig. 1-13 ARTICULAR DISC, FOSSA, AND CONDYLE (ANTERIOR VIEW). The disc is slightly thicker medially than laterally. *LP,* Lateral pole; *MP,* medial pole.

determined by the morphology of the condyle and mandibular fossa. During movement the disc is somewhat flexible and can adapt to the functional demands of the articular surfaces. Flexibility and adaptability do not imply that the morphology of the disc is reversibly altered during function, however. The disc maintains its morphology unless destructive forces or structural changes occur in the joint. If these changes occur, the morphology of the disc can be irreversibly altered, producing

biomechanical changes during function. These changes are discussed in later chapters.

The articular disc is attached posteriorly to a region of loose connective tissue that is highly vascularized and innervated (Fig. 1-14). This is known as the *retrodiscal tissue* or posterior attachment. Superiorly, it is bordered by a lamina of connective tissue that contains many elastic fibers, the superior retrodiscal lamina. The superior retrodiscal lamina attaches the articular disc posteriorly to

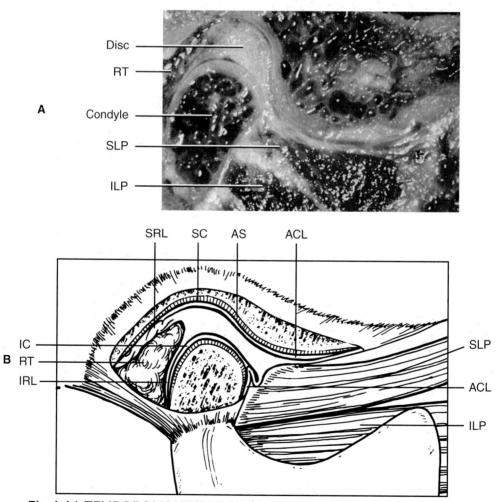

Fig. 1-14 TEMPOROMANDIBULAR JOINT. A, Lateral view. **B,** Diagram showing the anatomic components. *ACL,* Anterior capsular ligament (collagenous); *AS,* articular surface; *IC,* inferior joint cavity; *ILP,* inferior lateral pterygoid muscles; *IRL,* inferior retrodiscal lamina (collagenous); *RT,* retrodiscal tissues; *SC,* superior joint cavity; *SLP,* superior lateral pterygoid muscles; *SRL,* superior retrodiscal lamina (elastic). The discal (collateral) ligament has not been drawn. (**A,** *Courtesy Dr. Julio Turell, University of Montevideo, Uruguay.*)

the tympanic plate. At the lower border of the retrodiscal tissues is the inferior retrodiscal lamina, which attaches the inferior border of the posterior edge of the disc to the posterior margin of the articular surface of the condyle. The inferior retrodiscal lamina is composed chiefly of collagenous fibers, not elastic fibers like the superior retrodiscal lamina. The remaining body of the retrodiscal tissue is attached posteriorly to a large venous plexus, which fills with blood as the condyle moves forward.[3,4] The superior and inferior attachments of the anterior region of the disc are to the capsular ligament, which surrounds most of the joint. The superior attachment is to the anterior margin of the articular surface of the temporal bone. The inferior attachment is to the anterior margin of the articular surface of the condyle. Both these anterior attachments are composed of collagenous fibers. Anteriorly, between the attachments of the capsular ligament, the disc is also attached by tendinous fibers to the superior lateral pterygoid muscle.

The articular disc is attached to the capsular ligament not only anteriorly and posteriorly but also medially and laterally. This divides the joint into two distinct cavities. The upper or superior cavity is bordered by the mandibular fossa and the superior surface of the disc. The lower or inferior cavity is bordered by the mandibular condyle and the inferior surface of the disc. The internal surfaces of the cavities are surrounded by specialized endothelial cells that form a synovial lining. This lining, along with a specialized synovial fringe located at the anterior border of the retrodiscal tissues, produces synovial fluid, which fills both joint cavities. Thus the TMJ is referred to as a *synovial joint*. This synovial fluid serves two purposes. Because the articular surfaces of the joint are nonvascular, the synovial fluid acts as a medium for providing metabolic requirements to these tissues. Free and rapid exchange exists between the vessels of the capsule, the synovial fluid, and the articular tissues. The synovial fluid also serves as a lubricant between articular surfaces during function. The articular surfaces of the disc, condyle, and fossa are very smooth, so friction during movement is minimized. The synovial fluid helps to minimize this friction further.

Synovial fluid lubricates the articular surfaces by way of two mechanisms. The first is called *boundary* lubrication, which occurs when the joint is moved and the synovial fluid is forced from one area of the cavity into another. The synovial fluid located in the border or recess areas is forced on the articular surface, thus providing lubrication. Boundary lubrication prevents friction in the moving joint and is the primary mechanism of joint lubrication.

A second lubricating mechanism is called *weeping* lubrication. This refers to the ability of the articular surfaces to absorb a small amount of synovial fluid.[5] During function of a joint, forces are created between the articular surfaces. These forces drive a small amount of synovial fluid in and out of the articular tissues. This is the mechanism by which metabolic exchange occurs. Under compressive forces, therefore, a small amount of synovial fluid is released. This synovial fluid acts as a lubricant between articular tissues to prevent sticking. Weeping lubrication helps eliminate friction in the compressed but not moving joint. Only a small amount of friction is eliminated as a result of weeping lubrication; therefore prolonged compressive forces to the articular surfaces will exhaust this supply. The consequence of prolonged static loading of the joint structures is discussed in later chapters.

Histology of the Articular Surfaces

The articular surfaces of the mandibular condyle and fossa are composed of four distinct layers or zones (Fig. 1-15). The most superficial layer is called the *articular zone*. It is found adjacent to the joint cavity and forms the outermost functional surface. Unlike most other synovial joints, this articular layer is made of dense fibrous connective tissue rather than hyaline cartilage. Most of the collagen fibers are arranged in bundles and oriented nearly parallel to the articular surface.[6,7] The fibers are tightly packed and can withstand the forces of movement. It is thought that this fibrous connective tissue affords the joint several advantages over hyaline cartilage. Because fibrous connective tissue is generally less susceptible than hyaline cartilage to the effects of aging, it is less likely to break down over time. It also has a much

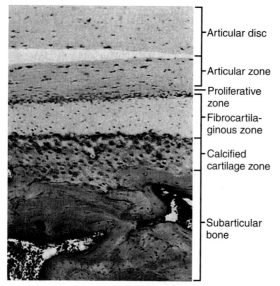

Articular disc

Articular zone

Proliferative zone

Fibrocartilaginous zone

Calcified cartilage zone

Subarticular bone

Fig. 1-15 Histologic section of a healthy mandibular condyle showing the four zones: articular, proliferative, fibrocartilaginous, and calcified. *(From Cohen B, Kramer IRH, editors: Scientific foundations of dentistry, London, 1976, William Heinemann.).*

evacuated, forming bone cells from within the medullary cavity. The surface of the extracellular matrix scaffolding provides an active site for remodeling activity while endosteal bone growth proceeds, as it does elsewhere in the body.

The articular cartilage is composed of chondrocytes and intercellular matrix.[9] The chondrocytes produce the collagen, proteoglycans, glycoproteins, and enzymes that form the matrix. Proteoglycans are complex molecules composed of a protein core and glycosaminoglycan chains. The proteoglycans are connected to a hyaluronic acid chain forming proteoglycan aggregates that make up a great protein of the matrix (Fig. 1-16). These aggregates are very hydrophilic and are intertwined throughout the collagen network. Because these aggregates tend to blind water, the matrix expands and the tension in the collagen fibrils counteracts the swelling pressure of the proteoglycan aggregates.[10] In this way the interstitial fluid contributes to support joint loading. The external pressure resulting from joint loading is in equilibrium with the internal pressure of the articular cartilage. As joint loading increases, tissue fluid flows outward until a new

better ability to repair than does hyaline cartilage.[8] The importance of these two factors is significant in TMJ function and dysfunction and is discussed more completely in later chapters.

The second zone, the *proliferative zone*, is mainly cellular. It is in this area that undifferentiated mesenchymal tissue is found. This tissue is responsible for the proliferation of articular cartilage in response to the functional demands placed on the articular surfaces during loading.

In the third zone, the *fibrocartilaginous zone*, the collagen fibrils are arranged in bundles in a crossing pattern, although some of the collagen is seen in a radial orientation. The fibrocartilage appears to be in a random orientation, providing a three-dimensional network that offers resistance against compressive and lateral forces.

The fourth and deepest zone is called the *calcified cartilage zone*. This zone comprises chondrocytes and chondroblasts distributed throughout the articular cartilage. In this zone the chondrocytes become hypertrophic, die, and have their cytoplasm

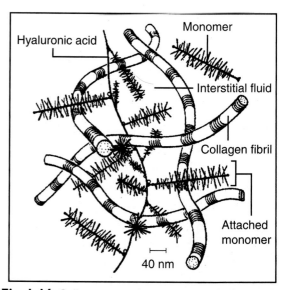

Hyaluronic acid

Monomer

Interstitial fluid

Collagen fibril

Attached monomer

40 nm

Fig. 1-16 Collagen network interacting with the proteoglycan network in the extracellular matrix forming a fiber reinforced composite. *(From Mow VC, Ratcliffe A: Cartilage and diarthrodial joints as paradigms for hierarchical materials and structures, Biomaterials 13:67-81, 1992.)*

equilibrium is achieved. As loading is decreased, fluid is reabsorbed and the tissue regains its original volume. Joint cartilage is nourished predominantly by diffusion of synovial fluid, which depends on this pumping action during normal activity.[11] This pumping action is the basis for the weeping lubrication that was discussed previously and is thought to be important in maintaining healthy articular cartilage.[12]

Innervation of the Temporomandibular Joint

As with all joints, the TMJ is innervated by the same nerve that provides motor and sensory innervation to the muscles that control it (the trigeminal nerve). Branches of the mandibular nerve provide the afferent innervation. Most innervation is provided by the auriculotemporal nerve as it leaves the mandibular nerve behind the joint and ascends laterally and superiorly to wrap around the posterior region of the joint.[13] Additional innervation is provided by the deep temporal and masseteric nerves.

Vascularization of the Temporomandibular Joint

The TMJ is richly supplied by a variety of vessels that surround it. The predominant vessels are the superficial temporal artery from the posterior; the middle meningeal artery from the anterior; and the internal maxillary artery from the inferior. Other important arteries are the deep auricular, anterior tympanic, and ascending pharyngeal arteries. The condyle receives its vascular supply through its marrow spaces by way of the inferior alveolar artery and also receives vascular supply by way of "feeder vessels" that enter directly into the condylar head both anteriorly and posteriorly from the larger vessels.[14]

LIGAMENTS

As with any joint system, ligaments play an important role in protecting the structures. The ligaments of the joint are composed of collagenous connective tissues that have particular lengths. They do not stretch. However, if extensive forces are applied to a ligament, whether suddenly or over a prolonged period of time, the ligament can be elongated. When this occurs, the function of

the ligament is compromised, thereby altering joint function. This alteration is discussed in future chapters that discuss pathology of the joint.

Ligaments do not enter actively into joint function but instead act as passive restraining devices to limit and restrict border movements. Three functional ligaments support the TMJ: (1) the collateral ligaments, (2) the capsular ligament, and (3) the temporomandibular (TM) ligament. Two accessory ligaments also exist: (4) the sphenomandibular and (5) the stylomandibular.

Collateral (Discal) Ligaments

The collateral ligaments attach the medial and lateral borders of the articular disc to the poles of the condyle. They are commonly called the *discal ligaments*, and there are two. The medial discal ligament attaches the medial edge of the disc to the medial pole of the condyle. The lateral discal ligament attaches the lateral edge of the disc to the lateral pole of the condyle (see Figs. 1-14 and 1-17).

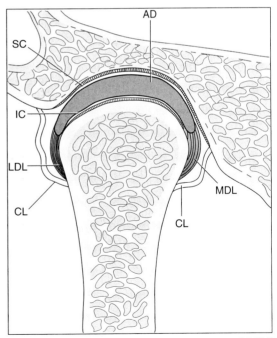

Fig. 1-17 TEMPOROMANDIBULAR JOINT (ANTERIOR VIEW). *AD,* Articular disc; *CL,* capsular ligament; *IC,* inferior joint cavity; *LDL,* lateral discal ligament; *MDL,* medial discal ligament; *SC,* superior joint cavity.

These ligaments are responsible for dividing the joint mediolaterally into the superior and inferior joint cavities. The discal ligaments are true ligaments, composed of collagenous connective tissue fibers; therefore they do not stretch. They function to restrict movement of the disc away from the condyle. In other words, they allow the disc to move passively with the condyle as it glides anteriorly and posteriorly. The attachments of the discal ligaments permit the disc to be rotated anteriorly and posteriorly on the articular surface of the condyle. Thus these ligaments are responsible for the hinging movement of the TMJ, which occurs between the condyle and the articular disc.

The discal ligaments have a vascular supply and are innervated. Their innervation provides information regarding joint position and movement. Strain on these ligaments produces pain.

Capsular Ligament

As previously mentioned, the entire TMJ is surrounded and encompassed by the capsular ligament (Fig. 1-18). The fibers of the capsular ligament are attached superiorly to the temporal bone along the borders of the articular surfaces of the mandibular fossa and articular eminence. Inferiorly, the fibers of the capsular ligament attach to the neck of the condyle. The capsular ligament acts to resist any medial, lateral, or inferior forces that tend to separate or dislocate the articular surfaces. A significant function of the capsular ligament is to encompass the joint, thus retaining the synovial fluid. The capsular ligament is well innervated and provides proprioceptive feedback regarding position and movement of the joint.

Temporomandibular Ligament

The lateral aspect of the capsular ligament is reinforced by strong, tight fibers that make up the lateral ligament, or TM ligament. The TM ligament is composed of two parts, an outer oblique portion and an inner horizontal portion (Fig. 1-19). The outer portion extends from the outer surface of the articular tubercle and zygomatic process posteroinferiorly to the outer surface of the condylar neck. The inner horizontal portion extends from the outer surface of the articular tubercle and zygomatic process posteriorly and horizontally to the lateral pole of the condyle and posterior part of the articular disc.

The oblique portion of the TM ligament resists excessive dropping of the condyle, therefore limiting the extent of mouth opening. This portion of the ligament also influences the normal opening movement of the mandible. During the initial phase of opening, the condyle can rotate around a fixed point until the TM ligament becomes tight as its point of insertion on the neck of the condyle is rotated posteriorly. When the ligament is taut, the neck of the condyle cannot rotate further. If the

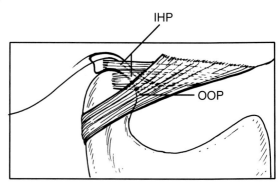

Fig. 1-19 TEMPOROMANDIBULAR LIGAMENT (LATERAL VIEW). Two distinct parts are shown: the outer oblique portion *(OOP)* and the inner horizontal portion *(IHP)*. The OOP limits normal rotational opening movement; the IHP limits posterior movement of the condyle and disc. *(Modified from Du Brul EL: Sicher's oral anatomy, ed 7, St Louis, 1980, Mosby.)*

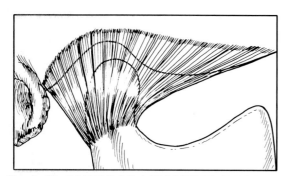

Fig. 1-18 CAPSULAR LIGAMENT (LATERAL VIEW). Note that it extends anteriorly to include the articular eminence and encompass the entire articular surface of the joint.

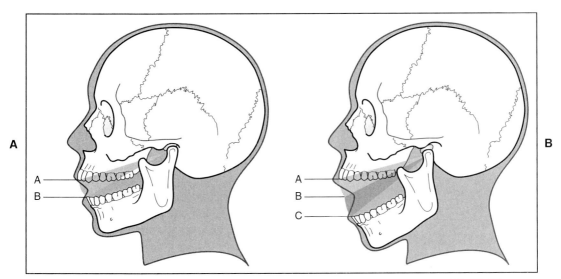

Fig. 1-20 EFFECT OF THE OUTER OBLIQUE PORTION OF THE TEMPOROMANDIBULAR (TM) LIGAMENT. A, As the mouth opens, the teeth can be separated about 20 to 25 mm (from A to B) without the condyles moving from the fossae. **B,** TM ligaments are fully extended. As the mouth opens wider, they force the condyles to move downward and forward out of the fossae. This creates a second arc of opening (from B to C).

mouth were to be opened wider, the condyle would need to move downward and forward across the articular eminence (Fig. 1-20). This effect can be demonstrated clinically by closing the mouth and applying mild posterior force to the chin. With this force applied, the patient should be asked to open the mouth. The jaw will easily rotate open until the teeth are 20 to 25 mm apart. At this point, resistance will be felt when the jaw is opened wider. If the jaw is opened still wider, a distinct change in the opening movement will occur, representing the change from rotation of the condyle around a fixed point to movement forward and down the articular eminence. This change in opening movement is brought about by the tightening of the TM ligament.

This unique feature of the TM ligament, which limits rotational opening, is found only in humans. In the erect postural position and with a vertically placed vertebral column, continued rotational opening movement would cause the mandible to impinge on the vital submandibular and retromandibular structures of the neck. The outer oblique portion of the TM ligament functions to resist this impingement.

The inner horizontal portion of the TM ligament limits posterior movement of the condyle and disc. When force applied to the mandible displaces the condyle posteriorly, this portion of the ligament becomes tight and prevents the condyle from moving into the posterior region of the mandibular fossa. The TM ligament therefore protects the retrodiscal tissues from trauma created by the posterior displacement of the condyle. The inner horizontal portion also protects the lateral pterygoid muscle from overlengthening or extension. The effectiveness of this ligament is demonstrated during cases of extreme trauma to the mandible. In such cases, the neck of the condyle will be seen to fracture before the retrodiscal tissues are severed or the condyle enters the middle cranial fossa.

Sphenomandibular Ligament
The sphenomandibular ligament is one of two TMJ accessory ligaments (Fig. 1-21). It arises from the spine of the sphenoid bone and extends downward to a small bony prominence on the medial surface of the ramus of the mandible, which is called the *lingula*. It does not have any significant limiting effects on mandibular movement.

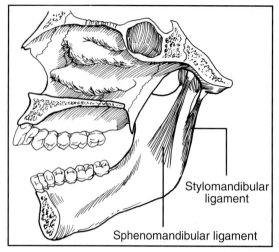

Stylomandibular
ligament

Sphenomandibular ligament

Fig. 1-21 Mandible, temporomandibular joint, and accessory ligaments.

Stylomandibular Ligament

The second accessory ligament is the stylomandibular ligament (see Fig. 1-21). It arises from the styloid process and extends downward and forward to the angle and posterior border of the ramus of the mandible. It becomes taut when the mandible is protruded but is most relaxed when the mandible is opened. The stylomandibular ligament therefore limits excessive protrusive movements of the mandible.

MUSCLES OF MASTICATION

The skeletal components of the body are held together and moved by the skeletal muscles. The skeletal muscles provide for the locomotion necessary for the individual to survive. Muscles are made of numerous fibers ranging from 10 to 80 μm in diameter. Each of these fibers in turn is made up of successively smaller subunits. In most muscles the fibers extend the entire length of the muscle, except for about 2% of the fibers. Each fiber is innervated by only one nerve ending, located near the middle of the fiber. The end of the muscle fiber fuses with a tendon fiber, and the tendon fibers in turn collect into bundles to form the muscle tendon that inserts into the bone. Each muscle

fiber contains several hundred to several thousand myofibrils. Each myofibril in turn has, lying side by side, about 1500 myosin filaments and 3000 actin filaments, which are large polymerized protein molecules that are responsible for muscle contraction. For a more complete description of the physiology of muscle contraction, other publications should be pursued.[15]

Muscle fibers can be characterized by type according to the amount of myoglobin (a pigment similar to hemoglobin). Fibers with higher concentrations of myoglobin are deeper red in color and capable of slow but sustained contraction. These fibers are called *slow muscle fibers* or *type I muscle fibers*. Slow fibers have a well-developed aerobic metabolism and are therefore resistant to fatigue. Fibers with lower concentrations of myoglobin are whiter and are called *fast muscle fibers* or *type II fibers*. These fibers have fewer mitochondria and rely more on anaerobic activity for function. Fast muscle fibers are capable of quick contraction but fatigue more rapidly.

All skeletal muscles contain a mixture of fast and slow fibers in varying proportions that reflect the function of that muscle. Muscles that are called on to respond quickly are made of predominately white fibers. Muscles that are mainly used for slow, continuous activity have higher concentrations of slow fibers.

Four pairs of muscles make up a group called the *muscles of mastication*: the masseter, temporalis, medial pterygoid, and lateral pterygoid. Although not considered to be muscles of mastication, the digastrics also play an important role in mandibular function and therefore are discussed in this section. Each muscle is discussed according to its attachment, the direction of its fibers, and its function.

Masseter

The masseter is a rectangular muscle that originates from the zygomatic arch and extends downward to the lateral aspect of the lower border of the ramus of the mandible (Fig. 1-22). Its insertion on the mandible extends from the region of the second molar at the inferior border posteriorly to include the angle. It has two portions, or heads: (1) The

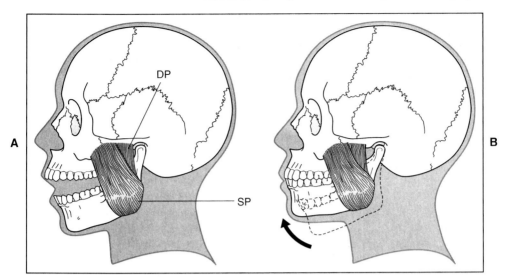

Fig. 1-22 A, Masseter muscle. *DP,* Deep portion; *SP,* superficial portion. **B,** Function: elevation of the mandible.

superficial portion consists of fibers that run downward and slightly backward, and (2) the *deep* portion consists of fibers that run in a predominantly vertical direction.

As fibers of the masseter contract, the mandible is elevated and the teeth are brought into contact. The masseter is a powerful muscle that provides the force necessary to chew efficiently. Its superficial portion may also aid in protruding the mandible. When the mandible is protruded and biting force is applied, the fibers of the deep portion stabilize the condyle against the articular eminence.

Temporalis
The temporalis is a large, fan-shaped muscle that originates from the temporal fossa and the lateral surface of the skull. Its fibers come together as they extend downward between the zygomatic arch and the lateral surface of the skull to form a tendon that inserts on the coronoid process and anterior border of the ascending ramus. It can be divided into three distinct areas according to fiber direction and ultimate function (Fig. 1-23). The anterior portion consists of fibers that are directed almost vertically. The middle portion contains fibers that run obliquely across the lateral aspect of the skull (slightly forward as they pass downward). The posterior portion consists of fibers that are

aligned almost horizontally, coming forward above the ear to join other temporalis fibers as they pass under the zygomatic arch.

When the temporal muscle contracts, it elevates the mandible and the teeth are brought into contact. If only portions contract, the mandible is moved according to the direction of those fibers that are activated. When the anterior portion contracts, the mandible is raised vertically. Contraction of the middle portion will elevate and retrude the mandible. Function of the posterior portion is somewhat controversial. Although it would appear that contraction of this portion will retrude the mandible, DuBrul[16] suggests that the fibers below the root of the zygomatic process are the only significant ones and therefore contraction will cause elevation and only slight retrusion. Because the angulation of its muscle fibers varies, the temporalis is capable of coordinating closing movements. Thus it is a significant positioning muscle of the mandible.

Pterygoideus Medialis
The medial (internal) pterygoid originates from the pterygoid fossa and extends downward, backward, and outward to insert along the medial surface of the mandibular angle (Fig. 1-24). Along with the masseter, it forms a muscular sling that supports

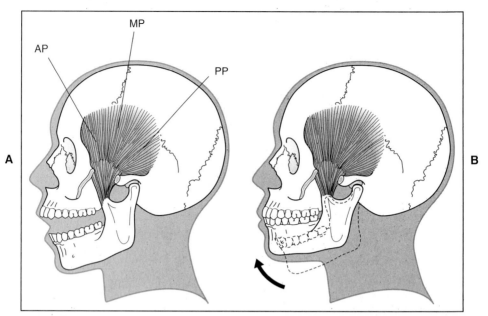

Fig. 1-23 A, Temporal muscle. *AP,* Anterior portion; *MP,* middle portion; *PP,* posterior portion. **B,** Function: elevation of the mandible. The exact movement by the location of the fibers or portion being activated.

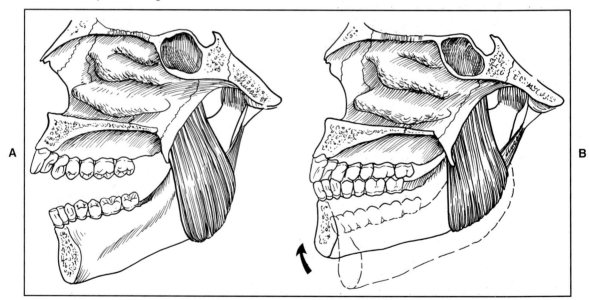

Fig. 1-24 A, Medial pterygoid muscle. **B,** Function: elevation of the mandible.

the mandible at the mandibular angle. When its fibers contract, the mandible is elevated and the teeth are brought into contact. This muscle is also active in protruding the mandible. Unilateral contraction will bring about a mediotrusive movement of the mandible.

Pterygoideus Lateralis

For many years the lateral (external) pterygoid was described as having two distinct portions or bellies: (1) an inferior and (2) a superior. Because the muscle appeared anatomically to be as one in structure and function, this description was acceptable until studies proved differently.[17,18] Now it is appreciated that the two bellies of the lateral pterygoid function quite differently. Therefore in this text the lateral pterygoid is divided and identified as two distinct and different muscles, which is appropriate because their functions are nearly opposite. The muscles are described as the inferior lateral and the superior lateral pterygoid.

Inferior Lateral Pterygoid. The inferior lateral pterygoid originates at the outer surface of the lateral pterygoid plate and extends backward, upward, and outward to its insertion primarily on the neck of the condyle (Fig. 1-25). When the right and left inferior lateral pterygoids contract simultaneously, the condyles are pulled down the articular eminences and the mandible is protruded. Unilateral contraction creates a mediotrusive movement of that condyle and causes a lateral movement of the mandible to the opposite side. When this muscle functions with the mandibular depressors, the mandible is lowered and the condyles glide forward and downward on the articular eminences.

Superior Lateral Pterygoid. The superior lateral pterygoid is considerably smaller than the inferior and originates at the infratemporal surface of the greater sphenoid wing, extending almost horizontally, backward, and outward to insert on the articular capsule, the disc, and the neck of the condyle (see Figs. 1-14 and 1-25). The exact attachment of the superior lateral pterygoid to the disc is somewhat debatable. Although some authors[19] suggest no attachment, most studies reveal the presence of a muscle-disc attachment.[14,20-24] The majority of the fibers of the superior lateral pterygoid (60% to 70%) attach to the neck of the condyle, with only 30% to 40% attaching to the disc. Importantly, the attachments are more predominant on the medial aspect than on the lateral. Approaching the joint structures from the lateral aspect would reveal little or no muscle attachment. This may explain the different findings in these studies.

Although the inferior lateral pterygoid is active during opening, the superior remains inactive, becoming active only in conjunction with the elevator muscles. The superior lateral pterygoid is especially active during the power stroke and when the teeth are held together. The *power stroke* refers to movements that involve closure of the mandible against resistance, such as in chewing or clenching the teeth together. The functional significance of the superior lateral pterygoid is discussed in more detail in the next section, which deals with the biomechanics of the TMJ.

The clinician should note that the pull of the lateral pterygoid on the disc and condyle is predominantly in an anterior direction; however, it also has

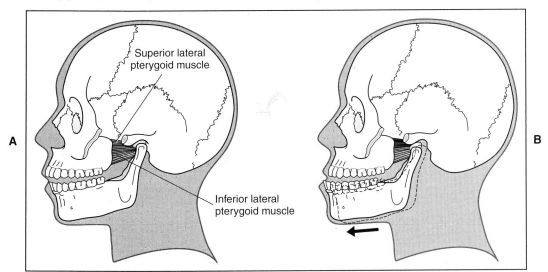

Fig. 1-25 A, Inferior and superior lateral pterygoid muscles. **B,** Function of the inferior lateral pterygoid: protrusion of the mandible.

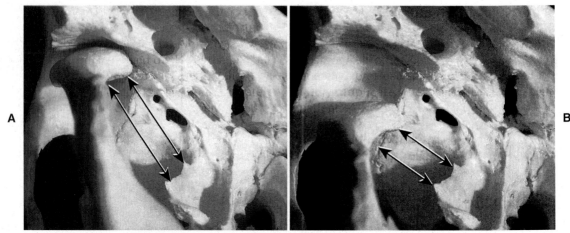

Fig. 1-26 A, When the condyle is in a normal relationship in the fossa, the attachments of the superior and inferior lateral pterygoid muscles create a medial and anterior pull on the condyle and disc *(arrows)*. **B,** As the condyle moves anteriorly from the fossa, the pull becomes more medially directed *(arrows)*.

a significantly medial component (Fig. 1-26). As the condyle moves more forward, the medial angulation of the pull of these muscles becomes even greater. In the wide-open mouth position, the direction of the muscle pull is more medial than anterior.

Interestingly, approximately 80% of the fibers that make up both lateral pterygoid muscles are slow muscle fibers (type I).[25,26] This suggests that these muscles are relatively resistant to fatigue and may serve to brace the condyle for long periods of time without difficulty.

Digastricus

Although the digastric is not generally considered a muscle of mastication, it does have an important influence on the function of the mandible. It is divided into two portions, or bellies (Fig. 1-27):

1. The *posterior belly* originates from the mastoid notch, just medial to the mastoid process; its fibers run forward, downward, and inward to the intermediate tendon attached to the hyoid bone.

2. The *anterior belly* originates at a fossa on the lingual surface of the mandible, just above the lower border and close to the midline; its fibers extend downward and backward to insert at the same intermediate tendon as does the posterior belly.

When the right and left digastrics contract and the hyoid bone is fixed by the suprahyoid and infrahyoid muscles, the mandible is depressed and pulled backward and the teeth are brought out of contact. When the mandible is stabilized, the digastric muscles with the suprahyoid and infrahyoid muscles elevate the hyoid bone, which is a necessary function for swallowing.

The digastrics are one of many muscles that depress the mandible and raise the hyoid bone (Fig. 1-28). Generally muscles that are attached from the mandible to the hyoid bone are called *suprahyoid*, and those attached from the hyoid bone to the clavicle and sternum are called *infrahyoid*. The suprahyoid and infrahyoid muscles play a major role in coordinating mandibular function, as do many of the other numerous muscles of the head and neck. It can be quickly observed that a study of mandibular function is not limited to the muscles of mastication. Other major muscles, such as the sternocleidomastoid and the posterior cervical muscles, play major roles in stabilizing the skull and enabling controlled movements of the mandible to be performed. A finely tuned dynamic balance exists among all of the head and neck muscles, and this must be appreciated for an understanding of the physiology of mandibular movement to occur. As a person yawns, the head is

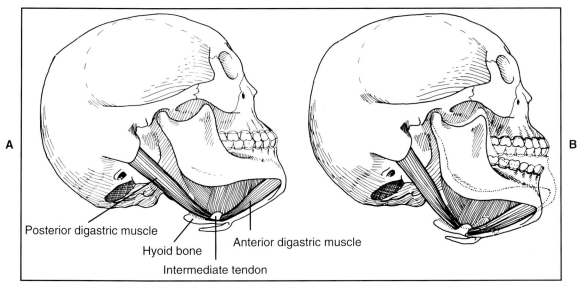

Posterior digastric muscle

Hyoid bone

Anterior digastric muscle

Intermediate tendon

Fig. 1-27 A, Digastric muscle. **B,** Function: depression of the mandible.

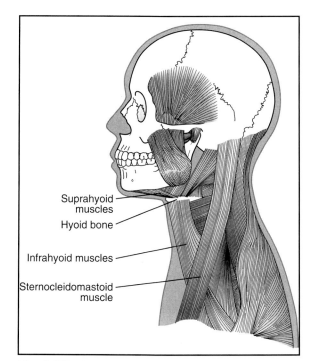

Suprahyoid muscles

Hyoid bone

Infrahyoid muscles

Sternocleidomastoid muscle

Fig. 1-28 Movement of the head and neck is a result of the finely coordinated efforts of many muscles. The muscles of mastication represent only part of this complex system.

brought back by contraction of the posterior cervical muscles, which raises the maxillary teeth. This simple example demonstrates that even normal functioning of the masticatory system uses many more muscles than just those of mastication. With an understanding of this relationship, one can see that any effect on the function of the muscles of mastication also has an effect on other head and neck muscles. A more detailed review of the physiology of the entire masticatory system is presented in Chapter 2.

BIOMECHANICS OF THE TEMPOROMANDIBULAR JOINT

The TMJ is an extremely complex joint system. The fact that two TMJs are connected to the same bone (the mandible) further complicates the function of the entire masticatory system. Each joint can simultaneously act separately and yet not completely without influence from the other. A sound understanding of the biomechanics of the TMJ is essential and basic to the study of function and dysfunction in the masticatory system.

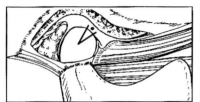 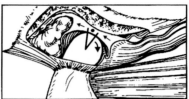 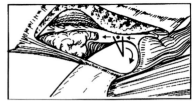

Fig. 1-29 Normal movement of the condyle and disc during mouth opening. As the condyle moves out of the fossa, the disc rotates posteriorly on the condyle around the attachment of the discal collateral ligaments. Rotational movement occurs predominately in the lower joint space, whereas translation occurs predominately in the superior joint space.

The TMJ is a compound joint. Its structure and function can be divided into two distinct systems:

1. One joint system is the tissues that surround the inferior synovial cavity (i.e., the condyle and the articular disc). Because the disc is tightly bound to the condyle by the lateral and medial discal ligaments, the only physiologic movement that can occur between these surfaces is rotation of the disc on the articular surface of the condyle. The disc and its attachment to the condyle are called the *condyle-disc complex*; this joint system is responsible for rotational movement in the TMJ.

2. The second system is made up of the condyle-disc complex functioning against the surface of the mandibular fossa. Because the disc is not tightly attached to the articular fossa, free sliding movement is possible between these surfaces in the superior cavity. This movement occurs when the mandible is moved forward (referred to as *translation*). Translation occurs in this superior joint cavity between the superior surface of the articular disc and the mandibular fossa (Fig. 1-29). Thus the articular disc acts as a nonossified bone contributing to both joint systems, and hence the function of the disc justifies classifying the TMJ as a true compound joint.

The articular disc has been referred to as a *meniscus*. However, it is not a meniscus at all. By definition, a meniscus is a wedge-shaped crescent of fibrocartilage attached on one side to the articular capsule and unattached on the other side, extending freely into the joint spaces. A meniscus does not divide a joint cavity, isolating the synovial fluid, nor does it serve as a determinant of joint movement. Instead, it functions passively to assist movement between the bony parts. Typical menisci are found in the knee joint. In the TMJ the disc functions as a true articular surface in both joint systems and is therefore more accurately termed an *articular disc*.

Now that the two individual joint systems have been described, the entire TMJ can be considered again. The articular surfaces of the joint have no structural attachment or union, yet contact must be maintained constantly for joint stability. Stability of the joint is maintained by constant activity of the muscles that pull across the joint, primarily the elevators. Even in the resting state, these muscles are in a mild state of contraction called *tonus* (this feature is discussed in Chapter 2). As muscle activity increases, the condyle is increasingly forced against the disc and the disc against the fossa, resulting in an increase in the interarticular pressure* of these joint structures.[27-29] In the absence of interarticular pressure, the articular surfaces will separate and the joint will technically dislocate.

The width of the articular disc space varies with interarticular pressure. When the pressure is low, as in the closed rest position, the disc space widens. When the pressure is high, as during clenching of the teeth, the disc space narrows. The contour and movement of the disc permit constant contact of the articular surfaces of the joint, which

---

*Interarticular pressure is the pressure between the articular surfaces of the joint.

is necessary for joint stability. As the interarticular pressure increases, the condyle seats itself on the thinner intermediate zone of the disc. When the pressure is decreased and the disc space is widened, a thicker portion of the disc is rotated to fill the space. Because the anterior and posterior bands of the disc are wider than the intermediate zone, technically the disc could be rotated either anteriorly or posteriorly to accomplish this task. The direction of the disc rotation is determined not by chance, but by the structures attached to the anterior and posterior borders of the disc.

Attached to the posterior border of the articular disc are the retrodiscal tissues, sometimes referred to as the *posterior attachment*. As previously mentioned, the superior retrodiscal lamina is composed of varying amounts of elastic connective tissue. Because this tissue has elastic properties and because in the closed mouth position it is somewhat folded over itself, the condyle can easily move out of the fossa without creating any damage to the superior retrodiscal lamina. When the mouth is closed (the closed joint position), the elastic traction on the disc is minimal to none. However, during mandibular opening, when the condyle is pulled forward down the articular eminence, the superior retrodiscal lamina becomes increasingly stretched, creating increased forces to retract the disc. In the full forward position, the posterior retractive force on the disc created by the tension of the stretched superior retrodiscal lamina is at a maximum. The interarticular pressure and the morphology of the disc prevent the disc from being overretracted posteriorly. In other words, as the mandible moves into a full forward position and during its return, the retraction force of the superior retrodiscal lamina holds the disc rotated as far posteriorly on the condyle as the width of the articular disc space will permit. This is an important principle in understanding joint function. Likewise, it is important to remember that the superior retrodiscal lamina is the only structure capable of retracting the disc posteriorly on the condyle, although this retractive force is only present during wide opening movements.

Attached to the anterior border of the articular disc is the superior lateral pterygoid muscle. When this muscle is active, the fibers that are attached to the disc pull anteriorly and medially. Therefore the superior lateral pterygoid is technically a protractor of the disc. Remember, however, that this muscle is also attached to the neck of the condyle. This dual attachment does not allow the muscle to pull the disc through the discal space. Protraction of the disc, however, does not occur during jaw opening. When the inferior lateral pterygoid is protracting the condyle forward, the superior lateral pterygoid is inactive and therefore does not bring the disc forward with the condyle. The superior lateral pterygoid is activated only in conjunction with activity of the elevator muscles during mandibular closure or a power stroke.

Understanding the features that cause the disc to move forward with the condyle in the absence of superior lateral pterygoid activity is important. The anterior capsular ligament attaches the disc to the anterior margin of the articular surface of the condyle (see Fig. 1-14). In addition, the inferior retrodiscal lamina attaches the posterior edge of the disc to the posterior margin of the articular surface of the condyle. Both ligaments are composed of collagenous fibers and will not stretch. Therefore a logical assumption is that they force the disc to translate forward with the condyle. Although logical, such an assumption is incorrect: These structures are not primarily responsible for movement of the disc with the condyle. Ligaments do not actively participate in normal joint function but only passively restrict extreme border movements. The mechanism by which the disc is maintained with the translating condyle is dependent on the morphology of the disc and the interarticular pressure. In the presence of a normally shaped articular disc, the articulating surface of the condyle rests on the intermediate zone, between the two thicker portions. As the interarticular pressure is increased, the discal space narrows, which more positively seats the condyle on the intermediate zone.

During translation, the combination of disc morphology and interarticular pressure maintains the condyle on the intermediate zone and the disc is forced to translate forward with the condyle. Therefore the morphology of the disc is extremely important in maintaining proper position during function. Proper morphology plus interarticular pressure results in an important self-positioning feature of the disc. Only when the morphology of the disc has been greatly altered does the ligamentous attachment of the disc affect joint function. When this occurs, the biomechanics of the joint is altered and dysfunctional signs begin. These conditions are discussed in detail in later chapters.

As with most muscles, the superior lateral pterygoid is constantly maintained in a mild state of contraction or tonus, which exerts a slight anterior and medial force on the disc. In the resting closed joint position, this anterior and medial force will normally exceed the posterior elastic retraction force provided by the nonstretched superior retrodiscal lamina. Therefore in the resting closed joint position, when the interarticular pressure is low and the disc space widened, the disc will occupy the most anterior rotary position

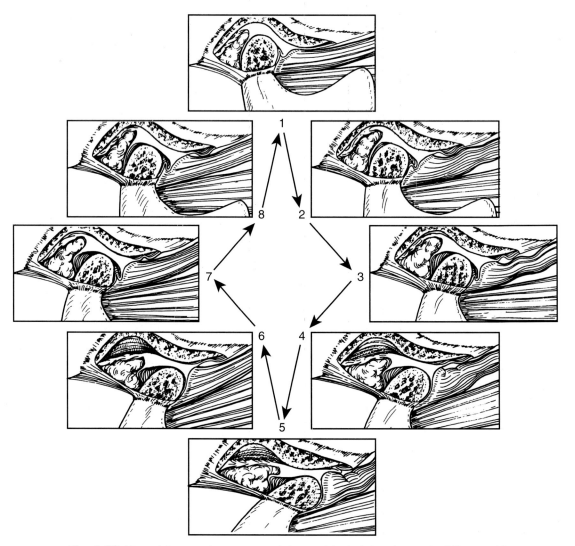

Fig. 1-30 Normal functional movement of the condyle and disc during the full range of opening and closing. The disc is rotated posteriorly on the condyle as the condyle is translated out of the fossa. The closing movement is the exact opposite of opening. The disc is always maintained between the condyle and the fossa.

on the condyle permitted by the width of the space. In other words, at rest with the mouth closed, the condyle will be positioned in contact with the intermediate and posterior zones of the disc.

This disc relationship is maintained during minor passive rotational and translatory mandibular movements. As soon as the condyle is moved forward enough to cause the retractive force of the superior retrodiscal lamina to be greater than the muscle tonus force of the superior lateral pterygoid, the disc is rotated posteriorly to the extent permitted by the width of the articular disc space. When the condyle is returned to the resting closed joint position, once again the tonus of the superior lateral pterygoid becomes the predominant force and the disc is repositioned forward as far as the disc space will permit (Fig. 1-30).

The functional importance of the superior lateral pterygoid muscle becomes obvious when observing the effects of the power stroke during unilateral chewing. When one bites down on a hard substance on one side (e.g., a tough steak), the TMJs are not equally loaded. This occurs because the force of closure is not applied to the joint but is instead applied to the food. The jaw is fulcrumed around the hard food, causing an increase in interarticular pressure in the contralateral joint and a sudden decrease in interarticular pressure in the ipsilateral (same side) joint.[30,31] This can lead to separation of the articular surfaces, resulting in dislocation of the ipsilateral joint. To prevent this dislocation, the superior lateral pterygoid becomes active during the power stroke, rotating the disc forward on the condyle so that the thicker posterior border of the disc maintains articular contact. Therefore joint stability is maintained during the power stroke of chewing. As the teeth pass through the food and approach intercuspation, the interarticular pressure is increased. As the interarticular pressure is increased in the joint, the disc space is decreased and the disc is mechanically rotated posteriorly so that the thinner intermediate zone fills the space. When the force of closure is discontinued, the resting closed joint position is once again assumed (see Fig. 1-30).

Understanding these basic concepts in TMJ function is essential to understanding joint dysfunction. Normal biomechanical function of the TMJ must follow the orthopedic principles just presented. Clinicians should remember the following:

1. Ligaments do not actively participate in normal function of the TMJ. They act as guide wires, restricting certain joint movements while permitting others. They restrict joint movements both mechanically and through neuromuscular reflex activity (see Chapter 2).
2. Ligaments do not stretch. If traction force is applied, they can become elongated (i.e., increase in length). (*Stretch* implies the ability to return to the original length.) Once ligaments have been elongated, normal joint function is often compromised.
3. The articular surfaces of the TMJs must be maintained in constant contact. This contact is produced by the muscles that pull across the joints (the elevators: temporal, masseter, and medial pterygoid).

A sound understanding of these principles is necessary for the evaluation and treatment of the various disorders that are presented throughout the remainder of this book.

References

1. Wink CS, St Onge M, Zimny ML: Neural elements in the human temporomandibular articular disc, *J Oral Maxillofac Surg* 50:334-337, 1992.
2. Ichikawa H, Wakisaka S, Matsuo S, Akai M: Peptidergic innervation of the temporomandibular disk in the rat, *Experientia* 45:303-304, 1989.
3. Westesson PL, Kurita K, Eriksson L, Katzberg RH: Cryosectional observations of functional anatomy of the temporomandibular joint, *Oral Surg Oral Med Oral Pathol* 68:247-255, 1989.
4. Sahler LG, Morris TW, Katzberg RW, Tallents RH: Microangiography of the rabbit temporomandibular joint in the open and closed jaw positions, *J Oral Maxillofac Surg* 48:831-834, 1990.
5. Shengyi T, Yinghua X: Biomechanical properties and collagen fiber orientation of TMJ discs in dogs: part 1. Gross anatomy and collagen fibers orientation of the disc, *J Craniomandib Disord* 5:28-34, 1991.
6. De Bont L, Liem R, Boering G: Ultrastructure of the articular cartilage of the mandibular condyle: aging and degeneration, *Oral Surg Oral Med Oral Pathol* 60:631-641, 1985.
7. De Bont L, Boering G, Havinga P, Leim RSB: Spatial arrangement of collagen fibrils in the articular cartilage of the mandibular condyle: a light microscopic and scanning electron microscopic study, *J Oral Maxillofac Surg* 42:306-313, 1984.

8. Robinson PD: Articular cartilage of the temporo-mandibular joint: can it regenerate? *Ann R Coll Surg Engl* 75:231-236, 1993.

9. Mow VC, Ratcliffe A, Poole AR: Cartilage and diarthrodial joints as paradigms for hierarchical materials and structures, *Biomaterials* 13:67-97, 1992.

10. Maroudas A: Balance between swelling pressure and collagen tension in normal and degenerate cartilage, *Nature* 260:808-809, 1976.

11. Mow VC, Holmes MH, Lai WM: Fluid transport and mechanical properties of articular cartilage: a review, *J Biomech* 17:377-394, 1984.

12. Stegenga B, de Bont LG, Boering G, van Willigen JD: Tissue responses to degenerative changes in the temporomandibular joint: a review, *J Oral Maxillofac Surg* 49:1079-1088, 1991.

13. Fernandes PR, de Vasconsellos HA, Okeson JP, Bastos RL, Maia ML: The anatomical relationship between the position of the auriculotemporal nerve and mandibular condyle, *Cranio* 21:165-171, 2003.

14. Tanaka TT: *TMJ microanatomy: an approach to current controversies*, Chula Vista, Calif, 1992, Clinical Research Foundation.

15. Guyton AC: *Textbook of medical physiology*, ed 8, Philadelphia, 1991, Saunders, p 1013.

16. Du Brul EL: *Sicher's oral anatomy*, ed 7, St Louis, 1980, Mosby.

17. McNamara JA: The independent functions of the two heads of the lateral pterygoid muscle in the human temporomandibular joint, *Am J Anat* 138:197-205, 1973.

18. Mahan PE, Wilkinson TM, Gibbs CH, Mauderli A, Brannon LS: Superior and inferior bellies of the lateral pterygoid muscle EMG activity at basic jaw positions, *J Prosthet Dent* 50:710-718, 1983.

19. Wilkinson TM: The relationship between the disk and the lateral pterygoid muscle in the human temporomandibular joint, *J Prosthet Dent* 60:715-724, 1988.

20. Dusek TO, Kiely JP: Quantification of the superior lateral pterygoid insertion on TMJ components, *J Dent Res* 70:421-427, 1991.

21. Carpentier P, Yung JP, Marguelles-Bonnet R, Meunissier M: Insertion of the lateral pterygoid: an anatomic study of the human temporomandibular joint, *J Oral Maxillofac Surg* 46:477-782, 1988.

22. Marguelles-Bonnet R, Yung JP, Carpentier P, Meunissier M: Temporomandibular joint serial sections made with mandible in intercuspal position, *J Craniomandib Pract* 7:97-106, 1989.

23. Tanaka TT: *Advanced dissection of the temporomandibular joint*, Chula Vista, Calif, 1989, Clinical Research Foundation.

24. Heylings DJ, Nielsen IL, McNeill C: Lateral pterygoid muscle and the temporomandibular disc, *J Orofac Pain* 9:9-16, 1995.

25. Ericksson PO: Special histochemical muscle-fiber characteristics of the human lateral pterygoid muscle, *Arch Oral Biol* 26:495-501, 1981.

26. Mao J, Stein RB, Osborn JW: The size and distribution of fiber types in jaw muscles: a review, *J Craniomandib Disord* 6:192-201, 1992.

27. Boyd RL, Gibbs CH, Mahan PE, Richmond AF, Laskin JL: Temporomandibular joint forces measured at the condyle of *Macaca arctoides*, *Am J Orthod Dentofacial Orthop* 97:472-479, 1990.

28. Mansour RM, Reynik RJ: In vivo occlusal forces and moments: I. Forces measured in terminal hinge position and associated moments, *J Dent Res* 54:114-120, 1975.

29. Smith DM, McLachlan KR, McCall WD: A numerical model of temporomandibular joint loading, *J Dent Res* 65:1046-1052, 1986.

30. Rassouli NM, Christensen LV: Experimental occlusal interferences. Part III. Mandibular rotations induced by a rigid interference, *J Oral Rehabil* 22:781-789, 1995.

31. Christensen LV, Rassouli NM: Experimental occlusal interferences. Part IV. Mandibular rotations induced by a pliable interference, *J Oral Rehabil* 22:835-844, 1995.

Functional Neuroanatomy and Physiology of the Masticatory System

CHAPTER 2

"You cannot successfully treat dysfunction unless you understand function."

—JPO

*T*he function of the masticatory system is complex. Discriminatory contraction of the various head and neck muscles is necessary to move the mandible precisely and allow effective functioning. A highly refined neurologic control system regulates and coordinates the activities of the entire masticatory system. It consists primarily of nerves and muscles; hence the term *neuromuscular system*. A basic understanding of the anatomy and function of the neuromuscular system is essential to understanding the influence that tooth contacts, as well as other conditions, have on mandibular movement.

This chapter is divided into three sections. The first section reviews in detail the basic neuroanatomy and function of the neuromuscular system. The second describes the basic physiologic activities of mastication, swallowing, and speech. The third section reviews important concepts and mechanisms that are necessary to understand orofacial pain. Grasping the concepts in these three sections should greatly enhance the clinician's ability to understand a patient's complaint and provide effective therapy.

ANATOMY AND FUNCTION OF THE NEUROMUSCULAR SYSTEM

For purposes of discussion, the neuromuscular system is divided into two major components: (1) the neurologic structures and (2) the muscles. The anatomy and function of each of these components is reviewed separately, although in many instances it is difficult to separate function. With an understanding of these components, basic neuromuscular function can be reviewed.

MUSCLES

Motor Unit

The basic component of the neuromuscular system is the motor unit, which consists of a number of muscle fibers that are innervated by one motor neuron. Each neuron joins with the muscle fiber at a motor endplate. When the neuron is activated, the motor endplate is stimulated to release small amounts of acetylcholine, which initiates depolarization of the muscle fibers. Depolarization causes the muscle fibers to shorten or contract.

The number of muscle fibers innervated by one motor neuron varies greatly according to the function of the motor unit. The fewer the muscle fibers per motor neuron, the more precise the movement. A single motor neuron may innervate only two or three muscle fibers, as in the ciliary muscles (which precisely control the lens of the eye). Conversely, one motor neuron may innervate hundreds of muscle fibers, as in any large muscle (e.g., the rectus femoris in the leg). A similar variation exists in the number of muscle fibers per motor neuron within the muscles of mastication. The inferior lateral pterygoid muscle has a relatively low muscle fiber/motor neuron ratio; therefore it is capable of the fine adjustments in length needed to adapt to horizontal changes in the mandibular position. In contrast, the masseter has a greater number of motor fibers per motor neuron, which corresponds to its more gross function of providing the force necessary during mastication.

Muscle

Hundreds to thousands of motor units along with blood vessels and nerves are bundled together by connective tissue and fascia to make up a muscle. The major muscles that control movement of the masticatory system were described in Chapter 1. To understand the effect these muscles have on each other and their bony attachments, one must observe the basic skeletal relationships of the head and neck. The skull is supported in position by the cervical spine. However, the skull is not centrally located or balanced over the cervical spine. In fact, if a dry skull were placed in its correct position on the cervical spine, it would be overbalanced to the anterior and quickly fall forward. Any balance becomes even more remote when the position of the mandible hanging below the anterior portion of the skull is considered. It can be easily seen that a balance of the skeletal components of the head and neck does not exist. Muscles are necessary to overcome this weight and mass imbalance. If the head is to be maintained in an upright position so that one can see forward, muscles that attach the posterior aspect of the skull to the cervical spine and shoulder region must contract. Some of the muscles that serve this function are the trapezius, sternocleidomastoideus, splenius capitis, and longus capitis. It is possible, however, for these muscles to overcontract and direct the line of vision too far upward. To counteract this action, an antagonistic group of muscles exists in the anterior region of the head: the masseter (joining the mandible to the skull), the suprahyoids (joining the mandible to the hyoid bone), and the infrahyoids (joining the hyoid bone to the sternum and clavicle). When these muscles contract, the head is lowered. Thus a balance of muscular forces exists that maintains the head in a desired position (Fig. 2-1). These muscles, plus others, also maintain proper side-to-side positioning and rotation of the head.

Muscle Function. The motor unit can carry out only one action: contraction or shortening.

The entire muscle, however, has three potential functions:

1. When a large number of motor units in the muscle are stimulated, contraction or an overall shortening of the muscle occurs. This type of shortening under a constant load is called *isotonic contraction*. Isotonic contraction occurs in the masseter when the mandible is elevated, forcing the teeth through a bolus of food.
2. When a proper number of motor units contract opposing a given force, the resultant function of the muscle is to hold or stabilize the jaw. This contraction without shortening is called *isometric contraction*, and it occurs in the masseter when an object is held between the teeth (e.g., a pipe or pencil).
3. A muscle can also function through *controlled relaxation*. When stimulation of the motor unit is discontinued, the fibers of the motor unit relax and return to their normal length. By control of this decrease in motor unit stimulation, a precise muscle lengthening can occur that allows smooth and deliberate movement. This type of controlled relaxation is observed in the masseter when the mouth opens to accept a new bolus of food during mastication.

Using these three functions, the muscles of the head and neck maintain a constant desirable head position. A balance exists between the muscles that function to raise the head and those that function to depress it. During even the slightest movement of the head, each muscle functions in harmony with others to carry out the desired movement. If the head is turned to the right, certain muscles must shorten (isotonic contraction), others must relax (controlled relaxation), and still others must stabilize or hold certain relationships (isometric contraction). A highly sophisticated control system is necessary to coordinate this finely tuned muscle balance.

These three types of muscle activities are present during routine function of the head and neck. Another type of muscle activity, *eccentric contraction*, can occur during certain conditions. This type of contraction is often injurious to the muscle tissue. *Eccentric contraction* refers to the lengthening of a muscle at the same time that it is contracting. An example of eccentric contraction occurs with the tissue damage associated during an extension-flexion

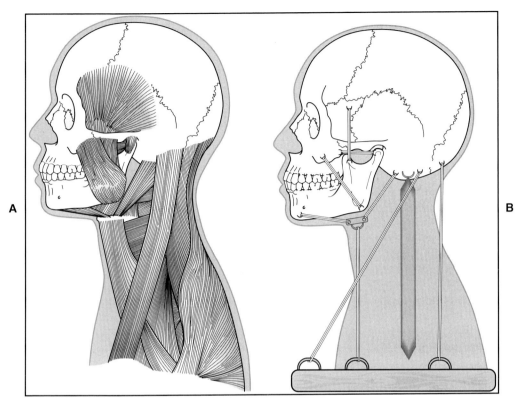

Fig. 2-1 Precise and complex balance of the head and neck muscles must exist to maintain proper head position and function. **A,** Muscle system. **B,** Each of the major muscles acts like an elastic band. The tension provided must precisely contribute to the balance that maintains the desired head position. If one elastic band breaks, the balance of the entire system is disrupted and the head position altered.

injury (whiplash injury). At the precise moment of a motor vehicle accident, the cervical muscles contract to support the head and resist movement. If, however, the impact is great, the sudden change in the inertia of the head causes it to move while the muscles contract trying to support it. The result is a sudden lengthening of the muscles while they are contracting. This type of sudden lengthening of muscles while contracting often results in injury and is discussed in later sections of the chapter devoted to muscle pain.

NEUROLOGIC STRUCTURES

Neuron

The basic structural unit of the nervous system is the neuron. The neuron is composed of a mass of protoplasm termed the *nerve cell body* and protoplasmic processes from the nerve cell body called *dendrites* and *axons*. The nerve cell bodies located in the spinal cord are found in the gray substance of the central nervous system (CNS). Cell bodies found outside the CNS are grouped together in *ganglia*. The axon (from the Greek word *axon*, meaning "axle" or "axis") is the central core that forms the essential conducting part of a neuron and is an extension of cytoplasm from a nerve cell. Many neurons group together to form a nerve fiber. These neurons are capable of transferring electrical and chemical impulses along their axes, enabling information to pass both in and out of the CNS. Depending on their location and function, neurons are designated by different terms. An *afferent* neuron conducts the nervous impulse toward the CNS, whereas an *efferent* neuron conducts it peripherally. *Internuncial neurons*, or *interneurons*, lie wholly within the CNS. Sensory or receptor neurons, afferent in type, receive and convey impulses from receptor organs. The first sensory neuron is called the *primary* or *first-order neuron*. *Second-* and *third-order* sensory neurons are internuncial. *Motor* or efferent neurons convey nervous impulses to produce muscular or secretory effects.

Nervous impulses are transmitted from one neuron to another only at a synaptic junction, or *synapse*, where the processes of two neurons are in close proximity. All afferent synapses are located within the gray substance of the CNS, so there are no anatomic peripheral connections between sensory fibers. All connections are within the CNS, and the peripheral transmission of a sensory impulse from one fiber to another is abnormal.

Information from the tissues outside the CNS must be transferred into the CNS and on to the higher centers in the brainstem and cortex for interpretation and evaluation. Once this information is evaluated, appropriate action must be taken.

The higher centers then send impulses down the spinal cord and back out to the periphery to an efferent organ for the desired action. The primary afferent neuron (first-order neuron) receives a stimulus from the sensory receptor. This impulse is carried by the primary afferent neuron into the CNS by way of the dorsal root to synapse in the dorsal horn of the spinal cord with a secondary (second-order) neuron (Fig. 2-2). The cell bodies of all the primary afferent neurons are located in the dorsal root ganglia. The impulse is then carried by the second-order neuron across the spinal cord to the anterolateral spinothalamic pathway, which ascends to the higher centers. Multiple *interneurons* (e.g., third order, fourth order) may be involved with the transfer of this impulse to the thalamus and cortex. Interneurons located in the dorsal horn may become involved with the impulse as it synapses with the second-order neuron. Some of these neurons may directly synapse with an efferent neuron that is directed back out the CNS by way of the ventral root to stimulate an efferent organ (e.g., a muscle).

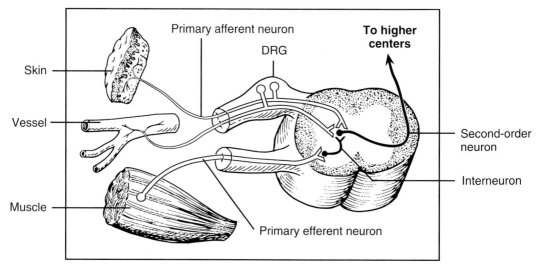

Fig. 2-2 DEPICTION OF THE PERIPHERAL NERVE INPUT INTO THE SPINAL CORD. First-order neurons (i.e., primary afferents) carry input into the dorsal horn to synapses with the second-order neurons. The second-order neuron then crosses over and ascends on to the higher centers. Small interneurons connect the primary afferent neuron with the primary motor (efferent) neuron allowing reflex arc activity. The dorsal root ganglion *(DRG)* contains the cell bodies of the primary afferent neurons. *(From Okeson JP: Bell's orofacial pains, ed 6, Chicago, 2005, Quintessence.)*

Brainstem and Brain

Once the impulses have been passed to the second-order neurons, these neurons carry them to the higher centers for interpretation and evaluation. Numerous centers in the brainstem and brain help give meaning to the impulses. The clinician should remember that numerous interneurons may be involved in transmitting the impulses on to higher centers. In fact, attempting to follow an impulse through the brainstem on to the cortex is no simple task. In order to intelligently discuss muscle function and pain in this text, certain functional regions of the brainstem and brain must be described. The clinician should keep in mind that the following descriptions provide an overview of several important functional components of

the CNS; other texts can provide a more complete discussion of the subject.[1,2]

Fig. 2-3 depicts the functional areas of the brainstem and brain that are reviewed in this section. Understanding these areas and their functions will help the clinician appreciate orofacial pain. The important areas reviewed are the spinal tract nucleus, reticular formation, thalamus, hypothalamus, limbic structures, and cortex. They are discussed in the order by which neural impulses pass on to the higher centers.

Spinal Tract Nucleus. Throughout the body, primary afferent neurons synapse with the second-order neurons in the dorsal horn of the spinal column. Afferent input from the face and oral structures, however, does not enter the spinal cord

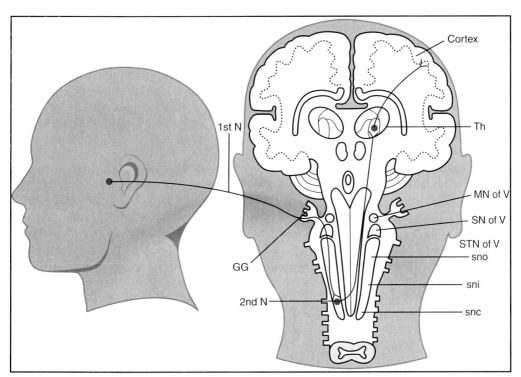

Fig. 2-3 DEPICTION OF THE TRIGEMINAL NERVE ENTERING THE BRAINSTEM AT THE LEVEL OF THE PONS. The primary afferent neuron *(1st N)* enters the brainstem to synapse with a second-order neuron *(2nd N)* in the trigeminal spinal tract nucleus *(STN of V).* The spinal tract nucleus is divided into three regions: subnucleus oralis *(sno)*, subnucleus interpolaris *(sni)*, and subnucleus caudalis *(snc)*. The trigeminal brainstem complex is also composed of the motor nucleus of V *(MN of V)* and the main sensory nucleus of V *(SN of V).* The cell bodies of the trigeminal nerve are located in the gasserian ganglion *(GG).* Once one second-order neuron receives the input, it is carried on to the thalamus *(Th)* for interpretation. *(Modified from Okeson JP: Bell's orofacial pains, ed 6, Chicago, 2005, Quintessence.)*

by way of spinal nerves. Instead, sensory input from the face and mouth is carried by way of the fifth cranial nerve, the trigeminal nerve. The cell bodies of the trigeminal afferent neurons are located in the large gasserian ganglion. Impulses carried by the trigeminal nerve enter directly into the brainstem in the region of the pons to synapse in the trigeminal spinal nucleus (see Fig. 2-3). This region of the brainstem is structurally similar to the dorsal horn of the spinal cord. In fact, it may be considered an extension of the dorsal horn and is sometimes referred to as the *medullary dorsal horn*.

The brainstem trigeminal nucleus complex consists of two main parts: (1) the main sensory trigeminal nucleus, which is rostrally located and receives periodontal and some pulpal afferents, and (2) the spinal tract of the trigeminal nucleus, which is more caudally located. The spinal tract is divided into three parts: (1) the subnucleus oralis; (2) the subnucleus interpolaris; and (3) the subnucleus caudalis, which corresponds to the medullary dorsal horn. Tooth pulp afferents go to all three subnuclei.[3] The subnucleus caudalis has especially been implicated in trigeminal nociceptive mechanisms on the basis of electrophysiologic observations of nociceptive neurons.[4,5] The subnucleus oralis appears to be a significant area of this trigeminal brainstem complex for oral pain mechanisms.[5-7]

Another component of the trigeminal brainstem complex is the motor nucleus of the fifth cranial nerve. This area of the complex is involved with interpretation of impulses that demand motor responses. Motor reflex activities of the face are initiated from this area in a similar manner to the spinal reflex activities in the rest of the body.[8]

Reticular Formation. After the primary afferent neurons synapse in the spinal tract nucleus, the interneurons transmit the impulses up to the higher centers. The interneurons ascend by way of several tracts passing through an area of the brainstem called the *reticular formation*. Within the reticular formation are concentrations of cells or *nuclei* that represent "centers" for various functions. The reticular formation plays an extremely important role in monitoring impulses that enter the brainstem. The reticular formation controls the overall activity of the brain by either enhancing the impulses on to the brain or by inhibiting the impulses. This portion of the brainstem has an extremely important influence on pain and other sensory input.

Thalamus. The thalamus is located in the center of the brain with the cerebrum surrounding it from the top and sides and the midbrain below (see Fig. 2-3). It is made up of numerous nuclei that function together to interrupt impulses. Almost all impulses from the lower regions of the brain, as well as from the spinal cord, are relayed through synapses in the thalamus before proceeding to the cerebral cortex. The thalamus acts as a relay station for most of the communication among the brainstem, cerebellum, and cerebrum. While impulses arise to the thalamus, the thalamus makes assessments and directs the impulses to appropriate regions in the higher centers for interpretation and response.

If one were to compare the human brain with a computer, the thalamus would represent the keyboard that controls the functions and directs the signals. The thalamus drives the cortex to activity and enables the cortex to communicate with the other regions of the CNS. Without the thalamus, the cortex is useless.

Hypothalamus. The hypothalamus is a small structure in the middle of the base of the brain. Although it is small, its function is great. The hypothalamus is the major center of the brain for controlling internal body functions, such as body temperature, hunger, and thirst. Stimulation of the hypothalamus excites the sympathetic nervous system throughout the body, increasing the overall level of activity of many internal parts of the body, especially increasing heart rate and causing blood vessel constriction. One can clearly see that this small area of the brain has some powerful effects on function of the individual. As discussed later, increased level of emotional stress can stimulate the hypothalamus to upregulate the sympathetic nervous system and greatly influence nociceptive impulses entering the brain. This simple statement should have extreme meaning to the clinician managing pain.

Limbic Structures. The word *limbic* means "border." The limbic system comprises the border structures of the cerebrum and the diencephalon.

The limbic structures function to control our emotional and behavioral activities. Within the limbic structures are centers or nuclei that are responsible for specific behaviors such as anger, rage, and docility. The limbic structures also control emotions such as depression, anxiety, fear, or paranoia. A pain-pleasure center apparently exists; on an instinctive level, the individual is driven toward behaviors that stimulate the pleasure side of the center. These drives are not generally perceived at a conscious level but more as a basic instinct. The instinct, however, will bring certain behaviors to a conscious level. For example, when an individual experiences chronic pain, behavior will be oriented toward withdrawal from any stimulus that may increase the pain. Often the sufferer will withdraw from life itself, and mood alterations such as depression will occur. It is believed that portions of the limbic structures interact and develop associations with the cortex, thereby coordinating the conscious cerebral behavioral functions with the subconscious behavioral functions of the deeper limbic system.

Impulses from the limbic system leading into the hypothalamus can modify any one or all of the many internal bodily functions controlled by the hypothalamus. Impulses from the limbic system feeding into the midbrain and medulla can control such behavior as wakefulness, sleep, excitement, and attentiveness. With this basic understanding of limbic function, one can quickly understand the impact it can have on the overall function of the individual. The limbic system certainly plays a major role in pain problems, as discussed in later chapters.

Cortex. The cerebral cortex represents the outer region of the cerebrum and is made up predominantly of gray matter. The cerebral cortex is the portion of the brain most frequently associated with the thinking process, even though it cannot provide thinking without simultaneous action of deeper structures of the brain. The cerebral cortex is the portion of the brain in which essentially all of one's memories are stored, and it is also the area most responsible for one's ability to acquire many muscle skills. Researchers still do not know the basic physiologic mechanisms by which the cerebral cortex stores either memories or knowledge of muscle skills.

In most areas the cerebral cortex is about 6 mm thick, and all together it contains an estimated 50 to 80 billion nerve cell bodies. Perhaps a billion nerve fibers lead away from the cortex, as well as comparable numbers leading into it, passing to other areas of the cortex, to and from deeper structures of the brain, and some all the way to the spinal cord.

Different regions of the cerebral cortex have been identified to have different functions. A motor area is primarily involved with coordinating motor function. A sensory area receives somatosensory input for evaluation. Areas for special senses, such as visual and auditory areas, are also found.

If one were to again compare the human brain with a computer, the cerebral cortex would represent the hard disc drive that stores all information of memory and motor function. Once again, one should remember that the thalamus (the keyboard) is the necessary unit that calls the cortex to function.

Sensory Receptors

Sensory receptors are neurologic structures or organs located in all body tissues that provide information to the CNS by way of the afferent neurons regarding the status of these tissues. As in other areas of the body, various types of sensory receptors are located throughout the tissues that make up the masticatory system. Specialized sensory receptors provide specific information to the afferent neurons and thus back to the CNS. Some receptors are specific for discomfort and pain. These are called *nociceptors*. Other receptors provide information regarding the position and movement of the mandible and associated oral structures. These are called *proprioceptors*. Receptors that carry information regarding the status of the internal organs are referred to as *interoceptors*. Constant input received from all of these receptors allows the cortex and brainstem to coordinate action of individual muscles or muscle groups to create appropriate response in the individual.

Like other systems, the masticatory system uses four major types of sensory receptors to monitor the status of its structures: (1) the muscle spindles, which are specialized receptor organs found in the muscle tissues; (2) the Golgi tendon organs, located in the tendons; (3) the pacinian corpuscles, located in tendons, joints, periosteum, fascia, and subcutaneous tissues; and (4) the nociceptors, found generally throughout all the tissues of the masticatory system.

Muscle Spindles. Skeletal muscles consist of two types of muscle fiber. The first are the extrafusal fibers, which are contractile and make up the bulk of the muscle; the other are the intrafusal fibers, which are only minutely contractile. A bundle of intrafusal muscle fibers bound by a connective tissue sheath is called a *muscle spindle* (Fig. 2-4). The muscle spindles primarily monitor tension within the skeletal muscles. They are interspersed throughout the muscles and aligned parallel with the extrafusal fibers. Within each spindle the nuclei of the intrafusal fibers are arranged in two distinct fashions: chainlike (nuclear chain type) and clumped (nuclear bag type).

Two types of afferent nerves supply the intrafusal fibers. They are classified according to their diameters. The larger fibers conduct impulses at a higher speed and have lower thresholds. Those that end in the central region of the intrafusal fibers are the larger group (Ia, A alpha) (discussed later in this chapter) and are said to be the primary endings (so-called annulospiral endings). Those that end in the poles of the spindle (away from the central region) are the smaller group (II, A beta) and are the secondary endings (so-called flower spray endings).

Because the intrafusal fibers of the muscle spindles are aligned parallel to the extrafusal fibers of the muscles, when the muscle is stretched, so also are the intrafusal fibers. This stretch is monitored at the nuclear chain and nuclear bag regions. The annulospiral and flower spray endings are activated by the stretch, and the afferent neurons carry these neural impulses to the CNS. The afferent neurons originating in the muscle spindles of the muscles of mastication have their cell bodies in the trigeminal mesencephalic nucleus.

The intrafusal fibers receive efferent innervation by way of fusimotor nerve fibers. These fibers are given the alphabetical classification of gamma

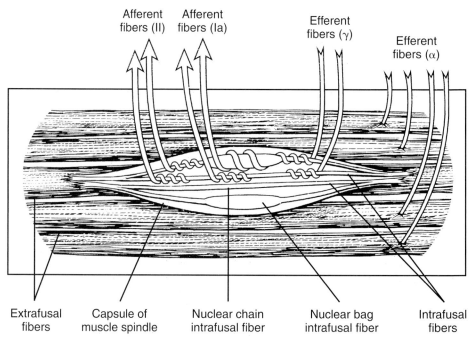

Fig. 2-4 Muscle spindle. *(Modified from Bell WE et al: Physiology and biochemistry, Edinburgh, 1972, Churchill Livingstone.)*

fibers or gamma efferents to distinguish them from the alpha nerve fibers, which supply the extrafusal fibers. Like other efferent fibers, the gamma efferent fibers originate in the CNS and, when stimulated, cause contraction of the intrafusal fibers. When the intrafusal fibers contract, the nuclear chain and nuclear bag areas are stretched, which is registered as though the entire muscle were stretched, and afferent activity is initiated. Thus there are two manners in which the afferent fibers of the muscle spindles can be stimulated: generalized stretching of the entire muscle (extrafusal fibers) and contraction of the intrafusal fibers by way of the gamma efferents. The muscle spindles can only register the stretch; they cannot differentiate between these two activities. Therefore the activities are recorded as the same activity by the CNS.

The extrafusal muscle fibers receive innervation by way of the alpha efferent motor neurons. Most of these have their cell bodies in the trigeminal motor nucleus. Stimulation of these neurons therefore causes the group of extrafusal muscle fibers (motor unit) to contract.

From a functional standpoint, the muscle spindle acts as a length-monitoring system. It constantly feeds back information to the CNS regarding the state of elongation or contraction of the muscle. When a muscle is suddenly stretched, both its extrafusal and intrafusal fibers elongate. The stretch of the spindle causes firing of the group I and group II afferent nerve endings leading back to the CNS. When the alpha efferent motor neurons are stimulated, the extrafusal fibers of the muscle contract and the spindle is shortened. This shortening brings about a decrease in the afferent output of the spindle. A total shutdown of the spindle activity would occur during muscle contraction if there were no gamma efferent system. As stated earlier, stimulation of the gamma efferents causes the intrafusal fibers of the muscle spindle to contract. This can elicit afferent activity from the spindle even when the muscle is contracting. Gamma efferent drive can therefore assist in maintaining muscle contraction.

The gamma efferent system is believed to act as a mechanism to sensitize the muscle spindles. Thus this fusimotor system acts as a biasing mechanism that alters the firing of the muscle spindle.

Clinicians should note that the gamma efferent mechanism is not as well investigated in the masticatory system as in other spinal cord systems. Although it appears to be active in most of the masticatory muscles, some apparently have no gamma efferents. The importance of the gamma efferent system is further emphasized in the discussion of muscle reflexes.

Golgi Tendon Organs. The Golgi tendon organs are located in the muscle tendon between the muscle fibers and their attachment to the bone. At one time they were thought to have a higher sensory threshold than the muscle spindles and therefore functioned solely to protect the muscle from excessive or damaging tension. It now appears that they are more sensitive and active in reflex regulation during normal function. They primarily monitor tension, whereas the muscle spindles primarily monitor muscle length.

The Golgi tendon organs occur in series with the extrafusal muscle fibers and not in parallel as with the muscle spindles. Each of these sensory organs consists of tendinous fibers surrounded by lymph spaces enclosed within a fibrous capsule. Afferent fibers enter near the middle of the organ and spread out over the extent of the fibers. Tension on the tendon stimulates the receptors in the Golgi tendon organ. Therefore contraction of the muscle also stimulates the organ. Likewise, an overall stretching of the muscle creates tension in the tendon and stimulates the organ.

Pacinian Corpuscles. The pacinian corpuscles are large oval organs made up of concentric lamellae of connective tissue. These organs are widely distributed, and because of their common location in the joint structures they are considered to serve principally for the perception of movement and firm pressure (not light touch).

At the center of each corpuscle is a core containing the termination of a nerve fiber. These corpuscles are found in the tendons, joints, periosteum, tendinous insertions, fascia, and subcutaneous tissue. Pressure applied to such tissues deforms the organ and stimulates the nerve fiber.

Nociceptors. Generally, nociceptors are sensory receptors that are stimulated by injury and transmit injury information to the CNS by way of the afferent nerve fibers. Nociceptors are located throughout most of the tissues in the masticatory system. Several general types exist: Some respond exclusively to noxious mechanical and thermal stimuli; others respond to a wide range of stimuli, from tactile sensations to noxious injury; still others are low-threshold receptors specific for light touch, pressure, or facial hair movement. The last type is sometimes called a *mechanoreceptor*.

The nociceptors primarily function to monitor the condition, position, and movement of the tissues in the masticatory system. When conditions exist that are either potentially harmful or actually cause injury to the tissue, the nociceptors relay this information to the CNS as sensations of discomfort or pain. The sensation of pain is discussed later in this chapter.

NEUROMUSCULAR FUNCTION

Function of the Sensory Receptors

The dynamic balance of the head and neck muscles previously described is possible through feedback provided by the various sensory receptors. When a muscle is passively stretched, the spindles inform the CNS of this activity. Active muscle contraction is monitored by both the Golgi tendon organs and the muscle spindles. Movement of the joints and tendons stimulates the pacinian corpuscles. All of the sensory receptors are continuously providing input to the CNS. The brainstem and thalamus are in charge of constantly monitoring and regulating body activities. Information concerning normal body homeostasis is dealt with at this level, and the cortex is not even brought into the regulatory process. If, however, incoming information has significant consequence to the person, the thalamus passes the information to the cortex for conscious evaluation and decision. The thalamus and brainstem therefore have a powerful influence on the function of an individual.

Reflex Action

A reflex action is the response resulting from a stimulus that passes as an impulse along an afferent neuron to a posterior nerve root or its cranial equivalent, where it is then transmitted to an efferent neuron leading back to the skeletal muscle. Although the information is sent to the higher centers, the response is independent of will and

occurs normally with no cortex or brainstem influence. A reflex action may be monosynaptic or polysynaptic. A monosynaptic reflex occurs when the afferent fiber directly stimulates the efferent fiber in the CNS. A polysynaptic reflex is present when the afferent neuron stimulates one or more interneurons in the CNS, which in turn stimulate the efferent nerve fibers.

Two general reflex actions are important in the masticatory system: (1) the myotatic reflex and (2) the nociceptive reflex. These are not unique to the masticatory muscles but are found in other skeletal muscles as well.

Myotatic (Stretch) Reflex. The *myotatic* or *stretch reflex* is the only monosynaptic jaw reflex. When a skeletal muscle is quickly stretched, this protective reflex is elicited and brings about a contraction of the stretched muscle.

The myotatic reflex can be demonstrated by observing the masseter while a sudden downward force is applied to the chin. This force can be applied with a small rubber hammer (Fig. 2-5). As the muscle spindles within the masseter suddenly stretch, afferent nerve activity is generated from the spindles. These afferent impulses pass into the brainstem to the trigeminal motor nucleus by way of the trigeminal mesencephalic nucleus, where the primary afferent cell bodies are located. These same afferent fibers synapse with the alpha efferent motor neurons leading directly back to the extrafusal fibers of the masseter. Stimulation of the alpha efferent by the Ia afferent fibers causes the muscle to contract. Clinically, this reflex can be demonstrated by relaxing the jaw muscles, allowing the teeth to separate slightly. A sudden downward tap on the chin will cause the jaw to be reflexly elevated. The masseter contracts, resulting in tooth contact.

The myotatic reflex occurs without specific response from the cortex and is important in determining the resting position of the jaw. If complete relaxation of all the muscles that support the jaw occurred, the forces of gravity would act to lower the jaw and separate the articular surfaces of the temporomandibular joint (TMJ). To prevent this dislocation, the elevator muscles (and other muscles) are maintained in a mild state of contraction called *muscle tonus*. This property of the elevator

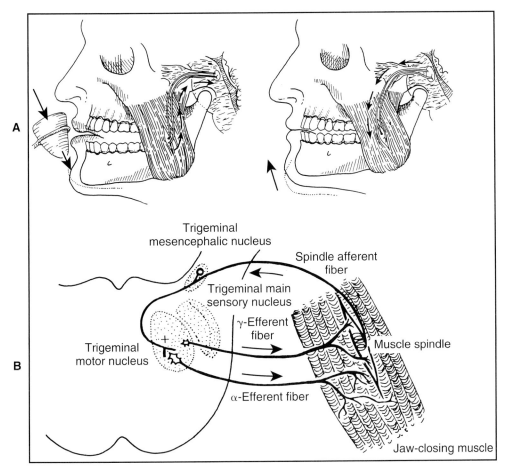

Fig. 2-5 A, Myotatic reflex is activated by a sudden application of downward force to the chin with a small rubber hammer. This results in contraction of the elevator muscles (masseter). This prevents further stretching and often causes an elevation of the mandible into occlusion. **B,** The pathway is as follows: Sudden stretching of the muscle spindle increases the afferent output from the spindle. The afferent impulses pass into the brainstem by way of the trigeminal mesencephalic nucleus. The afferent fibers synapse in the trigeminal motor nucleus with the alpha efferent motor neurons that lead directly back to the extrafusal fibers of the elevator muscle, which was stretched. The reflex information sent to the extrafusal fibers is to contract. The presence of the gamma efferent fibers is noted. Stimulation of these fibers can cause contraction of the intrafusal fibers of the spindle and thus sensitize the spindle to a sudden stretch. *(From Sessle BJ: Mastication, swallowing, and related activities. In Roth GI, Calmes R, editors: Oral biology, St Louis, 1981, Mosby.)*

muscles counteracts the effect of gravity on the mandible and maintains the articular surfaces of the joint in constant contact. The myotatic reflex is a principal determinant of muscle tonus in the elevator muscles. As gravity pulls down on the mandible, the elevator muscles are passively stretched, which also creates stretching of the muscle spindles. This information is reflexly passed from the afferent neurons originating in the spindles to the alpha motor neurons that lead back to the extrafusal fibers of the elevator muscles. Thus passive stretching causes a reactive contraction that relieves the stretch on the muscle spindle. Muscle tonus can also be influenced by afferent input from other sensory receptors, such as those from the skin or the oral mucosa.

The myotatic reflex and resulting muscle tonus can also be influenced by the higher centers via the fusimotor system. The cortex and brainstem can bring about increased gamma efferent activity to the intrafusal fibers of the spindle. As this activity increases, the intrafusal fibers contract, causing a partial stretching of the nuclear bag and nuclear chain areas of the spindles. This lessens the amount of stretch needed in the overall muscle before the spindle afferent activity is elicited. Therefore the higher centers can use the fusimotor system to alter the sensitivity of the muscle spindles to stretch. Increased gamma efferent activity increases the sensitivity of the myotatic (stretch) reflex, whereas decreased gamma efferent activity decreases the sensitivity of this reflex. The specific manner by which the higher centers influence gamma efferent activity is summarized later in this chapter.

When a muscle contracts, the muscle spindles are shortened, which causes the afferent activity output of these spindles to shut down. If the electrical potential of the afferent nerve activity is monitored, a silent period (no electrical activity) is noted during this contraction stage. Gamma efferent activity can influence the length of the silent period. High gamma efferent activity causes contraction of the intrafusal fibers, which lessens the time the spindle is shut down during a muscle contraction. Decreased gamma efferent activity lengthens this silent period.

Nociceptive (Flexor) Reflex. The *nociceptive* or *flexor reflex* is a polysynaptic reflex to noxious stimuli and therefore is considered to be protective. Examples are present in the large limbs (e.g., in withdrawal of a hand as it touches a hot object). In the masticatory system this reflex becomes active when a hard object is suddenly encountered during mastication (Fig. 2-6). As the tooth is forced down on the hard object, a sudden, noxious stimulus is generated by overloading the periodontal structures. The primary afferent nerve fibers carry the information to the trigeminal spinal tract nucleus, where they synapse with interneurons.

These interneurons travel to the trigeminal motor nucleus. The motor response taken during this reflex is more complicated than the myotatic reflex in that the activity of several muscle groups must be coordinated to carry out the desired motor response.[9,10] Not only must the elevator muscles be inhibited to prevent further jaw closure on the hard object, but the jaw opening muscles must be activated to bring the teeth away from potential damage.[11,12] As the afferent information from the sensory receptors reaches the interneurons, two distinct actions occur:

1. Excitatory interneurons leading to the efferent neurons in the trigeminal motor nucleus of the jaw-opening muscles are stimulated. This action causes these muscles to contract.
2. At the same time the afferent fibers stimulate inhibitory interneurons, which have the effect on the jaw-elevating muscles of causing them to relax.

The overall result is that the jaw quickly drops and the teeth are pulled away from the object causing the noxious stimulus. This process is called *antagonistic inhibition*, and it occurs in many nociceptive reflex actions throughout the body.

The myotatic reflex protects the masticatory system from sudden stretching of a muscle. The nociceptive reflex protects the teeth and supportive structures from damage created by sudden and unusually heavy functional forces. The Golgi tendon organs protect the muscle from overcontraction by eliciting inhibition stimuli directly to the muscle that they monitor. Numerous other types of reflex actions are found in the muscles of mastication. Many are complex and controlled in higher centers of the CNS. Reflex actions play a major role in functioning (e.g., mastication, swallowing, gagging, coughing, speaking).[3]

Reciprocal Innervation

The control of antagonistic muscles is of vital importance in reflex activity. It is of equal importance to the everyday function of the body. As in other muscle systems, each muscle that supports the head and in part controls function has an antagonist that counteracts its activity. This is the basis of the muscle balance previously described. Certain groups of muscles primarily elevate the

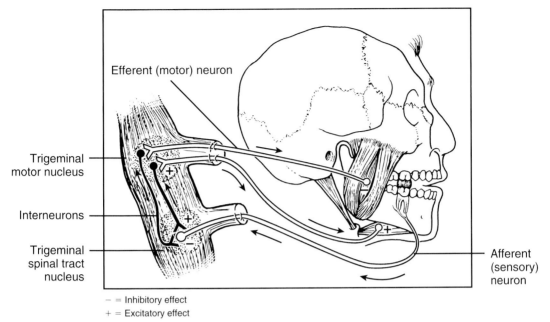

Efferent (motor) neuron

Trigeminal motor nucleus

Interneurons

Trigeminal spinal tract nucleus

Afferent (sensory) neuron

− = Inhibitory effect
+ = Excitatory effect

Fig. 2-6 The nociceptive reflex is activated by unexpectedly biting on a hard object. The noxious stimulus is initiated from the tooth and periodontal ligament being stressed. Afferent nerve fibers carry the impulse to the trigeminal spinal tract nucleus. The afferent neurons stimulate both excitatory and inhibitory interneurons. The interneurons synapse with the efferent neurons in the trigeminal motor nucleus. Inhibitory interneurons synapse with efferent fibers leading to the elevator muscles. The message carried is to discontinue contraction. The excitatory interneurons synapse with the efferent neurons that innervate the jaw-depressing muscles. The message sent is to contract, which brings the teeth away from the noxious stimulus.

mandible; other groups primarily depress it. For the mandible to be elevated by the temporal, medial pterygoid, or masseter muscles, the suprahyoid muscles must relax and lengthen. Likewise, for it to be depressed, the suprahyoids must contract while the elevators relax and lengthen.

The neurologic controlling mechanism for these antagonistic groups is known as *reciprocal innervation*. This phenomenon enables smooth and exact control of mandibular movement to be achieved. For the skeletal relationship of the skull, mandible, and neck to be maintained, each of the antagonistic muscle groups must remain in a constant state of mild tonus. This will overcome the skeletal imbalances of gravity and keep the head in what is termed the *postural position*. As discussed previously, muscle tonus plays an important role in the mandibular rest position, as well as in resistance to any passive displacement of the mandible. Muscles that are in full contraction activate most of the muscle fibers that can compromise blood flow, resulting in fatigue and pain. By contrast, muscle tonus requires contraction of a minimal number of muscle fibers, and the contracting fibers are constantly being rotated. This type of activity allows proper blood flow and does not produce fatigue.

Regulation of Muscle Activity

To create a precise mandibular movement, input from the various sensory receptors must be received by the CNS through the afferent fibers. The brainstem and cortex must assimilate and organize this input and elicit appropriate motor activities through the efferent nerve fibers. These motor activities involve the contraction of some muscle groups and the inhibition of others. It is generally thought that the gamma efferent system is permanently activated, though it does not necessarily set up movement. The gamma discharge keeps the alpha motor neurons reflexly prepared to receive impulses arising from the cortex or directly from the afferent impulses of the spindles. Most mandibular movements are probably controlled by a link between the gamma efferents, the spindle afferents, and the alpha motor neurons. This combined output produces the required contraction or inhibition of the muscles and allows the neuromuscular system to keep a check on itself.

Various conditions of the masticatory system greatly influence mandibular movement and function. The sensory receptors in the periodontal ligaments, periosteum, TMJs, tongue, and other soft tissues of the mouth continuously feed back information, which is processed and used to direct muscle activity. Noxious stimuli are reflexly avoided so that movement and function can occur with minimal injury to the tissues and structures of the masticatory system.

Influence from the Higher Centers

As previously mentioned, the brainstem and cortex function together to assess and evaluate incoming impulses. Although the cortex is the main determiner of action, the brainstem is in charge of maintaining homeostasis and controlling normally subconscious body functions. Within the brainstem is a pool of neurons that controls rhythmic muscle activities such as breathing, walking, and chewing. This pool of neurons is collectively know as the *central pattern generator* (CPG).[13-17] The CPG is responsible for the precise timing of activity between antagonistic muscles so that specific functions can be carried out. During the process of chewing, for example, the CPG initiates contraction of the suprahyoid and infrahyoid muscles at the precise time the elevator muscles are told to relax. This allows the mouth to open and accept food. Next the CPG initiates contraction of the elevator muscles while relaxing the suprahyoid and infrahyoid muscles, producing closure of the mouth onto the food. This process is repeated until the particle size of the food is small enough to be swallowed easily. For the CPG to be most efficient, it must receive constant sensory input

from the masticatory structures. Therefore the tongue, lips, teeth, and periodontal ligaments are constantly feeding back information that allows the CPG to determine the most appropriate and efficient chewing stroke.

Once an efficient chewing pattern that minimizes damage to any structure is found, it is learned and repeated. This learned pattern is called a *muscle engram*. Therefore chewing can be thought of as an extremely complex reflex activity that is primarily controlled by the CPG with input from numerous sensory receptors. Like many other reflex activities, chewing is a subconscious activity yet can be brought to conscious control at any time. Breathing and walking are other CPG reflex activities that generally occur at subconscious levels but can also be brought under voluntary control at will. The process of chewing is discussed in more detail later in this chapter.

Influence of the Higher Centers on Muscle Function. Generally when a stimulus is sent to the CNS, a complex interaction occurs to determine the appropriate response. The cortex, with influence from the thalamus, CPG, limbic structures, reticular formation, and hypothalamus, determines the action that will be taken in terms of direction and intensity. This action is often almost automatic, as in chewing. Although the patient is aware of it, there is no active participation in its execution. In the absence of any significant emotional state, the action is usually predictable and accomplishes the task efficiently. However, when the individual is experiencing higher levels of emotional states, such as fear, anxiety, frustration, or anger, the following major modifications of muscle activity can occur:

1. An increase in emotional stress excites the limbic structures and hypothalamic-pituitary-adrenal (HPA) axis activating the gamma efferent system.[18,19] With this increased gamma efferent activity comes contraction of the intrafusal fibers, resulting in partial stretching of the sensory regions of the muscle spindles. When spindles are partially stretched, less stretching of the overall muscle is necessary to elicit a reflex action. This affects the myotatic reflex and ultimately results in an increase in muscle tonus. The muscles also become more sensitive to external stimuli, which often leads to further

increases in muscle tonicity. These conditions lead to an increase in the interarticular pressure of the TMJ.

2. The increased gamma efferent activity may also increase the amount of irrelevant muscle activity. The reticular formation, with influence from the limbic system and HPA axis, can create additional muscle activity unrelated to the accomplishment of a specific task.[20] Often these activities assume the role of nervous habits such as biting on the fingernails or on pencils, clenching the teeth together, or bruxism. As discussed in Chapter 7, these activities can have dramatic effects on the function of the masticatory system.

MAJOR FUNCTIONS OF THE MASTICATORY SYSTEM

The neuroanatomy and physiology that have been discussed provide a mechanism by which important functional movements of the mandible can be executed. The three major functions of the masticatory system are (1) mastication, (2) swallowing, and (3) speech. In addition, secondary functions aid in respiration and the expression of emotions. All functional movements are highly coordinated, complex neuromuscular events. Sensory input from the structures of the masticatory system (i.e., teeth, periodontal ligaments, lips, tongue, cheeks, palate) is received and integrated in the CPG with existing reflex actions and learned muscle engrams to achieve a desired functional activity. Because the occlusion of the teeth plays a principal role in function of the masticatory system, a sound understanding of the dynamics of these major functional activities is essential.

MASTICATION

Mastication is defined as the act of chewing foods.[21] It represents the initial stage of digestion, when the food is broken down into small particle sizes for ease of swallowing. Mastication is most often an enjoyable activity that uses the senses of taste, touch, and smell. When a person is hungry, mastication is a pleasurable and satisfying act. When the stomach is full, feedback inhibits these positive feelings.

Mastication may have a relaxing effect by decreasing muscle tonus and fidgeting activities.[22] It has been described as having a soothing quality.[23] Mastication is a complex function that uses not only the muscles, teeth, and periodontal supportive structures, but also the lips, cheeks, tongue, palate, and salivary glands. This functional activity is generally automatic and practically involuntary, yet when desired, it can be readily brought under voluntary control.

Chewing Stroke
Mastication is made up of rhythmic and well-controlled separation and closure of the maxillary and mandibular teeth. This activity is under the control of the CPG located in the brainstem. Each opening and closing movement of the mandible represents a chewing stroke. The complete chewing stroke has what is described as a tear-shaped movement pattern. It can be divided into opening and closing movements. The closing movement has been further subdivided into the *crushing phase* and the *grinding phase* (Fig. 2-7). During mastication, similar chewing strokes are repeated over and over as the food is broken down. When the mandible is traced in the frontal plane during a single chewing stroke, the following sequence occurs: In the opening phase, it drops downward from the intercuspal position to a point where the incisal edges of the teeth are about 16 to 18 mm apart. It then moves laterally 5 to 6 mm from the midline as the

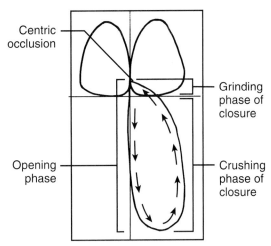

Fig. 2-7 Frontal view of the chewing stroke.

closing movement begins. The first phase of closure traps the food between the teeth and is called the *crushing phase*. As the teeth approach each other, the lateral displacement is lessened so that when the teeth are only 3 mm apart the jaw occupies a position only 3 to 4 mm lateral to the starting position of the chewing stroke. At this point the teeth are so positioned that the buccal cusps of the mandibular teeth are almost directly under the buccal cusps of the maxillary teeth on the side to which the mandible has been shifted. As the mandible continues to close, the bolus of food is trapped between the teeth. This begins the *grinding phase* of the closure stroke. During the grinding phase

the mandible is guided by the occlusal surfaces of the teeth back to the intercuspal position, which causes the cuspal inclines of the teeth to pass across each other, permitting shearing and grinding of the bolus of food.

If movement of a mandibular incisor is followed in the sagittal plane during a typical chewing stroke, it will be seen that during the opening phase the mandible moves slightly anteriorly (Fig. 2-8). During the closing phase it follows a slightly posterior pathway, ending in an anterior movement back to the maximum intercuspal position. The amount of anterior movement depends on the contact pattern of the anterior teeth[24] and the stage

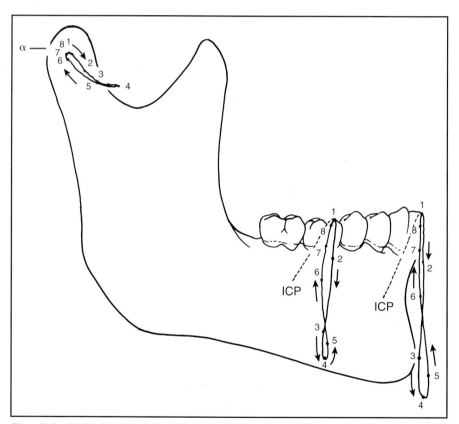

Fig. 2-8 CHEWING STROKE IN THE SAGITTAL PLANE OF THE WORKING SIDE. During opening, the incisor moves slightly anterior to the intercuspal position *(ICP)* and then returns from a slightly posterior position. The first molar has also been traced on the side to which the mandible moves (the working side). The molar begins with an anterior movement during the opening phase and a more posterior movement during the closing stroke. The working side condyle also moves posteriorly during the closing stroke *(α)* until final closure, when it shifts anteriorly to the intercuspal position. *(From Lundeen HC, Gibbs CH: Advances in occlusion, Boston, 1982, John Wright PSG.)*

of mastication. In the early stages, incising of food is often necessary. During incising the mandible moves forward a significant distance, depending on the alignment and position of the opposing incisors. After the food has been incised and brought into the mouth, less forward movement is necessary. In the later stages of mastication, crushing of the bolus is concentrated on the posterior teeth and little anterior movement occurs; yet even during the later stages of mastication, the opening phase is anterior to the closing stage.[25-27]

The movement of the mandibular first molar in the sagittal plane during a typical chewing stroke varies according to the side on which the person is chewing. If the mandible moves to the right side, then the right first molar moves in a pathway similar to that of the incisor. In other words, the molar moves slightly forward during the opening phase and closes on a slightly posterior pathway, moving anteriorly during the final closure as the tooth intercuspates. The condyle on the right side also follows this pathway, closing in a slightly posterior position with a final anterior movement into intercuspation (see Fig. 2-8).[25,27]

If the first molar is traced on the opposite side, it will be seen to follow a different pattern. When the mandible moves to the right side, the left mandibular first molar drops almost vertically, with little anterior or posterior movement until the complete opening phase has occurred. On closure the mandible moves anteriorly slightly and the tooth returns almost directly to intercuspation (Fig. 2-9). The condyle on the left side also follows a pathway similar to that of the molar. No final anterior movement into the intercuspal position in the pathway of either the molar or the condyle occurs.[25,27]

As with the anterior movement, the amount of lateral movement of the mandible relates to the stage of mastication. When food is initially introduced into the mouth, the amount of lateral

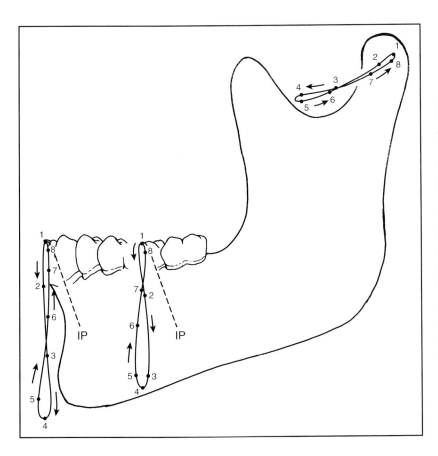

Fig. 2-9 CHEWING STROKE IN THE SAGITTAL PLANE OF THE NONWORKING SIDE. Note that the first molar initially drops from the intercuspal position *(IP)* almost vertically with little to no anterior or posterior movement. The final stage of the closing stroke is also almost completely vertical. The condyle on the nonworking side moves anteriorly during opening and follows almost the same pathway on its return. The nonworking side condyle is never situated posterior to the intercuspal position. *(From Lundeen HC, Gibbs CH: Advances in occlusion, Boston, 1982, John Wright PSG.)*

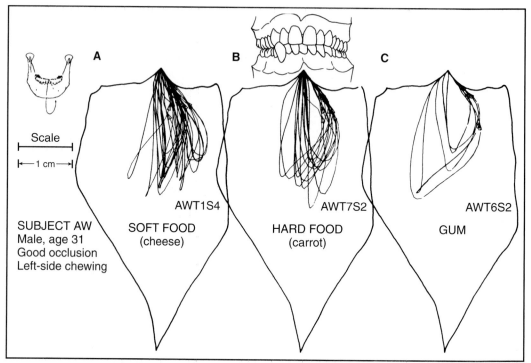

Fig. 2-10 CHEWING STROKE (FRONTAL VIEW). Chewing on a carrot (**B,** hard food) appears to create a broader stroke than chewing on cheese (**A,** soft food). Chewing gum (**C,** gum) produces an even broader and wider chewing stroke. *(From Lundeen HC, Gibbs CH: Advances in occlusion, Boston, 1982, John Wright PSG.)*

movement is great and then becomes less as the food is broken down. The amount of lateral movement also varies according to the consistency of the food (Fig. 2-10). The harder the food, the more lateral the closure stroke becomes.[25] The hardness of the food also has an effect on the number of chewing strokes necessary before a swallow is initiated: the harder the food, the more chewing strokes needed.[28] Interestingly, in some subjects the number of chewing strokes does not change with varying textures of food.[28] This might suggest that for some subjects the CPG is less influenced by sensory input and more by muscle engrams.

Although mastication can occur bilaterally, about 78% of observed subjects have a preferred side where the majority of chewing occurs.[29] This is normally the side with the greatest number of tooth contacts during lateral glide.[30,31] Persons who seem to have no side preference simply alternate their chewing from one side to the other. As mentioned in Chapter 1, chewing on one side leads to unequal

loading of the TMJs.[32-34] Under normal conditions this does not create any problem because of the stabilizing effect of the superior lateral pterygoids on the discs.

Tooth Contacts during Mastication

Early studies[35] suggested that the teeth do not actually contact during mastication. It was speculated that food between the teeth, along with the acute response of the neuromuscular system, prohibits tooth contacts. Other studies,[36,37] however, have revealed that tooth contacts do occur during mastication. When food is initially introduced into the mouth, few contacts occur. As the bolus is broken down, the frequency of tooth contacts increases. In the final stages of mastication, just before swallowing, contacts occur during each stroke.[38] Two types of contact have been identified: (1) *gliding*, which occurs as the cuspal inclines pass by each other during the opening and grinding phases of mastication, and (2) *single*, which occurs

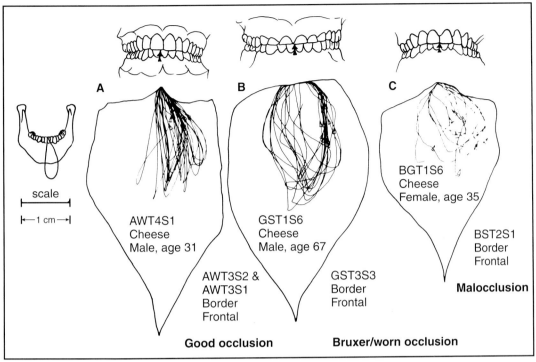

Fig. 2-11 BORDER AND CHEWING MOVEMENTS (FRONTAL VIEW) WITH LEFT SIDE WORKING. Note that the occlusal condition has a marked effect on the chewing stroke. **A,** Good occlusion. **B,** Worn occlusion (bruxism). **C,** Malocclusion. *(From Lundeen HC, Gibbs CH:* Advances in occlusion, *Boston, 1982, John Wright PSG.)*

in the maximum intercuspal position.[39] Apparently, all persons have some degree of gliding contacts. The mean percentage of gliding contacts that occur during chewing has been found to be 60% during the grinding phase and 56% during the opening phase.[40] The average length of time[40] for tooth contact during mastication is 194 ms. These contacts apparently influence or even dictate the initial opening and final grinding phase of the chewing stroke.[32] It has even been demonstrated that the occlusal condition can influence the entire chewing stroke. During mastication the quality and quantity of tooth contacts constantly relay sensory information back to the CNS regarding the character of the chewing stroke. This feedback mechanism allows for alteration in the chewing stroke according to the particular food being chewed. Generally, tall cusps and deep fossae promote a predominantly vertical chewing stroke, whereas flattened or worn teeth encourage a broader chewing stroke.

When the posterior teeth contact in undesirable lateral movement, the malocclusion produces an irregular and less repeatable chewing stroke (Fig. 2-11).[40]

When the chewing strokes of normal persons are compared with those of persons who have TMJ pain, marked differences can be seen.[41] Normal persons masticate with chewing strokes that are well rounded, are more repeated, and have definite borders. When the chewing strokes of persons with TMJ pain are observed, a less frequent repeat pattern is noted. The strokes are much shorter and slower and have an irregular pathway. These slower, irregular but repeatable pathways appear to relate to the altered functional movement of the condyle around which the pain is centered.

Forces of Mastication
The maximum biting force that can be applied to the teeth varies from individual to individual. It is generally found that males can bite with more force

than can females. In one study[42] it was reported that a female's maximum biting load ranges from 79 to 99 lb (35.8 to 44.9 kg), whereas a male's biting load varies from 118 to 142 lb (53.6 to 64.4 kg). The greatest maximum biting force reported is 975 lb (443 kg).[43]

It has also been noted that the maximum amount of force applied to a molar is usually several times that which can be applied to an incisor. In another study[44] the range of maximum force applied to the first molar was 91 to 198 lb (41.3 to 89.8 kg), whereas the maximum force applied to the central incisors was 29 to 51 lb (13.2 to 23.1 kg).

The maximum biting force appears to increase with age up to adolescence.[45,46] It has also been demonstrated[42,46-49] that individuals can increase their maximum biting force over time with practice and exercise. Therefore a person whose diet contains a high percentage of tough foods will develop a stronger biting force. This concept may explain why some studies[49] reveal an increased biting strength in the Eskimo population. Increased biting strength may also be attributed to facial skeletal relationships. Persons with marked divergence of the maxilla and mandible generally cannot apply as much force to the teeth as can persons with maxillary and mandibular arches that are relatively parallel.

The amount of force placed on the teeth during mastication varies greatly from individual to individual. A study by Gibbs et al.[50] reports that the grinding phase of the closure stroke averaged 58.7 lb on the posterior teeth. This represented 36.2% of the subject's maximum bite force. An earlier study that examined different food consistencies[51] suggested much less force. Anderson reported that chewing carrots produced approximately 30 lb (14 kg) of force on the teeth, whereas chewing meat produced only 16 lb (7 kg). It has also been demonstrated that tooth pain[52] or muscle pain[53] reduces the amount of forced used during chewing.

During chewing the greatest amount of force is placed on the first molar region.[54] With tougher foods, chewing occurs predominantly on the first molar and second premolar areas.[55-57] The biting force of subjects with complete dentures is only one fourth that of subjects with natural teeth.[57]

Role of the Soft Tissues in Mastication

Mastication could not be performed without the aid of adjacent soft tissue structures. As food is introduced into the mouth, the lips guide and control intake, as well as seal off the oral cavity. The lips are especially necessary when liquid is being introduced. The tongue plays a major role, not only in taste but also in maneuvering the food within the oral cavity for sufficient chewing. When food is introduced, the tongue often initiates the breaking-up process by pressing it against the hard palate. The tongue then pushes the food onto the occlusal surfaces of the teeth, where it can be crushed during the chewing stroke. During the opening phase of the next chewing stroke, the tongue repositions the partially crushed food onto the teeth for further breakdown. While it is repositioning the food from the lingual side, the buccinator muscle (in the cheek) is accomplishing the same task from the buccal side. The food is thus continuously replaced on the occlusal surfaces of the teeth until the particle size is small enough to be swallowed efficiently. The tongue is also effective in dividing food into portions that require more chewing and portions that are ready to be swallowed. After eating, the tongue sweeps the teeth to remove any food residue that has been trapped in the oral cavity.

SWALLOWING (DEGLUTITION)

Swallowing is a series of coordinated muscular contractions that moves a bolus of food from the oral cavity through the esophagus to the stomach. It consists of voluntary, involuntary, and reflex muscular activity. The decision to swallow depends on several factors: the degree of fineness of the food, the intensity of the taste extracted, and the degree of lubrication of the bolus. During swallowing the lips are closed, sealing the oral cavity. The teeth are brought up into their maximum intercuspal position, stabilizing the mandible.

Stabilization of the mandible is an important part of swallowing. The mandible must be fixed so that contraction of the suprahyoid and infrahyoid muscles can control proper movement of the hyoid bone needed for swallowing. The normal adult swallow that uses the teeth for mandibular stability has been called the *somatic swallow*. When teeth are not present, as in the infant, the mandible must be braced by other means. In the infantile swallow, or *visceral swallow*,[58] the mandible is braced by placing the tongue forward and between the dental arches or gum pads. This type of swallow occurs until the posterior teeth erupt.

As the posterior teeth erupt into occlusion, the occluding teeth brace the mandible and the adult swallow is assumed. Occasionally the normal transition from infantile swallow to adult swallow does not occur. This may be caused by lack of tooth support because of poor tooth position or arch relationship. The infantile swallow may also be maintained when discomfort occurs during tooth contact because of caries or tooth sensitivity. Overretention of the infantile swallow can result in labial displacement of the anterior teeth by the powerful tongue muscle. This may present clinically as an anterior open bite (no anterior tooth contacts). It should be noted, however, that the presence of a tongue-thrusting condition does not necessarily lead to altered tooth position.

In the normal adult swallow the mandible is stabilized by tooth contacts. The average tooth contact[40] during swallowing lasts about 683 ms. This is more than three times longer than during mastication. The force applied to the teeth[40] during swallowing is approximately 66.5 lb, which is 7.8 lb more than the force applied during mastication.

A common belief[59-62] has been that when the mandible is braced, it is brought into a somewhat posterior or retruded position. If the teeth do not fit well together in this position, an anterior slide occurs to the intercuspal position. Studies imply that when the teeth contact evenly and simultaneously in the retruded closing position, the muscles of mastication appear to function at lower levels of activity and more harmoniously during mastication.[63] In my opinion, the quality of the intercuspal position will determine the position of the mandible during swallowing, not a retruded relationship with fossa. Anterior slides are rarely seen during function. Muscle engrams and reflex activity maintain closure of the mandible into the intercuspal position.

Although swallowing is one continuous act, for purposes of discussion it is divided into three stages (Fig. 2-12).

First Stage

The first stage of swallowing is voluntary and begins with selective parting of the masticated food into a mass or bolus. This separation is performed mostly by the tongue. The bolus is placed on the dorsum of the tongue and pressed lightly against the hard palate. The tip of the tongue rests on the hard palate just behind the incisors. The lips are sealed, and the teeth are brought together. The presence of the bolus on the mucosa of the palate initiates a reflex wave of contraction in the tongue that presses the bolus backward. As the bolus reaches the back of the tongue, it is transferred to the pharynx.

Second Stage

Once the bolus has reached the pharynx, a peristaltic wave caused by contraction of the pharyngeal constrictor muscles carries it down to the esophagus. The soft palate rises to touch the posterior pharyngeal wall, sealing off the nasal passages. The epiglottis blocks the pharyngeal airway to the trachea and keeps the food in the esophagus. During this stage of swallowing the pharyngeal muscular activity opens the pharyngeal orifices of the eustachian tubes, which are normally closed.[23] These first two stages of swallowing together last an estimated 1 second.

Third Stage

The third stage of swallowing consists of passing the bolus through the length of the esophagus and into the stomach. Peristaltic waves carry the bolus down the esophagus. The waves take 6 to 7 seconds to carry the bolus through the length of the esophagus. As the bolus approaches the cardiac sphincter, the sphincter relaxes and lets the bolus enter the stomach. In the upper section of the esophagus, the muscles are mainly voluntary and can be used to return food to the mouth when necessary for more complete mastication. In the lower section the muscles are entirely involuntary.

Frequency of Swallowing

Studies[64] have demonstrated that the swallowing cycle occurs 590 times during a 24-hour period: 146 cycles during eating, 394 cycles between meals

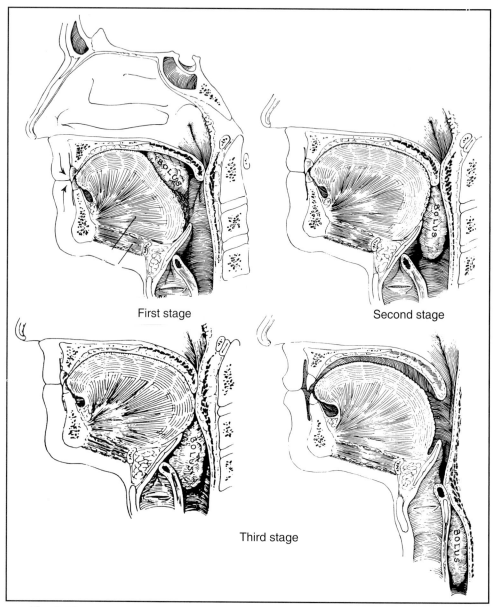

Fig. 2-12 Three stages of swallowing. *(From Silverman SI: Oral physiology, St Louis, 1961, Mosby.)*

while awake, and 50 cycles during sleep. Lower levels of salivary flow during sleep result in less need to swallow.[65]

SPEECH

Speech is the third major function of the masticatory system. It occurs when a volume of air is forced from the lungs by the diaphragm through the larynx and oral cavity. Controlled contraction and relaxation of the vocal cords or bands of the larynx create a sound with the desired pitch.[23] Once the pitch is produced, the precise form assumed by the mouth determines the resonance and exact articulation of the sound. Because speech is created by the release of air from the lungs, it occurs during

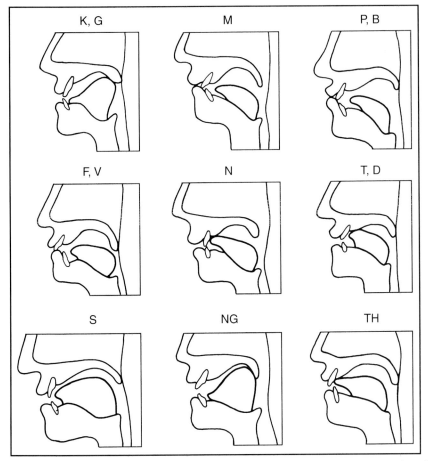

Fig. 2-13 Articulation of sounds created by specific positions of the lips, tongue, and teeth. *(From Jenkins GN: The physiology of the mouth, ed 4, Oxford, England, 1978, Blackwell Scientific.)*

the expiration stage of respiration. Inspiration of air is relatively quick and taken at the end of a sentence or pause. Expiration is prolonged, allowing a series of syllables, words, or phrases to be uttered.

Articulation of Sound

By varying the relationships of the lips and tongue to the palate and teeth, one can produce a variety of sounds.[23] Important sounds formed by the lips are the letters *m*, *b*, and *p*. During these sounds the lips come together and touch. The teeth are important in saying the *s* sound. The incisal edges of the maxillary and mandibular incisors closely approximate (but do not touch). The air is passed

between the teeth, and the *s* sound is created. The tongue and the palate are especially important in forming the *d* sound. The tip of the tongue reaches up to touch the palate directly behind the incisors.

Many sounds can also be formed by using a combination of these anatomic structures. For example, the tongue touches the maxillary incisors to form the *th* sound. The lower lip touches the incisal edges of the maxillary teeth to form the *f* and *v* sounds. For sounds such as *k* or *g*, the posterior portion of the tongue rises to touch the soft palate (Fig. 2-13).

During the early stages of life, people are taught proper articulation of sounds for speech. Tooth contacts do not occur during speech. If a malpositioned tooth contacts an opposing tooth during speech, sensory input from the tooth and periodontal ligament quickly relays the information to the CNS. The CNS perceives this as potentially damaging and immediately alters the speech pattern by way of the efferent nerve pathways. A new speech pattern that avoids the tooth contact is developed. This new pattern may result in a slight lateral deviation of the mandible to produce the desired sound without tooth contact.

Once speech is learned, it comes almost entirely under the unconscious control of the neuromuscular system. In that sense it can be thought of as a learned reflex.

MECHANISMS OF OROFACIAL PAIN

Pain, the physical sensation associated with injury or disease, is an extremely complex neurophysiologic process. When viewed superficially, it appears to be merely a protective reflex mechanism for the purpose of alarming the individual to harm or damage. It certainly does act in this manner, as can be seen when someone touches a hot object and reflexly pulls away (i.e., the nociceptive reflex), but this is obviously not the only type of pain. Often pain is felt in a body structure long after an injury has occurred, and therefore avoidance or protection from damage can not explain the occurrence of this pain.

PAIN MODULATION

For many years the degree and number of nociceptors stimulated were assumed to be responsible for the intensity of pain perceived by the CNS. This, however, is not found to be true clinically. In some patients small injuries create great pain, whereas in others only mild pain is reported with much greater injury. As pain has been studied, it has become increasingly clear that the degree of suffering does not relate well to the amount of tissue damage. Instead, the degree of suffering relates more closely to the patient's *perceived threat* of the injury and the amount of *attention given* to the injury.[66,67]

When this phenomenon was first appreciated, it defied contemporary pain theories. In 1965 the gate-control theory of pain modulation[68] was developed to explain the phenomenon, and in 1978 this theory was modified.[69] Pain modulation means that the impulses arising from a noxious stimulus, which are primarily carried by the afferent neurons from the nociceptors, can be altered before they reach the cortex for recognition. This alteration or modulation of sensory input can occur while the primary neuron synapses with the interneuron when it initially enters the CNS or while the input ascends to the brainstem and cortex. This influence may have an excitatory effect, which increases the noxious stimulus, or an inhibitory effect, which decreases the stimulus.

The conditions that influence the modulation of noxious input can be either psychologic or physical. Psychologic factors relate to the emotional state of the person (e.g., happy, sad, contented, depressed, anxious). In addition, prior conditioning influences the person's response to a noxious stimulus. Physical factors (e.g., rested or fatigued) also affect pain modulation. Tissue inflammation and hyperemia tend to enhance the sensation of pain. Likewise, the duration of the stimulus tends to affect pain in an excitatory manner. In other words, the longer a stimulus is felt, the greater the pain becomes.

At this point it is important to distinguish the differences among four terms: nociception, pain, suffering, and pain behavior:

1. *Nociception* refers to the noxious stimulus originating from the sensory receptor. This information is carried into the CNS by the primary neuron.
2. *Pain* is an unpleasant sensation perceived in the cortex, usually as a result of incoming nociceptive input. The presence or absence of nociceptive input, however, does not always relate closely to pain. As mentioned, the CNS can alter or modulate nociceptive input before it reaches the cortex for recognition. Therefore nociceptive input entering the CNS can be modified in such a manner that the cortex never perceives it as pain. This ability of the CNS to modulate noxious stimulation is an extremely important function. The modulation of nociception input can both increase and decrease the perception of pain.

3. *Suffering* refers to yet another phenomenon: how the human reacts to the perception of pain. When pain is perceived by the cortex, a complex interaction of many factors begins. Factors such as past experiences, expectations, perceived threat of the injury, and attention drawn to the injury determine to what degree the subject will suffer. Suffering, therefore, may not be proportionally related to nociception or pain. Patients experiencing little pain may suffer greatly, whereas others with significant pain may suffer less.

4. *Pain behavior* is still another term with a different meaning. *Pain behavior* refers to the individual's audible and visible actions that communicate suffering to others. Pain behavior is the only communication the clinician receives regarding the pain experience. This behavior is as unique as people themselves.

The clinician must recognize that the information related to the therapist by the patient is neither nociception nor pain nor even suffering. The patient only relates his or her pain behavior. Yet it is through this communication that the clinician must gain insight into the patient's problem; this is often a difficult task.

The body has at least three mechanisms by which pain can be modulated[70]: (1) the nonpainful cutaneous stimulation system, (2) the intermittent painful stimulation system, and (3) the psychologic modulating system.

Nonpainful Cutaneous Stimulation System

Nerve fibers carrying information to the CNS (afferent fibers) have various thicknesses. As mentioned earlier, the larger the diameter of the fiber, the faster the impulses it carries will travel. The afferents are divided into four major groups according to size: I (a and b), II, III, and IV. Another system uses standard capital letters with Greek letter subdivisions: A alpha, equivalent to group I; A beta, to group II; A delta, to group III; and C, to group IV. The A delta and C divisions are the main conductors of pain. The large A fibers (group I) carry the sensations of touch, motion, and position (proprioception). It has been postulated that if the larger fibers are stimulated at the same time as the smaller ones, the larger fibers will mask the input to the CNS of the smaller ones.[69] According to this theory, for

the effect to be great, the stimulation of the large fibers must be constant and below a painful level. The effect is immediate and usually vanishes after the large-fiber stimulus is removed.

Noxious input that reaches the spinal cord can also be altered at virtually each synapse in the ascending pathway to the cortex. This modulation of pain is attributed to various structures that have been collectively called the *descending inhibitory system*. The descending inhibitory system maintains an extremely important function in the CNS. The CNS receives a constant barrage of sensory impulses from all structures in the body. This sensory input is generated in the dorsal root ganglia and can be perceived as painful.[71] One role of the descending inhibitory system is to modulate this input so as not to be perceived by the cortex as pain. This system can be thought of as an intrinsic analgesic mechanism. The descending inhibitory system apparently uses several neurotransmitters, with one of the most important being serotonin.[72-74] This system is also likely to play an important role in other brainstem functions that have been previously discussed.

The descending inhibitory system assists the brainstem in actively suppressing input to the cortex. The importance of this function becomes obvious when one looks at the process of sleep. In order for an individual to sleep, the brainstem and descending inhibitory system must completely inhibit sensory input (e.g., sound, sight, touch) to the cortex. Without a well-functioning descending inhibitory system, sleep would be impossible. A poorly functioning descending inhibitory system is also likely to allow unwanted sensory input to ascend to the cortex and be perceived as painful. In this condition pain is perceived in the absence of noxious stimulation. This is precisely what is seen routinely in chronic pain management centers. In other words, patients report significant pain in the absence of apparent cause.

Transcutaneous electrical nerve stimulation (TENS) is an example of the nonpainful cutaneous stimulation system masking a painful sensation. Constant subthreshold impulses in larger nerves near the site of an injury or other lesion block the smaller nerves' input, preventing painful stimuli from reaching the brain. When the TENS is discontinued, however, the pain usually returns. (The use of TENS in the management of certain pain conditions is discussed in Chapter 11.)

Intermittent Painful Stimulation System

Another type of pain-modulation system can be evoked by the stimulation of areas of the body that have high concentrations of nociceptors and low electrical impedance. Stimulation of these areas may reduce pain felt at a distant site. This reduction is due to the release of endogenous opioids called *endorphins*. Endorphins are polypeptides produced in the body that seem to have effects as powerful as (possibly more powerful than) those of morphine in reducing pain.

Two basic types of endorphins have been identified: (1) the enkephalins and (2) the beta-endorphins. The enkephalins appear to be released in the cerebrospinal fluid and therefore act quickly and locally to reduce pain. The beta-endorphins are released like hormones by the hypophysis cerebri into the bloodstream. They are slower acting than the enkephalins, but their effect lasts longer.

For endorphins to be released, it appears that certain areas of the body must be intermittently stimulated to a level of pain. This is the basis for acupuncture: A needle placed in a specific area of the body having high concentrations of nociceptors and low electrical impedance is twisted approximately two times a second to create intermittent low levels of pain. The stimulation causes the release of certain enkephalins in the cerebrospinal fluid, and this reduces the pain felt in tissues innervated by that area. Beta-endorphins are released into the bloodstream by physical exercise, especially prolonged exercise, which may help explain why long-distance runners often experience a euphoric feeling after a run ("runner's high"). Because they are released into the bloodstream, beta-endorphins create an effect that is more generalized throughout the body and lasts longer than the enkephalins.

Psychologic Modulating System

At present the manner in which the psychologic modulating system functions is not well understood.

However, it is believed to exert great influence on the suffering that a person experiences. For example, certain psychologic states affect pain, some positively and some negatively. Increased levels of emotional stress can be strongly correlated with increased levels of pain.[75] Other conditions that seem to intensify the pain experience are anxiety, fear, depression, and despair. Certainly the amount of attention drawn to an injury, as well as the consequence of the injury, can greatly influence suffering. Patients who devote a great amount of attention to their pain are likely to suffer more. Conversely, patients who are able to direct attention away from their pain are likely to suffer less. Distractions such as psychologic or physical activities can often be helpful in reducing pain. Psychologic states such as confidence, assurance, tranquility, and serenity should be encouraged. Prior conditioning and experience also affect the degree of pain felt. (The psychologic modulating system is discussed in later chapters.)

Rationale

After one has grasped the concept of pain modulation, it is easy to see that pain is a great deal more than a mere sensation or reflex. It is the end result of a process that has been altered between its origins (the nociceptors) and its destination (the cortex) by both physical and psychologic factors. It may best be described as an experience rather than just a sensation, especially when it is of long duration. The experience of pain and eventually suffering may be the most important consideration in caring for patients.

TYPES OF PAIN

To better understand and treat pain, the clinician must be able to differentiate its *source* from its *site*. Although these words may sound similar, they are not the same. The site of pain is the location where the patient describes feeling it. The source of pain is the location where it is actually originating. Practitioners may be tempted to assume that these are identical, but they are not always. Pain with a site and source in the same location is *primary pain*. Primary pain is easily appreciated because it is likely the most common type of pain. A good example would be a toothache. The patient feels pain in a specific tooth, and a dental examination reveals this tooth to have a large carious lesion, which in fact is causing the pain. (The site and the source are the same.)

Not all pains are primary, however, and this can make the treatment of masticatory disorders problematic. Some pains have their site and source in different locations. In other words, where the patient feels the pain is not where the pain is originating. These are called *heterotopic pains*. Generally three types of heterotopic pain exist:

1. *Central pain*. When a tumor or other disturbance is present in the CNS, the pain is often felt not in the CNS but in peripheral structures. For example, some brain tumors can produce pain in the face, neck, and even the shoulder; and often accompanying this pain are systemic symptoms of nausea, muscle weakness, numbness, and balance disorders.

2. *Projected pain*. In this type, neurologic disturbances cause painful sensations to shoot down the peripheral distributions of the same nerve root that is involved in the disturbance. An example of projected pain would be entrapment of a nerve in the cervical region, which produces pain that is felt radiating down the arm to the hand and fingers.

3. *Referred pain*. With this type, the sensations are felt not in the involved nerve but in other branches of that nerve or even in an entirely different nerve. An example of referred pain is cardiac pain. When a patient suffers a myocardial infarction (heart attack), the pain is often felt in the neck and mandible, radiating down the left arm, rather than in the area of the heart.[76]

Referred pain is not a haphazard occurrence but seems to follow certain clinical rules:

1. The most frequent occurrence of referred pain is within a single nerve root, passing from one branch to another (e.g., a mandibular molar referring pain to a maxillary molar). In this case the mandibular branch of the fifth cranial nerve (trigeminal) is referring pain to the maxillary branch of the same nerve. This is a fairly common occurrence with dental pain. Generally, if the pain is referred to another distribution of the same nerve, it does so in a "laminated" manner.[77] This means that incisors refer to incisors, premolars to premolars, and molars to molars on the same side of the mouth. In other words, molars do not refer pain to incisors or incisors to molars.

2. Sometimes referred pain can be felt outside the nerve responsible for it. When this occurs, it generally moves cephalad (upward, toward the head) and not caudal.

3. In the trigeminal area, referred pain never crosses the midline unless it originates at the midline. For example, pain in the right TMJ will not cross over to the left side of the face. This is not true, however, in the cervical region or below; cervicospinal pain can be referred across the midline, although it normally stays on the same side as the source.

Heterotopic pain is a frequent finding in head and neck pain problems. For treatment to be effective, it must be directed at the source and not the site of the pain. When dealing with primary pain, the clinician should not find this a problem because the site and the source are the same. With heterotopic pain, however, a common mistake is to treat the site of the pain—and this will always fail to resolve the pain problem. An example of such misdirected effort would be treating jaw pain at the dental level for a patient who was having a heart attack. Remember, treatment must be aimed toward the *source* and not toward the *site* of pain.

Another rule to remember is that local provocation of the source of pain will cause an increase in symptoms, but local provocation of the site of pain will generally not increase symptoms. For example, if the TMJ is the source of pain, jaw movement (local provocation) will accentuate the pain; but if the cervical muscles are the source and the pain is referred to the region of the TMJ (a common situation), the patient will complain of TMJ pain but jaw function will not increase this pain. The same is true when cardiac pain is referred to the jaw. Jaw function does not increase the pain. Pain that is felt in the masticatory structures but is not accentuated by jaw function should be looked on with suspicion. It may be coming from another structure, and treatment rendered to the masticatory apparatus would not be indicated.

CENTRAL EXCITATORY EFFECT

Although referred pain has been clinically recognized for years, the precise mechanism by which it is created has not been scientifically documented. Apparently, certain input into the CNS, such as deep pain, can create an excitatory effect on other nonassociated interneurons. This phenomenon is called the *central excitatory effect*. It has been suggested that neurons carrying nociceptive input into the CNS can excite other interneurons in one of two possible ways:

1. The first explanation suggests that if the afferent input is constant and prolonged, it continuously bombards the interneuron, resulting in an accumulation of neurotransmitter substance at the synapses. If this accumulation becomes great, neurotransmitter substance can spill over to an adjacent interneuron, causing it also to become excited. From there, the impulses go to the brain centrally and the brain perceives nociception being transmitted by both neurons. The original excited neuron is, of course, providing input from a true source of pain (primary pain), but the other neuron is being only centrally excited. Therefore the pain perceived by the brain from this neuron is heterotopic pain (specifically, referred pain).

2. A second explanation of the central excitatory effect is that of convergence.[78-80] It is well documented that many incoming neurons can synapse on a single interneuron. That single interneuron may itself be one of many neurons that converge to synapse with the next ascending interneuron. As this convergence nears the brainstem and cortex, it can become increasingly difficult for the cortex to evaluate the precise location of the input. Under normal circumstances the cortex does an excellent job of differentiating sites. However, in the presence of continuous deep pain the convergence can confuse the cortex, resulting in the perception of pain in normal structures (heterotopic pain).

Importantly, the clinician should realize that all pains do not cause central excitatory effects.

The type of pain that can create these heterotopic pain effects is constant (not intermittent) and has its source in deep structures (not the skin or gingiva). Examples of structures that can produce *deep pain* are musculoskeletal, neural, vascular, and visceral structures.

Of particular interest is the relationship of the descending tract of the trigeminal nerve to the upper dorsal roots. This relationship explains how deep pain in the cervical region can commonly be referred to the face. Important to remember is that the sensory input from the trigeminal nerve synapses in the spinal V nucleus. Also important to appreciate is that the most caudal region of the spinal tract nucleus extends inferiorly into the region where the upper cervical nerves enter the spinal cord (cervical nerves 1 through 5). Therefore neurons from the trigeminal, as well as cranial nerves VII, IX, and X, share in the same neuron pool with neurons from the upper cervical spine.[81-83] This convergence of the trigeminal and cervical nerves is an anatomic and physiologic explanation for referred pain from the cervical region to the trigeminal. Fig. 2-14 depicts this condition.

As an example of the central excitatory effect, consider the cervicospinal muscles and the TMJ. Experiencing a cervicospinal extension-flexion injury (whiplash) in a motor vehicle accident is not uncommon.[84] If after several weeks the condition is not relieved, it becomes a source of constant deep pain. This pain input originates at the primary neurons, which synapse with interneurons, and the messages converge in the CNS. If at the synapse of an interneuron an overproduction of neurotransmitter substance (or a convergence effect) occurs, a nearby interneuron can be excited. From that point on to the brain, the centrally excited interneuron carries nociceptive information. If the afferent interneuron is supplying information from the tissues of the TMJ, the brain then interprets the information as pain in the TMJ. In other words, the overall interpretation of the pain experience is that pain is felt in the cervicospinal area, as well as in the TMJ (see Fig. 2-14). The cervicospinal area is the true (primary) source of the pain, and the TMJ is the site of referred (heterotopic) pain. Thus although it may be functioning normally, the TMJ seems painful because of this central excitatory effect.

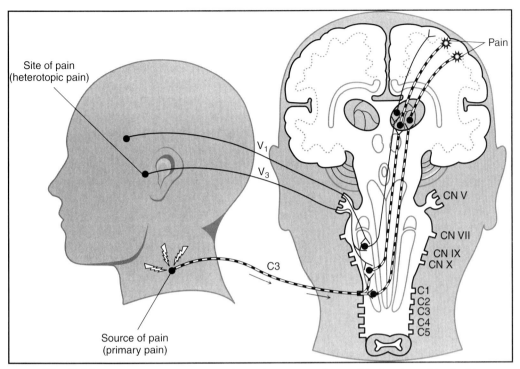

Fig. 2-14 Injury to the trapezius muscle results in tissue damage. Nociception arising in this cervical region is transmitted to the second-order neuron and relayed on to the higher centers for interruption. As this input becomes protracted, the adjacent converging neuron is also centrally excited, which relays additional nociception on to the higher centers. The sensory cortex now perceives two locations of pain. One area is the trapezius region that represents a true source of nociception (primary pain). The second area of perceived pain is felt in the temporomandibular joint area, which is only a site of pain, not a source of pain. This pain is heterotopic (referred). *(Modified from Okeson JP: Bell's orofacial pains, ed 6, Chicago, 2005, Quintessence.)*

Treatment of the masticatory apparatus will not resolve the complaints because the masticatory apparatus is only the site of the pain, not the source.

The previous illustration needs to be well appreciated by the dentist treating patients with facial pain disorders because it occurs frequently. Failure to recognize this condition will certainly lead to an improper diagnosis and mistreatment. The importance of this phenomenon cannot be overemphasized to the dentist treating pain. The implications of this central excitatory effect is discussed in future chapters.

Clinical Manifestations of the Central Excitatory Effect

Central excitatory effects can present several distinct clinical manifestations according to the type of interneuron affected (afferent, efferent, or autonomic).

When *afferent* interneurons are involved, referred pain is often reported. Referred pain is wholly dependent on the original source of the pain. In other words, local provocation of the *site* of the pain does not accentuate the sensation experienced by the patient. However, local provocation of the *source* both increases the pain at the source and often also increases the pain felt at the site. A local anesthetic blockade of the site does not affect the pain felt because this is not where the pain is originating. A local anesthetic blockade of the source masks both the source and the site of referred pain. Diagnostic blocking of the site and source of pain can be extremely useful when investigating pain problems (and is discussed in more detail in Chapter 10).

Another type of pain sensation that can be experienced when afferent interneurons are stimulated is *secondary hyperalgesia*.[85] To understand this condition, the term must be broken down and explained. *Hyper* implies raised or increased; *algesia* suggests a painful condition. The word, in fact, means increased sensitivity to painful stimulus. Primary hyperalgesia occurs when increased sensitivity results because of some local factor, such as a splinter in the finger. After a few hours the tissue around the splinter becomes quite sensitive to touch. This is primary hyperalgesia because the source of the problem (the splinter) is in the same location as the site of the heightened sensitivity. Secondary hyperalgesia is present when there is increased sensitivity of tissues without a local cause. A common location for secondary hyperalgesia is the scalp. Patients who experience constant deep pain will commonly report that "their hair hurts." When the scalp is examined, no local cause can be found. This is a fairly frequent situation in cases of head and neck pain.

Secondary hyperalgesia is slightly different from referred pain in that local anesthetic blocking at the source of the pain may not immediately arrest the symptoms. Instead, secondary hyperalgesia may linger for some time (12 to 24 hours) after the blockade is administered. This clinical feature can cause some confusion during diagnosis.

Until now only the central excitatory effect as a producer of pain symptoms has been considered. This is true when afferent interneurons are involved. If the central excitatory effect involves efferent interneurons, however, motor responses can be experienced. One type of efferent effect is the development of a localized area of hypersensitivity within the muscle tissues. These areas are called *trigger points*, and they are discussed in more detail in later chapters. Another common efferent effect secondary to constant deep pain is a reflex excitation of the muscle that slightly modifies its functional activity.[86] As previously discussed, the CPG regulates rhythmic activities of the mandible. Therefore when the mouth is opened, the depressing muscles are activated while the elevator muscles are relaxed. In the presence of pain, however, the CNS seems to respond differently. Stohler[87] has

demonstrated that when facial pain is experimentally introduced in normal subjects, the masseter muscle reveals an increase in electromyographic activity during opening of the mouth. This antagonistic muscle action causes a decrease in the velocity and degree of mouth opening. Experts believe that the CNS produces these effects so as to protect the threatened part.[8]

This phenomenon is called *protective co-contraction* because of simultaneous contraction of antagonistic muscle groups. Bell[88] recognized this CNS response as protective muscle splinting. Although this condition is a normal CNS response to deep pain, it can lead to muscle pain if it is prolonged. Protective co-contraction (muscle splinting) is normally experienced in the general location of the deep pain input, or cephalad to it (following the same rules as for referred pain). Thus pain felt in the cervical spine can produce a reflex muscle response in the trigeminal area, such as in the muscles of mastication.[89] This condition is not unusual and unfortunately fools many dentists into treating the muscles of mastication as the primary source of the pain. However, such treatment alone cannot resolve the problem because the origin of the protective co-contraction is the cervical spine. Cervicospinal pain must be addressed for effective elimination of the masticatory muscle pain problem.

Understanding the effect of deep pain on the masticatory muscles is extremely important for patient management. This topic is discussed with great detail in later chapters. One aspect of this pain, however, must be addressed at this time because it is vitally important in understanding muscle pain. As has already been stated, deep pain input can induce protective co-contraction. If co-contraction is protracted, muscle pain will result. Once muscle pain is present it represents a source of deep pain, which can continue to produce more co-contraction. The clinical result is a pain condition that is self-perpetuating. This condition then becomes wholly independent of the original source of pain. Previously this condition was called *cyclic muscle spasms*. Recent studies, however, fail to support the concept that the muscles are actually experiencing spasms.[8] Therefore this condition is more appropriately called *cyclic muscle pain*. This condition can become a diagnostic problem for the clinician because the patient continues to report suffering long after the original source of pain has resolved.

Because cyclic muscle pain is an important clinical problem to understand, the following example is given to illustrate some considerations in its management.

Case Report

A third molar is extracted, and during the ensuing week a localized osteitis (dry socket) develops. This becomes a source of constant deep pain that, by way of the central excitatory effect, produces protective co-contraction (muscle splinting) of the masseter and medial pterygoid muscle. The patient returns in 5 days complaining of the painful condition. Examination reveals a limited range of mandibular opening, caused not by the infection but by the secondary muscle response. If the source of the deep pain is resolved quickly (i.e., the local osteitis is eliminated), the protective co-contraction is resolved and normal mandibular opening will return. If the source is not quickly resolved, the protracted co-contraction may itself produce pain, which then perpetuates the protective co-contraction and establishes a cyclic muscle pain condition. In such a case, eliminating the original source of pain (the osteitis) will not eliminate the muscle pain. Treatment must now be directed specifically toward the masticatory muscle pain disorder, which has become wholly independent of the original source of pain. ▪

If central excitatory effects involve the autonomic neurons, characteristic manifestations will be seen. Because the autonomic system controls the dilation and constriction of blood vessels, variation in blood flow will appear as reddening or blanching of the involved tissues. Patients may complain of puffy eyelids or a dry eye. Sometimes the conjunctivae of the eye will redden. Even allergy-type symptoms may be reported (e.g., a stuffy or runny nose). Some patients may report a swelling of the face on the same side as the pain. Clinically significant swelling is rarely seen in temporomandibular disorders, yet this complaint is commonly reported by many patients and may represent slight edema secondary to autonomic effects.

The key to determining whether these symptoms are a result of the central excitatory effect is their unilaterality. Clinicians should remember that central excitatory effects do not cross the midline in the trigeminal area. Therefore the clinical manifestations will be seen only on the side of the constant deep pain. In other words, one eye will be red and the other normal, or one nostril may be discharging mucus and the other not. If the source of the autonomic problem were systemic (e.g., allergy), both eyes would be red and both nostrils discharging.

Understanding these central excitatory effects is basic to the management of facial pain problems. The role that such conditions play in the diagnosis and treatment of temporomandibular disorders is discussed in detail in later chapters.

Suggested Readings

Bell WE: *Temporomandibular disorders: classification, diagnosis, management*, ed 3, Chicago, 1990, Year Book Medical.

Okeson JP: *Bell's orofacial pains*, ed 6, Chicago, 2005, Quintessence.

References

1. Okeson JP: *Bell's orofacial pains*, ed 6, Chicago, 2005, Quintessence.
2. Guyton AC: *Textbook of medical physiology*, Philadelphia, 1991, Saunders, p 1013.
3. De Laat A: Reflexes elicitable in jaw muscles and their role during jaw function and dysfunction: a review of the literature. Part II. Central connections of orofacial afferent fibers, *Cranio* 5:246-253, 1987.
4. Dubner R, Bennett GJ: Spinal and trigeminal mechanisms of nociception, *Annu Rev Neurosci* 6:381-418, 1983.
5. Sessle BJ: The neurobiology of facial and dental pain: present knowledge, future directions, *J Dent Res* 66:962-981, 1987.
6. Hu JW, Dostrovsky JO, Sessle BJ: Functional properties of neurons in cat trigeminal subnucleus caudalis (medullary dorsal horn). I. Responses to oral-facial noxious and nonnoxious stimuli and projections to thalamus and subnucleus oralis, *J Neurophysiol* 45:173-192, 1981.
7. Sessle BJ: Recent insights into brainstem mechanisms underlying craniofacial pain, *J Dent Educ* 66:108-112, 2002.
8. Lund JP, Donga R, Widmer CG, Stohler CS: The pain-adaptation model: a discussion of the relationship between

chronic musculoskeletal pain and motor activity, *Can J Physiol Pharmacol* 69:683-694, 1991.

9. Tsai CM, Chiang CY, Yu XM, Sessle BJ: Involvement of trigeminal subnucleus caudalis (medullary dorsal horn) in craniofacial nociceptive reflex activity, *Pain* 81:115-128, 1999.

10. Tsai C: The caudal subnucleus caudalis (medullary dorsal horn) acts as an interneuronal relay site in craniofacial nociceptive reflex activity, *Brain Res* 826:293-297, 1999.

11. Stohler CS, Ash MM: Excitatory response of jaw elevators associated with sudden discomfort during chewing, *J Oral Rehabil* 13:225-233, 1986.

12. Manns AE, Garcia C, Miralles R, Bull R, Rocabado M: Blocking of periodontal afferents with anesthesia and its influence on elevator EMG activity, *Cranio* 9:212-219, 1991.

13. Lund JP, Dellow PG: The influence of interactive stimuli on rhythmical masticatory movements in rabbits, *Arch Oral Biol* 16:215-223, 1971.

14. Nozaki S, Iriki A, Nakamura Y: Localization of central rhythm generator involved in cortically induced rhythmical masticatory jaw-opening movement in the guinea pig, *Neurophysiology* 55:806-825, 1986.

15. Dellow PG, Lund JP: Evidence for central timing of rhythmical mastication, *J Physiol (Lond)* 215:1-13, 1971.

16. Lund JP: Mastication and its control by the brainstem, *Crit Rev Oral Biol Med* 2:33-64, 1991.

17. Yamashita S, Hatch JP, Rugh JD: Does chewing performance depend upon a specific masticatory pattern? *J Oral Rehabil* 26:547-553, 1999.

18. McBeth J, Chiu YH, Silman AJ, Ray D, Morriss R et al: Hypothalamic-pituitary-adrenal stress axis function and the relationship with chronic widespread pain and its antecedents, *Arthritis Res Ther* 7:R992-R1000, 2005.

19. Nyklicek I, Bosch JA, Amerongen AV: A generalized physiological hyperreactivity to acute stressors in hypertensives, *Biol Psychol* 70:44-51, 2005.

20. Nicholson RA, Lakatos CA, Gramling SE: EMG reactivity and oral habits among facial pain patients in a scheduled-waiting competitive task, *Appl Psychophysiol Biofeedback* 24:235-247, 1999.

21. *Dorland's illustrated medical dictionary*, ed 30, Philadelphia, 2003, Saunders, p 1104.

22. Hollingsworth HL: Chewing as a technique of relaxation, *Science* 90:385-387, 1939.

23. Jenkins GN: *The physiology and biochemistry of the mouth*, Oxford, England, 1974, Blackwell Scientific.

24. Nishigawa K, Nakano M, Bando E, Clark GT: Effect of altered occlusal guidance on lateral border movement of the mandible, *J Prosthet Dent* 68:965-969, 1992.

25. Lundeen HC, Gibbs CH: *Advances in occlusion*, Boston, 1982, John Wright PSG.

26. Schweitzer JM: Masticatory function in man, *J Prosthet Dent* 11:625-647, 1961.

27. Gibbs CH, Messerman T, Reswick JB, Derda HJ: Functional movements of the mandible, *J Prosthet Dent* 26:604-620, 1971.

28. Horio T, Kawamura Y: Effects of texture of food on chewing patterns in the human subject, *J Oral Rehabil* 16:177-183, 1989.

29. Pond LH, Barghi N, Barnwell GM: Occlusion and chewing side preference, *J Prosthet Dent* 55:498-500, 1986.

30. Beyron HL: Occlusal changes in the adult dentition, *J Am Dent Assoc* 48:674-686, 1954.

31. Beyron HL: Occlusal relations and mastication in Australian Aborigines, *Acta Odontol Scand* 22:597-678, 1964.

32. Throckmorton GS, Groshan GJ, Boyd SB: Muscle activity patterns and control of temporomandibular joint loads, *J Prosthet Dent* 63:685-695, 1990.

33. Christensen LV, Rassouli NM: Experimental occlusal interferences. Part IV. Mandibular rotations induced by a pliable interference, *J Oral Rehabil* 22:835-844, 1995.

34. Rassouli NM, Christensen LV: Experimental occlusal interferences. Part III. Mandibular rotations induced by a rigid interference, *J Oral Rehabil* 22:781-789, 1995.

35. Jankelson B, Hoffman GM, Hendron AJ: Physiology of the stomatognathic system, *J Am Dent Assoc* 46:375-386, 1953.

36. Anderson DJ, Picton DCA: Tooth contact during chewing, *J Dent Res* 36:21-26, 1957.

37. Ahlgren J: Mechanism of mastication, *Acta Odontol Scand* 24:44-45, 1966.

38. Adams SH, Zander HA: Functional tooth contacts in lateral and centric occlusion, *J Am Dent Assoc* 69:465-473, 1964.

39. Glickman I, Pameijer JH, Roeber FW, Brian MA: Functional occlusion as revealed by miniaturized radio transmitters, *Dent Clin North Am* 13:667-679, 1969.

40. Suit SR, Gibbs CH, Benz ST: Study of gliding tooth contacts during mastication, *J Periodontol* 47:331-334, 1975.

41. Mongini F, Tempia-Valenta G: A graphic and statistical analysis of the chewing movements in function and dysfunction, *J Craniomandib Pract* 2:125-134, 1984.

42. Brekhus PH: Stimulation of the muscles of mastication, *J Dent Res* 20:87-92, 1941.

43. Gibbs CH, Mahan PE, Mauderli A, Lundeen HC, Walsh EK: Limits of human bite strength, *J Prosthet Dent* 56:226-229, 1986.

44. Howell AH, Manly RS: An electronic strain gauge for measuring oral forces, *J Dent Res* 27:705-712, 1948.

45. Garner LD, Kotwal NS: Correlation study of incisive biting forces with age, sex, and anterior occlusion, *J Dent Res* 52:698-702, 1973.

46. Worner HK, Anderson MN: Biting force measurements in children, *Aust Dent J* 48:1-5, 1944.

47. Worner HK: Gnathodynamics: the measurement of biting forces with a new design of gnathodynamometer, *Aust Dent J* 43:381-386, 1939.

48. Kiliardis S, Tzakis MG, Carlsson GE: Effects of fatigue and chewing training on maximal bite force and endurance, *Am J Orthod Dentofacial Orthop* 107:372-378, 1995.

49. Waugh LM: Dental observation among Eskimos, *J Dent Res* 16:355-356, 1937.

50. Gibbs CH, Mahan PE, Lundeen HC, Brehan K: Occlusal forces during chewing: influence on biting strength and food consistency, *J Prosthet Dent* 46:561-567, 1981.

51. Anderson DJ: Measurement of stress in mastication. II, *J Dent Res* 35:671-673, 1956.

52. Goldreich H, Gazit E, Lieberman MA, Rugh JD: The effect of pain from orthodontic arch wire adjustment on masseter muscle electromyographic activity, *Am J Orthod Dentofacial Orthop* 106:365-370, 1994.

53. Bakke M, Michler L: Temporalis and masseter muscle activity in patients with anterior open bite and craniomandibular disorders, *Scand J Dent Res* 99:219-228, 1991.

54. Howell AH, Brudevold F: Vertical forces used during chewing of food, *J Dent Res* 29:133-136, 1950.

55. Brudevold F: A basic study of the chewing forces of a denture wearer, *J Am Dent Assoc* 43:45-51, 1951.

56. Lundgren D, Laurell L: Occlusal force pattern during chewing and biting in dentitions restored with fixed bridges of cross-arch extension, *J Oral Rehabil* 13:57-71, 1986.

57. Michael CG, Javid NS, Colaizzi FA, Gibbs CH: Biting strength and chewing forces in complete denture wearers, *J Prosthet Dent* 63:549-553, 1990.

58. Cleall JF: A study of form and function, *Am J Orthod* 51:566-594, 1965.

59. Gillings BRD, Kohl JT, Zander HA: Contact patterns using miniature radio transmitters, *J Dent Res* 42:177-180, 1963.

60. Graf H, Zander HA: Tooth contact patterns in mastication, *J Prosthet Dent* 13:1055-1066, 1963.

61. Butler JH, Zander HA: Evaluation of two occlusal concepts, *Periodont Acad Rev* 2:5-19, 1968.

62. Arstad T: Retrusion facets (book review), *J Am Dent Assoc* 52:519, 1956.

63. Ramfjord SP: Dysfunctional temporomandibular joint and muscle pain, *J Prosthet Dent* 11:353-362, 1961.

64. Flanagan JB: The 24-hour pattern of swallowing in man, *J Dent Res* 42(abstr #165):1072, 1963.

65. Schneyer LH, Pigman W, Hanahan L, Gilmore RW: Rate of flow of human parotid, sublingual and submaxillary secretions during sleep, *J Dent Res* 35:109-114, 1956.

66. Wall PD: On the relation of injury to pain, *Pain* 6:253-261, 1979.

67. Melzack R, Wall PD, Ty TC: Acute pain in an emergency clinic: latency of onset and descriptor patterns related to different injuries, *Pain* 14:33-43, 1982.

68. Melzack R, Wall PD: Pain mechanisms: a new theory, *Science* 150:971-979, 1965.

69. Wall PD: The gate control theory of pain mechanisms: a reexamination and restatement, *Brain* 101:1-18, 1978.

70. Okeson JP: *Bell's orofacial pains*, ed 6, Chicago, 2005, Quintessence, pp 63-94.

71. Wall PD, Devor M: Sensory afferent impulses originate from dorsal root ganglia as well as from the periphery in normal and nerve injured rats, *Pain* 17:321-339, 1983.

72. Basbaum AI: Descending control of pain transmission: possible serotonergic-enkephalinergic interactions, *Adv Exp Med Biol* 133:177-189, 1981.

73. Basbaum AT: Brainstem control of nociception: the contribution of the monoamines, *Pain* 11(Suppl):231-239, 1981.

74. Belcher G, Ryall RW, Schaffner R: The differential effects of 5-hydroxytryptamine, noradrenalin, and raphe stimulation on nociceptive and nonnociceptive dorsal horn interneurons in the cat, *Brain Res* 151:307-321, 1978.

75. Sternbach RA: Pain and "hassles" in the United States: findings of the Nuprin pain report, *Pain* 27:69-80, 1986.

76. Kreiner M, Okeson JP: Toothache of cardiac origin, *J Orofac Pain* 13:201-207, 1999.

77. Okeson JP: *Bell's orofacial pains*, ed 6, Chicago, 2005, Quintessence, p 72.

78. Milne RJ, Foreman RD, Giesler GJ: Viscerosomatic convergence into primate spinothalamic neurons: an explanation for referral of pelvic visceral pain. In Bonica JJ, Lindblom U, Iggo A, editors: *Advances in pain research pain therapy*, New York, 1983, Raven.

79. Sessle BJ, Hu JW, Amano N, Zhong G: Convergence of cutaneous, tooth pulp, visceral, neck and muscle afferents onto nociceptive and nonnociceptive neurones in trigeminal subnucleus caudalis (medullary dorsal horn) and its implications for referred pain, *Pain* 27:219-235, 1986.

80. Sessle BJ, Hu JW: Mechanisms of pain arising from articular tissues, *Can J Physiol Pharmacol* 69:617-626, 1991.

81. Kerr FWL: Structural relation of the trigeminal spinal tract to upper cervical roots and the solitary nucleus in the cat, *Exp Neurol* 4:134-148, 1961.

82. Kerr FWL: Facial, vagal and glossopharyngeal nerves in the cat: afferent connections, *Arch Neurol* 6:264-281, 1962.

83. Kerr FWL: The divisional organization of afferent fibers of the trigeminal nerve, *Brain* 86:721-732, 1963.

84. Barnsley L, Lord S, Bogduk N: Whiplash injury: a clinical review, *Pain* 58:283-307, 1994.

85. Cervero F, Meyer RA, Campbell JN: A psychophysical study of secondary hyperalgesia: evidence for increased pain to input from nociceptors, *Pain* 58:21-28, 1994.

86. Broton JG, Sessle BJ: Reflex excitation of masticatory muscles induced by algesic chemicals applied to the temporomandibular joint of the cat, *Arch Oral Biol* 33: 741-747, 1988.

87. Stohler C, Yamada Y, Ash MM: Antagonistic muscle stiffness and associated reflex behaviour in the pain-dysfunctional state, *Helv Odont Acta* 29:719-726, 1985.

88. Bell WE: *Temporomandibular disorders: classification, diagnosis, management*, ed 3, Chicago, 1990, Year Book Medical, pp 195-201.

89. Carlson CR, Okeson JP, Falace DA, Nitz AJ, Lindroth JE: Reduction of pain and EMG activity in the masseter region by trapezius trigger point injection, *Pain* 55:397-400, 1993.

Alignment and Occlusion of the Dentition

"Occlusion is the static relationship of the teeth and is basic to all aspects of dentistry."

—JPO

The alignment and occlusion of the dentition are extremely important in masticatory function. The basic activities of chewing, swallowing, and speaking depend greatly not only on the position of teeth in the dental arches but also on the relationship of opposing teeth as they are brought into occlusion. Tooth positions are determined not by chance, but by numerous controlling factors such as arch width and tooth size. They are also determined by various controlling forces, such as those provided by the surrounding soft tissues. This chapter is divided into three sections. The first section discusses the factors and forces that determine tooth position in the dental arches. The second section describes the normal relationship of the teeth as they are aligned within the arches (intraarch alignment). The third section describes the normal relationship of the arches to each other as they are brought into occlusion (interarch alignment).

FACTORS AND FORCES THAT DETERMINE TOOTH POSITION

The alignment of the dentition in the dental arches occurs as a result of complex multidirectional forces acting on the teeth during and after eruption. As the teeth erupt, they are directed into a position where opposing forces are in equilibrium. The major opposing forces that influence tooth position originate from the surrounding musculature. Labial to the teeth are the lips and cheeks, which provide relatively light but constant lingually directed forces. On the opposite side of the dental arches is the tongue, which provides labially and buccally directed forces to the lingual surface of the teeth. Both the forces applied labially by the lips and cheeks and lingually by the tongue are light but constant; these are the types of forces that over time can move teeth within the dental arches.

The labiolingual and buccolingual forces are equal in a tooth position in the oral cavity. In this so-called *neutral position*, or *space*, tooth stability is achieved (Fig. 3-1). If during eruption a tooth is positioned too far to the lingual or facial, the prevailing force (the tongue if in linguoversion, the lips and cheeks if in facioversion) will force that tooth into the neutral position. This normally occurs when there is adequate space for the tooth within the dental arch. If space is not adequate, the surrounding muscular forces are not usually sufficient to position the tooth in proper arch alignment. The tooth then remains outside the normal arch form, and crowding is observed. This crowding remains until additional outside force is provided to correct the tooth size and arch length discrepancy (i.e., orthodontia).

Even after eruption, any change or disruption in the magnitude, direction, or frequency of these muscular forces will tend to move the tooth into a position where the forces are again in equilibrium.

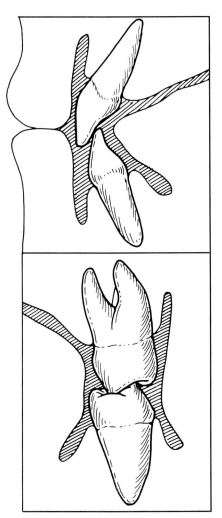

Fig. 3-1 NEUTRAL POSITION. This is the position of the tooth when the lingual forces are in equilibrium with the labial forces (lips and cheeks). It exists for both anterior and posterior teeth.

This type of disruption may result if the tongue is either unusually active or large. This can result in greater forces applied lingually to the teeth than labially by the lips. The neutral space is not lost but is merely displaced to the labial. This commonly leads to a labial flaring of the anterior teeth until they reach a position at which the labial and lingual forces are again in equilibrium. Clinically this presents as an anterior open bite (Fig. 3-2). If an individual with this condition is asked to swallow,

the tongue fills the anterior space (see Fig. 3-2, *B* and *D*). Originally it was assumed that the force applied by the tongue during this type of swallow was responsible for the labial displacement or flaring of the anterior teeth. Recent evidence does not substantiate this concept. In fact, the greater likelihood is that the anterior teeth are displaced labially by the constant resting or posturing position of the tongue and not the actual activity of swallowing.[1] The tongue thrusting forward during a swallow is more likely associated with the patient's attempt to seal the mouth, which is necessary for efficient swallowing.

The clinician should remember that these muscular forces are constantly acting on and regulating tooth function. Forces not directly derived from the oral musculature but associated with oral habits can also influence tooth position. Constantly biting on a pipe, for example, can alter tooth position. Musical instruments placed between the maxillary and mandibular teeth (e.g., a clarinet) may provide labial forces to the lingual surfaces of the maxillary anterior teeth, resulting in a labial flaring. When abnormal tooth position is identified, it is important to question for these types of habits. If the etiology of the position is not eliminated, correction of the tooth position will surely fail.

The proximal surfaces of the teeth are also subjected to a variety of forces. Proximal contact between adjacent teeth helps maintain the teeth in normal alignment. A functional response of the alveolar bone and the gingival fibers surrounding the teeth appears to result in a mesial drifting of the teeth toward the midline. During mastication a slight buccolingual, as well as vertical, movement of the teeth over time also results in wear of the proximal contact areas. When these areas are worn, the mesial drifting helps maintain contact between adjacent teeth and thus stabilizes the arch. Mesial drift becomes most apparent when the surface of a posterior tooth is destroyed by caries or an entire tooth is extracted. With the loss of proximal contact, the tooth distal to the extraction site will drift mesially into the space, which (especially in the molar area) usually causes this tooth to tip into the space.

Another important factor that helps to stabilize tooth alignment is occlusal contact, which prevents

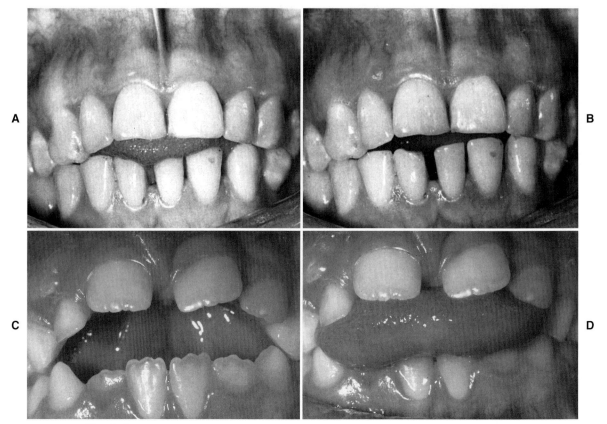

Fig. 3-2 A, An anterior open bite in an adult associated with a large and active tongue. **B,** During a swallow the tongue is seen to fill the anterior space so that the mouth can be sealed for swallowing. **C,** A young individual who has developed an anterior open bite secondary to an active tongue. **D,** During a swallow the tongue is seen to fill the anterior space, allowing the individual to swallow. *(Courtesy Dr. Preston E. Hicks, University of Kentucky College of Dentistry, Lexington.)*

the extrusion or supereruption of teeth, thus maintaining arch stability. Each time the mandible is closed, the unique occlusal contact pattern reemphasizes and maintains tooth position. If a portion of the occlusal surface of a tooth is lost or altered, the dynamics of the periodontal supportive structures will allow shifting of the tooth. Unopposed teeth are likely to supererupt until occlusal contact is established. Therefore when a tooth is lost, not only is the distal tooth likely to move mesially, but the unopposed tooth is also likely to erupt, seeking an occlusal contact (Fig. 3-3). Therefore it becomes apparent that the proximal and occlusal contacts are important in maintaining tooth alignment and arch integrity. The effect of one missing

tooth can be dramatic in the loss of stability of the dental arches.

INTRAARCH TOOTH ALIGNMENT

Intraarch tooth alignment refers to the relationship of the teeth to each other within the dental arch. This section describes the normal intraarch characteristics of the maxillary and mandibular teeth.

The *plane of occlusion* is the plane that would be established if a line were drawn through all the buccal cusp tips and incisal edges of the mandibular teeth (Fig. 3-4), then broadened into a plane to include the lingual cusp tips and continuing across

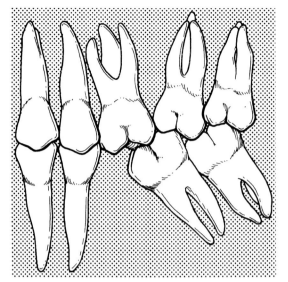

Fig. 3-3 The loss of a single tooth can have significant effects on the stability of both arches. Note that with loss of the mandibular first molar, the mandibular second and third molars tip mesially, the mandibular second premolar moves distally, and the opposing maxillary first molar is supererupted.

the arch to include the opposite side buccal and lingual cusp tips. When the plane of occlusion is examined, it becomes apparent that it is not flat. The two temporomandibular joints, which rarely function with identical simultaneous movements, determine much of the movement that is detectible. Because most jaw movements are complex, with the centers of rotation constantly shifting, a flat

occlusal plane will not permit simultaneous functional contact in more than one area of the dental arch. Therefore the occlusal planes of the dental arches are curved in a manner that permits maximum utilization of tooth contacts during function. The curvature of the occlusal plane is primarily a result of the fact that the teeth are positioned in the arches at varying degrees of inclination.

When examining the arches from the lateral view, the mesiodistal axial relationship can be seen. If lines are extended through the long axes of the roots occlusally through the crowns (Fig. 3-5), the angulation of the teeth with respect to the alveolar bone can be observed. In the mandibular arch both the anterior and posterior teeth are mesially inclined. The second and third molars are more inclined than the premolars. In the maxillary arch a different pattern of inclination exists (Fig. 3-6). The anterior teeth are generally mesially inclined, with the most posterior molars being distally inclined. If from the lateral view an imaginary line is drawn through the buccal cusp tips of the posterior teeth (molars and premolars), a curved line following the plane of occlusion will be established (see Fig. 3-4, *A*) that is convex for the maxillary arch and concave for the mandibular arch. These convex and concave lines match perfectly when the dental arches are placed into occlusion. This curvature of the dental arches was first described by von Spee[2] and is therefore referred to as the *curve of Spee.*

When observing the dental arches from the frontal view, the buccolingual axial relationship

A 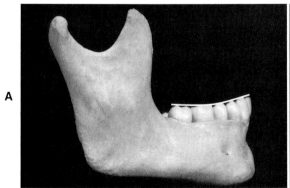 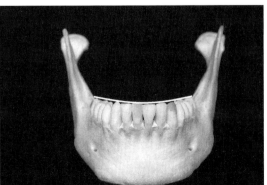 B

Fig. 3-4 PLANE OF OCCLUSION. A, Curve of Spee. **B,** Curve of Wilson.

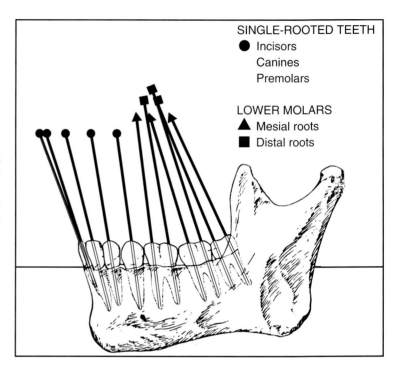

Fig. 3-5 ANGULATION OF THE MANDIBULAR TEETH. Note that both the anterior and posterior teeth are inclined mesially. *(From Dempster WT, Adams WJ, Duddles RA: Arrangement in the jaws of the roots of the teeth, J Am Dent Assoc 67:779-797, 1963.)*

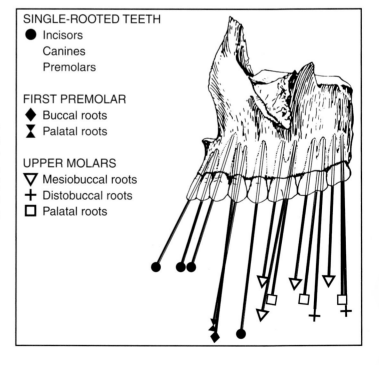

Fig. 3-6 ANGULATION OF THE MAXILLARY TEETH. The anterior teeth are mesially inclined, whereas the most posterior teeth become more distally inclined with reference to the alveolar bone. *(From Dempster WT, Adams WJ, Duddles RA: Arrangement in the jaws of the roots of the teeth, J Am Dent Assoc 67: 77-7979, 1963.)*

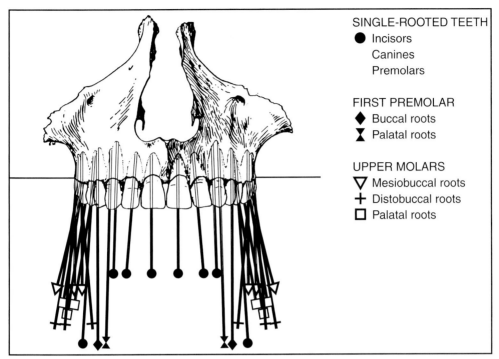

Fig. 3-7 ANGULATION OF THE MAXILLARY TEETH. Note that all the posterior teeth are slightly inclined buccally. *(From Dempster WT, Adams WJ, Duddles RA: Arrangement in the jaws of the roots of the teeth,* J Am Dent Assoc 67:779-797, 1963.)

can be seen. Generally the posterior teeth in the maxillary arch have a slightly buccal inclination (Fig. 3-7). In the mandibular arch the posterior teeth have a slightly lingual inclination (Fig. 3-8). If a line is drawn through the buccal and lingual cusp tips of both the right and the left posterior teeth, a curved plane of occlusion will be observed (see Fig. 3-4, *B*). The curvature is convex in the maxillary arch and concave in the mandibular arch. Again, if the arches are brought into occlusion, the tooth curvatures will match perfectly. This curvature in the occlusal plane observed from the frontal view is called the *curve of Wilson*.

Early in dentistry, observers sought to develop some standardized formulas that would describe intraarch relationships. Bonwill,[3] one of the first to describe the dental arches, noted that an equilateral triangle existed between the centers of the condyles and the mesial contact areas of the mandibular central incisors. He depicted this as having 4-inch sides. In other words, the distance from the mesial contact area of the mandibular

central incisor to the center of either condyle was 4 inches, and the distance between the centers of the condyles was 4 inches. In 1932 Monson[4] used Bonwill's triangle and proposed a theory that a sphere existed with a radius of 4 inches, the center of which was an equal distance from the occlusal surfaces of the posterior teeth and from the centers of the condyles. Although these concepts were roughly correct, they were oversimplifications and would not hold true in all instances. Reaction to such simplistic theories stimulated investigators to both oppose and defend these ideas. From such controversies developed the theories of occlusion that are used in dentistry today.

The occlusal surfaces of the teeth are made up of numerous cusps, grooves, and sulci. During function these occlusal elements permit effective breaking up of the food and mixing with saliva to form a bolus that is easily swallowed. For discussion purposes, the occlusal surfaces of the posterior teeth can be divided into several areas.

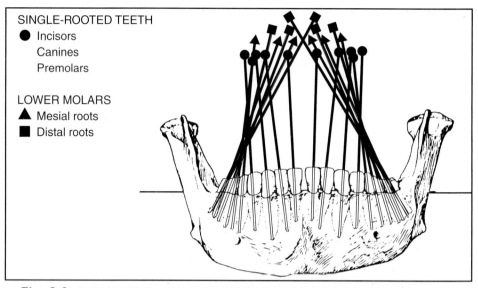

Fig. 3-8 ANGULATION OF THE MANDIBULAR TEETH. Note that all the posterior teeth are slightly inclined lingually. *(From Dempster WT, Adams WJ, Duddles RA: Arrangement in the jaws of the roots of the teeth, J Am Dent Assoc 67:779-797, 1963.)*

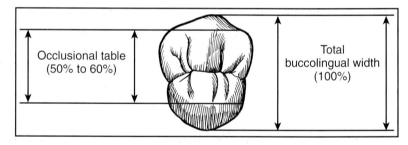

Fig. 3-9 Occlusal table of a maxillary premolar.

The area of the tooth between the buccal and lingual cusp tips of the posterior teeth is called the *occlusal table* (Fig. 3-9). The major forces of mastication are applied on this area. The occlusal table represents approximately 50% to 60% of the total buccolingual dimension of the posterior tooth and is positioned over the long axis of the root structure. It is considered the *inner aspect* of the tooth because it falls between the cusp tips. Likewise, the occlusal area outside the cusp tips is called the *outer aspect*. The inner and outer aspects of the tooth are made up of inclines that extend from the cusp tips to either the central fossa (CF) areas or the height of the contour on the lingual or labial surfaces of the teeth. Thus these inclines are called *inner* and *outer inclines* (Fig. 3-10). Inner and outer

inclines are further identified by describing the cusp of which they are a part. For example, the inner incline of the buccal cusp of the maxillary right first premolar identifies a specific area in the dental arch. Tooth inclines are also identified with respect to the surface toward which they are directed (i.e., mesial or distal). Mesially inclined surfaces are those that face the mesial portion of the tooth, and distally inclined surfaces are those that face the distal portion (Fig. 3-11).

INTERARCH TOOTH ALIGNMENT

Interarch tooth alignment refers to the relationship of the teeth in one arch to those in the other. When the

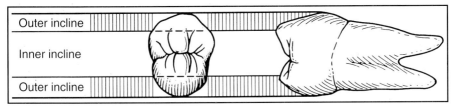

Fig. 3-10 Inner and outer inclines of a maxillary premolar.

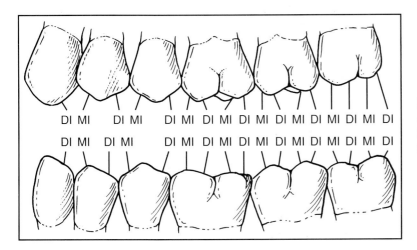

Fig. 3-11 MESIAL INCLINES (MI) AND DISTAL INCLINES (DI). An incline adjacent to each posterior cusp tip is demonstrated.

two arches come into contact, as in mandibular closure, the occlusal relationship of the teeth is established. This section describes the normal interarch characteristics of the maxillary and mandibular teeth in occlusion.

The maxillary and mandibular teeth occlude in a precise and exact manner. The distance of a line that begins at the distal surface of the third molar, extends mesially through all of the proximal contact areas around the entire arch, and ends at the distal surface of the opposite third molar represents the *arch length*. Both arches have approximately the same length, with the mandibular arch being only slightly smaller (maxillary arch, 128 mm; mandibular arch, 126 mm).[5] This slight difference is a result of the narrower mesiodistal distance of the mandibular incisors compared with the maxillary incisors. The *arch width* is the distance across the arch. The width of the mandibular arch is slightly less than that of the maxillary arch; thus when the arches occlude, each maxillary tooth is more

facially positioned than the occluding mandibular tooth.

Because the maxillary teeth are more facially positioned (or at least have more facial inclination), the normal occlusal relationship of the posterior teeth is for the mandibular buccal cusps to occlude along the CF areas of the maxillary teeth. Likewise, the maxillary lingual cusps occlude along the CF areas of the mandibular teeth (Fig. 3-12). This occlusal relationship protects the surrounding soft tissue. The buccal cusps of the maxillary teeth prevent the buccal mucosa of the cheek and lips from falling between the occlusal surface of the teeth during function. Likewise, the lingual cusps of the mandibular teeth help keep the tongue from getting between the maxillary and mandibular teeth.

The role of the tongue, cheeks, and lips, of course, is important during function because they continuously replace the food on the occlusal surfaces of the teeth for more complete breakdown.

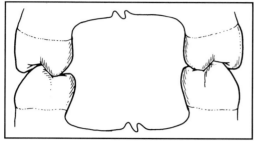

Fig. 3-12 NORMAL BUCCOLINGUAL ARCH RELA-TIONSHIP. The mandibular buccal cusps occlude in the central fossae of the maxillary teeth, and the maxillary lingual cusps occlude in the central fossae of the mandibular teeth.

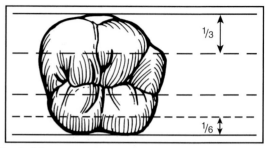

Fig. 3-14 MANDIBULAR FIRST MOLAR. The position of the centric and noncentric cusp tips are demonstrated with respect to the entire buccolingual width of the tooth.

The normal buccolingual relationship helps maximize the efficiency of the musculature while minimizing any trauma to the soft tissue (from cheek or tongue biting). Occasionally, because of discrepancies in skeletal arch size or eruption patterns, the teeth occlude in such a manner that the maxillary buccal cusps contact in the CF area of the mandibular teeth. This relationship is referred to as a *crossbite* (Fig. 3-13).

The buccal cusps of the mandibular posterior teeth and the lingual cusps of the maxillary posterior teeth occlude with the opposing CF areas. These cusps are called the *supporting cusps*, or *centric cusps*, and are primarily responsible for maintaining the distance between the maxilla and mandible. This distance supports the vertical facial height and is called the *vertical dimension of occlusion*. These cusps also play a major role in mastication because contact occurs on both the inner and outer aspects

of the cusps. The centric cusps are broad and rounded. When viewed from the occlusal, their tips are located approximately one third the distance into the total buccolingual width of the tooth (Fig. 3-14).

The buccal cusps of the maxillary posterior teeth and the lingual cusps of the mandibular posterior teeth are called the *guiding* or *noncentric cusps*. These are relatively sharp, with definite tips that are located approximately one sixth the distance into the total buccolingual width of the tooth (see Fig. 3-14). A small area of the noncentric cusps can have functional significance. This area is located on the inner incline of the noncentric cusps near the CF of the tooth and either contacts with or is close to a small portion of the outer aspect of the opposing centric cusp. The small area of the centric cusp (about 1 mm) is the only area in which an outer aspect has any functional significance. This area has therefore been called the *functional outer aspect*. A small outer aspect on each centric cusp can function against the inner incline of the noncentric cusp (Fig. 3-15). Because this area assists in the shearing of food during mastication, the noncentric cusps have also been called the *shearing cusps*.

The major role of the noncentric cusps is to minimize tissue impingement, as already mentioned, and to maintain the bolus of food on the occlusal table for mastication. The noncentric cusps also give the mandible stability so that when the teeth are in full occlusion a tight, definite occlusal relationship results. This relationship of

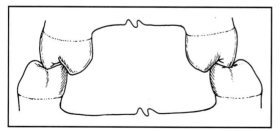

Fig. 3-13 POSTERIOR CROSSBITE. When this condition exists, the mandibular lingual cusps occlude in the central fossae of the maxillary teeth and the maxillary buccal cusps occlude in the central fossae of the mandibular teeth.

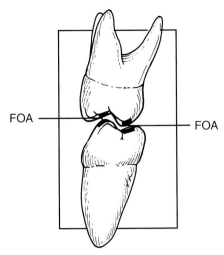

Fig. 3-15 The functional outer aspect *(FOA)* of the centric cusp is the only area of an outer incline with functional significance.

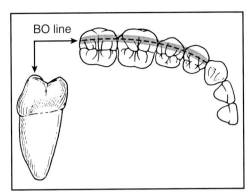

Fig. 3-16 Buccoocclusal *(BO)* line of the left mandibular arch.

the teeth in their maximum intercuspation is called the *maximum intercuspal position* (ICP). If the mandible moves laterally from this position, the noncentric contact will contact and guide it. In the same manner, if the mouth is opened and then closed, the noncentric cusps will help guide the mandible back to the ICP. In addition, during mastication these cusps finish the guiding contacts that provide feedback to the neuromuscular system, which controls the chewing stroke. Therefore the noncentric cusps are also appropriately referred to as *guiding cusps*.

BUCCOLINGUAL OCCLUSAL CONTACT RELATIONSHIP

When the dental arches are viewed from the occlusal, certain landmarks can be visualized, making it helpful to understand the interocclusal relationship of the teeth.
1. If an imaginary line is extended through all the buccal cusp tips of the mandibular posterior teeth, the buccoocclusal (BO) line is established. In a normal arch this line flows smoothly and continuously, revealing the general arch form. It also represents the demarcation between the inner and outer aspects of the buccal cusps (Fig. 3-16).

2. Likewise, if an imaginary line is extended through the lingual cusps of the maxillary posterior teeth, the linguoocclusal (LO) line is observed. This line reveals the general arch form and represents the demarcation between the outer and inner aspects of these centric cusps (Fig. 3-17).
3. If a third imaginary line is extended through the central developmental grooves of the maxillary and mandibular posterior teeth, the CF line is established. In the normal well-aligned arch, this line is continuous and reveals the arch form (Fig. 3-18).

Once the CF line is established, it is worthwhile to note an important relationship of the proximal

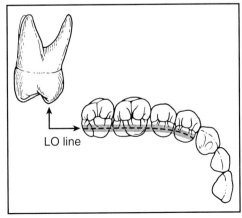

Fig. 3-17 Linguoocclusal *(LO)* line of the right maxillary arch.

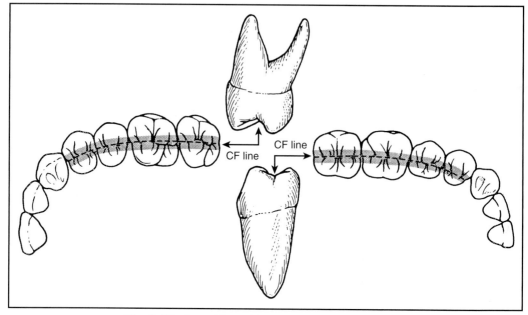

Fig. 3-18 Central fossa *(CF)* line of the left dental arches.

contact areas. These areas are generally located slightly buccal to the CF line (Fig. 3-19), which allows for a greater lingual embrasure area and a smaller buccal embrasure area. During function, then, the larger lingual embrasure will act as a major spillway for the food being masticated. As the teeth are brought into contact, the majority of the food will be shunted to the tongue, which is more efficient in returning food to the occlusal table than is the buccinator and perioral musculature.

Buccal embrasure area

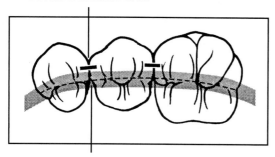

Lingual embrasure area

Fig. 3-19 The proximal contact areas between posterior teeth are generally located buccal to the central fossa line.

To visualize the buccolingual relationships of the posterior teeth in occlusion, one must simply match up the appropriate imaginary lines. As depicted in Fig. 3-20, the BO line of the mandibular teeth occludes with the CF line of the maxillary teeth. Simultaneously, the LO line of the maxillary teeth occludes with the CF line of the mandibular teeth.

MESIODISTAL OCCLUSAL CONTACT RELATIONSHIP

As just mentioned, occlusal contacts occur when the centric cusps contact the opposing CF line. Viewed from the facial, these cusps typically contact in one of two areas: (1) CF areas and (2) marginal ridge and embrasure areas.

The contacts between cusp tips and the CF areas have been likened to the grinding of a pestle in a mortar. When two unlike curved surfaces meet, only certain portions come into contact at a given time, leaving other areas free of contact to act as spillways for the substance being crushed. As the mandible shifts during mastication, different areas contact, creating different spillways. This shifting increases the efficiency of mastication.

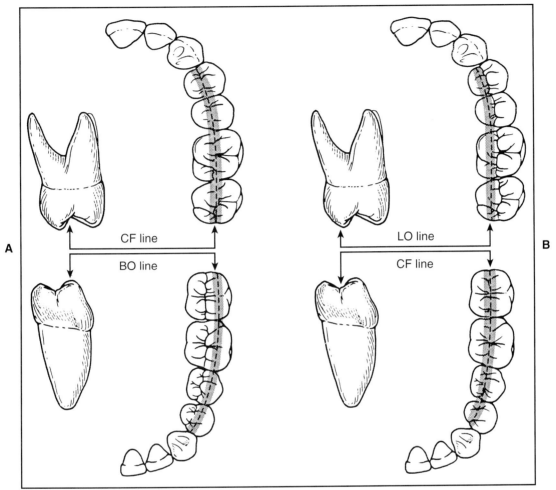

Fig. 3-20 NORMAL OCCLUDING RELATIONSHIP OF THE DENTAL ARCHES. A, The buccal cusps (centric) of the mandibular teeth occlude in the central fossae *(CF)* of the maxillary teeth. **B,** The lingual cusps (centric) of the maxillary teeth occlude in the central fossae of the mandibular teeth. *BO,* Buccoocclusal; *LO,* linguoocclusal.

The second type of occlusal contact is between cusp tips and marginal ridges. Marginal ridges are slightly raised convex areas at the mesial and distal borders of the occlusal surfaces that join with the interproximal surface of the teeth. The most elevated portion of the marginal ridge is only slightly convex. Therefore the type of contact is best depicted by the cusp tip contacting a flat surface. In this relationship the cusp tip can penetrate through food easily, and spillways are provided in all directions. As the mandible moves laterally, the actual contact area shifts, increasing efficiency of the chewing stroke. Note that the exact cusp tip is not solely responsible for occlusal contact. A circular area around the true cusp tip with a radius of about 0.5 mm provides the contact area with the opposing tooth surface.

When the normal interarch tooth relationship is viewed from the lateral, it can be seen that each tooth occludes with two opposing teeth. However, there are two exceptions to this rule: the mandibular central incisors and the maxillary third molars. In these cases the teeth occlude with only one opposing tooth. Therefore throughout the arch any given tooth is found to occlude with its namesake in the opposing arch plus an adjacent tooth.

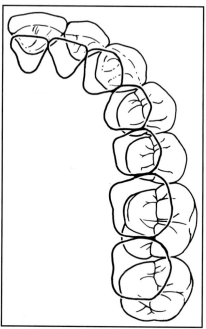

Fig. 3-21 INTERARCH RELATIONSHIP OF THE MAXILLARY AND MANDIBULAR TEETH. (The mandibular teeth are only outlined.) Each mandibular posterior tooth is situated slightly lingual and mesial to its counterpart.

This one-tooth-to-two-teeth relationship helps distribute occlusal forces to several teeth and ultimately over the entire arch. It also helps maintain some arch integrity, even when a tooth is lost, because stabilizing occlusal contacts are still maintained on all the remaining teeth.

In the normal relationship the mandibular teeth are positioned slightly lingual and mesial to their counterparts. This is true of both the posterior and anterior teeth (Fig. 3-21). In examining the common contact patterns of the dental arches, it is helpful to study the posterior teeth and anterior teeth separately.

COMMON OCCLUSAL RELATIONSHIPS OF THE POSTERIOR TEETH

In examining the occlusal relationships of the posterior teeth, much attention is centered around the first molar. The mandibular first molar is normally situated slightly mesial to the maxillary first molar.

Class I

The following characteristics identify the most typical molar relationship found in the natural dentition, first described by Angle[6] as a *Class I* relationship:

1. The mesiobuccal cusp of the mandibular first molar occludes in the embrasure area between the maxillary second premolar and first molar.
2. The mesiobuccal cusp of the maxillary first molar is aligned directly over the buccal groove of the mandibular first molar.
3. The mesiolingual cusp of the maxillary first molar is situated in the CF area of the mandibular first molar.

In this relationship each mandibular tooth occludes with its counterpart and the adjacent mesial tooth. (For example, the mandibular second premolar contacts both the maxillary second premolar and the maxillary first premolar.) The contacts between molars occur on both cusp tips and fossae and cusp tips and marginal ridges.

Two variations in the occlusal contact patterns can result with respect to the marginal ridge areas. In some instances a cusp contacts the embrasure area (and often both adjacent marginal ridges) directly, resulting in two contacts on the area of the cusp tip (Fig. 3-22). In other instances the cusp tip is positioned such that it contacts only one marginal ridge, resulting in only one contact on the cusp tip. The latter situation is used in describing the common molar relationships. Fig. 3-23 depicts the buccal view and typical occlusal contact pattern of a Class I molar relationship.

Class II

In some patients the maxillary arch is large or advanced anteriorly, or the mandibular arch is small or positioned posteriorly. These conditions will result in the mandibular first molar being positioned distal to the Class I molar relationship (Fig. 3-24), described as a *Class II* molar relationship. It is often depicted by the following characteristics:

1. The mesiobuccal cusp of the mandibular first molar occludes in the CF area of the maxillary first molar.
2. The mesiobuccal cusp of the mandibular first molar is aligned with the buccal groove of the maxillary first molar.

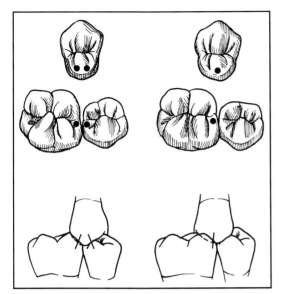

Fig. 3-22 Some centric cusps occlude in the embrasures between opposing teeth. This causes two contacts surrounding the cusp tip *(top)*. Others occlude in an embrasure area and contact only one opposing marginal ridge *(bottom)*.

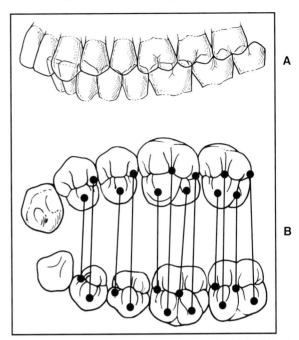

Fig. 3-24 INTERARCH RELATIONSHIPS OF A CLASS II MOLAR OCCLUSION. A, Buccal. **B,** Occlusal showing typical contact areas.

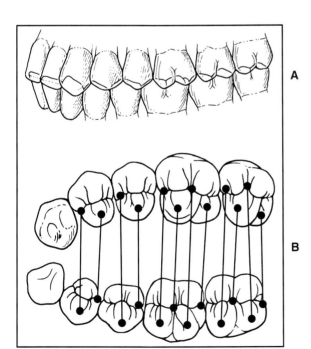

Fig. 3-23 INTERARCH RELATIONSHIPS OF A CLASS I MOLAR OCCLUSION. A, Buccal. **B,** Occlusal showing typical contact areas.

3. The distolingual cusp of the maxillary first molar occludes in the CF area of the mandibular first molar.

When compared with the Class I relationship, each occlusal contact pair is situated distally, approximately the mesiodistal width of a premolar.

Class III

A third type of molar relationship, often found corresponding to a predominant growth of the mandible, is termed *Class III*. In this relationship, growth positions the mandibular molars mesial to the maxillary molars as seen in Class I (Fig. 3-25). The Class III characteristics are as follows:

1. The distobuccal cusp of the mandibular first molar is situated in the embrasure between the maxillary second premolar and first molar.
2. The mesiobuccal cusp of the maxillary first molar is situated over the embrasure between the mandibular first and second molar.
3. The mesiolingual cusp of the maxillary first molar is situated in the mesial pit of the mandibular second molar.

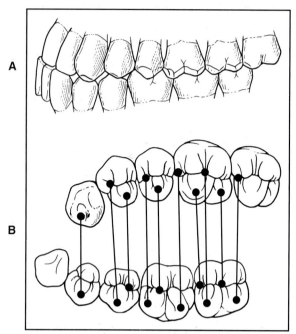

Fig. 3-25 INTERARCH RELATIONSHIPS OF A CLASS III MOLAR OCCLUSION. A, Buccal. **B,** Occlusal showing typical contact areas.

Again, each occlusal contact pair is situated just mesial to the contact pair in a Class I relationship, about the width of a premolar.

The most commonly found molar relationship is the Class I. Although the conditions described for Class II and Class III are fairly uncommon, Class II and Class III *tendencies* are quite common. A Class II or III tendency describes a condition that is not Class I yet is not extreme enough to satisfy the description of Class II or III. The anterior teeth and their occlusal contacts can also be affected by growth patterns.

COMMON OCCLUSAL RELATIONSHIPS OF THE ANTERIOR TEETH

Like the maxillary posterior teeth, the maxillary anterior teeth are normally positioned labial to the mandibular anterior teeth. Unlike the posterior teeth, however, both maxillary and mandibular anterior teeth are inclined to the labial, ranging 12 to 28 degrees from a vertical reference line.[7] Although a

great amount of variation occurs, the normal relationship will find the incisal edges of the mandibular incisors contacting the lingual surfaces of the maxillary incisors. These contacts commonly occur in the lingual fossae of the maxillary incisors approximately 4 mm gingival to the incisal edges. In other words, when viewed from the labial, 3 to 5 mm of the mandibular anterior teeth are hidden by the maxillary anterior teeth (Fig. 3-26). Because the crowns of the mandibular anterior teeth are approximately 9 mm in length, a little more than half the crown is still visible from the labial view.

The labial inclination of the anterior teeth is indicative of a function different from that of the posterior teeth. As previously mentioned, the main function of the posterior teeth is to aid in effectively breaking up food during mastication while maintaining the vertical dimension of occlusion. The posterior teeth are aligned such that the heavy vertical forces of closure can be placed on them with no adverse effect to either the teeth or their supportive structures. The labial inclination of the maxillary anterior teeth and the manner in which the mandibular teeth occlude with them do not favor resistance to heavy occlusal forces. If heavy forces occur on the anterior teeth during mandibular closure, the tendency is to displace the maxillary teeth labially. Therefore in a normal occlusion, contacts on the anterior teeth in the ICP are much lighter than on the posterior teeth. An absence of contacts on the anterior teeth in the ICP is not uncommon. The purpose of the anterior teeth, then, is not to maintain the vertical dimension of occlusion but to guide the mandible

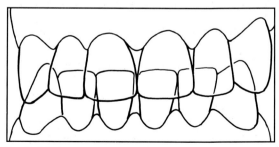

Fig. 3-26 Normally the maxillary anterior teeth overlap the mandibular anterior teeth almost half the length of the mandibular crowns.

through the various lateral movements. The anterior tooth contacts that provide guidance of the mandible are called the *anterior guidance.*

The anterior guidance plays an important role in the function of the masticatory system. Its characteristics are dictated by the exact position and relationship of the anterior teeth, which can be examined both horizontally and vertically. The horizontal distance by which the maxillary anterior teeth overlap the mandibular anterior teeth, known as the *horizontal overlap* (sometimes called *overjet*) (Fig. 3-27), is the distance between the labial incisal edge of the maxillary incisor and the labial surface of the mandibular incisor in the ICP. The anterior guidance can also be examined in the vertical plane,

known as the *vertical overlap* (sometimes called *overbite*). The vertical overlap is the distance between the incisal edges of the opposing anterior teeth. As previously mentioned, the normal occlusion has approximately 3 to 5 mm of vertical overlap. An important characteristic of the anterior guidance is determined by the intricate interrelationship of both these factors.

Another important function of the anterior teeth is that of performing the initial acts of mastication. The anterior teeth function to incise food as it is introduced into the oral cavity. Once it has been incised, it is quickly carried to the posterior teeth for a more complete breakdown. The anterior teeth also play a significant role in speech, lip support, and aesthetics.

In some persons this normal anterior tooth relationship does not exist. Variations can result from different developmental and growth patterns. Some of the relationships have been identified by using specific terms (Fig. 3-28). When a person has an underdeveloped mandible (Class II molar relationship), the mandibular anterior teeth often contact at the gingival third of the lingual surfaces of the maxillary teeth. This anterior relationship is termed a *deep bite* (deep overbite). If in an anterior Class II relationship the maxillary central and laterals are at a normal labial inclination, it is considered to be a *division 1.* When the maxillary incisors are lingually inclined, the anterior relationship is termed a *Class II, division 2.* An extreme deep bite can result in contact with the gingival tissue palatal to the maxillary incisors.

In other persons in whom there may be pronounced mandibular growth, the mandibular anterior teeth are often positioned forward and contact with the incisal edges of the maxillary anterior teeth (molar Class III relationship). This is termed an *end-to-end* (or *edge-to-edge*) relationship. In extreme cases the mandibular anterior teeth can be positioned so far forward that no contact occurs in the ICP (i.e., Class III).

Another anterior tooth relationship is one that actually has a negative vertical overlap. In other words, with the posterior teeth in maximum intercuspation, the opposing anterior teeth do not overlap or even contact each other. This anterior relationship is termed an *anterior open bite.* In a person

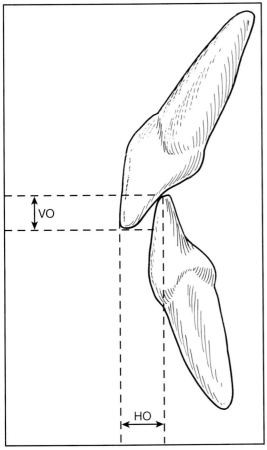

Fig. 3-27 Normal interarch relationships of the anterior teeth showing two types of overlap. *HO,* Horizontal; *VO,* vertical.

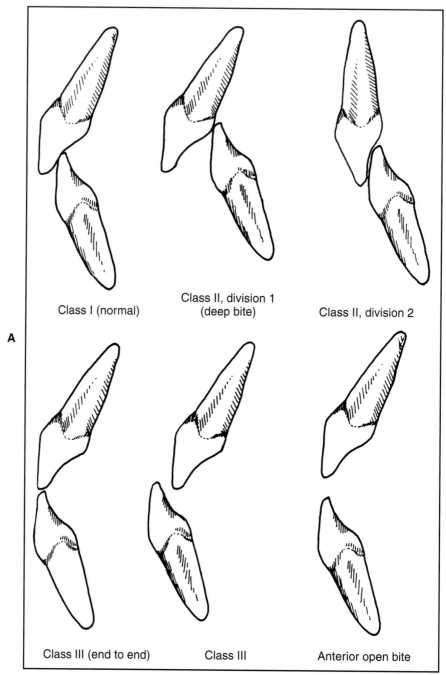

Class I (normal)

Class II, division 1 (deep bite)

Class II, division 2

A

Class III (end to end)

Class III

Anterior open bite

Fig. 3-28 A, Six variations of anterior tooth relationships.

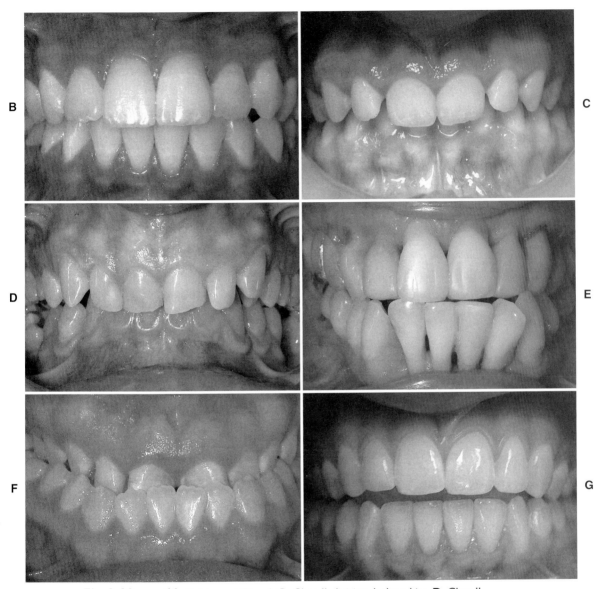

Fig. 3-28, cont'd B, Normal Class I. **C,** Class II, division 1, deep bite. **D,** Class II, division 2. **E,** Class III, end to end. **F,** Class III. **G,** Anterior open bite.

with an anterior open bite, no anterior tooth contacts may occur during mandibular movement.

OCCLUSAL CONTACTS DURING MANDIBULAR MOVEMENT

To this point, only the static relationships of the posterior and anterior teeth have been discussed.

Remember, however, that the masticatory system is extremely dynamic. The temporomandibular joints and associated musculature permit the mandible to move in all three planes (sagittal, horizontal, and frontal). Along with these movements come potential tooth contacts. An understanding of the types and location of tooth contacts that occur during the basic mandibular movements

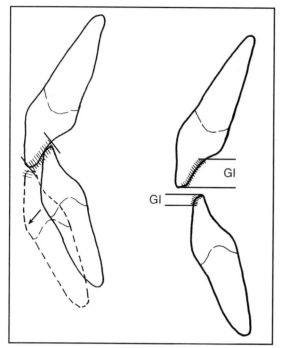

Fig. 3-29 The guiding inclines *(GI)* of the maxillary teeth are the surfaces responsible for the characteristics of anterior guidance.

is important. The term *eccentric* has been used to describe any movement of the mandible from the ICP that results in tooth contact. Three basic eccentric movements are discussed: (1) protrusive, (2) laterotrusive, and (3) retrusive.

Protrusive Mandibular Movement

A *protrusive mandibular movement* occurs when the mandible moves forward from the ICP. Any area of a tooth that contacts an opposing tooth during protrusive movement is considered to be protrusive contact. In a normal occlusal relationship the predominant protrusive contacts occur on the anterior teeth, between the incisal and labial edges of the mandibular incisors against the lingual fossa areas and incisal edges of the maxillary incisors. These are considered the guiding inclines of the anterior teeth (Fig. 3-29). On the posterior teeth the protrusive movement causes the mandibular centric cusps (buccal) to pass anteriorly across the occlusal surfaces of the maxillary teeth (Fig. 3-30). Posterior protrusive contacts occur between the distal inclines of the maxillary lingual cusps and the mesial inclines of the opposing

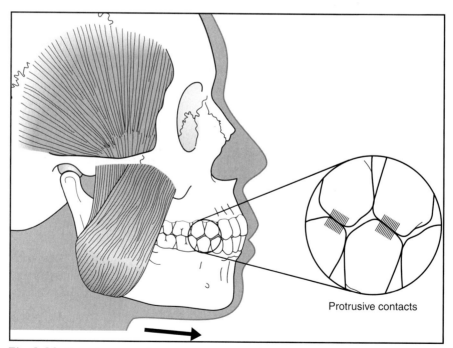

Protrusive contacts

Fig. 3-30 Posterior protrusive contacts can occur between the distal inclines of maxillary teeth and the mesial inclines of mandibular teeth.

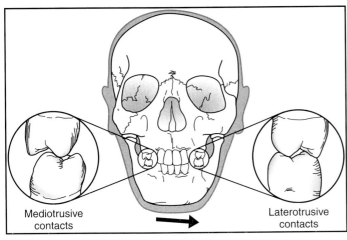

Mediotrusive contacts

Laterotrusive contacts

Fig. 3-31 LEFT LATEROTRUSIVE MOVE-MENT. Contacts can occur between the inner inclines of the maxillary buccal cusps and the outer inclines of the mandibular buccal cusps; they can also occur between the outer inclines of the maxillary lingual cusps and the inner inclines of the mandibular lingual cusps. Mediotrusive contacts can occur between the inner inclines of the maxillary lingual cusps and the inner inclines of the mandibular buccal cusps. When the mandible is moved to the right, similar contacts can occur on the contralateral teeth.

fossae and marginal ridges. Posterior protrusive contacts can also occur between the mesial inclines of the mandibular buccal cusps and the distal inclines of the opposing fossae and marginal edges.

Laterotrusive Mandibular Movement

During a *lateral mandibular movement* the right and left mandibular posterior teeth move across their opposing teeth in different directions.

If, for example, the mandible moves laterally to the left (Fig. 3-31), the left mandibular posterior teeth will move laterally across their opposing teeth. However, the right mandibular posterior teeth will move medially across their opposing teeth. The potential contact areas for these teeth are in different locations and are therefore designated by different names. Looking more closely at the posterior teeth on the left side during a left lateral movement reveals that contacts can occur on two incline areas. One is between the inner inclines of the maxillary buccal cusps and the outer inclines of the mandibular buccal cusps. The other is between the outer inclines of the maxillary lingual cusps and the inner inclines of the mandibular lingual cusps. Both these contacts are termed *laterotrusive*. To differentiate those occurring between opposing lingual cusps from those occurring between opposing buccal cusps, the term *lingual-to-lingual laterotrusive* contact is used to describe the former. The term *working contact* is also commonly used for both these laterotrusive contacts. Because most function occurs on the side to which the

mandible is shifted, the term *working contact* is appropriate.

During the same left lateral movement the right mandibular posterior teeth are passing in a medial direction across their opposing teeth. The potential sites for occlusal contacts are between the inner inclines of the maxillary lingual cusps and the inner inclines of the mandibular buccal cusps. These are called *mediotrusive contacts*. During a left lateral movement most function occurs on the left side, and therefore the right side has been designated the nonworking side. Thus these mediotrusive contacts are also called *nonworking contacts*. In earlier literature the term *balancing contact* was used.

If the mandible moves laterally to the right, the potential sites of contact will be identical with but reversed from those occurring in left lateral movement. The right side now has laterotrusive contacts, and the left side has mediotrusive contacts. These contact areas are on the same inclines as in the left lateral movement but on the teeth in the opposite side of the arch.

As previously mentioned, the anterior teeth play an important guiding role during left and right lateral mandibular movement. In a normal occlusal relationship the maxillary and mandibular canines contact during right and left lateral movements and therefore have laterotrusive contacts. These occur between the labial surfaces and incisal edges of the mandibular canines and the lingual fossae and incisal edges of the maxillary canines.

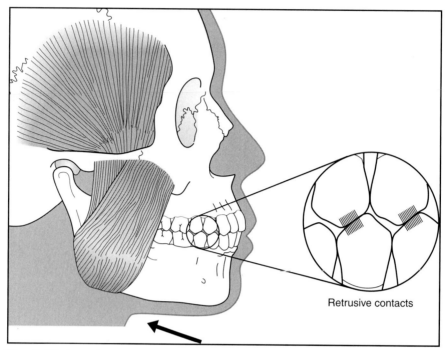

Fig. 3-32 Posterior retrusive contacts can occur between the mesial inclines of the maxillary teeth and the distal inclines of the mandibular teeth.

Like the protrusive contacts, they are considered the guiding inclines.

In summary, the laterotrusive (working) contacts on the posterior teeth occur on the inner inclines of the maxillary buccal cusps opposing the outer inclines of the mandibular buccal cusps and the outer inclines of the maxillary lingual cusps opposing the inner inclines of the mandibular lingual cusps. Mediotrusive (nonworking) contacts occur on the inner inclines of the maxillary lingual cusps opposing the inner inclines of the mandibular buccal cusps.

Retrusive Mandibular Movement

A *retrusive movement* occurs when the mandible moves posteriorly from the ICP. Compared with the other movements, a retrusive movement is quite small (1 or 2 mm). A retrusive movement is restricted by the ligamentous structures mentioned in Chapter 1. During a retrusive movement the mandibular buccal cusps move distally across the occlusal surface of their opposing maxillary teeth (Fig. 3-32). Areas of potential contact occur

between the distal inclines of the mandibular buccal cusps (centric) and the mesial inclines of the opposing fossae and marginal ridges. In the maxillary arch, retrusive contacts occur between the mesial inclines of the opposing central fossae and marginal ridges. Retrusive contacts occur on the reverse inclines of the protrusive contacts because the movement is exactly opposite.

Summary of Occlusal Contacts

When two opposing posterior teeth occlude in a normal manner (maxillary lingual cusps contacting the opposing central fossae and mandibular buccal cusps contacting the opposing central fossae), the potential contact area during any mandibular eccentric movement falls in a predictable area of the occlusal surface of the tooth. Each incline of the centric cusp can potentially provide eccentric contact with the opposing tooth. The inner incline of the noncentric cusp can also contact an opposing tooth during a specific eccentric movement. Fig. 3-33 depicts the occlusal contacts that might occur on the maxillary and mandibular first molars.

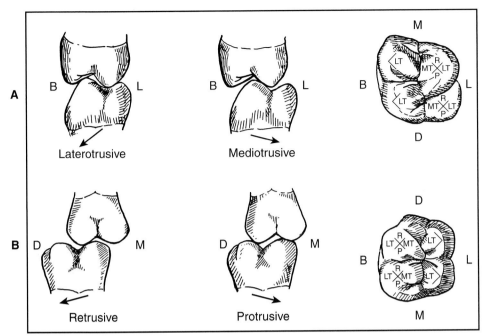

Fig. 3-33 A, Potential sites of contact during eccentric movements (lateral and proximal view). **B,** Potential sites of eccentric contacts surrounding the cusps of the maxillary and mandibular first molars (occlusal view). The contacts are demonstrated. *LT,* Laterotrusive; *MT,* mediotrusive; *P,* protrusive; *R,* retrusive.

Remember that these areas are only potential contact areas because all posterior teeth do not contact during all mandibular movements. In some instances a few teeth contact during a specific mandibular movement, which disarticulates the remaining teeth. If, however, a tooth contacts an opposing tooth during a specific mandibular movement, this diagram depicts the area of contact.

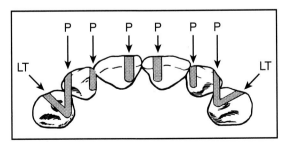

Fig. 3-34 Common sites for eccentric contacts on the maxillary anterior teeth. *LT,* Laterotrusive; *P,* protrusive.

When the anterior teeth occlude in a usual manner, the potential sites of contact during various mandibular movements are also predictable and are depicted in Fig. 3-34.

Suggested Readings

Ash MM, Nelson SJ: *Wheeler's dental anatomy, physiology, and occlusion,* ed 8, St Louis, 2003, Saunders.

Kraus BS, Jordan RE, Abrams L: *Dental anatomy and occlusion,* Baltimore, 1973, Waverly.

Moyer RE: *Handbook of orthodontics for the student and general practitioner,* ed 3, Chicago, 1973, Year Book Medical.

References

1. Sarver DM, Proffit WR: Special considerations in diagnosis and treatment planning. In Graber T, Vanarsdall R, Vig K, editors: *Orthodontics: current principles and techniques,* ed 4, St Louis, 2005, Mosby, pp 3-70.

2. Von Spee FG: *Prosthetic dentistry*, Chicago, 1928, Medico-Dental Publishing, pp 49-54.

3. Bonwill WGA: Geometrical and mechanical laws of articulation, *Trans Odontol Soc Pa* 119-133, 1885.

4. Monson GS: Applied mechanics to the theory of mandibular movements, *Dent Cosmos* 74:1039-1053, 1932.

5. Ash MM, Nelson SJ: *Wheeler's dental anatomy, physiology, and occlusion*, ed 8, St Louis, 2003, Saunders, pp 29-64.

6. Angle EH: Classification of malocclusion, *Dent Cosmos* 41:248-264, 1899.

7. Kraus BS, Jordon RE, Abrahams L: *Dental anatomy and occlusion*, Baltimore, 1973, Waverly, pp 226-230.

Mechanics of Mandibular Movement

4

CHAPTER

"Nature has blessed us with a marvelously dynamic masticatory system, allowing us to function and therefore exist."

—JPO

*M*andibular movement occurs as a complex series of interrelated three-dimensional rotational and translational activities. It is determined by the combined and simultaneous activities of both temporomandibular joints (TMJs). Although the TMJs cannot function entirely independently of each other, they also rarely function with identical concurrent movements. To better understand the complexities of mandibular movement, it is beneficial first to isolate the movements that occur within a single TMJ. The types of movement that occur are discussed first, and then the three-dimensional movements of the joint are divided into movements within a single plane.

TYPES OF MOVEMENT

Two types of movement occur in the TMJ: rotational and translational.

ROTATIONAL MOVEMENT

Dorland's Illustrated Medical Dictionary defines *rotation* as "the process of turning around an axis; movement of a body about its axis, called the *axis of rotation*."[1] In the masticatory system, rotation occurs when the mouth opens and closes around a fixed point or axis within the condyles. In other words, the teeth can be separated and then occluded with no positional change of the condyles (Fig. 4-1).

In the TMJ, rotation occurs as movement within the inferior cavity of the joint. Thus it is movement between the superior surface of the condyle and the inferior surface of the articular disc. Rotational movement of the mandible can occur in all three reference planes: horizontal, frontal (vertical), and sagittal. In each plane it occurs around a point, called the *axis*. The axis of rotation for each plane is described and illustrated.

Horizontal Axis of Rotation
Mandibular movement around the horizontal axis is an opening and closing motion. It is referred to as a *hinge movement*, and the horizontal axis around which it occurs is therefore referred to as the *hinge axis* (Fig. 4-2). The hinge movement is probably the only example of mandibular activity in which a "pure" rotational movement occurs. In all other movements, rotation around the axis is accompanied by translation of the axis.

When the condyles are in their most superior position in the articular fossae and the mouth is purely rotated open, the axis around which movement occurs is called the *terminal hinge axis*. Rotational movement around the terminal hinge can be readily demonstrated but rarely occurs during normal function.

Frontal (Vertical) Axis of Rotation
Mandibular movement around the frontal axis occurs when one condyle moves anteriorly out of

the terminal hinge position while the vertical axis of the opposite condyle remains in the terminal hinge position (Fig. 4-3). Because of the inclination of the articular eminence, which dictates that the frontal axis tilt as the moving or orbiting condyle travels anteriorly, this type of isolated movement does not occur naturally.

Sagittal Axis of Rotation

Mandibular movement around the sagittal axis occurs when one condyle moves inferiorly while the other remains in the terminal hinge position (Fig. 4-4). Because the ligaments and musculature of the TMJ prevent an inferior displacement of the condyle (dislocation), this type of isolated movement

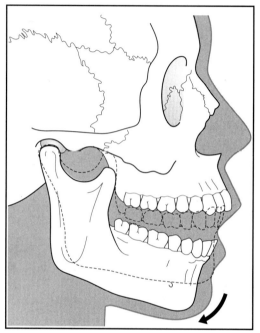

Fig. 4-1 Rotational movement about a fixed point in the condyle.

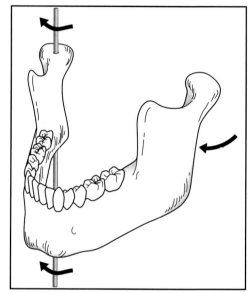

Fig. 4-3 Rotational movement around the frontal (vertical) axis.

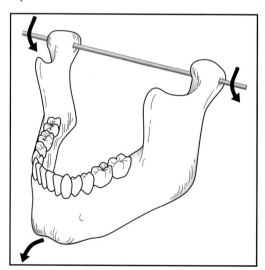

Fig. 4-2 Rotational movement around the horizontal axis.

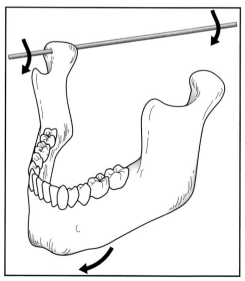

Fig. 4-4 Rotational movement around the sagittal axis.

does not occur naturally. It does occur in conjunction with other movements, however, when the orbiting condyle moves downward and forward across the articular eminence.

TRANSLATIONAL MOVEMENT

Translation can be defined as a movement in which each point of the moving object has simultaneously the same velocity and direction. In the masticatory system it occurs when the mandible moves forward, as in protrusion. The teeth, condyles, and rami all move in the same direction and to the same degree (Fig. 4-5).

Translation occurs within the superior cavity of the joint between the superior surface of the articular disc and the inferior surface of the articular fossa (i.e., between the disc-condyle complex and the articular fossa).

During most normal movements of the mandible, both rotation and translation occur simultaneously[2] (i.e., while the mandible is rotating around one or more of the axes, each of the axes is translating, or changing its orientation in space). This results in complex movements that are extremely difficult

to visualize. In this chapter, to simplify the task of understanding them, we consider the mandible as it moves in each of the three reference planes.

SINGLE-PLANE BORDER MOVEMENTS

Mandibular movement is limited by the ligaments and the articular surfaces of the TMJs, as well as by the morphology and alignment of the teeth. When the mandible moves through the outer range of motion, reproducible describable limits called *border movements* result. The border and typical functional movements of the mandible are described for each reference plane.

SAGITTAL PLANE BORDER AND FUNCTIONAL MOVEMENTS

Mandibular motion viewed in the sagittal plane can be seen to have four distinct movement components (Fig. 4-6):
1. Posterior opening border
2. Anterior opening border
3. Superior contact border
4. Functional

The range of posterior and anterior opening border movements is determined, or limited, primarily by ligaments and the morphology of the TMJs. Superior contact border movements are determined

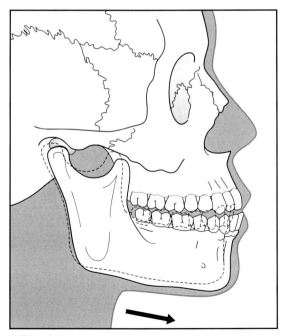

Fig. 4-5 Translational movement of the mandible.

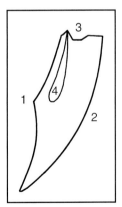

Fig. 4-6 Border and functional movements in the sagittal plane. *1*, Posterior opening border; *2*, anterior opening border; *3*, superior contact border; *4*, typical functional.

by the occlusal and incisal surfaces of the teeth. Functional movements are not considered border movements because they are not determined by an outer range of motion. They are determined by the conditional responses of the neuromuscular system (see Chapter 2).

Posterior Opening Border Movements

Posterior opening border movements in the sagittal plane occur as two-stage hinging movements. In the first stage (Fig. 4-7) the condyles are stabilized in their most superior positions in the articular fossae (i.e., the terminal hinge position). The most superior condylar position from which a hinge axis movement can occur is the centric relation (CR) position. The mandible can be lowered (mouth opening) in a pure rotational movement without translation of the condyles. Theoretically, a hinge movement (pure rotation) can be generated from any mandibular position anterior to CR; for this to occur, however, the condyles must be stabilized so that translation of the horizontal axis does

not occur. Because this stabilization is difficult to establish, posterior opening border movements that use the terminal hinge axis are the only repeatable hinge axis movements of the mandible.

In CR the mandible can be rotated around the horizontal axis to a distance of only 20 to 25 mm as measured between the incisal edges of the maxillary and mandibular incisors. At this point of opening, the temporomandibular ligaments tighten, after which continued opening results in an anterior and inferior translation of the condyles. As the condyles translate, the axis of rotation of the mandible shifts into the bodies of the rami, resulting in the second stage of the posterior opening border movement (Fig. 4-8). The exact location of the axes of rotation in the rami is likely to be the area of attachment of the sphenomandibular ligaments. During this stage, in which the mandible is rotating around a horizontal axis passing through the rami, the condyles are moving anteriorly and inferiorly and the anterior portion of the mandible is moving posteriorly and inferiorly.

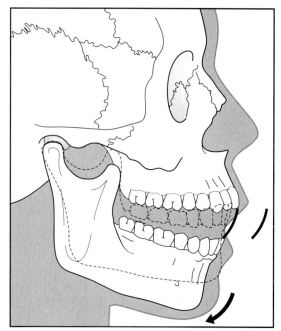

Fig. 4-7 ROTATIONAL MOVEMENT OF THE MANDIBLE WITH THE CONDYLES IN THE TERMINAL HINGE POSITION. This pure rotational opening can occur until the anterior teeth are some 20 to 25 mm apart.

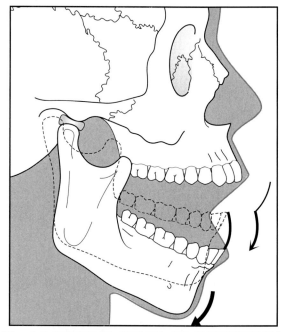

Fig. 4-8 SECOND STAGE OF ROTATIONAL MOVEMENT DURING OPENING. The condyle is translated down the articular eminence as the mouth rotates open to its maximum limit.

Maximum opening is reached when the capsular ligaments prevent further movement at the condyles. Maximum opening is in the range of 40 to 60 mm when measured between the incisal edges of the maxillary and mandibular teeth.

Anterior Opening Border Movements

With the mandible maximally opened, closure accompanied by contraction of the inferior lateral pterygoids (which keep the condyles positioned anteriorly) will generate the anterior closing border movement (Fig. 4-9). Theoretically, if the condyles were stabilized in this anterior position, a pure hinge movement could occur as the mandible was closing from the maximally opened to the maximally protruded position. Because the maximum protrusive position is determined in part by the stylomandibular ligaments, as closure occurs, tightening of the ligaments produces a posterior movement of the condyles. Condylar position is most anterior in the maximally open but not the maximally protruded position. The posterior movement of the condyle from the maximally open position to the maximally protruded position produces eccentricity in the anterior border movement. Therefore it is not a pure hinge movement.

Superior Contact Border Movements

Whereas the border movements previously discussed are limited by ligaments, the superior contact border movement is determined by the characteristics of the occluding surfaces of the teeth. Throughout this entire movement, tooth contact is present. Its precise delineation depends on (1) the amount of variation between CR and maximum intercuspation, (2) the steepness of the cuspal inclines of the posterior teeth, (3) the amount of vertical and horizontal overlap of the anterior teeth, (4) the lingual morphology of the maxillary anterior teeth, and (5) the general interarch relationships of the teeth. Because this border movement is solely tooth determined, changes in the teeth will result in changes in the nature of the border movement.

In the CR position, tooth contacts are normally found on one or more opposing pairs of posterior teeth. The initial tooth contact in terminal hinge closure (CR) occurs between the mesial inclines of a maxillary tooth and the distal inclines of a mandibular tooth (Fig. 4-10). If muscular force is applied to the mandible, a superoanterior movement or shift will result until the intercuspal position (ICP) is reached (Fig. 4-11). Additionally, this CR-to-maximum-intercuspation slide may have a lateral component. The slide from CR to ICP is present in approximately 90% of the population, and the average distance is 1.25 ± 1 mm.[3]

In the ICP the opposing anterior teeth usually contact. When the mandible is protruded from

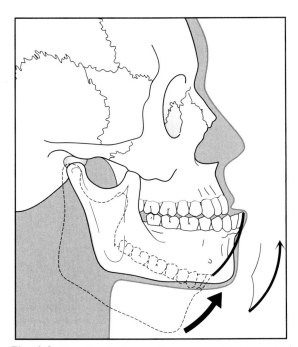

Fig. 4-9 Anterior closing border movement in the sagittal plane.

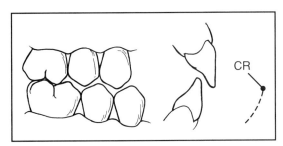

Fig. 4-10 Common relationship of the teeth when the condyles are in the centric relation *(CR)* position.

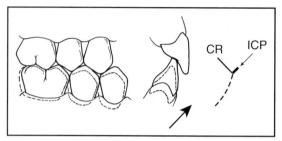

Fig. 4-11 Force applied to the teeth when the condyles are in centric relation *(CR)* will create a superoanterior shift of the mandible intercuspal position *(ICP)*.

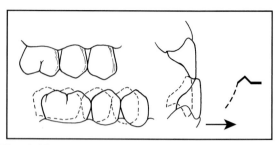

Fig. 4-13 Horizontal movement of the mandible as the incisal edges of maxillary and mandibular teeth pass across each other.

maximum intercuspation, contact between the incisal edges of the mandibular anterior teeth and the lingual inclines of the maxillary anterior teeth results in an anteroinferior movement of the mandible (Fig. 4-12). This continues until the maxillary and mandibular anterior teeth are in an edge-to-edge relationship, at which time a horizontal pathway is followed. The horizontal movement continues until the incisal edges of the mandibular teeth pass beyond the incisal edges of the maxillary teeth (Fig. 4-13). At this point the mandible moves in a superior direction until the posterior teeth contact (Fig. 4-14). The occlusal surfaces of posterior teeth then dictate the remaining pathway to the maximum protrusive movement, which joins with the most superior position of the anterior opening border movement (Fig. 4-15).

When a person has no discrepancy between CR and maximum intercuspation, the initial description

of the superior contact border movement is altered. From CR there is no superior slide to the ICP. The beginning protrusive movement immediately engages the anterior teeth and the mandible moves inferiorly, as detected by the lingual anatomy of the maxillary anterior teeth (Fig. 4-16).

Functional Movements

Functional movements occur during functional activity of the mandible. They usually take place within the border movements and therefore are considered free movements. Most functional activities require maximum intercuspation and therefore typically begin at and below the ICP. When the mandible is at rest, it is found to be located approximately 2 to 4 mm below the ICP (Fig. 4-17).[4,5] This position has been called the *clinical rest position*. Some studies suggest that it is quite variable.[6,7] It has also been determined that this so-called

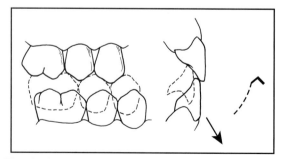

Fig. 4-12 As the mandible moves forward, contact of the incisal edges of the edges of the mandibular anterior teeth with the lingual surfaces of the maxillary anterior teeth creates an inferior movement.

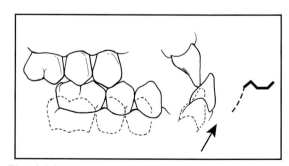

Fig. 4-14 Continued forward movement of the mandible results in a superior movement as the anterior teeth pass beyond the end-to-end position, resulting in posterior tooth contacts.

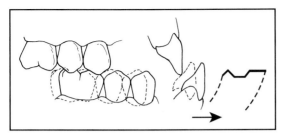

Fig. 4-15 Continued forward movement is determined by the posterior tooth surfaces until the maximum protrusive movement, as established by the ligaments, is reached. This maximum forward position joins the most superior point of the anterior opening border movement.

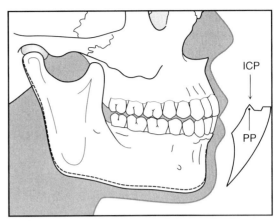

Fig. 4-17 The mandible in postural position *(PP)* is located some 2 to 4 mm below the intercuspal position *(ICP)*.

clinical rest position is not the position at which the muscles have their least amount of electromyographic activity.[7] The muscles of mastication are apparently at their lowest level of activity when the mandible is positioned approximately 8 mm inferior and 3 mm anterior to the ICP.[7]

At this point the force of gravity pulling the mandible down is in equilibrium with the elasticity and resistance to stretching of the elevator muscles and other soft tissues supporting the mandible. Therefore this position is best described as the clinical rest position. In it the interarticular pressure of the joint becomes low and dislocation is approached. Because function cannot readily occur from this position, the myotatic reflex, which counteracts the forces of gravity and maintains the jaw in the more functionally ready position 2 to 4 mm below the ICP, is activated. In this position the teeth can be quickly and effectively brought together for immediate function. The increased levels of electromyographic muscle activity in this position are indicative of the myotatic reflex.

Because this is not a true resting position, the position in which the mandible is maintained is more appropriately termed the *postural position*.

If the chewing stroke is examined in the sagittal plane, the movement will be seen to begin at the ICP and drop downward and slightly forward to the position of desired opening (Fig. 4-18). It then returns in a straighter pathway slightly posterior to the opening movement (as described in Chapter 2).

Postural Effects on Functional Movement. When the head is positioned erect and upright,

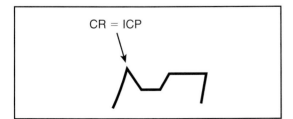

Fig. 4-16 The superior contact border movement when the condyles are in centric relation position *(CR)* is the same as the maximum intercuspal position *(ICP)* of the teeth.

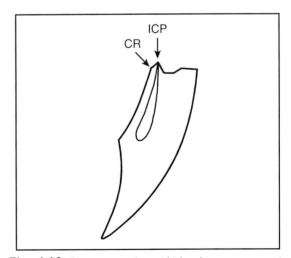

Fig. 4-18 Chewing stroke with border movements in the sagittal plane. *CR,* Centric relation; *ICP,* intercuspal position.

the postural position of the mandible is located 2 to 4 mm below the ICP. If the elevator muscles contract, the mandible will be elevated directly into the ICP. However, if the face is directed approximately 45 degrees upward, the postural position of the mandible will be altered to a slightly retruded position. This change is related to the stretching and elongation of the various tissues that are attached to and support the jaw.[8]

If the elevator muscles contract with the head in this position, the path of closure will be slightly posterior to the path of closure in the upright position. Tooth contact therefore will occur posterior to the ICP (Fig. 4-19). Because this tooth position is usually unstable, a slide results, shifting the mandible to maximum intercuspation.

It has been stated that the normal head position during eating is with the face directed downward 30 degrees.[9] This is referred to as the *alert feeding position*. In it the mandible shifts slightly anteriorly to the upright postural position. If the elevator muscles contract with the head in this position, the path of closure will be slightly anterior to that in the upright position. Tooth contacts therefore will occur anterior to the maximum ICP. Such an alteration in closure leads to heavy anterior tooth contacts. The alert feeding position can be significant in considering the functional relationships of teeth.

A 45-degree head extension is also a significant position because this is often the head posture assumed during drinking. In this posture the mandible is maintained more posterior to maximum intercuspation, and therefore closure with the head back often results in tooth contacts posterior to the ICP.

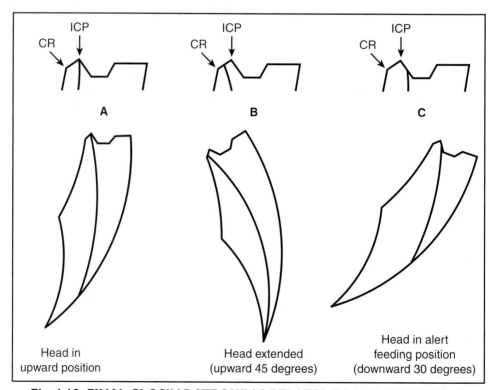

Fig. 4-19 FINAL CLOSING STROKE AS RELATED TO HEAD POSITION.
A, With the head upright the teeth are elevated directly into maximum intercuspation from the postural position. **B,** With the head raised 45 degrees, the postural position of the mandible becomes more posterior. When the teeth occlude, tooth contacts occur posterior to the intercuspal position *(ICP)*. **C,** With the head angled forward 30 degrees (alert feeding position), the postural position of the mandible becomes more anterior. When the teeth occlude, tooth contacts occur anterior to maximum intercuspation. *CR,* Centric relation.

HORIZONTAL PLANE BORDER AND FUNCTIONAL MOVEMENTS

Traditionally a device known as a *Gothic arch tracer* has been used to record mandibular movement in the horizontal plane. It consists of a recording plate attached to the maxillary teeth and a recording stylus attached to the mandibular teeth (Fig. 4-20). As the mandible moves, the stylus generates a line on the recording plate that coincides with this movement. The border movements of the mandible in the horizontal plane can therefore be easily recorded and examined.

When mandibular movements are viewed in the horizontal plane, a rhomboid-shaped pattern can be seen that has four distinct movement components (Fig. 4-21) plus a functional component:

1. Left lateral border
2. Continued left lateral border with protrusion
3. Right lateral border
4. Continued right lateral border with protrusion

Left Lateral Border Movements

With the condyles in the CR position, contraction of the right inferior lateral pterygoid will cause the right condyle to move anteriorly and medially (also inferiorly). If the left inferior lateral pterygoid

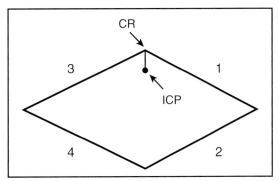

Fig. 4-21 Mandibular border movements in the horizontal plane. *1,* Left lateral; *2,* continued left lateral with protrusion; *3,* right lateral; *4,* continued right lateral with protrusion; *CR,* centric relation; *ICP,* intercuspal position.

stays relaxed, the left condyle will remain situated in CR and the result will be a left lateral border movement (i.e., the right condyle orbiting around the frontal axis of the left condyle). The left condyle is therefore called the *rotating condyle* because the mandible is rotating around it. The right condyle is called the *orbiting condyle* because it is orbiting around the rotating condyle. The left condyle is also called the *working condyle* because it is on the working side. Likewise, the right condyle is called the *non-working condyle* because it is located on the non-working side. During this movement the stylus will generate a line on the recording plate that coincides with the left border movement (Fig. 4-22).

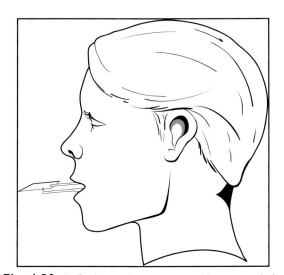

Fig. 4-20 A Gothic arch tracer is used to record the mandibular border movements in the horizontal plane. As the mandible moves, the stylus attached to the mandibular teeth generates a pathway on the recording table attached to the maxillary teeth.

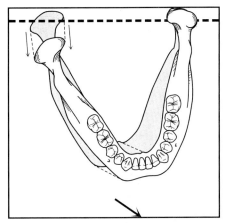

Fig. 4-22 Left lateral border movement recorded in the horizontal plane.

Continued Left Lateral Border Movements with Protrusion

With the mandible in the left lateral border position, contraction of the left inferior lateral pterygoid muscle along with continued contraction of the right inferior lateral pterygoid muscle will cause the left condyle to move anteriorly and to the right. Because the right condyle is already in its maximum anterior position, the movement of the left condyle to its maximum anterior position will cause a shift in the mandibular midline back to coincide with the midline of the face (Fig. 4-23).

Right Lateral Border Movements

Once the left border movements have been recorded on the tracing, the mandible is returned to CR and the right lateral border movements are recorded.

Contracting of the left inferior lateral pterygoid muscle will cause the left condyle to move anteriorly and medially (also inferiorly). If the right inferior lateral pterygoid muscle stays relaxed, the right condyle will remain situated in the CR position. The resultant mandibular movement will be right lateral border (e.g., the left condyle orbiting around the frontal axis of the right condyle). The right condyle in this movement is therefore called the *rotating condyle* because the mandible is rotating around it. The left condyle during this movement is

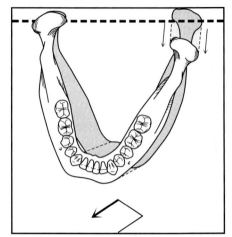

Fig. 4-24 Right lateral border movement recorded in the horizontal plane.

called the *orbiting condyle* because it is orbiting around the rotating condyle. During this movement the stylus will generate a line on the recording plate that coincides with the right lateral border movement (Fig. 4-24).

Continued Right Lateral Border Movements with Protrusion

With the mandible in the right lateral border position, contraction of the right inferior lateral pterygoid muscle along with continued contraction of the left inferior lateral pterygoid will cause the right condyle to move anteriorly and to the left. Because the left condyle is already in its maximum anterior position, the movement of the right condyle to its maximum anterior position will cause a shift back in the mandibular midline to coincide with the midline of the face (Fig. 4-25). This completes the mandibular border movement in the horizontal plane.

Lateral movements can be generated by varying levels of mandibular opening. The border movements generated with each increasing degree of opening will result in succeedingly smaller tracings until, at the maximally open position, little or no lateral movement can be made (Fig. 4-26).

Functional Movements

As in the sagittal plane, functional movements in the horizontal plane most often occur near the ICP.

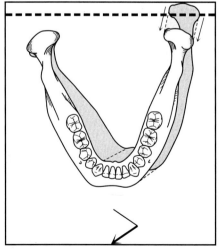

Fig. 4-23 Continued left lateral border movement with protrusion recorded in the horizontal plane.

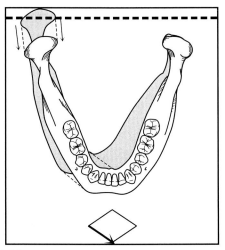

Fig. 4-25 Continued right lateral border movement with protrusion recorded in the horizontal plane.

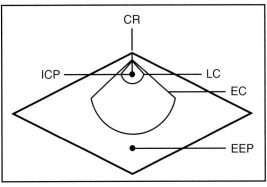

Fig. 4-27 Functional range within the horizontal border movements. *CR*, Centric relation; *EC*, area used in the early stages of mastication; *EEP*, end-to-end position of the anterior teeth; *ICP*, intercuspal position; *LC*, area used in the later stages of mastication just before swallowing occurs.

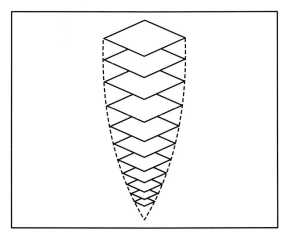

Fig. 4-26 MANDIBULAR BORDER MOVEMENTS IN THE HORIZONTAL PLANE RECORDED AT VARIOUS DEGREES OF OPENING. Note that the borders come closer together as the mouth is opened.

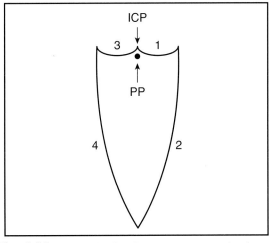

Fig. 4-28 Mandibular border movements in the frontal plane. *1*, Left lateral superior; *2*, left lateral opening; *3*, right lateral superior; *4*, right lateral opening; *ICP*, intercuspal position; *PP*, postural position.

FRONTAL (VERTICAL) BORDER AND FUNCTIONAL MOVEMENTS

When mandibular motion is viewed in the frontal plane, a shield-shaped pattern can be seen that has four distinct movement components (Fig. 4-28) along with the functional component:
1. Left lateral superior border
2. Left lateral opening border

During chewing the range of jaw movement begins some distance from the maximum ICP, but as the food is broken down into smaller particle sizes, jaw action moves closer and closer to the ICP. The exact position of the mandible during chewing is dictated by the existing occlusal configuration (Fig. 4-27).

3. Right lateral superior border
4. Right lateral opening border

Although the mandibular border movements in the frontal plane have not been traditionally "traced," an understanding of them is useful in visualizing mandibular activity three dimensionally.

Left Lateral Superior Border Movements

With the mandible in maximum intercuspation, a lateral movement is made to the left. A recording device will disclose an inferiorly concave path being generated (Fig. 4-29). The precise nature of this path is primarily determined by the morphology and interarch relationships of the maxillary and mandibular teeth that are in contact during this movement. Of secondary influence are the condyle-disc-fossa relationships and morphology of the working or rotating side TMJ. The maximum lateral extent of this movement is determined by the ligaments of the rotating joint.

Left Lateral Opening Border Movements

From the maximum left lateral superior border position, an opening movement of the mandible produces a laterally convex path. As maximum opening is approached, ligaments tighten and produce a medially directed movement that causes a shift back in the mandibular midline to coincide with the midline of the face (Fig. 4-30).

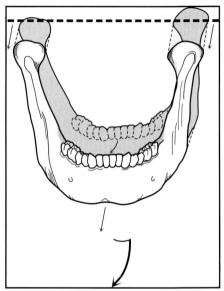

Fig. 4-30 Left lateral opening border movement recorded in the frontal plane.

Right Lateral Superior Border Movements

Once the left frontal border movements are recorded, the mandible is returned to maximum intercuspation. From this position a lateral movement is made to the right (Fig. 4-31) that is similar to the left lateral superior border movement. Slight differences may occur because of tooth contacts involved.

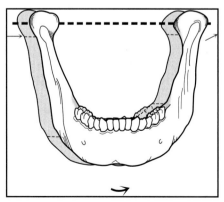

Fig. 4-29 Left lateral superior border movement recorded in the frontal plane.

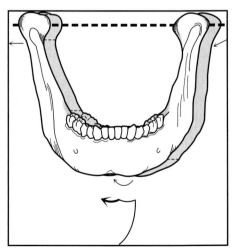

Fig. 4-31 Right lateral superior border movement recorded in the frontal plane.

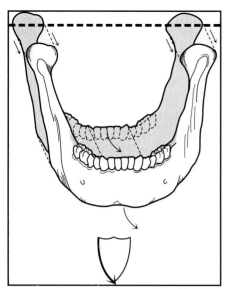

Fig. 4-32 Right lateral opening border movement recorded in the frontal plane.

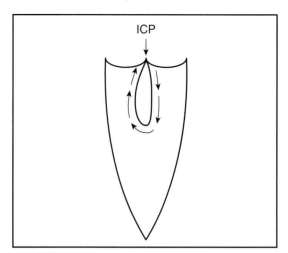

Fig. 4-33 Functional movement within the mandibular border movement recorded in the frontal plane. *ICP*, Intercuspal position.

Right Lateral Opening Border Movements

From the maximum right lateral border position, an opening movement of the mandible produces a laterally convex path similar to that of the left opening movement. As maximum opening is approached, ligaments tighten and produce a medially directed movement that causes a shift back in the mandibular midline to coincide with the midline of the face to end this left opening movement (Fig. 4-32).

Functional Movements

As in the other planes, functional movements in the frontal plane begin and end at the ICP. During chewing, the mandible drops directly inferiorly until the desired opening is achieved. It then shifts to the side on which the bolus is placed and rises up. As it approaches maximum intercuspation, the bolus is broken down between the opposing teeth. In the final millimeter of closure, the mandible quickly shifts back to the ICP (Fig. 4-33).

ENVELOPE OF MOTION

By combining mandibular border movements in the three planes (sagittal, horizontal, and frontal), a three-dimensional envelope of motion can be produced (Fig. 4-34) that represents the maximum range of movement of the mandible. Although the envelope has this characteristic shape, differences will be found from person to person. The superior surface of the envelope is determined by tooth contacts, whereas the other borders are primarily determined by ligaments and joint anatomy that restrict or limit movement.

THREE-DIMENSIONAL MOVEMENT

To demonstrate the complexity of mandibular movement, a seemingly simple right lateral excursion will be used. As the musculature begins to contract and move the mandible to the right, the left condyle is propelled out of its CR position. As the left condyle is orbiting anteriorly around the frontal axis of the right condyle, it encounters the posterior slope of the articular eminence, which causes an inferior movement of the condyle around the sagittal axis with resultant tilting of the frontal axis. Additionally, contact of the anterior teeth produces a slightly greater inferior movement in the anterior part of the mandible than in the posterior part, which results in an opening movement around the horizontal axis. Because the left condyle is moving anteriorly and

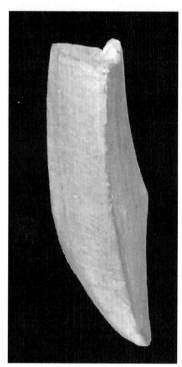

Fig. 4-34 Model of the envelope of motion.

inferiorly, the horizontal axis is shifting anteriorly and inferiorly.

This example illustrates that during a simple lateral movement, motion occurs around each axis (sagittal, horizontal, and vertical), and simultaneously each axis tilts to accommodate the movement occurring around the other axes. All this happens within the envelope of motion and is intricately controlled by the neuromuscular system to avoid injury to any of the oral structures.

Suggested Readings

Pietro AJ: Concepts of occlusion. A system based on rotational centers of the mandible, *Dent Clin North Am* 607-620, 1963.

Posselt U: *The physiology of occlusion and rehabilitation,* ed 2, Philadelphia, 1968, FA Davis.

References

1. *Dorland's illustrated medical dictionary,* ed 30, Philadelphia, 2003, Saunders, p 1643.
2. Lindauer SJ, Sabol G, Isaacaso RJ, Davidovitch M: Condylar movement and mandibular rotation during jaw opening, *Am J Orthod Dentofacial Orthop* 107:573-577, 1995.
3. Posselt U: Movement areas of the mandible, *J Prosthet Dent* 7:375-385, 1957.
4. Garnick J, Ramfjord SP: An electromyographic and clinical investigation, *J Prosthet Dent* 12:895-911, 1962.
5. Schweitzer JM: *Oral rehabilitation,* St Louis, 1951, Mosby, pp 514-518.
6. Atwood DA: A critique of research of the rest position of the mandible, *J Prosthet Dent* 16:848-854, 1966.
7. Rugh JD, Drago CJ: Vertical dimension: a study of clinical rest position and jaw muscle activity, *J Prosthet Dent* 45:670-675, 1981.
8. DuBrul EL: *Sicher's oral anatomy,* St Louis, 1980, Mosby.
9. Mohl ND: Head posture and its role in occlusion, *N Y State Dent J* 42:17-23, 1976.

Criteria for Optimum Functional Occlusion

CHAPTER 5

"The clinician managing the masticatory structures needs to understand basic orthopedic principles."

—JPO

*D*orland's Illustrated Medical Dictionary defines *occlude* as "to close tight, as to bring the mandibular teeth into contact with the teeth in the maxilla."[1] In dentistry, *occlusion* refers to the relationship of the maxillary and mandibular teeth when they are in functional contact during activity of the mandible. The question that arises is: What is the best functional relationship or occlusion of the teeth? This question has stimulated much discussion and debate. Over the years, several concepts of occlusion have been developed and have gained varying degrees of popularity. It might be interesting to follow the development of these concepts.

HISTORY OF THE STUDY OF OCCLUSION

The first description of the occlusal relationships of the teeth was made by Edward Angle in 1899.[2] Occlusion became a topic of interest and much discussion in the early years of modern dentistry as the restorability and replacement of teeth became more feasible. The first significant concept developed to describe optimum functional occlusion was called *balanced occlusion*.[3] This concept advocated bilateral and balancing tooth contacts during all lateral and protrusive movements. Balanced occlusion was developed primarily for complete dentures, with the rationale that this

type of bilateral contact would aid in stabilizing the denture bases during mandibular movement. The concept was widely accepted, and with advances in dental instrumentation and technology it carried over into the field of fixed prosthodontics.[4,5]

As total restoration of the dentition became more feasible, controversy arose regarding the desirability of balanced occlusion in the natural dentition. After much discussion and debate, the concept of unilateral eccentric contact was subsequently developed for the natural dentition.[6,7] This theory suggested that laterotrusive contacts (working contacts), as well as protrusive contacts, should occur only on the anterior teeth. It was during this time that the term *gnathology* was first used. The study of gnathology has come to be known as the exact science of mandibular movement and resultant occlusal contacts. The gnathologic concept was popular not only for use in restoring teeth but also as a treatment goal in attempting to eliminate occlusal problems. It was accepted so completely that patients with any other occlusal configuration were considered to have a malocclusion and often were treated merely because their occlusion did not conform to the criteria thought to be ideal.

In the late 1970s the concept of dynamic individual occlusion emerged. This concept centers around the health and function of the masticatory system and not on any specific occlusal configuration.[8] If the structures of the masticatory system are functioning efficiently and without pathology, the occlusal configuration is considered physiologic and acceptable regardless of specific tooth contacts.

Therefore no change in the occlusion is indicated. After examination of numerous patients with a variety of occlusal conditions and no apparent occlusal-related pathology, the merit of this concept becomes evident.

The problem facing dentistry today is apparent when a patient with the signs and symptoms of occlusal-related pathology comes to the dental office for treatment. The dentist must determine which occlusal configuration is most likely to eliminate this pathology. What occlusion is least likely to create any pathologic effects for most people over the longest time? What is the optimum functional occlusion? Although many concepts exist, the study of occlusion is so complex that these questions have not been satisfactorily answered.

In an attempt to determine which conditions seem least likely to cause any pathologic effects, this chapter examines certain anatomic and physiologic features of the masticatory system. An accumulation of these features will represent the optimum functional occlusion, which, although it may not have a high incidence in the general population, should represent to the clinician the treatment goals when attempting to either eliminate occlusion-related disorders or restore a mutilated dentition.

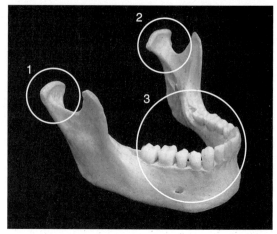

Fig. 5-1 When the mandible is elevated, force is applied to the cranium in three areas: *(1 and 2)* the temporomandibular joints and *(3)* the teeth.

CRITERIA FOR THE OPTIMUM FUNCTIONAL OCCLUSION

As discussed, the masticatory system is an extremely complex and interrelated system of muscles, bones, ligaments, teeth, and nerves. To simplify a discussion of this system is difficult yet necessary before the basic concepts that influence the function and health of all the components can be understood.

The mandible is a bone that is attached to the skull by ligaments and suspended in a muscular sling. When the elevator muscles (the masseter, the medial pterygoid, and the temporalis) function, their contraction raises the mandible such that contact is made and force is applied to the skull in three areas: the two temporomandibular joints (TMJs) and the teeth (Fig. 5-1). Because these muscles have the capability of providing

heavy forces, the potential for damage to occur at the three sites is high. Thus these areas need to be examined closely to determine the optimum orthopedic relationship that will prevent, minimize, or eliminate any breakdown or trauma. The joints and teeth will be examined separately.

OPTIMUM ORTHOPEDICALLY STABLE JOINT POSITION

The term *centric relation* (CR) has been used in dentistry for many years. Although over the years it has had a variety of definitions, it is generally considered to designate the position of the mandible when the condyles are in an orthopedically stable position. Earlier definitions described CR as the most retruded position of the condyles.[9-11] Because this position is determined mainly by the ligaments of the TMJ, it has been called a *ligamentous position*. It became useful to the prosthodontist because it was a reproducible mandibular position that could be used during the construction of complete dentures.[11] At the time it was considered the most reliable reference point obtainable in an edentulous patient for accurately recording the relationship between the mandible and maxilla and ultimately for controlling the occlusal contact pattern.

The popularity of CR grew and soon carried over into the field of fixed prosthodontics. Its usefulness in fixed prosthodontics was substantiated both by its reproducibility and by early research studies associated with muscle function.[12,13]

Conclusions from the early electromyographic (EMG) studies suggested that the muscles of mastication function more harmoniously and with less intensity when the condyles are in CR at the time that the teeth are in maximum intercuspation.[12-14] For many years the dental profession generally accepted these findings and concluded that CR was a sound physiologic position. More recent understanding of the biomechanics and function of the TMJ, however, has questioned the retruded position of the condyle as the most orthopedically stable position in the fossa.

Today the term *CR* is somewhat confusing because the definition has changed. Whereas earlier definitions[11,15] described the condyles as being in their most retruded or posterior positions, more recently[16] it has been suggested that the condyles are in their most superior position in the articular fossae. Some clinicians[17,18] suggest that none of these definitions of CR is the most physiologic position and that the condyles should ideally be positioned downward and forward on the articular eminences. The controversy regarding the most physiologic position of the condyles will continue until conclusive evidence exists that one position is more physiologic than the others.

Nevertheless, in the midst of this controversy, dentists must provide needed treatment for their patients. The use of a stable, orthopedic position is essential to treatment. Therefore it is necessary to examine and evaluate all available information if one is to draw intelligent conclusions on which to base treatment.

In establishing the criteria for the optimum orthopedically stable joint position, the anatomic structures of the TMJ must be closely examined. As previously described, the articular disc is composed of dense fibrous connective tissue devoid of nerves and blood vessels.[19] This allows it to withstand heavy forces without damage or the inducement of painful stimuli. The purpose of the disc is to separate, protect, and stabilize the condyle in the mandibular fossa during functional movements.

Positional stability of the joint, however, is not determined by the articular disc. As in any other joint, positional stability is determined by the muscles that pull across the joint and prevent dislocation of the articular surfaces. The directional forces of these muscles determine the optimum orthopedically stable joint position. This is an orthopedic principle that is true for all joints. Muscles stabilize joints. Therefore each mobile joint has a *musculoskeletally stable* (MS) position.

When pursuing the most stable position for the TMJs, the muscles that pull across the joints must be considered. The major muscles that stabilize the TMJs are the elevators. The direction of the force placed on the condyles by the masseters and medial pterygoids is superoanterior (Fig. 5-2). Although the temporal muscles have fibers that are oriented posteriorly, they nevertheless predominantly elevate the condyles in a straight superior direction.[20] These three muscle groups are primarily responsible for joint position and stability; however, the inferior lateral pterygoids also make a contribution.

In the postural position, without any influence from the occlusal condition, the condyles are stabilized by muscle tonus of the elevators and the inferior lateral pterygoids. The temporal muscles

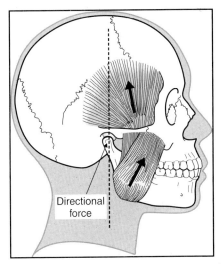

Fig. 5-2 The directional force of the primary elevator muscles (temporalis, masseter, and medial pterygoid) is to seat the condyles in the fossae in a superoanterior position.

position the condyles superiorly in the fossae. The masseters and medial pterygoids position the condyles superoanteriorly. Tonus in the inferior lateral pterygoids positions the condyles anteriorly against the posterior slopes of the articular eminences.

By way of summary, then, the most orthopedically stable joint position as dictated by the muscles is when the condyles are located in their most superoanterior position in the articular fossae, fully seated and resting against the posterior slopes of the articular eminences. This description is not complete, however, until the position of the articular discs is considered. Optimum joint relationship is achieved only when the articular discs are properly interposed between the condyles and the articular fossae. The position of the discs in the resting joints is influenced by the interarticular pressures, the morphology of the discs themselves, and the tonus in the superior lateral pterygoid muscles. This last causes the discs to be rotated on the condyles as far forward as the discal spaces (determined by interarticular pressure) and the thickness of the posterior border of the discs will allow.

The complete definition of the most orthopedically stable joint position therefore is when the condyles are in their most superoanterior position in the articular fossae, resting against the posterior slopes of the articular with the discs properly interposed. The condyles assume this position when the elevator muscles are activated with no occlusal influences. This position is therefore considered to be the most MS position of the mandible.

In this MS position, the articular surfaces and tissues of the joints are aligned such that forces applied by the musculature do not create any damage. When a dried skull is examined, the anterior and superior roof of the mandibular fossa can be seen to be quite thick and physiologically able to withstand heavy loading forces.[19,20] Therefore during rest and function, this position is both anatomically and physiologically sound.

The MS position is now described in the *Glossary of Prosthodontic Terms* as CR.[21] Although earlier definitions[9-11] of CR emphasized the most retruded position of the condyles, most clinicians have come to appreciate that seating the condyle in the

superoanterior position is far more orthopedically acceptable.

The controversy arises as to whether there is an anteroposterior range in the most superior position of the condyle. Dawson[16] suggested that there is not, which implies that if the condyles move either anteriorly or posteriorly from the most superior position, they will also move inferiorly. This may be accurate in the young, healthy joint, but one must realize that not all joints are the same. Posterior force applied to the mandible is resisted in the joint by the inner horizontal fibers of the temporomandibular (TM) ligament. The most superoposterior position of the condyles is therefore, by definition, a ligamentous position. If this ligament is tight, little difference may exist among the most superior retruded position, the most superior position (i.e., Dawson's position), and the superoanterior (MS) position. However, if the TM ligament is loose or elongated, an anteroposterior range of movement can occur while the condyle remains in its most superior position (Fig. 5-3). The more posterior the force placed on the mandible, the more elongation of the ligament will occur and the more posterior will be the condylar position. The degree of anteroposterior

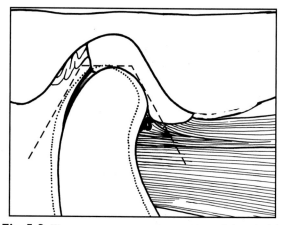

Fig. 5-3 The most superoanterior position of the condyle *(solid line)* is musculoskeletally the most stable position of the joint. However, if the inner horizontal fibers of the temporomandibular ligament allow for some posterior movement of the condyle, posterior force will displace the mandible from this to a more posterior, less stable position *(dotted line).* The two positions are at the same superior level.

freedom varies according to the health of the joint structures. A healthy joint appears to permit little posterior condylar movement from the MS position.[22] Unfortunately, the health of the joint may be difficult to clinically assess.

Studies of the mandibular chewing cycle demonstrate that in healthy subjects the rotating (working) condyle moves posterior to the intercuspal position (ICP) during the closing portion of the cycle (see Chapter 2). Therefore some degree of condylar movement posterior to the ICP is normal during function. In most joints this movement is small (1 mm or less). However, if changes occur in the structures of the joint (e.g., elongation of the TM ligament, joint disorders), the anteroposterior range of movement can be increased. The clinician should note that the most superior and posterior (or retruded) position for the condyle is not a physiologically or anatomically sound position (Fig. 5-4). In this position, force can be applied to the posterior aspect of the disc, inferior retrodiscal lamina, and retrodiscal tissues. Because the retrodiscal tissues are highly vascularized and well supplied with sensory nerve fibers,[23] anatomically they are not structured to accept force. Therefore when force is applied to this area, there is a great potential for eliciting pain and/or causing breakdown.[24-28]

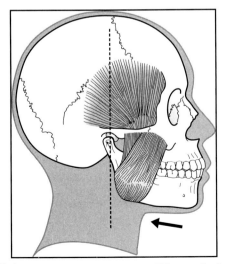

Fig. 5-4 Posterior force to the mandible can displace the condyle from the musculoskeletally stable position.

When the dried skull is examined from an anatomic standpoint, the posterior aspect of the mandibular fossa is seen to be quite thin and apparently not meant for stress bearing. This feature further emphasizes the fact that the superior posterior condylar position does not appear to be the optimum functional position of the joint.

Interestingly, as discussed in Chapter 1, ligaments do not actively participate in joint function. They exist to act as limiting structures for certain extended or border joint movements. Nevertheless, for years in dentistry the idea of using this border ligamentous position as an optimum functional position for the condyles was discussed. Such a border relationship would not be considered optimum for any other joint. Why would this orthopedic principle be any different for the TMJ?

Because it is sometimes clinically difficult to determine the extracapsular and intracapsular condition of the joint, it is advisable not to place posterior force on the mandible when attempting to locate the MS position of the joint. The major emphasis should be on guiding or directing the condyles to their most superoanterior position in the fossae. This can be accomplished either by a bilateral mandibular guiding technique or by the musculature itself (as discussed in later chapters). For the remainder of this text, CR will be defined as the most superoanterior position of the condyles in the articular fossae with the discs properly interposed. It can thus be seen that CR and the MS position are the same. This definition of CR is becoming widely accepted.[21]

Another concept of mandibular stability[18] suggests that a different position is optimal for the condyles. In this concept the condyles are described as being in their optimum position when they are translated to some degree down the posterior slopes of the articular eminences (Fig. 5-5). As the condyles are positioned downward and forward, the disc complexes follow; thus forces to the bone are dissipated effectively. Examination of the dried skull reveals that this area of the articular eminence is quite thick and able to physiologically withstand force. Therefore this position, like the most superoanterior position, appears to be anatomically capable of accepting forces. In fact, this is a normal protrusive movement of

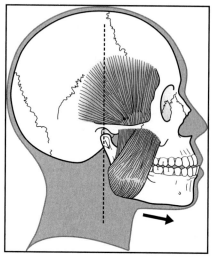

Fig. 5-5 Forward movement of the mandible brings the condyles down the articular eminences. Increased muscle activity is likely.

the mandible. The major differences between this position and the MS position lie in muscle function and mandibular stability.

To position the condyles downward and forward on the posterior slopes of the articular eminences, the inferior lateral pterygoid muscles must contract. This is compatible with a protrusive movement. However, as soon as the elevator muscles are contracted, the force applied to the condyles by these muscles is in a superior and slightly anterior direction. This directional force will tend to drive the condyles to the superoanterior position as already described (i.e., MS position). If the maximum ICP were developed in this more forward position, a discrepancy would exist between the most stable occlusal position and the most stable joint position. Therefore in order for the patient to open and close in the ICP (which is, of course, necessary to function), the inferior lateral pterygoid muscles must maintain a contracted state to keep the condyles from moving up to the most superoanterior positions. Therefore this position represents a "muscle-stabilized" position, not an MS position. Assuming that this position would require more muscle activity to maintain mandibular stability is logical. Because muscle pain is the most common complaint of patients with

masticatory disorders, it would not seem favorable to develop an occlusal condition that may actually increase muscle activity. Therefore it does not appear that this position is compatible with muscular rest,[29] and it cannot be considered the most physiologic or functional position.

Another concept that has been proposed to help the dentist locate the most optimal condylar position is through the use of electrical stimulation and subsequent relaxation of elevator muscles. In this concept the elevator muscles are electrically pulsed or stimulated at regular intervals in an attempt to produce relaxation. This technique has been used by physical therapists for years with good success in reducing muscle tension and pain. Therefore there may be good rationale to use electrical stimulation to reduce muscle pain, even though data are scarce (see Chapter 11). The followers of this concept believe that if this pulsation is done in an upright-head position, the elevator muscles will continue to relax until their EMG activity reaches the lowest level possible, which they describe as *rest*. This rest represents the point at which the forces of gravity pulling down on the mandible equal the elasticity of the muscles and ligaments that support the mandible (viscoelastic tone). In most cases this means that the mandible is positioned downward and forward to the seated superoanterior position. The fact that this is the position of lowest EMG activity does not mean this is a reasonable position from which the mandible should function. As discussed in this text, the rest position (lowest EMG activity) may be found at 8 to 9 mm of mouth opening, whereas the postural position is located 2 to 4 mm below the ICP in readiness to function.[30,31] Assuming that the ideal mandibular position is at the lowest point of EMG activity is a naive thought and certainly not substantiated with data. However, followers of this philosophy believe that it is at this position the occlusion should be established.

At least three important considerations question the likelihood that this position is an ideal mandibular position. The first is related to the fact that this position is almost always found to be downward and forward to the seated condylar position. If the teeth are restored in this position and the elevator muscles contract, the condyles will be seated superiorly, leaving only posterior teeth to occlude. The only way the occlusal position can be maintained is to maintain the inferior lateral pterygoid muscles in a partial state of contraction bracing the condyles against the posterior slope of the articular eminences. This, of course, represents a "muscle-braced" position and not an MS position, as previously discussed.

Another consideration in finding a desirable mandibular position by pulsing the elevator muscles is that this position is almost always found to be at an increased vertical dimension. The highest force that can be generated by the elevator muscles is at 4 to 6 mm of tooth separation.[32] It is at this distance that the elevator muscles are most efficient in breaking through food substances. Building the teeth into maximum intercuspation at this vertical dimension would likely cause a great increase of forces to the teeth and periodontal structures, increasing the potential for breakdown.

A third consideration in using this technique is that once the muscles are relaxed, the mandibular position can be greatly influenced by gravity. Therefore the patient's head position can change the acquired maxillary/mandibular relationship. If the patient moves his or her head forward or back or even tilts it to the right or left, the mandibular position will likely change. It would not appear that this type of variation is reliable when restoring the teeth.

Another concern with this technique is that basically each individual, whether healthy or with a mandibular disorder, will assume an open and forward position of the mandible following muscle pulsation. Therefore this technique is not helpful in distinguishing patients from normal healthy controls. When this occurs, healthy individuals could be considered for unnecessary therapy, which may be quite extensive.

In summary, from an anatomic standpoint, one can conclude that the most superior and anterior position of the condyles resting on the discs against the posterior slopes of the articular eminences is the most orthopedically sound position. From a muscle standpoint it also appears that this MS position of the condyles is optimal. An additional value is that it also has the prosthodontic advantage of being reproducible. Because the condyles are in a superior border position, a repeatable terminal hinge movement can be executed (see Chapter 9).

OPTIMUM FUNCTIONAL TOOTH CONTACTS

The MS position just described has been considered only in relation to the influencing factors of the joint and muscles. As previously discussed, the occlusal contact pattern strongly influences the muscular control of mandibular position. When closure of the mandible in the MS position creates an unstable occlusal condition, the neuromuscular system quickly feeds back appropriate muscle action to locate a mandibular position that will result in a more stable occlusal condition. Therefore the MS position of the joints can be maintained only when it is in harmony with a stable occlusal condition. The stable occlusal condition should allow for effective functioning while minimizing damage to any components of the masticatory system. The clinician should remember that the musculature is capable of applying much greater force to the teeth than is necessary for function.[33,34] Thus it is important to establish an occlusal condition that can accept heavy forces with a minimal likelihood of damage and at the same time be functionally efficient.

The optimum occlusal condition can be determined by considering the following situations:

1. A patient has only the right maxillary and mandibular first molars present. As the mouth closes, these two teeth provide the only occlusal stops for the mandible (Fig. 5-6). Assuming that 40 lb of force is applied during function, it can be seen that all this force will be applied to these two teeth. Because contact is only on the right side, the mandibular position will be unstable and the forces of occlusion provided by the musculature will likely cause an overclosure on the left side and a shift in the mandibular position to that side.[35,36] This condition does not provide the mandibular stability necessary to function effectively (orthopedic instability). If heavy forces are applied to the teeth and joints in this situation, breakdown to

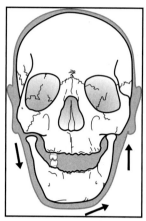

Fig. 5-6 When only right-side occlusal contacts are present, activity of the elevator muscles tends to pivot the mandible using the tooth contacts as a fulcrum. The result is an increase in joint force to the left temporomandibular joint (TMJ) and a decreased force to the right TMJ.

the joints, teeth, and supporting structure is a significant risk.[8,37-39]

2. Another patient has only the four first molars present. When the mouth is closed, both right and left side molars contact (Fig. 5-7). This occlusal condition is more favorable than the previous because when force is applied by the musculature, the bilateral molar contacts provide a more stable mandibular position. Although only minimal tooth surfaces accept the 40 lb of force provided during function, the additional teeth help lessen the force applied to each tooth (20 lb per tooth). Therefore this type of occlusal condition provides more mandibular stability while decreasing force to each tooth.

3. A third patient has only the four first molars and four second premolars present. When the mouth is closed in the MS position, all eight teeth contact evenly and simultaneously (Fig. 5-8). The additional teeth provide more stabilization of the mandible. The increase in the number of teeth occluding also decreases the forces to each tooth, thereby minimizing potential damage. (The 40 lb of force during function are now distributed to four pairs of teeth, resulting in only 10 lb on each tooth.)

Understanding the progression of these illustrations leads to the conclusion that the optimum occlusal condition during mandibular closure would be provided by even and simultaneous contact of all possible teeth. This type of occlusal relationship furnishes maximum stability for the mandible while minimizing the amount of force

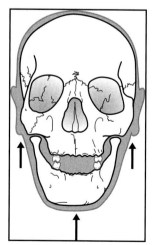

Fig. 5-7 With bilateral occlusal contacts, stability of the mandible is achieved.

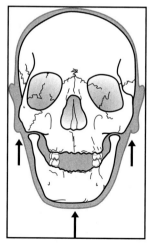

Fig. 5-8 Bilateral occlusal contacts continue to maintain mandibular stability. As the number of occluding teeth increases, the force to each tooth decreases.

placed on each tooth during function. Therefore the criteria for optimum functional occlusion developed to this point are described as even and simultaneous contact of all possible teeth when the mandibular condyles are in their most superoanterior position, resting against the posterior slopes of the articular eminences, with the discs properly interposed. In other words, the MS position of the condyles (i.e., CR position) coincides with the maximum ICP of the teeth. This is considered orthopedic stability.

Stating that the teeth must contact evenly and simultaneously is not descriptive enough to develop optimum occlusal conditions. The exact contact pattern of each tooth must be more closely examined so that a precise description of the optimum relationship can be derived. To evaluate this better, the actual direction and amount of force applied to each tooth needs to be closely examined.

Direction of Force Placed on the Teeth

When studying the supportive structures that surround the teeth, it is possible to make certain observations:

First, osseous tissues do not tolerate pressure forces.[10,23,40] In other words, if force is applied to bone, the bony tissue will resorb. Because the teeth are constantly receiving occlusal forces, a periodontal ligament (PDL) is present between the root of the tooth and the alveolar bone to help control these forces. The PDL is composed of collagenous connective tissue fibers that suspend the tooth in the bony socket. Most of these fibers run obliquely from the cementum, extending occlusally to attach in the alveolus (Fig. 5-9).[40] When force is applied to the tooth, the fibers support it and tension is created at the alveolar attachment. Pressure is a force that osseous tissue cannot accept, but tension (pulling) actually stimulates osseous formation. Therefore the PDL is capable of converting a destructive force (pressure) into an acceptable force (tension). In a general sense it can be thought of as a natural shock absorber controlling the forces of occlusion on the bone.

A second observation is how the PDL accepts various directions of occlusal force. When a tooth is contacted on a cusp tip or a relatively flat surface

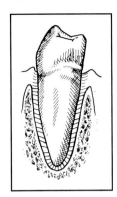

Fig. 5-9 PERIODONTAL LIGAMENT. Most fibers run obliquely from the cementum to the bone. (The width of the periodontal ligament has been greatly enlarged for illustrative purposes.)

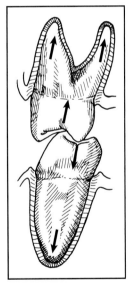

Fig. 5-10 When cusp tips contact flat surfaces, the resultant force is directed vertically through the long axes of the teeth *(arrows)*. This type of force is accepted well by the periodontal ligament.

such as the crest of a ridge or the bottom of a fossa, the resultant force is directed vertically through its long axis. The fibers of the PDL are aligned such that this type of force can be well accepted and dissipated (Fig. 5-10).[40] When a tooth

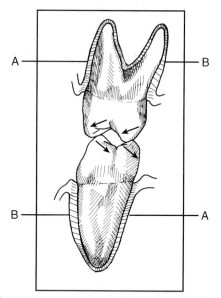

Fig. 5-11 When opposing teeth contact on inclines, the direction of force is not through the long axes of the teeth. Instead, tipping forces are created *(arrows)* that tend to cause compression *(A)* of certain areas of the periodontal ligament and elongation *(B)* of other areas.

is contacted on an incline, however, the resultant force is not directed through its long axis. Instead, a horizontal component is incorporated and tends to cause tipping (Fig. 5-11). Therefore when horizontally directed forces are applied to a tooth, many of the fibers of the PDL are not properly aligned to control them. As the tooth tips, some areas of the PDL are compressed while others are pulled or elongated. Overall, the forces are not effectively dissipated to the bone.[41-43]

The clinician should remember that vertical forces created by tooth contacts are well accepted by the PDL, but horizontal forces cannot be effectively dissipated.[42] These forces may create pathologic bone responses or even elicit neuromuscular reflex activity in an attempt to avoid or guard against incline contacts.[37]

By way of summary, then, if a tooth is contacted such that the resultant forces are directed through its long axis (vertically), the PDL is quite efficient in accepting the forces and breakdown is less likely. If a tooth is contacted in such a manner that horizontal forces are applied to the supportive structures, however, the likelihood of pathologic effects is greater.

The process of directing occlusal forces through the long axis of the tooth is known as *axial loading*. Axial loading can be achieved by two methods:

1. The first method is through the development of tooth contacts on either cusp tips or relatively flat surfaces that are perpendicular to the long axis of the tooth. These flat surfaces can be the crests of marginal ridges or the bottoms of fossae. With this type of contact the resultant forces will be directed through the long axis of the tooth (Fig. 5-12, *A*).[37,44]

2. The second method (called *tripodization*) requires that each cusp contacting an opposing fossa be developed such that it produces three contacts surrounding the actual cusp tip. When this is achieved, the resultant force is directed through the long axis of the tooth (Fig. 5-12, *B*).[45]

Both methods eliminate off-axis forces, thereby allowing the PDL to accept effectively potentially damaging forces to the bone and essentially reduce them.

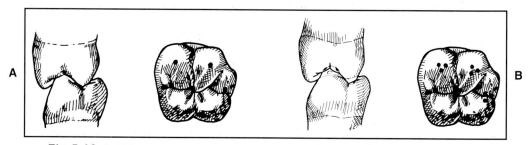

Fig. 5-12 Axial loading can be accomplished by **(A)** cusp tip–to–flat surface contacts or **(B)** reciprocal incline contacts (called *tripodization*).

Amount of Force Placed on the Teeth

The criteria for optimum occlusion have now been developed: First, even and simultaneous contact of all possible teeth should occur when the mandibular condyles are in their most superoanterior position resting on the posterior slopes of the articular eminences with the discs properly interposed. Second, each tooth should contact in such a manner that the forces of closure are directed through the long axis of the tooth.

One important aspect that has been left undiscussed relates to the complexity of the TMJ. The TMJ permits lateral and protrusive excursions, which allow the teeth to contact during different types of eccentric movements. These lateral excursions allow horizontal forces to be applied to the teeth. As already stated, horizontal forces are not well accepted by the supportive structures and the neuromuscular system, yet the complexity of the joint requires that some teeth bear the burden of these unacceptable forces. Thus several factors must be considered when identifying which tooth or teeth can best accept these horizontal forces.

The lever system of the mandible can be compared with a nutcracker. When a nut is being cracked, it is placed between the levers of the nutcracker and force is applied. If it is extremely hard, it is placed closer to the fulcrum to increase the likelihood of its being cracked. This demonstrates that greater forces can be applied to an object as its position nears the fulcrum. The same can be said of the masticatory system (Fig. 5-13). If a hard nut is to be cracked between the teeth, the most desirable position is not between the anterior teeth but between the posterior teeth, because as the nut is positioned closer to the fulcrum (the TMJ) and the area of the force vectors (the masseter and medial pterygoid muscles), greater force can be applied to the posterior than to the anterior teeth.[46-48]

The jaw, however, is more complex. Whereas the fulcrum of the nutcracker is fixed, that of the masticatory system is free to move. As a result, when heavy forces are applied to an object on the posterior teeth, the mandible is capable of shifting downward and forward to obtain the occlusal relationship that will best complete the desired task. This shifting of the condyles creates an unstable mandibular position. Additional muscle groups such as the inferior and superior lateral pterygoids and the temporals are then called on to stabilize the mandible, resulting in a more complex system than that of a simple nutcracker. Understanding this concept and realizing that heavy forces

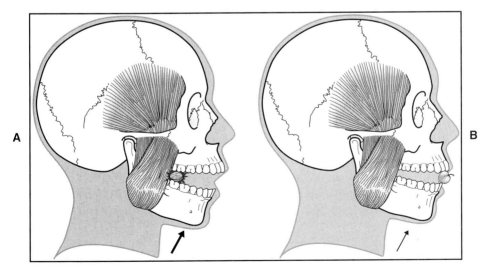

Fig. 5-13 The amount of force that can be generated between the teeth depends on the distance from the temporomandibular joint and the muscle force vectors. Much more force can be generated on the posterior teeth (**A**) than on the anterior teeth (**B**).

applied to the teeth can create pathologic changes lead to an obvious conclusion: The damaging horizontal forces of eccentric movement must be directed to the anterior teeth, which are positioned farthest from the fulcrum and the force vectors. Because the amount of force that can be applied to the anterior teeth is less than that which can be applied to the posterior teeth, the likelihood of breakdown is minimized.[48-50]

When all the anterior teeth are examined, it becomes apparent that the canines are best suited to accept the horizontal forces that occur during eccentric movements.[37,49,51,52] They have the longest and largest roots and therefore the best crown/root ratio.[53] They are also surrounded by dense compact bone, which tolerates the forces better than does the medullary bone found around posterior teeth.[54] Another advantage of the canines centers on sensory input and the resultant effect on the muscles of mastication. Apparently, fewer muscles are active when canines contact during eccentric movements than when posterior teeth contact.[55,56] Lower levels of muscular activity would decrease forces to the dental and joint structures, minimizing pathosis. Therefore when the mandible is moved in a right or left laterotrusive excursion, the maxillary and mandibular canines are appropriate teeth to contact and dissipate the horizontal forces while disoccluding or disarticulating the posterior teeth. When this condition exists, the patient is said to have *canine guidance* or *canine rise* (Fig. 5-14).

Many patients' canines, however, are not in the proper position to accept the horizontal forces; other teeth must contact during eccentric movements. The most favorable alternative to canine guidance is called *group function*. In group function, several teeth on the working side contact during the laterotrusive movement. The most desirable group function consists of the canine, premolars, and sometimes the mesiobuccal cusp of the first molar (Fig. 5-15). Any laterotrusive contacts more posterior than the mesial portion of the first molar are not desirable because of the increased amount of force that can be created as the contact gets closer to the fulcrum (TMJ).

The clinician should remember that the buccal cusp–to–buccal cusp contacts are more desirable

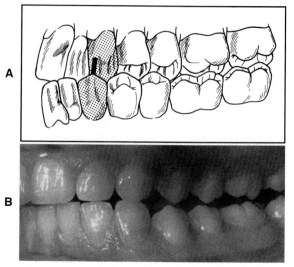

Fig. 5-14 CANINE GUIDANCE. A, Laterotrusive movement. **B,** Clinical appearance.

during laterotrusive movements than are lingual cusp–to–lingual cusp contacts (lingual to lingual working) (Fig. 5-16, *A*).

The laterotrusive contacts (either canine guidance or group function) need to provide adequate guidance to disocclude the teeth on the opposite side of the arch (mediotrusive or nonworking side) immediately (Fig. 5-16, *B*). Mediotrusive contacts

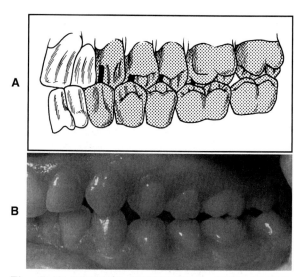

Fig. 5-15 GROUP FUNCTION GUIDANCE. A, Laterotrusive movement. **B,** Clinical appearance.

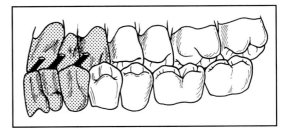

Fig. 5-17 Protrusive movement with anterior guidance.

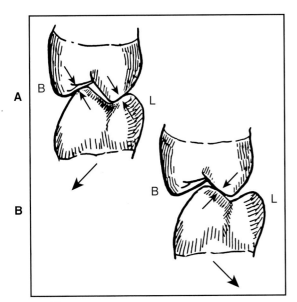

Fig. 5-16 A, Posterior teeth during a laterotrusive movement. Contacts can occur between opposing buccal *(B)* and lingual *(L)* cusps. When group function guidance is desirable, the buccal-to-buccal contacts are used. Lingual-to-lingual contacts are not desirable during eccentric movement. **B,** Posterior teeth during a mediotrusive movement. Contacts occur between the lingual cusps of maxillary teeth and the buccal cusps of mandibular teeth.

can be destructive to the masticatory system because of the amount and direction of the forces that can be applied to the joint and dental structures.* Some studies have suggested that mediotrusive contacts are perceived by the neuromuscular system differently from other types of occlusal contact. EMG studies[59,60] demonstrate that all tooth contacts are by nature inhibitory. In other words, the presence of tooth contacts tends to shut down or inhibit muscle activity. This results from the proprioceptors and nociceptors in the PDL, which when stimulated create inhibitory responses. Yet other EMG studies[61] suggest that the presence of mediotrusive contacts on posterior teeth increases muscle activity. Although the increase in muscle activity can be demonstrated, the rationale for its presence is unclear. (These concepts are discussed in more

detail in Chapter 7.) What is clear, however, is that mediotrusive contacts should be avoided in developing an optimum functional occlusion.

When the mandible moves forward into protrusive contact, damaging horizontal forces can be applied to the teeth. As with lateral movements, the anterior teeth can best receive and dissipate these forces.[48,49] Therefore during protrusion the anterior and not the posterior teeth should contact (Fig. 5-17). The anterior teeth should provide adequate contact or guidance to disarticulate the posterior teeth. Posterior protrusive contacts appear to provide unfavorable forces to the masticatory system because of the amount and direction of the force that is applied.*

During this discussion it has become evident that the anterior and posterior teeth function quite differently. The posterior teeth function effectively in accepting forces applied during closure of the mouth. They accept these forces well, primarily because their position in the arch is such that the force can be directed through their long axes and thus dissipated efficiently. The anterior teeth, however, are not positioned well in the arches to accept heavy forces. They are normally positioned at a labial angle to the direction of closure, so axial loading is nearly impossible.[53,55] If the maxillary anterior teeth receive heavy occlusal contacts during closure, there is a great likelihood that their supportive structures will not be able to tolerate the forces and they will be displaced labially. This is a common finding in patients who have lost posterior tooth support (posterior bite collapse) (Fig. 5-18).

---

*References 12, 13, 47, 52, 57, 58.

*References 12, 13, 47, 52, 57, 58.

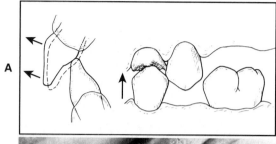

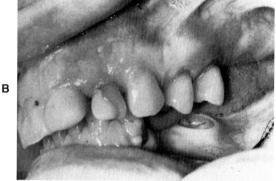

Fig. 5-18 A, Heavy occlusal contacts on the anterior teeth can occur when posterior tooth support is lost. The maxillary anterior teeth are not aligned properly to accept the mandibular closing forces. These contacts often lead to labial displacement or flaring of the maxillary anterior teeth. **B,** Posterior bite collapse. The posterior teeth have been lost, resulting in flaring of the anterior teeth. The labial flaring has led to increased interdental spacing proximal to the maxillary lateral incisor.

Anterior teeth, unlike posterior teeth, are in proper position to accept the forces of eccentric mandibular movements. Generally, therefore, it may be stated that posterior teeth function most effectively in stopping the mandible during closure, whereas anterior teeth function most effectively in guiding the mandible during eccentric movements. With an appreciation of these roles it becomes apparent that posterior teeth should contact slightly more heavily than anterior teeth when the teeth are occluded in the ICP. This condition is described as *mutually protected occlusion.*[51,52]

Postural Considerations and Functional Tooth Contacts

As discussed in Chapter 4, the postural position of the mandible is that which is maintained during periods of inactivity. It is generally 2 to 4 mm

below the ICP and can be influenced to some degree by head position. The degree to which it is affected by head position and the resulting occlusal contacts must be considered when developing an optimum occlusal condition.[62,63] In the normal upright head position, as well as the alert feeding position (head forward approximately 30 degrees), the posterior teeth should contact more heavily than the anterior teeth (mutually protected occlusion). If an occlusal condition is established with the patient reclined in a dental chair, the mandibular postural position and resultant occlusal condition may be slightly posteriorly oriented. When the patient sits up or assumes the alert feeding position, any change in the postural position and its effect on occlusal contacts must be evaluated. If in the upright head position or the alert feeding position the patient's mandible assumes a slightly anterior postural position, activity of the elevator muscles will result in heavy anterior tooth contacts. When this occurs, the anterior contacts must be reduced until the posterior teeth again contact more heavily during normal closure. This concept is called the *anterior envelope of function.* When this slight change in mandibular position is not considered, the resulting heavy anterior tooth contacts can lead to the development of functional wear patterns on the anterior teeth. This is not true for all patients, but it is difficult to predict which patient will show this response. This is especially important to the restorative dentist who wants to minimize forces to anterior restorations, such as porcelain crowns. Failure to understand and evaluate this position can lead to crown fractures.

SUMMARY OF OPTIMUM FUNCTIONAL OCCLUSION

On the basis of the concepts presented in this chapter, a summary of the most favorable functional occlusal conditions can be derived. The following conditions appear to be the least pathogenic for the greatest number of patients over the longest time:

1. When the mouth closes, the condyles are in their most superoanterior position (i.e., MS position), resting on the posterior slopes of

the articular eminences with the discs properly interposed. In this position there is even and simultaneous contact of all posterior teeth. The anterior teeth also contact but more lightly than the posterior teeth.

2. All tooth contacts provide axial loading of occlusal forces.
3. When the mandible moves into laterotrusive positions, adequate tooth-guided contacts on the laterotrusive (working) side are present to disocclude the mediotrusive (nonworking) side immediately. The most desirable guidance is provided by the canines (canine guidance).
4. When the mandible moves into a protrusive position, adequate tooth-guided contacts on the anterior teeth are present to disocclude all posterior teeth immediately.
5. In the upright head position and alert feeding position, posterior tooth contacts are heavier than anterior tooth contacts.

References

1. *Dorland's illustrated medical dictionary*, ed 30, Philadelphia, 2003, Saunders, p 1298.
2. Angle EH: Classification of malocclusion, *Dent Cosmos* 41:248-264, 1899.
3. Sears VH: Balanced occlusions, *J Am Dent Assoc* 12:1448-1453, 1925.
4. Young JL: Physiologic occlusion, *J Am Dent Assoc* 13:1089-1093, 1926.
5. Meyer FS: Cast bridgework in functional occlusion, *J Am Dent Assoc* 20:1015-1019, 1933.
6. Schuyler C: Correction of occlusion: disharmony of the natural dentition, *N Y Dent J* 13:455-463, 1947.
7. Stallard H, Stuart C: Concepts of occlusion, *Dent Clin North Am* November:591-601, 1963.
8. Ramfjord SP, Ash MM: *Occlusion*, ed 3, Philadelphia, 1983, Saunders, pp 129-136.
9. Boucher CO: *Current clinical dental terminology*, St Louis, 1963, Mosby.
10. Posselt U: Studies in the mobility of the human mandible, *Acta Odontol Scand* 10(Suppl):19-27, 1952.
11. Boucher CO: *Swenson's complete dentures*, St Louis, 1970, Mosby, p 112.
12. Ramfjord SP: Dysfunctional temporomandibular joint and muscle pain, *J Prosthet Dent* 11:353-362, 1961.
13. Ramfjord S: Bruxism: a clinical and electromyographic study, *J Am Dent Assoc* 62:21-28, 1961.
14. Brill N: Influence of occlusal patterns on movement of the mandible, *J Prosthet Dent* 12:255-261, 1962.
15. Posselt U: *Physiology of occlusion and rehabilitation*, Philadelphia, 1968, FA Davis, p 60.
16. Dawson PE: *Evaluation, diagnosis and treatment of occlusal problems*, St Louis, 1989, Mosby, pp 28-34.
17. Jankelson B, Swain CW: Physiological aspects of masticatory muscle stimulation: the myomonitor, *Quintessence Int* 3:57-62, 1972.
18. Gelb H: *Clinical management of head, neck and TMJ pain and dysfunction*, Philadelphia, 1977, Saunders.
19. DuBrul EL: *Sicher's oral anatomy*, St Louis, 1980, Mosby, p 178.
20. Moffet BC: Articular remodeling in the adult human temporomandibular joint, *Am J Anat* 115:119-127, 1969.
21. Van Blarcom CW, Campbell SD, Carr AB et al: *The glossary of prosthodontic terms*, ed 7, St Louis, 1999, Mosby, p 58.
22. Wu CZ, Chou SL, Ash MM: Centric discrepancy associated with TM disorders in young adults, *J Dent Res* 69:334-337, 1990.
23. DuBrul EL: *Sicher's oral anatomy*, St Louis, 1980, Mosby.
24. Jankelson B, Adib F: Effect of variation in manipulation force on the repetitiveness of centric relations registration: a computer-based study, *J Am Dent Assoc* 113:59-62, 1987.
25. Isberg A, Isacsson G: Tissue reactions associated with internal derangement of the temporomandibular joint. A radiographic, cryomorphologic, and histologic study, *Acta Odontol Scand* 44:160-164, 1986.
26. Farrar WB, McCarty WL: *A clinical outline of temporomandibular joint diagnosis and treatment*, Montgomery, Ala, 1983, Normandie Publications.
27. Dolwick MF: *Diagnosis and etiology of internal derangements of the temporomandibular joint: President's Conference on the Examination, Diagnosis, and Management of TM Disorders*, Chicago, 1983, American Dental Association, pp 112-117.
28. Stegenga B, de Bont LG, Boering G: Osteoarthrosis as the cause of craniomandibular pain and dysfunction: a unifying concept, *J Oral Maxillofac Surg* 47:249-256, 1989.
29. Maruyama T, Nishio K, Kotani M, Miyauchi S, Kuroda T: The effect of changing the maxillomandibular relationship by a bite plane on the habitual mandibular opening and closing movement, *J Oral Rehabil* 11:455-465, 1984.
30. Rugh JD, Drago CJ: Vertical dimension: a study of clinical rest position and jaw muscle activity, *J Prosthet Dent* 45:670-675, 1981.
31. Manns A, Zuazola RV, Sirhan RM, Quiroz M, Rocabado M: Relationship between the tonic elevator mandibular activity and the vertical dimension during the states of vigilance and hypnosis, *Cranio* 8:163-170, 1990.
32. Manns A, Miralles R, Santander H, Valdivia J: Influence of the vertical dimension in the treatment of myofascial pain-dysfunction syndrome, *J Prosthet Dent* 50:700-709, 1983.
33. Gibbs CH, Mahan PE, Lundeen HC, Brehan K: Occlusal forces during chewing: influence on biting strength and food consistency, *J Prosthet Dent* 46:561-567, 1981.
34. Bates JF: Masticatory function—a review of the literature. II. Speed of movements of the mandible, rate of chewing, and forces developed in chewing, *J Oral Rehabil* 2:249-256, 1975.

35. Shore NA, Schaefer MC: Temporomandibular joint dysfunction, *Quintessence Int* 10:9-14, 1979.
36. Tsukasa I, Gibbs C, Marguelles-Bonnet R, Lupkiewicz S, Young HM et al: Loading on the temporomandibular joint with five occlusal conditions, *J Prosthet Dent* 56:478-484, 1986.
37. Guichet NE: *Occlusion: a teaching manual*, Anaheim, Calif, 1977, The Denar Corporation.
38. Mongi F: Anatomical and clinical evaluation of the relationships between the temporomandibular joint and occlusion, *J Prosthet Dent* 38:539-547, 1977.
39. Polson AM, Zander HA: Occlusal traumatism. In Lundeen HC, Gibbs CH, editors: *Advances in occlusion*, Boston, 1982, John Wright PSG, pp 143-148.
40. Goldman HM, Cohen WD: *Periodontal therapy*, St Louis, 1968, Mosby, p 45.
41. Zander HA, Muhlemann HR: The effects of stress on the periodontal structures, *Oral Surg Oral Med Oral Pathol* 9:380-387, 1956.
42. Glickman I: Inflammation and trauma from occlusion, *J Periodontol* 34:5-15, 1963.
43. McAdam D: Tooth loading and cuspal guidance in canine and group function occlusion, *J Prosthet Dent* 35:283-297, 1976.
44. Kemper JT, Okeson JP: *Introduction to occlusal anatomy. A waxing manual*, Lexington, 1982, University of Kentucky Press.
45. Lundeen H: *Introduction to occlusal anatomy*, Lexington, 1969, University of Kentucky Press.
46. Howell AH, Manly RS: An electronic strain gauge for measuring oral forces, *J Dent Res* 27:705-712, 1948.
47. Manns A, Miralles R, Valdivia J, Bull R: Influence of variation in anteroposterior occlusal contacts on electromyographic activity, *J Prosthet Dent* 61:617-623, 1989.
48. Lee RL: *Anterior guidance advances in occlusion*, Boston, 1982, John Wright PSG, pp 51-80.
49. Standlee JP: Stress transfer to the mandible during anterior guidance and group function at centric movements, *J Prosthet Dent* 34:35-45, 1979.
50. Korioth TWP, Hannam AG: Effect of bilateral asymmetric tooth clenching on load distribution at the mandibular condyle, *J Prosthet Dent* 64:62-78, 1990.
51. Williamson EH, Eugene H: Williamson on occlusion and TMJ dysfunction. (Part 2) (interviewed by Sidney Brandt), *J Clin Orthod* 15:393-404, 1981.
52. Lucia VA: *Modern gnathology concepts*, St Louis, 1961, Mosby.
53. Kraus BS, Jordon RE, Abrahams L: *Dental anatomy and occlusion*, Baltimore, 1973, Waverly Press, p 226.
54. Goldman HM, Cohen WD: *Periodontal therapy*, St Louis, 1968, Mosby.
55. Ash MM, Nelson SJ: *Wheeler's dental anatomy, physiology, and occlusion*, ed 8, St Louis, 2003, Saunders, pp 29-64.
56. Williams EH, Lundquist DO: Anterior guidance: its effect on the electromyographic activity of the temporal and masseter muscles, *J Prosthet Dent* 49:816-825, 1983.
57. Ramfjord SP, Ash MM: *Occlusion*, ed 3, Philadelphia, 1983, Saunders.
58. Dawson PE: *Evaluation, diagnosis and treatment of occlusal problems*, St Louis, 1989, Mosby.
59. Ahlgren J: The silent period in the EMG of the jaw muscles during mastication and its relationship to tooth contacts, *Acta Odontol Scand* 27:219-234, 1969.
60. Schaerer P, Stallard RE, Zander HA: Occlusal interferences and mastication: an electromyographic study, *J Prosthet Dent* 17:438-450, 1967.
61. Williamson EH, Lundquist DO: Anterior guidance: its effect on electromyographic activity of the temporal and masseter muscles, *J Prosthet Dent* 49:816-823, 1983.
62. Koidis PT, Novak M, Magiliotou MC, Burch JG: Influence of postural position on occlusal contact strain patterns, *J Dent Res* 65:189, 1986 (abstract).
63. Mohl ND: Head posture and its role in occlusion, *N Y State Dent J* 42:17-23, 1976.

Determinants of Occlusal Morphology

CHAPTER 6

"Developing teeth that successfully permit efficient masticatory function is basic to dentistry and survival."

—JPO

In health the occlusal anatomy of the teeth functions in harmony with the structures controlling the movement patterns of the mandible. The structures that determine these patterns are the temporomandibular joints (TMJs) and the anterior teeth. During any given movement the unique anatomic relationships of these structures combine to dictate a precise and repeatable pathway. To maintain harmony of the occlusal condition, the posterior teeth must pass close to but must not contact their opposing teeth during mandibular movement. Importantly, the clinician should examine each of these structures carefully and appreciate how the anatomic form of each can determine the occlusal morphology necessary to achieve an optimum occlusal relationship. The structures that control mandibular movement are divided into two types: (1) those that influence the movement of the posterior portion of the mandible and (2) those that influence the movement of the anterior portion of the mandible. The TMJs are considered the *posterior controlling factors* (PCFs), and the anterior teeth are considered the *anterior controlling factors* (ACFs). The posterior teeth are positioned between these two controlling factors and thus can be affected by both to varying degrees.

POSTERIOR CONTROLLING FACTORS (CONDYLAR GUIDANCE)

As the condyle moves out of the centric relation position, it descends along the articular eminence of the mandibular fossa. The rate at which it moves inferiorly as the mandible is being protruded depends on the steepness of the articular eminence. If the surface is quite steep, the condyle will take a steep, vertically inclined path. If it is flatter, the condyle will take a path that is less vertically inclined. The angle at which the condyle moves away from a horizontal reference plane is referred to as the *condylar guidance angle*.

Generally, the condylar guidance angle generated by the orbiting condyle when the mandible moves laterally is larger than when the mandible protrudes straightforward. This is because the medial wall of the mandibular fossa is generally steeper than the articular eminence of the fossa directly anterior to the condyle.

The two TMJs provide the guidance for the posterior portion of the mandible and are largely responsible for determining the character of mandibular movement posteriorly. They have therefore been referred to as the PCFs *of the mandibular movement*. The condylar guidance is considered to be a fixed factor because it is unalterable in the healthy patient. It can be altered, however, under certain conditions (trauma, pathosis, or a surgical procedure).

ANTERIOR CONTROLLING FACTORS (ANTERIOR GUIDANCE)

Just as the TMJs determine or control the manner in which the posterior portion of the mandible moves, so the anterior teeth determine how the anterior portion moves. As the mandible protrudes or moves laterally, the incisal edges of the mandibular teeth occlude with the lingual surfaces of the maxillary anterior teeth. The steepness of these lingual surfaces determines the amount of vertical movement of the mandible. If the surfaces are quite steep, the anterior aspect of the mandible will take a steep-incline path. If the anterior teeth have little vertical overlap, they will provide little vertical guidance during mandibular movement.

The anterior guidance is considered to be a variable rather than a fixed factor. It can be altered by dental procedures such as restorations, orthodontia, and extractions. It can also be altered by pathologic conditions such as caries, habits, and tooth wear.

UNDERSTANDING THE CONTROLLING FACTORS

To understand the influence of mandibular movement on the occlusal morphology of posterior teeth, one must consider the factors that influence mandibular movement. As discussed in Chapter 4, mandibular movement is determined by the anatomic characteristics both of the TMJs posteriorly and of the anterior teeth anteriorly. Variations in the anatomy of the TMJs and the anterior teeth can lead to changes in the movement pattern of the mandible. If the criteria for optimum functional occlusion are to be fulfilled, the morphologic characteristics of each posterior tooth must be in harmony with those of its opposing tooth or teeth during all eccentric mandibular movements. Therefore the exact morphology of the tooth is influenced by the pathway it travels across its opposing tooth or teeth.

The relationship of a posterior tooth to the controlling factors influences the precise movement of that tooth. This means that the nearer a tooth is to the TMJ, the more the joint anatomy will influence its eccentric movement and the less the anatomy of the anterior teeth will influence its movement. Likewise, the nearer a specific tooth is to the anterior teeth, the more the anatomy of the anterior teeth will influence its movement and the less the anatomy of the TMJs will influence that movement.

The occlusal surfaces of posterior teeth consist of a series of cusps with both vertical and horizontal dimensions. Cusps are made up of convex ridges that vary in steepness (vertical dimension) and direction (horizontal dimension).

Mandibular movement has both a vertical and a horizontal component, and it is the relationship between these components or the ratio that is significant in the study of mandibular movement. The vertical component is a function of the superoinferior movement, and the horizontal component a function of the anteroposterior movement. If a condyle moves downward two units as it moves forward two units, it moves away from a horizontal reference plane at an angle of 45 degrees. If it moves downward two units and forward one unit, it moves away from this plane at an angle of approximately 64 degrees. The angle of deviation from the horizontal reference plane is what clinicians study in mandibular movement.

Fig. 6-1 represents the mandible as it moves four units in the horizontal plane and zero units in the vertical plane, resulting in a deviation away from horizontal of 0 degrees. Fig. 6-2 shows the mandible moving four units in the horizontal and four units in the vertical plane. The result here is a deviation away from horizontal of 45 degrees.

In Fig. 6-3 the mandible moves four units in the horizontal plane, but in the vertical plane the PCF moves four units and the ACF moves six units. This results in a 45-degree movement of the PCF and a 57-degree movement of the ACF. Points between the factors will deviate by different amounts from the horizontal plane depending on their proximity to each factor. The nearer a point is to the PCF, for example, the more its movement will approach 45 degrees (because of the greater influence of the PCF on its movement). Likewise, the nearer a

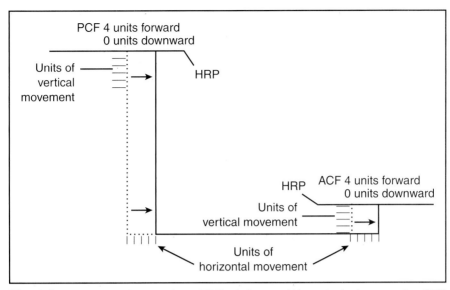

Fig. 6-1 Horizontal reference plane *(HRP)* of the mandible at both the posterior *(PCF)* and the anterior *(ACF)* controlling factor. The mandible moves horizontally four units from a position marked by the dotted line. No vertical movement occurs. The solid line represents the position of the mandible after the movement has taken place.

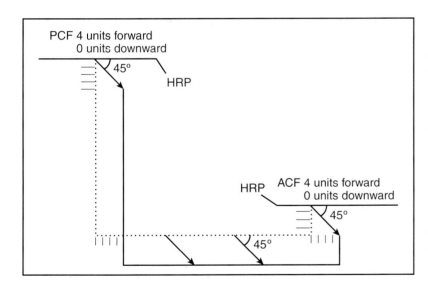

Fig. 6-2 Movement of the mandible four units horizontally and four units vertically at both the posterior *(PCF)* and the anterior *(ACF)* controlling factor. When the mandible moves four units down, it moves four units forward at the same time. The net result is that it is at a 45-degree angle from the horizontal reference planes. Because both the PCFs and the ACFs are causing the mandible to move at the same rate, each point on the mandible is at a 45-degree angle from the horizontal reference plane at the end of a mandibular excursion.

point is to the ACF, the more its movement will approach 57 degrees (because of the greater influence of the ACF on its movement). A point equidistant between the factors will move away from horizontal at an angle of approximately 51 degrees (which is midway between 45 and 57 degrees), and one that is 25% closer to the ACF than to the PCF will move away from horizontal at an angle of 54 degrees (one fourth of the way between 57 and 45 degrees).

To examine the influence of any anatomic variation on the movement pattern of the mandible, it

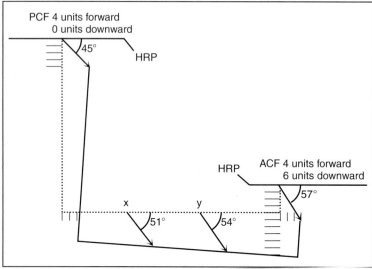

Fig. 6-3 RESULTANT MOVEMENT OF THE MANDIBLE WHEN THE CON-TROLLING FACTORS ARE NOT IDENTICAL. The posterior controlling factor *(PCF)* causes the posterior portion of the mandible to move four units forward (horizontally) and four units downward (vertically). However, the anterior controlling factor *(ACF)* causes the anterior portion of the mandible to move four units forward and six units downward. Therefore the posterior portion of the mandible is moving away from the reference plane at a 45-degree angle, and the anterior portion is moving away at a 57-degree angle. A point *(x)* that is equidistant from the controlling factors will move at a 51-degree angle from the reference plane. Another point *(y)* that is one fourth closer to the ACF than to the PCF will move at a 54-degree angle. Thus it can be seen that the nearer the point is to a controlling factor, the more its movement is influenced by the factor.

is necessary to control all factors except the one being examined. Remember that the significance of the anterior and condylar guidances lies in how they influence posterior tooth shape. Because the occlusal surface can be affected in two manners (height and width), it is logical to separate the structural influence on mandibular movement into factors that influence the vertical components and those that influence the horizontal components. The anatomy of the occlusal surface is also influenced by its relationship with the tooth that passes across it during movement. Therefore the location of the tooth to the center of rotation is also discussed.

distance it extends into the depth of an opposing fossa are determined by three factors:
1. The ACF of mandibular movement (i.e., anterior guidance)
2. The PCF of mandibular movement (i.e., condylar guidance)
3. The nearness of the cusp to these controlling factors

The posterior centric cusps are generally developed to disocclude during eccentric mandibular movements but to contact in the intercuspal position. For this to occur, they must be long enough to contact in the intercuspal position but not so long that they contact during eccentric movements.

VERTICAL DETERMINANTS OF OCCLUSAL MORPHOLOGY

Factors that influence the heights of cusps and the depths of fossae are the vertical determinants of occlusal morphology. The length of a cusp and the

EFFECT OF CONDYLAR GUIDANCE (ANGLE OF THE EMINENCE) ON CUSP HEIGHT

As the mandible is protruded, the condyle descends along the articular eminence. Its descent in relation to a horizontal reference plane is determined by the steepness of the eminence. The steeper the eminence, the more the condyle is forced to move inferiorly as it shifts anteriorly. This results in greater vertical movement of the condyle, mandible, and mandibular teeth.

In Fig. 6-4 the condyle moves away from a horizontal reference plane at a 45-degree angle. To simplify visualization, anterior guidance is illustrated at an equal angle. The cusp tip of premolar A will move away from a horizontal reference plane at a 45-degree angle. To avoid eccentric contact between premolar A and premolar B in a protrusive movement, cuspal inclination must be less than 45 degrees.

In Fig. 6-5, condylar guidance and anterior guidance are presented as being 60 degrees to the horizontal reference planes. With these steeper vertical determinants, premolar A will move away

from premolar B at a 60-degree angle, resulting in longer cusps. Therefore a steeper angle of the eminence (condylar guidance) allows for steeper posterior cusps.

EFFECT OF ANTERIOR GUIDANCE ON CUSP HEIGHT

Anterior guidance is a function of the relationship between the maxillary and mandibular anterior teeth. As presented in Chapter 3, it consists of the vertical and horizontal overlaps of the anterior teeth. To illustrate its influence on mandibular movement and therefore on the occlusal shape of posterior teeth, some combinations of vertical and horizontal overlap appear in Fig. 6-6.

Parts A, B, and C present anterior relationships that maintain equal amounts of vertical overlap.

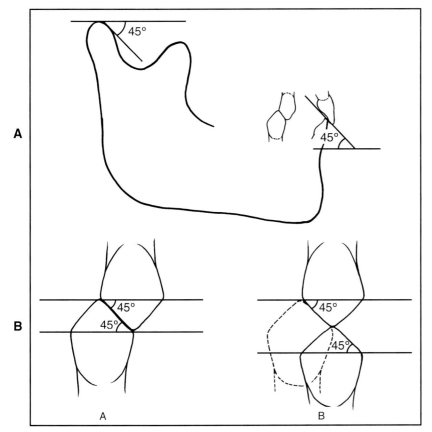

Fig. 6-4 A, The posterior and anterior controlling factors are the same, causing the mandible to move away from the reference plane at a 45-degree angle. **B,** For premolar *A* to be disoccluded from premolar *B* during a protrusive movement, the cuspal inclines must be less than 45 degrees.

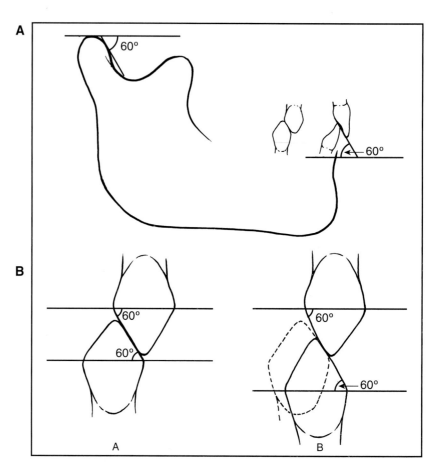

Fig. 6-5 A, Posterior and anterior controlling factors are identical and cause the mandible to move away from the reference plane at a 60-degree angle. **B,** For premolar A to be disoccluded from premolar B during a protrusive movement, the cuspal inclines must be less than 60 degrees. Thus it can be seen that steeper posterior and anterior controlling factors allow for steeper posterior cusps.

By comparing the changes in horizontal overlap, one can see that as the horizontal overlap increases, the anterior guidance angle decreases.

Parts D, E, and F present anterior relationships that maintain equal amounts of horizontal overlap but varying amounts of vertical overlap. By comparing the changes in vertical overlap, one can see that as the vertical overlap increases, the anterior guidance angle increases.

Because mandibular movement is determined to a great extent by anterior guidance, changes in the vertical and horizontal overlaps of the anterior teeth cause changes in the vertical movement patterns of the mandible. An increase in horizontal overlap leads to a decreased anterior guidance angle, less vertical component to mandibular movement, and flatter posterior cusps. An increase in vertical overlap produces an increased anterior guidance angle,

a more vertical component to mandibular movement, and steeper posterior cusps.

EFFECT OF THE PLANE OF OCCLUSION ON CUSP HEIGHT

The plane of occlusion is an imaginary line touching the incisal edges of the maxillary anterior teeth and the cusps of the maxillary posterior teeth. The relationship of the plane to the angle of the eminence influences the steepness of the cusps. When the movement of a mandibular tooth is viewed in relation to the plane of occlusion rather than in relation to a horizontal reference plane, the influence of the plane of occlusion can be seen.

In Fig. 6-7, condylar guidance and anterior guidance are combined to produce a 45-degree movement of a mandibular tooth when compared with

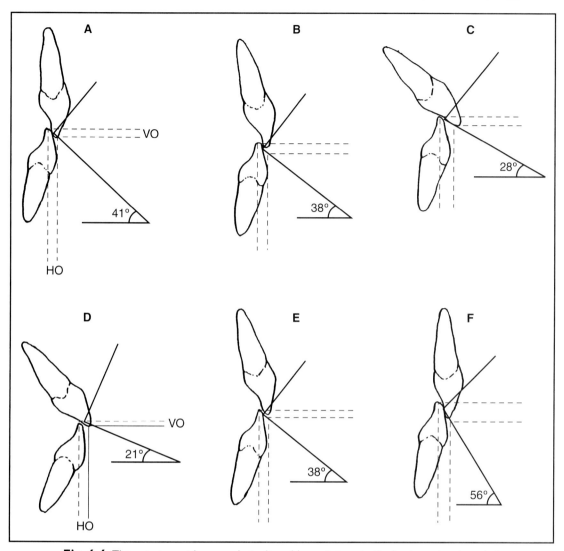

Fig. 6-6 The anterior guidance angle is altered by variations in the horizontal and vertical overlap. In **A** to **C** the horizontal overlap *(HO)* varies, whereas the vertical overlap *(VO)* remains constant. When the HO increases, the anterior guidance angle decreases. In **D** to **F** the VO varies, whereas the HO remains constant. As VO increases, the anterior guidance angle increases.

the horizontal reference plane. However, when the 45-degree movement is compared with one plane of occlusion (PO$_A$), it can be seen that the tooth is moving away from the plane at only a 25-degree angle, which results in the need for flatter posterior cusps so that posterior tooth contact will be avoided. When the tooth movement is compared

with the plane of occlusion (PO$_B$), it can be seen that the movement away from this plane is 60 degrees. Therefore the posterior teeth can have longer cusps, and we have determined that as the plane of occlusion becomes more nearly parallel to the angle of the eminence, the posterior cusps must be made shorter.

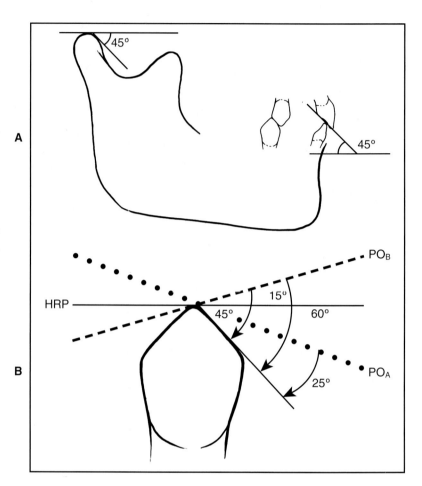

Fig. 6-7 A, The anterior and posterior controlling factors create a mandibular movement of 45 degrees from the horizontal reference plane. **B,** The tooth moves at a 45-degree angle from the reference plane *(HRP)*. However, if one plane of occlusion *(PO$_A$)* is angled, the tooth will move away from the reference plane at only 25 degrees. Therefore the cusp must be relatively flat to be disoccluded during protrusive movement. When the angle at which the tooth moves during a protrusive movement is compared with another plane of occlusion *(PO$_B$)*, a much greater discrepancy is evident (45 + 15 = 60 degrees). This allows for taller and steeper posterior cusps.

EFFECT OF THE CURVE OF SPEE ON CUSP HEIGHT

When viewed from the lateral, the *curve of Spee* is an anteroposterior curve extending from the tip of the mandibular canine along the buccal cusp tips of the mandibular posterior teeth. Its curvature can be described in terms of the length of the radius of the curve. With a short radius, the curve will be more acute than with a longer radius (Fig. 6-8).

The degree of curvature of the curve of Spee influences the height of the posterior cusps that will function in harmony with mandibular movement. In Fig. 6-9 the mandible is moving away from a horizontal reference plane at a 45-degree angle. Movement away from the maxillary posterior teeth will vary depending on the curvature of the curve

of Spee. Given a short radius, the angle at which the mandibular teeth move away from the maxillary teeth will be greater than with a long radius.

The orientation of the curve of Spee, as determined by the relationship of its radius to a horizontal reference plane, will also influence how the cusp height of an individual posterior tooth is affected. In Fig. 6-10, *A,* the radius of the curve forms a 90-degree angle with a constant horizontal reference plane. Molars (which are located distal to the radius) will have shorter cusps, whereas premolars (located mesial) will have longer cusps. In Fig. 6-10, *B,* the radius forms a 60-degree angle with a horizontal reference plane (rotating the curve of Spee more forward). By moving the curve more forward with respect to the horizontal plane, one can see that all the posterior teeth (premolars

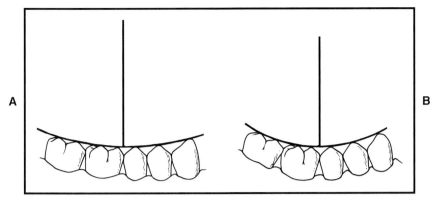

Fig. 6-8 CURVE OF SPEE. A, A longer radius causes a flatter plane of occlusion. **B,** A shorter radius causes a more acute plane of occlusion.

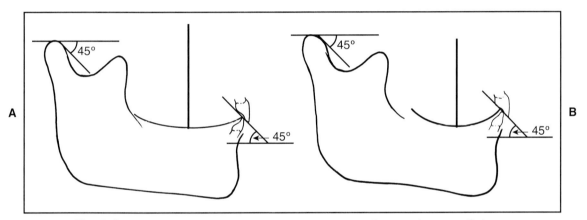

Fig. 6-9 The mandible is moving away from a horizontal reference plane at a 45-degree angle. The flatter the plane of occlusion **(A)**, the greater will be the angle at which the mandibular posterior teeth move away from the maxillary posterior teeth and therefore the taller the cusp can be. The more acute the plane of occlusion **(B)**, the smaller will be the angle of the mandibular posterior tooth movement and the flatter the teeth can be.

and molars) will have shorter cusps. In Fig. 6-10, *C*, if the perpendicular line from the constant horizontal reference plane is rotated posteriorly (curve of Spee placed more posteriorly), one can see that the posterior teeth (especially the molars) can have longer cusps.

EFFECT OF MANDIBULAR LATERAL TRANSLATION MOVEMENT ON CUSP HEIGHT

The mandibular lateral translation movement is a bodily side shift of the mandible that occurs during lateral movements (previously called *Bennett movement*). During a lateral excursion the orbiting condyle moves downward, forward, and inward in the mandibular fossa around axes located in the opposite (rotating) condyle. The degree of inward movement of the orbiting condyle is determined by two factors: (1) morphology of the medial wall of the mandibular fossa and (2) inner horizontal portion of the temporomandibular (TM) ligament, which attaches to the lateral pole of the rotating condyle. If the TM ligament of the rotating condyle is tight and the medial wall is close to the orbiting condyle, a pure arcing movement will be made

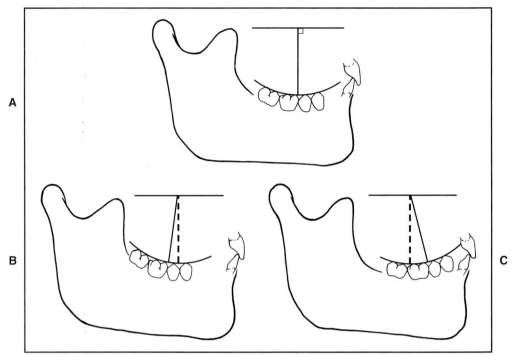

Fig. 6-10 ORIENTATION OF THE CURVE OF SPEE. A, Radius perpendicular to a horizontal reference plane. Posterior teeth located distal to the radius will need shorter cusps than those located mesial to the radius. **B,** If the plane of occlusion is rotated more posteriorly, it can be seen that more posterior teeth will be positioned distal to the perpendicular from the reference plane and can have shorter cusps. **C,** If the plane is rotated more anteriorly, it can be seen that more posterior teeth will be positioned mesial to the perpendicular and can have taller cusps.

around the axis of rotation in the rotating condyle. When this condition exists, no lateral translation of the mandible occurs (and therefore no mandibular lateral translation movement) (Fig. 6-11). Such a condition rarely occurs. Most often there is some looseness of the TM ligament, and the medial wall of the mandibular fossa lies medial to an arc around the axis of the rotating condyle (Fig. 6-12). When this occurs, the orbiting condyle is moved inwardly to the medial wall and produces a mandibular lateral translation movement.

The lateral translation movement has three attributes: amount, timing, and direction. The *amount* and *timing* are determined in part by the degree to which the medial wall of the mandibular fossa departs medially from an arc around the axis in the rotating condyle. They are also determined by the degree of lateral movement of the rotating

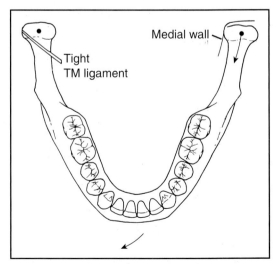

Fig. 6-11 With proximity of the medial wall and a tight temporomandibular *(TM)* ligament, there is no lateral translation movement.

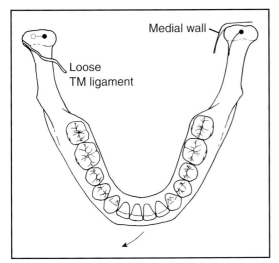

Fig. 6-12 When there is distance between the medial wall and medial pole of the orbiting condyle and the temporomandibular *(TM)* ligament allows some movement of the rotating condyle, a lateral translation movement occurs.

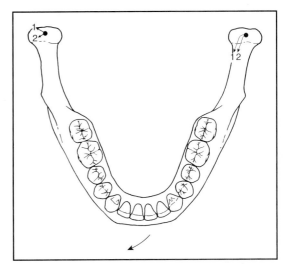

Fig. 6-14 The direction of the lateral translation movement is determined by the direction taken by the rotating condyle. When the rotating condyle follows pathway 1, the central fossa of the teeth will need to be wider than pathway 2 to disengage the opposing teeth.

condyle permitted by the TM ligament. The more medial the wall from the medial pole of the orbiting condyle, the greater the amount of lateral translation movement (Fig. 6-13); and the looser the TM ligament attached to the rotating condyle,

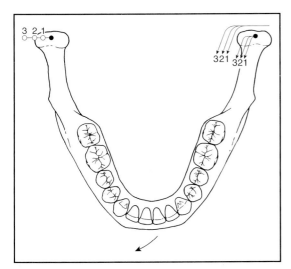

Fig. 6-13 The more medial the medial wall is from the condyle, the greater will be the lateral translation movement. Therefore when the medial wall is in position 3, it will allow more lateral translation of the mandible than in position 1.

the greater the lateral translation movement. The *direction* of lateral translation movement depends primarily on the direction taken by the rotating condyle during the bodily movement (Fig. 6-14).

Effect of the Amount of Lateral Translation Movement on Cusp Height

As just stated, the amount of lateral translation movement is determined by the tightness of the inner horizontal portion of the TM ligament attached to the rotating condyle, as well as the degree to which the medial wall of the mandibular fossa departs from the medial pole of the orbiting condyle. The looser this ligament and the greater its departure, the greater the amount of mandibular translation movement. As the lateral translation movement increases, the bodily shift of the mandible dictates that the posterior cusps be shorter to permit lateral translation without creating contact between the maxillary and mandibular posterior teeth (Fig. 6-15).

Effect of the Direction of the Lateral Translation Movement on Cusp Height

The direction of shift of the rotating condyle during a lateral translation movement is determined by the morphology and ligamentous attachments of

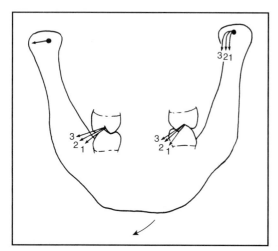

Fig. 6-15 The greater the lateral translation movement, the shorter is the posterior cusp. Pathway 3 will require shorter cusps than pathway 1.

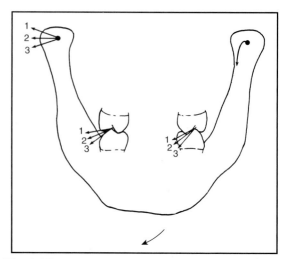

Fig. 6-17 The more superior the lateral translation movement of the rotating condyle (*1*), the shorter the posterior cusp. The more inferior the lateral translation movement (*3*), the taller the cusp.

the TM joint undergoing rotation. The movement occurs within a 60-degree (or less) cone, the apex of which is located at the axis of rotation (Fig. 6-16). Therefore in addition to lateral movement, the rotating condyle may also move in (1) a superior, (2) an inferior, (3) an anterior, or (4) a posterior direction. Furthermore, combinations of these can occur. In other words, shifts may be laterosuperoanterior, lateroinferoposterior, and so on.

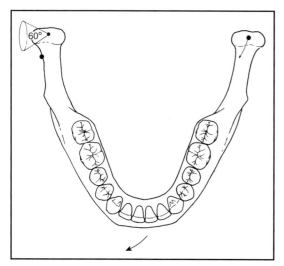

Fig. 6-16 The rotating condyle is capable of moving laterally within the area of a 60-degree cone during lateral translation movement.

Of importance as a determinant of cusp height and fossa depth is the vertical movement of the rotating condyle during a lateral translation movement (e.g., the superior and inferior movements) (Fig. 6-17). Thus a laterosuperior movement of the rotating condyle will require shorter posterior cusps than will a straight lateral movement; likewise, a lateroinferior movement will permit longer posterior cusps than will a straight lateral movement.

Effect of the Timing of the Lateral Translation Movement on Cusp Height

Timing of the lateral translation movement is a function of the medial wall adjacent to the orbiting condyle and the attachment of the TM ligament to the rotating condyle. These two conditions determine when this movement occurs during a lateral excursion. Of the three attributes of the lateral translation movement (amount, direction, and timing), the last has the greatest influence on the occlusal morphology of the posterior teeth. If the timing occurs late and the maxillary and mandibular cusps are beyond functional range, the amount and direction of the lateral translation movement will have little, if any, influence on occlusal morphology. However, if the timing of this

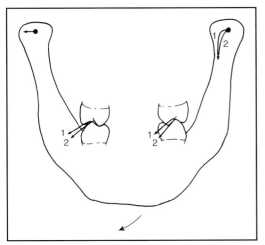

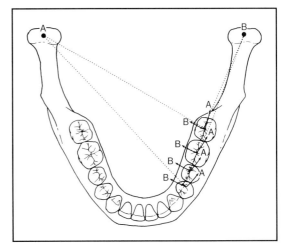

Fig. 6-18 TIMING OF THE LATERAL TRANS-LATION MOVEMENT. *1,* Immediate lateral translation movement (immediate side shift); *2,* progressive lateral translation movement (progressive side shift). The more immediate the lateral translation, the shorter the posterior cusp.

Fig. 6-19 The pathway that the cusp of a tooth follows in passing over the opposing tooth is a factor of its distance (radius) from the rotating condyle. Mediotrusive pathway *(A)* and laterotrusive pathway *(B).*

movement occurs early in the laterotrusive movement, the amount and direction of the lateral translation movement will markedly influence occlusal morphology.

When the lateral translation movement occurs early, a shift is seen even before the condyle begins to translate from the fossa. This is called an *immediate lateral translation movement* or *immediate side shift* (Fig. 6-18). If it occurs in conjunction with an eccentric movement, the movement is known as a *progressive lateral translation movement* or *progressive side shift.* The more immediate the side shift, the shorter the posterior teeth.

HORIZONTAL DETERMINANTS OF OCCLUSAL MORPHOLOGY

Horizontal determinants of occlusal morphology include relationships that influence the direction of ridges and grooves on the occlusal surfaces. Because cusps pass between ridges and over grooves during eccentric movements, the horizontal determinants also influence the placement of cusps.

Each centric cusp tip generates both laterotrusive and mediotrusive pathways across its opposing tooth. Each pathway represents a portion of the arc formed by the cusp rotating around the rotating condyle (Fig. 6-19). The angles formed by these pathways can be compared and will be found to vary depending on the relationship of the angle to certain anatomic structures.

EFFECT OF DISTANCE FROM THE ROTATING CONDYLE ON RIDGE AND GROOVE DIRECTION

Because the position of a tooth varies in relation to the axis of rotation of the mandible (i.e., rotating condyle), variation will occur in the angles formed by the laterotrusive and mediotrusive pathways. The greater the distance of the tooth from the axis of rotation (rotating condyle), the wider the angle formed by the laterotrusive and mediotrusive pathways (Fig. 6-20). This is consistent regardless of whether maxillary or mandibular teeth are being viewed. Actually, the angles are increased in size as the distance from the rotating condyle is increased because the mandibular pathways are being generated more mesially (see Fig. 6-20, A) and the maxillary pathways are being generated more distally (see Fig. 6-20, B).

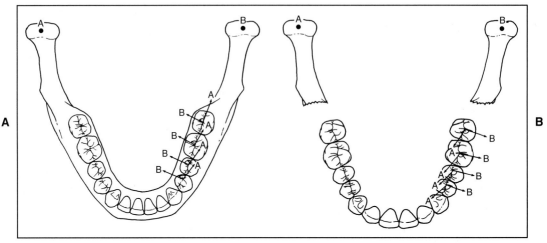

Fig. 6-20 The greater the distance of the tooth from the rotating condyle, the wider the angle formed by the laterotrusive and mediotrusive pathways. This is true for both mandibular **(A)** and maxillary **(B)** teeth. *A,* Mediotrusive pathway; *B,* laterotrusive pathway.

EFFECT OF DISTANCE FROM THE MIDSAGITTAL PLANE ON RIDGE AND GROOVE DIRECTION

The relationship of a tooth to the midsagittal plane will also influence the laterotrusive and mediotrusive pathways generated on the tooth by an opposing centric cusp. As the tooth is positioned farther from the midsagittal plane, the angles formed by the laterotrusive and mediotrusive pathways will increase (Fig. 6-21).

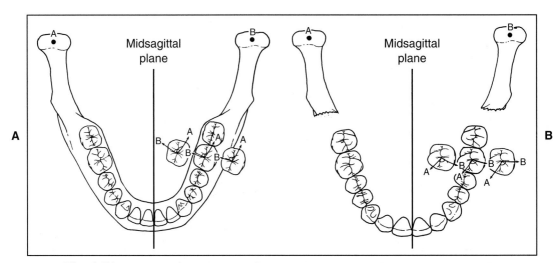

Fig. 6-21 The greater the distance of the tooth from the midsagittal plane, the wider the angle formed by the laterotrusive and mediotrusive pathways. This is true for both **(A)** mandibular and **(B)** maxillary teeth. *A,* Mediotrusive pathway; *B,* laterotrusive pathway.

EFFECT OF DISTANCE FROM THE ROTATING CONDYLES AND FROM THE MIDSAGITTAL PLANE ON RIDGE AND GROOVE DIRECTION

It has been demonstrated that a tooth's position in relation to the rotating condyle and the midsagittal plane influences the laterotrusive and mediotrusive pathways. The combination of the two positional relationships is what determines the exact pathways of the centric cusp tips. Positioning the tooth a greater distance from the rotating condyle, but nearer the midsagittal plane, would cause the latter determinant to negate the influence of the former. The greatest angle between the laterotrusive and mediotrusive pathways would be generated by teeth positioned in the dental arch at a great distance from both the rotating condyle and the midsagittal plane. Conversely, the smallest angles would be generated by teeth nearer to both the rotating condyle and the midsagittal plane.

Because of the curvature of the dental arch, the following can be seen: Generally, as the distance of a tooth from the rotating condyle increases, its distance from the midsagittal plane decreases. However, because the distance from the rotating condyle generally increases faster than the decrease in distance from the midsagittal plane, generally the teeth toward the anterior region (e.g., premolars) will have larger angles between the laterotrusive and mediotrusive pathways than will the teeth located more posteriorly (molars) (Fig. 6-22).

EFFECT OF MANDIBULAR LATERAL TRANSLATION MOVEMENT ON RIDGE AND GROOVE DIRECTION

The influence of the lateral translation movement has already been discussed as a vertical determinant of occlusal morphology. This movement also influences the directions of ridges and grooves. As the amount of it increases, the angle between the laterotrusive and mediotrusive pathways generated by the centric cusp tips increases (Fig. 6-23).

The direction that the rotating condyle shifts during a lateral translation movement influences the direction of laterotrusive and mediotrusive

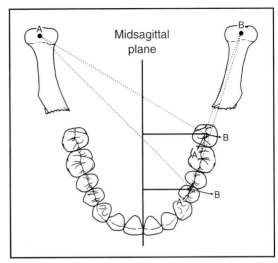

Fig. 6-22 The more anterior the tooth in the dental arch, the wider the angle formed by the *(A)* mediotrusive and *(B)* laterotrusive pathways.

pathways and resultant angles (Fig. 6-24). If the rotating condyle shifts in a lateral and anterior direction, the angle between the laterotrusive and mediotrusive pathways will decrease on both maxillary and mandibular teeth. If the condyle shifts laterally and posteriorly, the angles generated will increase.

EFFECT OF INTERCONDYLAR DISTANCE ON RIDGE AND GROOVE DIRECTION

In considering the influence of the intercondylar distance on the generation of laterotrusive and mediotrusive pathways, it is important to consider how a change in intercondylar distance influences the relationship of the tooth to the rotating condyle and midsagittal plane. As the intercondylar distance increases, the distance between the condyle and the tooth in a given arch configuration increases. This tends to cause wider angles between the laterotrusive and mediotrusive pathways. However, as the intercondylar distance increases, the tooth is placed nearer the midsagittal plane relative to the rotating condyle–midsagittal plane distance. This tends to decrease the angles

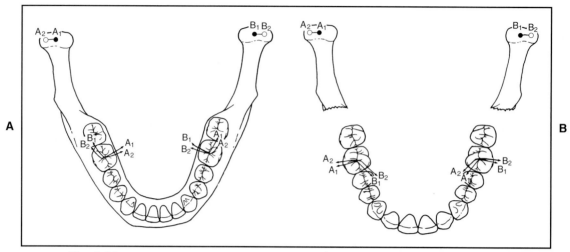

Fig. 6-23 As the amount of lateral translation movement increases, the angle between the **(A)** mediotrusive and **(B)** laterotrusive pathways generated by the centric cusp tips increases. This is true for both mandibular *(A)* and maxillary *(B)* teeth.

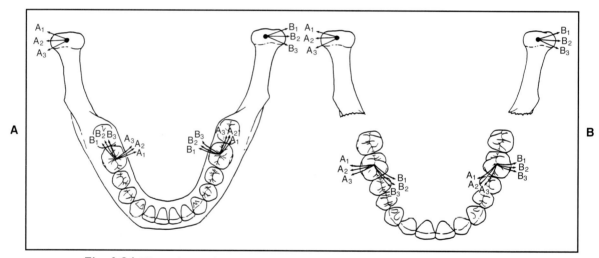

Fig. 6-24 Effect of anterolateral and posterolateral translation movement of the rotating condyle. The more anterolateral the movement of the rotating condyle, the smaller the angle formed by the mediotrusive and laterotrusive pathways (A_3 and B_3). The more posterolateral the movement of the rotating condyle, the wider the angle formed by the mediotrusive and laterotrusive pathways (A_1 and B_1). This is true for both mandibular **(A)** and maxillary **(B)** teeth.

generated (Fig. 6-25). The latter factor negates the influence of the former to the extent that the net effect of increasing the intercondylar distance is to decrease the angle between the laterotrusive and mediotrusive pathways. The decrease, however, is most often minimal and therefore the least influenced of the determinants.

A summary of the vertical and horizontal determinants of occlusal morphology can be found in Tables 6-1 and 6-2.

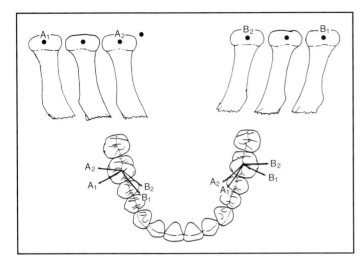

Fig. 6-25 The greater the intercondylar distances, the smaller the angle formed by the laterotrusive and mediotrusive pathways. The greater the intercondylar distances, the smaller the angle formed by the laterotrusive and mediotrusive cusp pathways (A_1 and B_1). The smaller the intercondylar distance, the wider the angle between the laterotrusive and mediotrusive cusp pathways (A_2 and B_2).

TABLE 6-1

Vertical Determinants of Occlusal Morphology (Cusp Height and Fossa Depth)

Factors	Conditions	Effects
Condylar guidance	Steeper the guidance	Taller the posterior cusps
Anterior guidance	Greater the vertical overlap	Taller the posterior cusps
	Greater the horizontal overlap	Shorter the posterior cusps
Plane of occlusion	More parallel the plane to condylar guidance	Shorter the posterior cusps
Curve of Spee	More acute the curve	Shorter the most posterior cusps
Lateral translation movement	Greater the movement	Shorter the posterior cusps
	More superior the movement of rotating condyle	Shorter the posterior cusps
	Greater the immediate side shift	Shorter the posterior cusps

TABLE 6-2

Horizontal Determinants of Occlusal Morphology (Ridge and Groove Direction)

Factors	Conditions	Effects
Distance from rotating condyle	Greater the distance	Wider the angle between laterotrusive and mediotrusive pathways
Distance from midsagittal plane	Greater the distance	Wider the angle between laterotrusive and mediotrusive pathways
Lateral translation movement	Greater the movement	Wider the angle between laterotrusive and mediotrusive pathways
Intercondylar distance	Greater the distance	Smaller the angle between laterotrusive and mediotrusive pathways

RELATIONSHIP BETWEEN ANTERIOR AND POSTERIOR CONTROLLING FACTORS

Attempts have been made to demonstrate a correlation between the vertical and horizontal relationships of the condylar guidance with the lingual concavities of the maxillary anterior teeth (vertical and horizontal relationships of anterior guidance). One philosophy suggests that anterior guidance should be consistent with condylar guidance. Consideration is directed primarily toward the PCFs that regulate steepness of the condylar movement (e.g., angle of the eminence and lateral translation movement). This philosophy suggests that as condylar movement becomes more horizontal (decrease in articular eminence angle with increase in lateral translation), the lingual concavities of the maxillary anterior teeth will increase to reflect a similar movement characteristic.

However, scientific evidence to support a correlation between the ACFs and PCFs is negligible.

Instead, studies seem to indicate that the angle of the articular eminence is not related to any specific occlusal relationship.[1-3] In other words, the ACFs and the PCFs are independent of each other. They are independent, yet they still function together in dictating mandibular movement. This is an important concept because the ACFs can be influenced by dental procedures. Alteration of the ACFs can play an important part in the treatment of occlusal disturbances in the masticatory system.

References

1. Moffett BC: The temporomandibular joint. In Sharry JJ, editor: *Complete denture prosthodontics*, New York, 1962, McGraw-Hill, pp 213-230.
2. Ricketts RM: Variations of the temporomandibular joint as revealed by cephalometric laminagraphy, *Am J Orthod* 36:877-892, 1950.
3. Angle JL: Factors in temporomandibular form, *Am J Anat* 83:223-234, 1948.

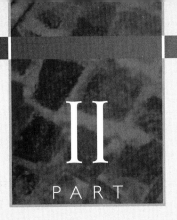

II
PART

Etiology and Identification of Functional Disturbances in the Masticatory System

It is realistic to assume that the more complex a system, the greater the likelihood that breakdown will occur. As discussed in Part I, the masticatory system is extremely complex. It is remarkable to think that in most instances it functions without major complications for the lifetime of the individual. When breakdown does occur, however, it can produce a situation as complicated as the system itself.

Part II consists of four chapters that discuss the etiology and identification of the major functional disturbances of the masticatory system. With a sound understanding of normal function comes the understanding of dysfunction.

Etiology of Functional Disturbances in the Masticatory System

7

CHAPTER

"The clinician who looks only at occlusion is missing as much as the clinician who never looks at occlusion."

—JPO

In the preceding six chapters a detailed description of the optimum anatomy and physiology of occlusion was presented. The discussion ranged from the exact contact and movement of a single tooth to the function of all structures that make up the masticatory system. The optimum functional occlusion was also presented. When less than ideal conditions exist, the clinician must question the prevalence of this condition and the consequences that arise from it. This chapter addresses various functional disturbances in the masticatory system and reviews the specific relationships of the etiologic factors that cause these disturbances.

TERMINOLOGY

Over the years functional disturbances of the masticatory system have been identified by a variety of terms. The variety of terms has contributed to some of the confusion in this area. In 1934 James Costen[1] described a group of symptoms that centered around the ear and temporomandibular joint (TMJ). Because of his work, the term *Costen syndrome* developed. Later the term *temporomandibular joint disturbances* became popular, and then in 1959 Shore[2] introduced the term *temporomandibular joint dysfunction syndrome*. Later came the term *functional temporomandibular joint disturbances*, coined by Ramfjord

and Ash.[3] Some terms described the suggested etiologic factors, such as *occlusomandibular disturbance*[4] and *myoarthropathy of the temporomandibular joint*.[5] Others stressed pain, such as *pain-dysfunction syndrome*,[6] *myofascial pain-dysfunction syndrome*,[7] and *temporomandibular pain-dysfunction syndrome*.[8]

Because the symptoms are not always isolated to the TMJ, some authors believe that the previous terms are too limited and that a broader, more collective term should be used, such as *craniomandibular disorders*.[9] Bell[10] suggested the term *temporomandibular disorders* (TMDs), which has gained popularity. This term does not merely suggest problems that are isolated to the joints but includes all disturbances associated with the function of the masticatory system.

The wide variety of terms used has contributed to the great amount of confusion that exists in this already complicated field of study. Lack of communication and coordination of research efforts often begins with differences in terminology. In an attempt to coordinate efforts, the American Dental Association[11] adopted the term *temporomandibular disorders*. In this text, temporomandibular disorders (TMDs) is the term used to include all functional disturbances of the masticatory system.

HISTORY OF TEMPOROMANDIBULAR DISORDERS

The dental profession was generally first drawn into the area of TMDs with an article written by

Dr. James Costen,[1] an otolaryngologist, in 1934. On the basis of 11 cases, Costen first suggested to the profession that changes in the dental condition were responsible for various ear symptoms. Not long after Costen's article, clinicians began to question the accuracy of his conclusions regarding etiology and treatment.[12-15] Although most, if not all, of Costen's original proposals have been disproved, the dental profession's interest was certainly stimulated by his work. In the late 1930s and through the 1940s, only a few dentists became interested in managing these pain problems. The most common therapies provided at that time were bite-raising appliances, which were first suggested and described by Costen himself.[16,17] In the late 1940s and into the 1950s, the dental profession began to question bite-raising appliances as the therapy of choice for mandibular dysfunction.[15,18] It was at this time that the profession began to look more closely at occlusal interferences as the major etiologic factor in TMD complaints.[19,20]

Scientific investigation of TMDs first began in the 1950s. Early scientific studies suggested that the occlusal condition could influence masticatory muscle function. Electromyographic studies were used to correlate such relationships.[20-22] In the late 1950s the first textbooks were written describing masticatory dysfunctions.[2,8,23] The most common conditions described at that time were masticatory muscle pain disorders. The cause of these disorders was generally thought to be occlusal disharmony. Occlusion and (later) emotional stress were accepted as the major etiologic factors of functional disorders of the masticatory system through the 1960s and into the 1970s. Then in the 1970s an explosion of interest in TMDs took place. Also at this time information reached the profession concerning pain disorders arising from intracapsular sources.[24] This information reoriented the profession's thinking and direction in the area of TMDs. It was not until the 1980s that the profession began to recognize fully and appreciate the complexity of TMDs. This complexity now has the profession striving to find its proper role in the management of TMDs and orofacial pains.[25]

EPIDEMIOLOGIC STUDIES OF TEMPOROMANDIBULAR DISORDERS

For the study of TMDs to have a place in the practice of dentistry, it must first be shown to represent a significant problem in the general population. Second, it must relate to structures that are treated by the dentist. If signs and symptoms of masticatory dysfunction are common in the general population, then TMDs become an important problem that needs to be addressed. Studies that examine these signs and symptoms are discussed.

If TMD symptoms do prove to be common, then one must next ask, "What is the etiology of TMD, and can it be treated by dental therapies?" The question of etiology needs to be discussed at this time because it is basic in understanding the dentist's role in managing TMDs. The question of therapy will be addressed in later chapters. Many dentists believe that the occlusion of the teeth is the primary cause of TMD symptoms. This question has been highly debated in dentistry since the days of Costen. If occlusion does play a significant role in the etiology of TMDs, the dentist can and should play an important role in the management of these disorders. On the other hand, if occlusion plays no role in TMDs, any attempt by the dentist to alter the occlusal condition is misdirected and should be avoided. It becomes obvious that this question is important to the dental profession. One of the goals of this chapter is to explore the scientific studies that give us insight into this most important question.

The prevalence of signs and symptoms associated with TMDs can best be appreciated by examining epidemiologic studies. *Dorland's Illustrated Medical Dictionary* describes epidemiology as "the study of the factors determining and influencing the frequency and distribution of disease, injury, and other health-related events and their causes in a defined human population for the purpose of establishing programs to prevent and control their development and spread."[26] Numerous epidemiologic studies have examined the prevalence of TMDs in given populations. A few of these are summarized[27-43] in Table 7-1. In each study patients were questioned regarding symptoms and then

TABLE 7-1

Signs and Symptoms of Temporomandibular Disorders in Investigated Populations

Author	No. of Individuals	No. of Women/Men	Age (yr)	Population	PREVALENCE (%) At Least One Symptom	At Least One Clinical Sign
Solberg et al., 1979[27]	739	370/369	19-25	American university students	26	76
Osterberg and Carlsson, 1979[28]	384	198/186	70	Retired Swedish	59	37
Swanljung and Rantanen, 1979[29]	583	341/256	18-64	Finnish workers	58	86
Ingervall et al., 1980,[30] 1981[31]	389	0/389	21-54	Swedish reservists	15	60
Nilner and Lassing, 1981[31]	440	218/222	7-14	Swedish children	36	72
Nilner, 1981[32]	309	162/147	15-18	Swedish children	41	77
Egermark-Eriksson et al., 1981[33]	136	74/62	7	Swedish children	39	33
	131	61/70	11		67	46
	135	59/76	15		74	61
Rieder et al., 1983[34]	1040	653/387	13-86	American private practice	33	50
Gazit et al., 1984[35]	369	181/188	10-18	Israeli children	56	44
Pullinger et al., 1988[36]	222	102/120	19-40	Dental hygiene and dental students	39	48
Agerberg and Inkapool, 1990[37]	637	323/314	18-64	Swedish adults	14	88
De Kanter et al., 1993[38]	3468	1815/1653	15-74	Dutch nationals	22	45
Magnusson et al., 1993[39]	293	164/129	17-25	Swedish young adults	43	—
Glass et al., 1993[40]	534	317/217	18-65	Kansas City adults	46	—
Tanne et al., 1993[41]	323	146/86	3-29	Prospective orthodontic patients	16	15
Nourallah and Johansson, 1995[42]	105	0/105	23	Saudi dental students	20	56
Hiltunen et al., 1995[43]	342	243/99	76-86	Finnish older adults	80	—
					TOTAL SYMPTOMS: 41%	TOTAL SIGNS: 56%

examined for common clinical signs associated with TMDs. The results are found under "Prevalence" in the right-hand column of Table 7-1. The number represents the percentage of patients who had at least one clinical symptom or one clinical sign that relates to TMDs. These studies suggest that signs and symptoms of TMDs are common in these populations. In fact, an average of 41% of these populations reported at least one symptom associated with TMDs, and an average of 56% showed at least one clinical sign. Because these studies ranged through many age and sex distributions, it is probably safe to assume that a similar percentage also exists in the general population. According to these studies, it would seem that a conservative estimate of the percentage of people in the general population with some type of TMD is between 40% and 60%. This figure is so high that it might lead one to doubt the validity of the studies. After all, half the patients seen in dental offices do not appear to be suffering from TMDs.

To appreciate these percentages better, the clinician needs to examine the studies more closely. The Solberg et al.[27] study can be helpful in appreciating the prevalence of TMDs. In this study the investigators examined 739 university students (aged 18 to 25) who were reporting to a student health clinic for enrollment in a health insurance program. A questionnaire was completed, and a short clinical examination was performed to identify any signs or symptoms related to TMDs. A *sign* was considered to be any clinical finding associated with a TMD. A *symptom* was any sign of which the patient was aware and therefore reported. The clinical examination revealed that 76% of the students had one or more signs associated with TMDs. The questionnaire, however, revealed that only 26% of the students reported having a symptom that related to TMDs. In other words, 50% of the group had signs that were not reported as symptoms. Signs that are present but unknown to the patient are called *subclinical*. It was also reported that only 10% of the total group had symptoms that were severe enough to cause the patient to seek treatment. Only 5% comprised a group that would be typically described as TMD patients seen in dental offices with severe problems. These kinds of findings are more readily

accepted as factual. In other words, one of every four patients in a general population will report some awareness of TMD symptoms, yet less than 10% of the population believe that their problem is severe enough to seek treatment.[44-49] The greatest factor that seems to determine whether they will seek care is the degree of pain they are experiencing.[50] It must not be forgotten, however, that all these studies report an average of 40% to 60% of the population as having at least one detectable sign that is associated with TMDs. Other studies have also confirmed these findings.[51-59]

Interestingly, although children and young adults reveal an increase in signs of TMDs as they age, this population rarely complains of any significant symptoms.[60] In a similar finding, patients who are 60 years of age or older also rarely complain of TMD symptoms.[61-64] Epidemiologic studies reveal that the most TMD symptoms are reported in the 20 to 40 age population.[38,62,65] The possible rationale for this finding is discussed in later chapters.

These studies reveal that the prevalence of functional disorders in the masticatory system is high, especially in certain populations. Because it is documented that occlusal contact patterns influence function of the masticatory system (see Chapter 2), a logical assumption is that the occlusal contact pattern may also influence functional disturbances. If this relationship is correct, it makes the study of occlusion a significant and important part of dentistry. The relationship between occlusion and TMDs, however, is not a simple one. Table 7-2 summarizes 57 epidemiologic studies of a variety of populations that attempted to look at the relationship between occlusion and the signs and symptoms associated with TMDs.[35,36,41,66-120] In this table, if a significant relationship was found between occlusal factors and TMDs, it is described in the right column. When no relationship was found, "no" appears in the column. The clinician should note that 22 of these studies found no relationship between occlusal factors and TMD symptoms, whereas 35 studies did find a relationship. The fact that these studies do not consistently report a common relationship explains why the subject of occlusion and TMDs has received so much controversy and debate.

TABLE 7-2

Studies That Investigated the Relationship between Occlusion and the Signs and Symptoms of Temporomandibular Disorders

Author	No. of Individuals	No. of Women/Men	Age (yr)	Population	Relationship between Occlusion and TMD	Type of Occlusal Condition Related
Williamson and Simmons, 1979[66]	53	27/26	9-30	Orthodontic patients	No	None
De Boever and Adriaens, 1983[67]	135	102/33	12-68	TMJ pain and dysfunctional patients	No	None
Egermark-Eriksson et al., 1983[68]	402	194/208	7-15	Random of sample children	Yes	Occlusal interferences, anterior open bites, anterior crossbite, Classes II and III
Gazit et al., 1984[35]	369	181/188	10-18	Israeli school children	Yes	Class II, III, crossbite, open bite, crowding
Brandt, 1985[69]	1342	669/673	6-17	Canadian school children	Yes	Overbite, overjet, open bite
Nesbitt et al., 1985[70]	81	43/38	22-43	Growth study patients	Yes	Class II, open bite, deep bite
Thilander, 1985[71]	661	272/389	20-54	Random sample in Sweden	Yes	Class III, crossbite
Budtz-Jorgenson et al., 1985[72]	146	81/65	>60	Older adults	Yes	Lost teeth
Bernal and Tsamtsouris, 1986[73]	149	70/79	3-5	American preschool children	Yes	Anterior crossbite
Nilner, 1986[74]	749	380/369	7-18	Swedish children adolescents	Yes	Centric slides, nonworking contacts
Stringert and Worms, 1986[75]	62	57/5	16-55	Subjects with structural and functional changes of TMJ versus control	No	None
Riolo et al., 1987[76]	1342	668/667	6-17	Random sample of children	Yes	Class II
Kampe et al., 1987[77]	29	—	16-18	Adolescents	Yes	Unilateral RCP
Kampe and Hannerz, 1987[78]	225	—	16-18	Adolescents	Yes	Occlusal interferences
Gunn et al., 1988[79]	151	84/67	6-18	Migrant children	No	None
Seligman et al., 1988[159]	222	102/120	19-41	Dental and dental hygiene students	Yes	Class II, Division 2, lack of RCP-ICP slide, asymmetric slide
Seligman and Pullinger, 1989[80]	418	255/159	18-72	Patients and nonpatient controls	Yes	Class II, Division I, asymmetric slide, RCP-ICP slides >1 mm, anterior open bite
Dworkin et al., 1990[81]	592	419/173	18-75	HMO members	No	None
Linde and Isacsson, 1990[82]	158	127/137	15-76	Patients with disc displacement and myofascial pain	Yes	Asymmetric RCP-ICP slide, unilateral RCP
Kampe et al., 1991[83]	189	—	18-20	Young adults	No	None

Study	N	Gender	Age	Population	Controls	Occlusal findings
Steele et al., 1991[84]	72	51/21	7-69	Patients with migraine headaches	No	None
Takenoshita et al., 1991[85]	79	42/37	15-65	TMD patients	No	None
Pullinger and Seligman, 1991[86]	319	216/103	18-72	Patients and asymptomatic controls	Yes	Increased overjet and anterior open bite with osteoarthrosis
Wanman and Agerberg, 1991[87]	264	Not given	19	Swedish young adults	Yes	Reduced number of occlusal contacts in ICP, long slide length
Cacchiotti et al., 1991[88]	81	46/35	19-40	Patients and nonpatient controls	No	None
Egermark and Thilander, 1992[89]	402	194/208	7-15	Swedish students	Yes	RCP-ICP slide length, unilateral RCP, occlusal interferences
Glaros et al., 1992[90]	81	—	12-36	Matched non-TMD patients	No	None
Huggare and Raustia, 1992[91]	32	28/4	14-44	TMD patients and controls	No	None
Kirveskari et al., 1992[92]	237	115/122	5,10	Finnish children	Yes	Occlusal interferences
Kononen, 1992[93]	104	0/104	18-70	Finnish men with Reiter's disease and matched controls	Yes	Loss of teeth
Kononen et al., 1992[94]	244	117/127	21-80	Matched groups of rheumatoid arthritis, psoriatic arthritis, ankylosing spondylitic patients, and controls	Yes	Longer RCP-ICP slide length, mediotrusive interferences, lost teeth, asymmetric slide
List and Helkimo, 1992[95]	74	58/22	19-71	Patients with myofascial pain	No	None
Shiau and Chang, 1992[96]	2033	872/1161	17-32	Taiwanese university students	Yes	Balancing interference group function, presence of restorations
Al Hadi, 1993[97]	600	189/311	—	Dental students	Yes	Group function, occlusal interferences, overjet >6 mm
Pullinger and Seligman, 1993[98]	418	287/131	18-72	Patients and asymptomatic controls	No	None (attrition)
Pullinger et al., 1993[99]	560	403/157	12-80	TMD patients differentiated into five disease groups and asymptomatic controls	Yes	Unilateral lingual crossbite, >4 missing posterior teeth, RCP-ICP slide >4 mm, first molars retrusive >8 mm, anterior open bite, overjet >5 mm
Scholte et al., 1993[100]	193	152/41	Mean 33	Random patients with TMD	Yes	Lost molar support
Tanne et al., 1993[41]	305	186/119	—	Orthodontic patients	Yes	Anterior open bite, crossbite, deep overbite
Wadhwa et al., 1993[101]	102	69/33	13-25	Teenagers and young adults	No	None (angle classification)

Continued

Contributions to this table from Dr. James McNamara, University of Michigan, Ann Arbor; and Dr. Donald Seligman, Los Angeles.[120]

HMO, Health maintenance organization; *ICP,* intercuspal position; *RCP,* retruded contact position; *TMD,* temporomandibular disorder; *TMJ,* temporomandibular joint.

TABLE 7-2

Studies That Investigated the Relationship between Occlusion and the Signs and Symptoms of Temporomandibular Disorders—cont'd

Author	No. of Individuals	No. of Women/Men	Age (yr)	Population	Relationship between Occlusion and TMD	Type of Occlusal Condition Related
Keeling et al., 1994[102]	3428	1789/1639	6-12	Florida school children	No	None
Magnusson et al., 1994[103]	12	78/46	25	Former Swedish students	Yes	Attrition, balancing contacts
Tsolka et al., 1994[104]	61	61/0	20-40	Female TMD patients and matched controls	Yes	Overjet
Vanderas, 1994[105]	386	—	6-12	Caucasian children	No	None
Bibb et al., 1995[106]	429	249/180	>65	Random older adults	No	None (posterior tooth support)
Castro, 1995[107]	63	34/29	—	TMD patients	Yes	Balancing side interferences
Hochman et al., 1995[108]	96	—	20-31	Israeli young adults	No	None
Lobbezoo-Scholte et al., 1995[109]	522	423/99	Mean 34	TM patients	Yes	Balancing side interferences
Olsson and Lindqvist, 1995[110]	—	—	—	Orthodontic patients	Yes	Angle Class II, Division I, deep bite, anterior open bite
Mauro et al., 1995[111]	125	—	Mean 36	TMD patients	No	None
Tsolka et al., 1995[112]	92	80/12	Age-matched	TMD patients and controls	Yes	Angle Class II, Division I
Westling, 1995[113]	193	96/97	17	Swedes	Yes	RCP-ICP slides >1 mm
Sato et al., 1996[114]	643	345/298	>70	Swedes	No	None
Raustia et al., 1995[115]	49	34/15	Mean 24	TMD patients and nonpatient controls	Yes	Overbite, asymmetric RCP-ICP slides, midline discrepancy
Seligman and Pullinger, 1996[116]	567	567/0	17-78	Two sets of female TMD patients and asymptomatic controls	Yes	Anterior open bite, unreplaced missing posterior teeth, RCP-ICP slide length, large overjet, laterotrusive attrition
Conti et al., 1996[117]	310	52/48	Mean 20	High school and university students	No	None
Ciancaglini et al., 1999[118]	483	300/183	Mean 45	Epidemiologic nonpatient survey	No	None (posterior support)
Seligman and Pullinger, 2000[119]	171	171/0	Mean 35	Female patients with intracapsular TMD and asymptomatic controls	Yes	Anterior open bite, crossbite, anterior attrition, RCP-ICP slide length, overjet

In fact, if occlusal factors were either the main cause of TMDs or if occlusion had nothing to do with TMDs, one would assume that more agreement in the findings would be seen. In addition, one might conclude that if occlusion were the major etiologic factor in TMDs, the profession would have confirmed this many years ago. On the other hand, if occlusion has nothing to do with TMDs, the profession would have also likewise already confirmed this conclusion. Apparently neither of these conclusions is true. Instead, the confusion and controversy concerning the relationship between occlusion and TMDs continues. The general message is that no simple cause-and-effect relationship explains the association between occlusion and TMDs.

When considering the 35 studies that did find a relationship between occlusion and TMDs, the clinician may ask, "What was the significant occlusal relationship that was found to be related to TMD symptoms?" As indicated in Table 7-2, no consistent occlusal conditions were reported in these studies. In fact, a variety of conditions were reported, the incidences of which vary greatly from study to study. These findings make it even more difficult to understand the relationship between occlusion and TMDs.

Most clinicians would also agree that the occlusal conditions found in these studies do not always lead to TMD symptoms. In fact, these findings are commonly found in symptom-free populations. To appreciate the role of occlusion in TMDs, the clinician must better understand the many factors that can influence function of this extremely complex system.

DEVELOPMENT OF FUNCTIONAL DISTURBANCES IN THE MASTICATORY SYSTEM

Even though signs and symptoms of disturbances in the masticatory system are common, understanding etiology can be complex. No single cause accounts for all signs and symptoms. Interestingly, if one refers to a medical textbook for suggested treatments of a disorder and only one therapy is listed, one will find that this treatment is usually effective. On the other hand, if the textbook lists multiple treatments for the same disorder, the therapist can assume that none of the suggested therapies will always be effective. Two explanations for these findings exist: (1) Either the disorder has multiple etiologies and no single treatment can affect all the etiologies, or (2) the disorder is not a single problem but represents an umbrella term under which there are multiple disorders. Regarding TMDs, both explanations are true. Certainly a multitude of conditions can affect masticatory function. Also, according to the structures involved, a variety of disorders can result. To simplify how TMD symptoms develop, the following formula is suggested:

Normal function + Event > Physiologic tolerance
⇒ TMD symptoms

Under normal conditions the masticatory system functions as described in Chapter 2. Occasionally, some type of an event interrupts normal function of the masticatory system. Many events are tolerated by the system with no consequence; therefore no clinical effect is noticed. However, if the event is significant, it can exceed the physiologic tolerance of the individual, creating a response by the system. The response of the system can be seen as a variety of clinical symptoms associated with TMDs. To explain this formula, each factor is discussed in more detail.

NORMAL FUNCTION

As discussed in Chapter 2, the masticatory system is a complex unit designed to carry out the tasks of chewing, swallowing, and speaking. These functions are basic to life. These tasks are carried out by the complex neuromuscular control system. As previously discussed, the brainstem (specifically the central pattern generator) regulates muscle action by way of muscle engrams that are appropriately selected according to sensory input received from the peripheral structures. When sudden, unexpected sensory input is received, protective reflex mechanisms are activated, creating a decrease in muscle activity in the area of the input. This nociceptive reflex is discussed in Chapter 2.

For a more complete review of normal function, refer to Chapter 2.

EVENTS

During normal function of the masticatory system, events can occur that may influence function. These events can be of either local or systemic origin.

Local Events

A local event may represent any change in sensory or proprioceptive input, such as the placement of an improperly occluding crown.[121] A local event may also be secondary to trauma involving local tissues. An example of such trauma is a postinjection response following local anesthesia. Trauma can also arise from opening the mouth too wide (i.e., strain) or unaccustomed use. An example of unaccustomed use is periodic episodes of bruxism. *Bruxism* refers to subconscious, nonfunctional grinding or gnashing of the teeth. This commonly occurs during sleep but may also occur during the day. Bruxism can play a significant role in TMDs and is discussed in detail later in this chapter.

Another factor representing an event that influences function of the masticatory system is constant deep pain input. This phenomenon is discussed in Chapter 2, but its clinical significance now becomes relative. Pain felt in masticatory or associated structures often alters normal muscle function by way of the central excitatory effects previously discussed. The clinician must appreciate this relationship to properly understand the patient's pain experience and how best to manage the pain complaint. The clinician should also realize that any pain, even of unknown cause (idiopathic pain), can produce this effect.

Systemic Events

For some patients the events that alter normal function occur at a systemic level, meaning the entire body and/or central nervous system (CNS) is involved. When this occurs, dental therapies are unlikely to be effective, frustrating the dentist who only treats teeth and occlusion. One of the most common types of systemic alteration is an increased level of emotional stress. The influence of emotional stress in TMDs is important and is discussed in more detail later.

PHYSIOLOGIC TOLERANCE

The clinician should realize that all individuals do not respond in the same manner to the same event. This variation reflects what might be thought of as the individual's physiologic tolerance. Each patient has the ability to tolerate certain events without any adverse effect. Physiologic tolerance is not something that has been well investigated scientifically. A patient's physiologic tolerance can likely be influenced by both local and systemic factors.

Local Factors

How the masticatory system responds to local factors is influenced in part by its orthopedic stability. Chapter 5 discusses the conditions of the masticatory system that provide the most stable orthopedic relationship between the mandible and maxilla. It can be summarized as follows: When the mandible closes with the condyles in their most superoanterior position, resting against the posterior slopes of the articular eminences with the discs properly interposed, there is even and simultaneous contact of all possible teeth directing forces through the long axes of those teeth. From that position, when the mandible moves eccentrically, the anterior teeth contact and disocclude the posterior teeth.

When these conditions exist, the masticatory system is best able to tolerate local and systemic events. On the other hand, when orthopedic stability is poor, relatively insignificant events can often disrupt function of the system. This is likely to be one way in which the occlusal condition of the teeth influence symptoms associated with TMDs. Orthopedic instability may result from conditions that are related to the occlusion, the joints, or both. The lack of occlusal stability may be associated with genetic, developmental, or iatrogenic causes. TMJ instability may also be related to alterations in the normal anatomic form, such as a disc displacement or an arthritic condition. Instability may likewise arise from a lack of harmony between the stable intercuspal position (ICP) of the teeth and the musculoskeletally stable (MS) position of the joints.

Systemic Factors

Multiple systemic factors likely influence a patient's physiologic tolerance. Although clinically apparent, scientific investigation in this area is sparse. Each patient possesses some unique characteristics that make up his or her constitution. These constitutional factors are likely influenced by genetics, gender, and diet. Systemic factors are also influenced by the presence of other conditions such as acute or chronic diseases or even the overall physical condition of the patient. Even the effectiveness of the pain modulation systems discussed in Chapter 2 can influence the individual's response to an event. For example, if the descending inhibitory system does not effectively modulate nociceptive input, the system becomes more vulnerable to encountered events.

TEMPOROMANDIBULAR SYMPTOMS

When an event exceeds an individual's physiologic tolerance, the system begins to reveal certain changes. Each structure of the masticatory system can tolerate a certain amount of functional change. When functional change exceeds a critical level, alteration of the tissues begins. This level is known as the *structural tolerance*. Each component of the masticatory system has a specific structural tolerance. If the structural tolerance of any component is exceeded, breakdown will occur. The initial breakdown is seen in the structure with the lowest structural tolerance. Therefore the breakdown site varies from individual to individual. Structural tolerances are influenced by factors such as anatomic form, previous trauma, and local tissue conditions. To appreciate the variation of breakdown sites, one must merely consider the structures of the masticatory system as links of a chain. A chain is as strong as its weakest link. When it is stretched, the weakest link breaks first, causing separation of the rest of the chain. When an event exceeds the individual's physiologic tolerance, the weakest structure in the masticatory system will show the first signs of breakdown. The potential sites of breakdown are the muscles, the TMJs, the

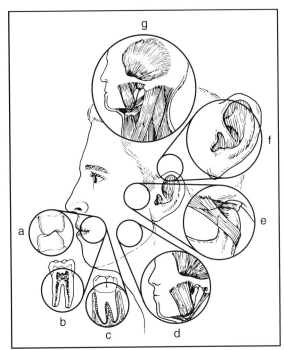

Fig. 7-1 When the masticatory system is overloaded, a variety of structures can reveal breakdown leading to symptoms. Some of the more common symptoms are *(a)* tooth wear, *(b)* pulpitis, *(c)* tooth mobility, *(d)* masticatory muscle pain, *(e)* temporomandibular joint pain, *(f)* ear pain, and *(g)* headache pain.

supportive structures of the teeth, and the teeth themselves (Fig. 7-1).

If the weakest structures (lowest structural tolerance) in the system are the muscles, the individual commonly experiences muscle tenderness and pain during mandibular movements. This is reported as limited jaw movement with related pain. If the TMJs are the weakest link, joint tenderness and pain will often be reported. The joint can also produce sounds such as clicking or grating. Sometimes the muscles and joints tolerate the changes, but because of increased activity of the muscles (bruxism), the weakest link is either the supportive structures of the teeth or the teeth themselves. Teeth then show mobility or wear. Common symptoms of the various TMDs are reviewed in Chapter 8.

ETIOLOGIC CONSIDERATIONS OF TEMPOROMANDIBULAR DISORDERS

As discussed earlier, the etiology of TMDs is complex and multifactorial. Numerous factors can contribute to TMDs. Factors that increase the risk of TMDs are called *predisposing factors*. Factors that cause the onset of TMDs are called *initiating factors*, and factors that interfere with healing or enhance the progression of TMDs are called *perpetuating factors*. In some instances a single factor may serve one or all of these roles.[9,122] The successful management of TMDs depends on identifying and controlling these contributing factors.

For the dentist attempting to manage a TMD patient, it is critical to appreciate the major etiologic factors that may be associated with the condition. This is essential for selecting proper and effective therapy. Therefore it is appropriate to begin a thorough discussion of the major etiologic factors that lead to TMDs. Proper identification of the correct factor is basic for therapeutic success. A review of the scientific literature reveals five major factors associated with TMDs. These factors are the occlusal condition, trauma, emotional stress, deep pain input, and parafunctional activities. The order in which these factors are discussed is not in order of their relative importance. In fact, the importance of any of these factors varies greatly from patient to patient. Each factor is reviewed in detail in this section. Occlusion is discussed first because of its unique place in dentistry. The clinician should be aware that the most important cause may not be the occlusal condition. Automatically making this assumption can lead to major treatment failures.

OCCLUSAL CONDITION

One contributing factor to TMDs that has been strongly debated for years is the occlusal condition. Early in the development of this field, the profession was convinced that occlusion was the most important contributing factor in TMD. More recently, many researchers argued that occlusal factors play little to no role in TMDs. Certainly the research data discussed previously in this chapter do not present overwhelming evidence for either

side of this debate. The relationship of occlusal factors in TMDs, however, is an extremely critical issue in dentistry. If occlusal factors are related to TMDs, the dentist is the only health care professional who can provide proper therapy. On the other hand, if occlusal factors are not related to TMDs, the dentist should refrain from treating TMDs with occlusal changes. One can understand the importance of this issue and therefore how highly emotional the debate has become.

The clinician should remember that the debate regarding the role of occlusion in TMDs does not reflect the importance of occlusion in dentistry. Occlusion is the foundation of dentistry. Sound occlusal relationships and stability are basic to successful masticatory function. Achieving sound occlusal stability should always be the primary goal of the dentist whose therapy will alter the occlusal condition. Yet the role of occlusion as an etiologic factor in TMDs is not the same in all patients. This section attempts to extrapolate and assimilate information from the available research documentation regarding this relationship. The clinician should remember that occlusal factors are not the only etiologic factors that can contribute to TMDs and not lose sight of the other four major etiologic factors discussed later.

When evaluating the relationship between occlusal factors and TMDs, the occlusal condition should be considered both statically and dynamically. To date, most occlusal studies have assessed the static relationship of the teeth. The studies cited previously considered the significance or nonsignificance of occlusal factors relative to the TMDs as isolated static factors. The findings are not impressive regarding any single factor being consistently associated with a TMD. Perhaps the clue to understanding the relationship between occlusal factors and TMDs is to investigate the relationship, if any, of a combination of factors in any given patient. Pullinger, Seligman, and Gornbein[99] attempted to do this by using a blinded multifactorial analysis to determine the weighted influence of each factor acting in combination with the other factors. The interaction of 11 occlusal factors was considered in randomly collected but strictly defined diagnostic groups compared with asymptomatic controls.

Pullinger et al.[99] concluded that no single occlusal factor was able to differentiate patients from healthy subjects. Four occlusal features, however, occurred mainly in TMD patients and were rare in normal subjects: (1) the presence of a skeletal anterior open bite, (2), retruded contact position (RCP)/ICP slides of greater than 2 mm, (3) overjets of greater than 4 mm, and (4) five or more missing and unreplaced posterior teeth. Unfortunately, all of these signs are rare not only in healthy individuals but also in patient populations as well, indicating limited diagnostic usefulness of these features.

Pullinger et al.[99,123] concluded that many occlusal parameters traditionally believed to be influential contribute only minor amounts to the change in risk in the multiple factor analysis used in their study. They reported that although the relative odds for disease were elevated with several occlusal variables, clear definition of disease groups was evident only in selective extreme ranges and involved only a few subjects. Thus they concluded that occlusion cannot be considered the most important factor in the definition of TMD.

The multifactorial analysis of Pullinger et al.[99,123] suggests that, except for a few defined occlusal conditions, there is a relatively minor relationship between occlusal factors and TMDs. It should be noted, however, that these studies report on the static relationship of the teeth, as well as the contact pattern of the teeth during various eccentric movements. This represents the traditional approach to evaluating occlusion. Perhaps these static relationships can provide only limited insight into the role of occlusion and TMD.

DYNAMIC FUNCTIONAL RELATIONSHIPS BETWEEN OCCLUSION AND TEMPOROMANDIBULAR DISORDERS

When considering the dynamic functional relationship between the mandible and the cranium, it appears that the occlusal condition can affect some TMDs in at least two ways. The first relates to how the occlusal condition affects orthopedic stability of the mandible as it loads against the cranium. The second is how acute changes in the occlusal condition can influence mandibular function, thus leading to TMD symptoms. Each condition is discussed separately.

Effects of Occlusal Factors on Orthopedic Stability

As described in Chapter 5, orthopedic stability exists when the stable ICP of the teeth is in harmony with the MS position of the condyles in the fossae. When this condition exists, functional forces can be applied to the teeth and joints without tissue injury. However, when this condition does not exist, opportunities for overloading and injury can be present. When orthopedic instability exists and the teeth are not in occlusion, the condyles are maintained in their MS positions by the elevator muscles (Fig. 7-2, *A*). However, when orthopedic instability exists and the teeth are brought into contact, only one tooth may contact (Fig. 7-2, *B*). This represents an unstable occlusal position, even though each condyle remains in a stable joint position. The individual must either maintain the stable joint position and only occlude on one tooth or bring the teeth into a more stable occlusal position, which may compromise joint stability. Because occlusal stability is basic to function (chewing, swallowing, and speaking), the priority is to achieve occlusal stability and the mandible is shifted to a position that maximizes occlusal contacts (the ICP). When this occurs, the shift can force one or both condyles from its MS position, resulting in orthopedic instability (Fig. 7-2, *C*). What this means is that when the teeth are in a stable position for loading, the condyles are not (or vice versa).

When orthopedic instability exists, however, merely bringing the teeth into occlusion may not create a problem because loading forces are minimal. Problems arise when such an orthopedically unstable condition is loaded by the elevator muscles or by extrinsic forces (trauma). Because the ICP represents the most stable position for the teeth, loading is accepted by the teeth without consequence. If the condyles are also in a stable relationship in the fossae, loading occurs with no adverse effect to the joint structures. If, however, loading occurs when a joint is not in a stable relationship with the disc and fossa, unusual movement can occur in an attempt to gain stability. This movement,

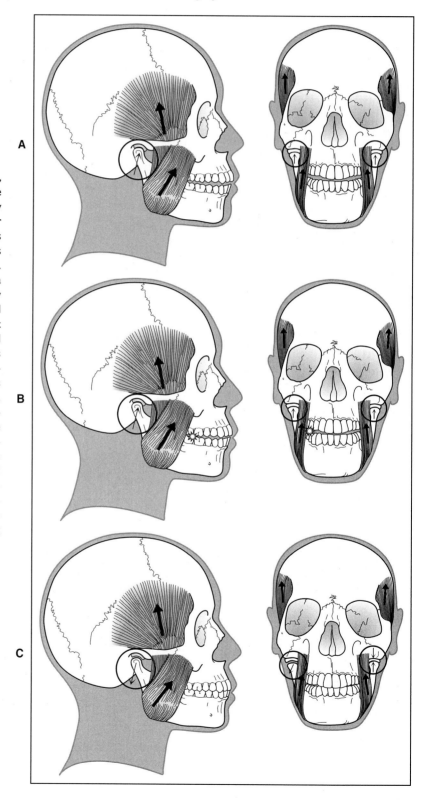

Fig. 7-2 A, With the teeth apart, the elevator muscles maintain the condyles in their musculoskeletally stable positions (i.e., superoanterior resting against the posterior slopes of the articular eminences). In this situation there is joint stability. **B,** When the mouth is closed, a single tooth contact does not allow the entire dental arch to gain full intercuspation. At this moment there is occlusal instability but still joint stability. Because the condyles and teeth do not fit in a stable relationship at the same time, this is orthopedic instability (see Chapter 5). **C,** To gain the occlusal stability necessary for functional activities, the mandible is shifted and the intercuspal position is achieved. At this moment the patient achieves occlusal stability, but the condyles may no longer be orthopedically stable. This orthopedic instability may not pose a problem unless unusual loading occurs. If loading begins, the condyles will seek out stability and the unusual movement can lead to strains on the condyle/disc complex, resulting in an intracapsular disorder.

although small, is often a translatory shift between disc and condyle. Movement such as this can lead to strain to the discal ligaments and eventually elongation of the discal ligaments and thinning of the disc. These changes can lead to a group of intracapsular disorders that are discussed in detail in the next chapter.

Two factors determine whether an intracapsular disorder will develop: (1) the degree of orthopedic instability and (2) the amount of loading. Orthopedic instabilities with discrepancies of 1 or 2 mm are not likely significant enough to create a problem. However, as the discrepancy between the MS position of the condyles and the maximum intercuspation of the teeth becomes greater, the risk of intracapsular disorders increases.[99,123]

The second factor that determines whether the patient will develop a TMD is the amount of loading. Therefore bruxing patients with orthopedic instability represent a higher risk for developing problems than nonbruxers with the same orthopedic instability. Also, forceful unilateral chewing can provide the mechanics that lead to sudden intracapsular disorders (see Chapter 8). These variables may help explain why patients with similar occlusal conditions may not develop similar disorders. In fact, when the static occlusal relationships of two patients are compared, the patient with the more significant malocclusion may not always be the patient who develops the disorder. Considering the dynamic functional aspect of the occlusion as it relates to the joint position is likely to provide more important information regarding the relative risk of developing a TMD.

Perhaps a different view of occlusion and TMDs needs to be considered to help describe this important relationship. The term *dental malocclusion* refers to the specific relationship of the teeth to each other, but it does not necessarily reflect any risk factors for the development of functional disturbances in the masticatory system (i.e., TMDs). Dentists have observed dental malocclusions for years (e.g., an open bite, an Angle Class II). However, this dental malocclusion does not relate well to TMDs, as depicted by the literature. These dental malocclusions are only important when viewed in relationship to the joint position. Therefore merely looking in the mouth or viewing hand-held study

casts does not provide insight as to the relative risk factor for TMDs. Only by observing the occlusal relationship with respect to the stable joint position can one appreciate the degree of *orthopedic instability* that is present. Orthopedic instability is the critical factor that needs to be considered when accessing relative risk factors for TMDs. The clinician should remember that a small discrepancy of 1 to 2 or 3 mm is epidemiologically normal and apparently not a risk factor. Small discrepancies appear to be well within the individual's ability to adapt (physiologic tolerance). Shifts of greater than 3 mm present more significant risk factors for TMDs.*

Effects of Acute Changes in the Occlusal Condition and Temporomandibular Disorder

A second manner by which the occlusal condition can affect TMD symptoms is through a sudden or acute change. As discussed in Chapter 2, the occlusal contact patterns of the teeth have significant influence on the activity of masticatory muscles.[125-128] In addition, introducing a slightly high contact between the teeth can induce masticatory muscle pain in some individuals.[129-131] The questions that must be asked are, "How do occlusal contacts influence muscle activity?" and "What type of muscle activity can lead to TMD symptoms?" In order to answer these important questions, one must distinguish between different types of masticatory muscle activities.

Activities of the Masticatory System. Activities of the masticatory muscles can be divided into two basic types: (1) *functional* (described in Chapter 2), which include chewing, speaking, and swallowing; and (2) *parafunctional* (i.e., nonfunctional), which include clenching or grinding of the teeth (i.e., bruxism) and various oral habits. The term *muscle hyperactivity* has also been used to describe any increased muscular activity over and above that necessary for function. Muscle hyperactivity thus includes not only the parafunctional activities of clenching, bruxing, and other oral habits but also any general increase in

---

*References 74, 80, 87, 99, 120, 122-124.

the level of muscle tonus. Some muscle hyperactivity may not even involve tooth contact or jaw movement but merely represent an increase in the static tonic contraction of the muscle.

Functional and parafunctional activities are quite different clinical entities. The former are controlled muscle activities that allow the masticatory system to perform necessary functions with minimum damage to any structure. Protective reflexes are constantly present, guarding against potential damaging tooth contacts. Interfering tooth contacts during function have inhibitory effects on functional muscle activity (see Chapter 2). Therefore functional activities are directly influenced by the occlusal condition.

Parafunctional activities appear to be controlled by an entirely different mechanism. Instead of being inhibited by tooth contacts, earlier concepts suggested that parafunctional activities were actually provoked by certain tooth contacts.[132-134] Although recently these concepts have for the most part been disproved, some occlusal relationships remain in question. Interestingly, the dental profession theorized etiologies and treated parafunctional activity for many years before it was actually scientifically observed and investigated in the natural environment.[135-139] A more complete description of parafunctional activity is presented later.

Occlusal Contacts and Muscle Hyperactivity. Muscle hyperactivity is an inclusive term referring to any increased level of muscle activity that is not associated with a functional activity. This includes not only bruxism and clenching but also any increase in muscle tonicity related to habits, posture, or increased emotional stress (discussed in the next section). As discussed in Chapter 2, the occlusal contact patterns of the teeth will influence the precise functional activity of the masticatory muscles. However, does this mean that occlusal contacts are related to masticatory muscle pain? Some studies* reveal a positive relationship between occlusal factors and masticatory symptoms, whereas others[67,105,147-155] show no relationship. Although it has been demonstrated that specific

occlusal contact patterns can influence specific muscle groups when subjects voluntarily clench and move in eccentric positions,[125,127,128,156-158] it has likewise been demonstrated that the occlusal contact pattern of the teeth does *not* influence nocturnal bruxism.[130,159-162] Altering the occlusal condition, however, does affect muscle function,[131,145,163] and the introduction of an experimental interference can even lead to painful symptoms.[164-166] Yet introducing an experimental interference does not increase bruxism as the profession believed to be true for years.[130] In a similar sense, eliminating occlusal interferences does not seem to significantly alter TMD symptoms,[160,167-169] yet in a few long-term studies the elimination of occlusal interferences in a relatively symptom-free population seemed to lower the incidence of developing future TMD symptoms.[170-172]

The idea that a high occlusal contact could increase muscle activity such as bruxism must be questioned in view of the orthopedic principles discussed in Chapters 1 and 2. When a ligament is elongated, the nociceptive reflex is activated, causing a shutdown of the muscles that pull across the involved joint. In the case of the mouth, the ligament is the periodontal ligament (PDL). When a tooth is contacted heavily, the PDL is overloaded, causing the nociceptive reflex to shut down the muscles that pull across the joint (i.e., the elevator muscles [temporalis, masseter, medial pterygoid]).[173] Therefore it would seem a direct violation of orthopedic principles to assume that heavy contact of a tooth could cause bruxism and/or clenching,[174] yet this same occlusal contact can create painful muscle symptoms.

After reviewing the literature, it becomes obvious that the precise effect of the occlusal condition on muscle hyperactivity has not been clearly established. It appears to be related to some types of muscle hyperactivity and not others. Yet this confusing issue is the essence of how dental therapy either fits or does not fit into the management of masticatory pain disorders. Perhaps a close review of a few scientific studies will help illustrate the important relationship among occlusion, muscle hyperactivity, and TMDs.

Williamson and Lundquist,[175] in studying the effect of various occlusal contact patterns on the

---

*References 27, 68, 74, 92, 112, 140-146.

temporal and masseter muscles, reported that when subjects with bilateral occlusal contacts during a laterotrusive excursion were asked to move in that direction, all four muscles remained active. If, however, the mediotrusive contacts were eliminated, only the working side muscles remained active. This means that when the mediotrusive contact is eliminated, the masseter and temporal muscles on the mediotrusive side are no longer active during the mediotrusive movement. The study further demonstrates that if a group function guidance exists, both the masseter and the temporal muscles on the working side are active during a laterotrusive movement. If, however, only the canines make contact during a laterotrusive movement (canine guidance), then only the temporal muscle on the ipsilateral side is active during the laterotrusive movement. This study points out the merit of canine guidance over group function and mediotrusive tooth contact. Along with other studies,[125,127,156-158,176] it also demonstrates that certain occlusal conditions can affect muscle groups that are activated during a particular mandibular movement. In other words, certain posterior occlusal contacts can increase activity of the elevator muscles. Thus the study substantiates the concept that the occlusal condition can increase muscle activity.

Before too much emphasis is placed on such studies, other evidence must be considered. Rugh et al.[130] decided to challenge the concept that a premature occlusal contact could cause bruxism. They deliberately placed a high crown in 10 subjects and observed its effects on nocturnal bruxism. Although much of the dental profession was certain that this would lead to increased levels of bruxism, it did not. In fact, most of the subjects had a significant *reduction* in bruxism during the first two to four nights, followed by a return to normal bruxing levels. The conclusion from this study and from others[160,161] would suggest that premature occlusal contacts do not increase bruxing activity. In other words, a high posterior occlusal contact does not necessarily increase muscle activity.

At first, these studies might appear to lead to opposite conclusions. However, both are sound and their results have been duplicated, demonstrating their reliability and accuracy. Therefore one should examine them more closely to appreciate how they contribute to the understanding of TMDs. Careful evaluation will reveal that these two studies actually investigate two different muscle activities. The first study assesses the effects of occlusal contacts on conscious and controlled, voluntary, mandibular movements. The other study assesses the effects on subconscious and uncontrolled, involuntary, muscle activity (nocturnal bruxism). These activities are quite different. Whereas the first is generated for functional use at a peripheral level (outside the CNS), the second is initiated and regulated at the CNS level. Muscle activity generated at the peripheral level has the benefit of the nociceptive reflex. In other words, influence from the peripheral structures (i.e., the teeth) has an inhibitory effect on it. In contrast, nocturnal bruxing seems to be generated at the CNS level and stimulation of the CNS has an excitatory effect on this activity (i.e., sleep stage, emotional stress [discussed later]). Thus the former study suggests that tooth contacts greatly influence the muscle response during functional activities of the masticatory system, but the latter study implies that tooth contacts have little effect on nocturnal bruxism.

Perhaps this type of muscle response explains why in the study by Rugh et al.[130] a significant reduction of nocturnal bruxism occurred during the first two to four nights of wearing the crown. As the subjects went to sleep and began bruxing events, their teeth came together and contacted the poorly fitting crown. This resulted in significant peripheral input to the CNS that was inhibitory and initially seemed to shut down the CNS-induced bruxing activity. After a few days of accommodation, the high crown was no longer perceived as damaging or noxious to the system and the inhibitory effect was reduced. Then the bruxing began again. This same phenomenon (altered peripheral sensory input causing decreased CNS activity) is likely to occur in other instances. For example, if the bruxing activity of a patient undergoing orthodontic treatment is monitored at night, it will almost always be found that immediately after an arch wire is activated, bruxism decreases or even stops.[177-179] This occurs because the teeth become so sensitive that any tooth contact initiates a painful sensory peripheral input, which in turn decreases bruxing events.

As the patient accommodates the tooth movement and tooth sensitivity decreases, the bruxing events resume. Therefore any immediate changing in peripheral sensory input has an effect of inhibiting CNS-induced activity. This inhibitory effect is likely the mechanism by which occlusal appliance therapy decreases bruxism (as is discussed more completely in later chapters).

Closer evaluation of the study by Rugh et al.[130] also reveals that a significant percentage of the subjects wearing the poorly fitting crown reported an increase in muscle pain. This was not associated with increased bruxism, as many would have predicted. Rather, it was more likely produced by increased tonus of the elevator muscles in their attempt to protect the mandible from closing on the poorly fitting crown. In other words, a sudden occlusal change that disrupts the ICP can lead to a protective response of the elevator muscles known as *protective co-contraction*. If this response is maintained, it can result in pain. This has been demonstrated in other studies.[164,165] Studies[87,165,166] also support the importance of a sound ICP for mandibular stability. Importantly, the clinician should remember that the increased tonus and the high crown do not cause an increase in bruxing activity.

How Do Occlusal Interferences Affect Muscle Symptoms? The question regarding occlusal interferences and muscle symptoms is basic to dentistry. If occlusal interferences create muscle symptoms, then the dentist needs to be the main provider of care for many TMDs. On the other hand, if occlusal contacts are not related to symptoms, the dentist needs to refrain from providing dental therapies. The studies that have just been reviewed suggest that tooth contacts affect different muscle functions in different ways. Two different types of muscle activities might be affected by an occlusal interference: functional or parafunctional. The clinician should remember that functional activity is greatly influenced by peripheral input (inhibitory), whereas parafunctional activity is predominantly influenced by CNS input (excitatory). Another factor that influences the muscle response is the acuteness or chronicity of the interference. In other words, an acute change in the occlusal condition will precipitate protective co-contraction. This protective response may produce muscle symptoms, which are discussed in the next chapter. At the same time, the acute change in the occlusal condition has an inhibitory effect on parafunctional activity.

As an occlusal interference becomes chronic, muscle response is altered. A chronic occlusal interference may affect functional activity in one of two ways:

1. The most common way is to alter muscle engrams so as to avoid the potentially damaging contact and get on with the task of function. This alteration is likely to be controlled by the central pattern generator discussed in Chapter 2 and represents an adaptive response. This is the most common way the body accommodates the altered sensory input.

2. Another form of adaptation relates to tooth movement to accommodate the heavy loading. Dentists should be thankful that most patients can adapt to change and do not show prolonged signs of dysfunction. However, if altered muscle engrams cannot adapt, continued muscle co-contraction can produce a muscle pain disorder that is discussed in the next chapter. A chronic occlusal interference seems to have little effect, however, on parafunctional activity. Although the acute interference seems to inhibit bruxing events, once the individual has accommodated the change, bruxing returns.

The type of the occlusal interference is also an important feature. The traditional types of interferences that were thought to create TMD symptoms were the mediotrusive (nonworking), posterior laterotrusive (working), and posterior protrusive contacts. Studies reveal, however, that these contacts are present in TMD patients, as well as in controls, and are not strongly related to TMD symptoms.[124] A significant centric relation slide may be related if it adversely affects orthopedic stability. As previously discussed, however, the slide must be significant (2 mm or greater). The contacts that seem to have the major impact on muscle function are those that significantly alter the ICP.[87,180] Experiments have demonstrated that introducing a high contact that interferes with closure into the ICP often produces muscle symptoms.[163-166]

The significance of these responses is paramount to treatment. For example, if a patient presents with early morning muscle tightness and pain, bruxism should be suspected. The treatment of choice is likely to be an occlusal appliance that will alter CNS-induced activity (described in Chapter 12). Alteration of the occlusal condition is generally not indicated because it is not an etiologic factor. On the other hand, if a patient reports that the pain problem began immediately following an alteration in the occlusion (i.e., placement of a crown) and is present much of the time, the occlusal condition should be suspected as a potential etiologic factor. Proper assessment should be made to determine the most appropriate therapy. In this sense, the clinician should appreciate that the patient's history may be more important than the examination. The examination is likely to reveal occlusal interferences in both patients, yet in only one patient is the occlusal condition related to the symptoms. The importance of history and examination are discussed in Chapter 9.

By way of summary, a good sound occlusal condition is paramount for healthy muscle function during chewing, swallowing, speaking, and mandibular posture. Disturbances in the occlusal condition can lead to increased muscle tonus (co-contraction) and symptoms.[181] Nocturnal bruxism, however, appears to be relatively unrelated to tooth contacts and is more closely related to others factors that will soon be discussed (CNS activity). It is vital for the clinician to understand these differences when establishing a diagnosis and developing an appropriate treatment plan for the patient.

Summary: How Occlusion Relates to Temporomandibular Disorders

In summary, the occlusal condition can affect TMDs by way of two mechanisms. One mechanism relates to the introduction of acute changes in the occlusal condition. Although acute changes can create a protective muscle co-contraction response leading to a muscle pain condition (see Chapter 8), most often new muscle engrams are developed and the patient adapts with little consequence. The second manner in which the occlusal condition can affect TMDs is in the presence of orthopedic instability. The orthopedic instability must be considerable, and it must be combined with significant loading forces. A simple way to remember these relationships is as follows: *Problems with bringing the teeth into occlusion are answered by the muscles. However, once the teeth are in occlusion, problems with loading the masticatory structures are answered in the joints.* The importance of these relationships is stressed throughout the remainder of this text. These relationships are, in fact, how dentistry relates to TMD. Therefore if one of these two conditions exists, dental therapy is likely indicated. Conversely, if neither of these conditions exists, dental therapy is contraindicated.

TRAUMA

Certainly, trauma to the facial structures can lead to functional disturbances in the masticatory system. Ample evidence supports this concept.[182-196] Trauma seems to have a greater impact on intracapsular disorder than muscular disorders. Trauma can be divided into two general types: *macrotrauma* and *microtrauma*. Macrotrauma is considered any sudden force that can result in structural alterations, such as a direct blow to the face. *Microtrauma* refers to any small force that is repeatedly applied to the structures over a long period of time. Activities such as bruxism or clenching can produce microtrauma to the tissues that are being loaded (i.e., teeth, joints, or muscles).[197] The specific types and effects of trauma are discussed in Chapter 8.

EMOTIONAL STRESS

A common systemic event that can influence masticatory function is an increase in the level of emotional stress experienced by the patient. As described in Chapter 2, the emotional centers of the brain influence muscle function. The hypothalamus, the reticular system, and particularly the limbic system are primarily responsible for the emotional state of the individual. These centers influence muscle activity in many ways, one of which is through the gamma efferent pathways. Stress can affect the body by activating the hypothalamus, which in turn prepares the body to respond (the autonomic nervous system). The hypothalamus, through complex neural pathways, increases the activity of the gamma efferents, which cause the intrafusal fibers of the muscle spindles to contract. This sensitizes the spindle so that any slight stretching of the muscle will cause a reflex contraction. The overall effect is an increase in tonicity of the muscle.[198]

The therapist must understand and appreciate emotional stress because it commonly plays an important role in TMD. The patient's emotional state is largely dependent on the psychologic stress being experienced. Stress is described by Selye[199] as "the nonspecific response of the body to any demand made upon it." Psychologic stress is an intricate part of life and not an unusual emotional disturbance isolated to institutionalized patients. Stress can be likened to a force that each one experiences. Contrary to popular belief, stress is not always bad. It is often a motivational force driving people to accomplish a task and achieve success. Circumstances or experiences that create stress are known as *stressors*. These can be unpleasant (e.g., losing one's job) or pleasant (e.g., leaving for a vacation). As far as the body is concerned, whether the stressor is pleasant or unpleasant is not significant.[199] The important fact to remember is that the body reacts to the stressor by creating certain demands for readjustment or adaptation (the fight-or-flight response). These demands are related in degree to the intensity of the stressor.

A simple way of describing stress is to consider it as a type of energy. When a stressful situation is encountered, energy is generated within the body and must be released in some way. Two types of releasing mechanisms exist: (1) *external* and (2) *internal*. The external stress-releasing mechanism is represented by activities such as shouting, cursing, hitting, or throwing objects. External stress-releasing mechanisms are quite natural, as revealed by a young child throwing a temper tantrum. However, because society has classified some of these behaviors as undesirable, other stress-releasing mechanisms (e.g., physical exercise) must be learned. It would appear that this type of release is a healthy way in which to deal with stress (discussed in later chapters).

The internal stress-releasing mechanism is used when a person releases the stress internally and develops a psychophysiologic disorder such as irritable bowel syndrome, hypertension, certain cardiac arrhythmia disorder, asthma, or an increase in the tonicity of the head and neck musculature. As accurate documentation regarding the prevalence of increased muscle tension is accumulated, it may be learned that this type of stress-releasing mechanism is by far the most common. The clinician should remember that the perception of the stressor, in both type and intensity, varies greatly from person to person. What may be stressful for one person quite possibly represents no stress for another. Therefore it is difficult to judge the intensity of a given stressor on a given patient.

Increased levels of emotional stress experienced by the patient increase not only the tonicity of head and neck muscles[198] but also the levels of nonfunctional muscle activity such as bruxism or tooth clenching.

Another systemic factor that can influence an individual's physiologic tolerance to certain events is his or her sympathetic activity or tone. The autonomic nervous system constantly monitors and regulates numerous subconscious systems that maintain homeostasis. One of the functions of the autonomic system is to regulate blood flow within the body. The sympathetic nervous system is closely related to the fight-or-flight reflex activated by stressors. Therefore in the presence of stress the capillary blood flow in the outer tissues is constricted, permitting increased blood flow to the more important musculoskeletal structures and internal organs. The result is a cooling of the skin such as the hands. Prolonged activity of the sympathetic nervous system can affect certain tissues such as the muscles. It has been suggested that sympathetic activity can increase muscle tone,[200,201] thereby producing a painful muscle condition. Increased sympathetic activity or tone therefore represents an etiologic factor that can influence TMD symptoms.

Emotional stress can also influence TMD symptoms by reducing the patient's physiologic tolerance. This is likely to occur because of increased sympathetic tone. This effect often represents the individual's learned response to various stressors.

This learned sympathetic response to stress plays an important role in chronic pain, as discussed in later chapters.

DEEP PAIN INPUT

Although often overlooked, a common concept is that sources of deep pain input can cause altered muscle function. This idea has been discussed in detail in Chapter 2. Deep pain input can centrally excite the brainstem, producing protective co-contraction.[202] This represents a normal healthy manner in which the body responds to injury or threat of injury. Therefore it is reasonable to find a patient who is suffering with pain, such as toothache (i.e., necrotic pulp), to have limited mouth opening. This represents the body's response to protect the injured part by limiting its use. This clinical finding is common in many toothache patients. Once the tooth pain is resolved, normal mouth opening returns. The limited mouth opening is merely a secondary response to the experience of the deep pain. If the clinician does not recognize this phenomenon, however, he or she may conclude that the limited mouth opening is a primary TMD problem and treatment would be misdirected. Any source of constant deep pain input can represent an etiologic factor that may lead to limited mouth opening and therefore clinically present as TMD. Tooth pain, sinus pain, and ear pain can create this response. Even pain sources remote to the face, such as cervical pain input, can lead to this condition (see Chapter 2). Too often, dentists do not appreciate this phenomenon and begin treating a patient for TMD complaints. Only after treatment failure is the cervical pain condition identified as being responsible for creating the facial pain and limited mouth opening. Understanding how this occurs is basic to treatment and emphasizes the importance of making the correct diagnosis (see Chapters 9 and 10).

PARAFUNCTIONAL ACTIVITIES

As previously discussed, *parafunctional activity* refers to any activity that is not considered functional (chewing, speaking, and swallowing). This includes bruxing, clenching, and certain oral habits.

Some of these activities may be responsible for creating TMD symptoms.[119,203] For purposes of discussion, parafunctional activity can be subdivided into two general types: (1) that which occurs through the day (diurnal) and (2) that which occurs at night (nocturnal).

Diurnal Activity

Parafunctional activity during the day consists of clenching and grinding, as well as many oral habits that are often performed without the individual even being aware of them (e.g., cheek and tongue biting; finger and thumb sucking; unusual postural habits; occupation-related activities such as biting on pencils, pins, or nails or holding objects under the chin [a telephone or violin]). During daily activities, individuals commonly place their teeth together and apply force.[204] This type of diurnal activity may be seen in someone who is concentrating on a task or performing a strenuous physical chore. The masseter muscle contracts periodically in a manner that is totally irrelevant to the task at hand. Such irrelevant activity, already described in Chapter 2, is commonly associated with many daytime tasks (e.g., driving a car, reading, writing, typing, lifting heavy objects). Some diurnal activities are closely related to the task being accomplished, such as a skin diver biting on the mouth piece or a musician playing certain musical instruments.[205,206]

The clinician must recognize that most parafunctional activities occur at a subconscious level. In other words, individuals are often not even aware of their clenching or cheek-biting habits. Therefore merely questioning the patient is not a reliable way to assess the presence or absence of these activities.[207] In many instances, once the clinician makes the patient aware of the possibility of these diurnal activities, he or she will recognize them and can then decrease them. This is the best treatment strategy that can be provided and is discussed more in later treatment chapters.

Nocturnal Activity

Data from various sources have suggested that parafunctional activity during sleep is quite common and seems to take the form of single episodes (referred to as *clenching*) and rhythmic contractions (known as *bruxing*). Whether these activities result from different etiologic factors or are the same phenomenon in two different presentations is not known. In many patients both activities occur and are sometimes difficult to separate. For that reason clenching and bruxism are often referred to as *bruxing events*.

Sleep. To best understand nocturnal bruxism, the clinician should first have an appreciation of the sleep process. Sleep is investigated by monitoring the brain wave activity (electroencephalogram) of an individual during sleep. This monitoring is called a *polysomnogram*. A polysomnogram reveals two basic types of brain wave activities that appear to cycle during a night of sleep: (1) *alpha* and (2) *delta*. Alpha waves are relatively fast (about 10 waves per second) and are the predominant waves observed during the early stages of sleep or light sleep. Delta waves are slower waves (0.5 to 4 waves per second) and are observed during the deeper stages of sleep. The sleep cyclic is divided into four stages that are free of rapid eye movement (non-REM) followed by a period of REM. Stages 1 and 2 represent the early phases of light sleep and are made up of groups of fast alpha waves along with a few beta waves and "sleep spindles." Stages 3 and 4 represent the deeper stages of sleep with the predominance of the slower beta waves.

During a normal cycle of sleep, a subject will pass from the light stages of 1 and 2 into the deeper stages of 3 and 4. The subject will then pass through a stage of sleep that is quite different from the others. This stage appears as a desynchronized activity in which other physiologic events occur, such as muscle twitching of the extremities and facial muscles, alterations in heart and breathing rates, and rapid movement of the eyes beneath the eyelids.[208] Because of this last characteristic, this phase has been called *REM sleep*. Dreaming occurs most commonly during REM sleep. After the REM period the person typically moves back into a lighter stage, and the cycle repeats itself throughout the night. Each complete cycle of sleep takes from 60 to 90 minutes, resulting in an average of 4 to 6 cycles of sleep per night. A REM phase usually occurs following stage 4 sleep and lasts from 5 to 15 minutes. Interestingly, 80% of people who are awakened during REM sleep can recall the

dream they were experiencing.[209] Only 5% of those awakened during non-REM phases can recall what they were dreaming (some can recall partially).

Approximately 80% of the sleep period of an adult is made up of non-REM sleep, with only 20% being REM sleep.[210] Because REM and non-REM sleep appear to be so different, it is thought that their functions are also quite different. Non-REM sleep is thought to be important in restoring function of the body systems. During this phase of sleep there is an increase in synthesis of vital macromolecules (e.g., proteins, RNA). REM sleep, on the other hand, seems to be important in restoring function of the cortex and brainstem activities. Experts believe that during this phase of sleep, emotions are dealt with and smoothed out. It is a time at which recent experiences are brought into perspective with old pathways.

The importance of these two types of sleep is evident from studies that attempt to deprive individuals of one or the other. When an individual is experimentally deprived of REM sleep, certain emotional states become predominant.[211] Individuals show greater anxiety and irritability. They also have difficulty concentrating. It would appear that REM sleep is important for *psychic rest*. A different finding is revealed when an individual is deprived of non-REM sleep.[212] When a normal subject is experimentally deprived of non-REM sleep for several nights, the subject will often begin to complain of musculoskeletal tenderness, aching, and stiffness. This may result from the individual's inability to restore metabolic requirements. In other words, non-REM sleep is important for *physical rest*. The clinician who treats TMDs must have an appreciation of the relationship between sleep and muscle pain. This relationship is discussed further in later chapters.

Stages of sleep and bruxing events. Controversy surrounds the stages of sleep during which bruxing occurs. Some studies[213,214] suggest that it takes place mainly during the REM stage, whereas others suggest that bruxism never occurs during REM sleep.[215-217] Still other studies[218-222] report that bruxing events occur during both REM and non-REM sleep, but most events seem to be associated with the lighter stage 1 and 2 non-REM sleep. Bruxing events appear to be associated with a change from deeper to lighter sleep, as can be demonstrated by directing a flashing light toward a sleeping person's face. Such stimulation has been shown to induce tooth grinding.[216] The same reaction was observed following sonic and tactical stimulation. Thus this and other studies have indicated that bruxing may be closely associated with the arousal phases of sleep.[219,220]

Duration of bruxing events. Sleep studies also reveal that the number and duration of bruxing events during sleep vary greatly, not only among persons but also within the same person. Kydd and Daly[223] reported that a group of 10 bruxists rhythmically clenched their teeth for a total mean duration of 11.4 minutes per night. These clenches commonly occurred in single episodes lasting 20 to 40 seconds. Reding et al.[218] reported the average bruxing event as lasting only 9 seconds (range 2.7 to 66.5 seconds), with a total average bruxing time of 40 seconds per hour. Clarke and Townsend[224] reported that bruxing events occurred an average of only five times during an entire sleep period, with an average duration of about 8 seconds per event. Trenouth[225] reported that a TMJ-bruxism group spent 38.7 minutes with their teeth together during an 8-hour period. In the same study a control group only spent 5.4 minutes with their teeth together during an 8-hour period. In three separate studies of normal subjects, Okeson et al.[219-221] found bruxing events averaged from 5 to 6 seconds.

Experts are uncertain as to the number and duration of bruxing events that can create muscle symptoms. Certainly great variation exists from patient to patient. Christensen[226-228] demonstrated that pain was produced in jaw muscles of subjects after 20 to 60 seconds of voluntary clenching. Therefore it would appear that bruxing events can induce symptoms in some individuals, although the specific nature of the symptoms and how much activity was involved were not reported.

Intensity of bruxing events. The intensity of bruxing events has not been studied well, but Clarke et al.[229] demonstrated an interesting finding. They found that an average bruxing event involved 60% of the maximum clenching power before the person went to sleep. This is a significant amount of force because the maximum clench far exceeds the normal forces that are used during mastication or any other functional activity. Interestingly, in this study 2 of the 10 patients exerted forces during bruxing events that actually exceeded the maximum force they could apply to the teeth during a voluntary clench. In these individuals a bruxing event during sleep would clearly be more likely to create problems than even a maximum clench during the waking period. In a more recent study, Rugh[230] demonstrated that 66% of nocturnal bruxing events were greater than the force of chewing, but only 1% of the events exceeded the force of a voluntary maximum clench.

Although some individuals demonstrate only diurnal muscle activity,[204] it is more common to find people with nocturnal activity.[135,136,231] In reality a certain amount of nocturnal bruxism is present in most normal subjects.[219-221] The clinician should remember, however, that both diurnal and nocturnal parafunctional activities occur at a subconscious level and therefore unawareness of the activity is common.

Sleep position and bruxing events. In a few studies sleep position and bruxing events have been studied. Before these investigations, researchers speculated that subjects did more bruxing while sleeping on their sides compared with sleeping on their backs.[232] Studies that actually documented sleep position and bruxing events do not substantiate this speculation. Instead, all studies report that either more bruxing events occur on the back than the side or no difference is observed.[219-221,233] Reports indicate that bruxing patients alter their sleeping positions more than nonbruxing subjects.[234]

Bruxing events and masticatory symptoms. An important question regarding nocturnal bruxism that has not been adequately addressed is the type and duration of bruxing events that cause masticatory symptoms. Ware and Rugh[222] studied a group of bruxism patients without pain and a group with pain and found that the latter group had a significantly higher number of bruxing events during REM sleep than did the former. Both groups, however, bruxed more than a control group. This study suggested that there might be two types of bruxism patient: one bruxing more during REM sleep and one bruxing more during the non-REM phases. Other studies by these authors[222,235] showed that the amount of sustained contraction occurring in bruxism was commonly much higher during REM than non-REM phases of sleep. These findings help explain the conflicting literature on sleep stages and bruxism and also may explain why some patients awake with pain but others with clinical evidence of bruxism report no pain.[236]

Muscle Activities and Masticatory Symptoms

As one begins to appreciate parafunctional activity, one also begins to understand how this type of muscle activity can represent a cause of some types of TMDs. Functional activity, on the other hand, does not seem to have the same risk factors. Five common factors will illustrate why these different muscle activities pose different TMD risk factors (Table 7-3).

Forces of Tooth Contacts. In evaluating the effect of tooth contacts on the structures of the masticatory system, two factors must be considered: the magnitude and duration of the contacts. A reasonable way to compare the effects of functional and parafunctional contacts is to evaluate the amount of force placed on the teeth in pounds per second per day for each activity.

Both chewing and swallowing activities must be evaluated (normally no tooth contacts occur during speech). Estimates[237] indicate that during each chewing stroke an average of 58.7 lb of force is applied to the teeth for 115 ms. This yields 6.75 lb/sec/chew.[238] In view of the fact that an estimated 1800 chews occur during an average day,[239]

one can see that the total occlusal force-time activity would be 12,150 lb/sec/day. The forces of swallowing must also be considered. Persons swallow some 146 times a day while eating.[240] Because an estimated 66.5 lb of force is applied to the teeth for 522 ms during each swallow,[238] this comes to 5068 lb/sec/day. Thus the total force-time activity for chewing and swallowing is about 17,200 lb/sec/day.

Tooth contacts during parafunctional activity are more difficult to evaluate because little is known regarding the amount of forces applied to the teeth. A significant amount of force over a given period can be recorded during nocturnal bruxism.[135,136,231] Rugh and Solberg[135] established that a significant amount of muscle activity consists of contractions that are greater than those used merely in swallowing and are sustained for 1 second or more. Each second is considered a unit of activity. Normal nocturnal muscle activities (parafunctional) average about 20 units per hour. If a conservative estimate of 80 lb of force per second is used for each unit, then the normal nocturnal activity for 8 hours is 12,800 lb/sec/night. This is less than the force applied to the teeth during function. These forces are those of normal activity and not of the bruxing patient. A patient who exhibits bruxing behavior can easily produce 60 units of activity per hour. If 80 lb of force is applied per second, 38,400 lb/sec/night is produced, which is three times the amount from functional activity per day. Consider also that 80 lb of force represents only half the average

TABLE **7-3**

Comparison of Functional and Parafunctional Activities Using Five Common Factors

Factor	Functional Activity	Parafunctional Activity
Forces of tooth contacts	17,200 lb/sec/day	57,600 lb/sec/day, possibly more
Direction of applied forces to teeth	Vertical (well tolerated)	Horizontal (not well tolerated)
Mandibular position	Centric occlusion (relatively stable)	Eccentric movements (relatively unstable)
Type of muscle contraction	Isotonic (physiologic)	Isometric (nonphysiologic)
Influence of protective reflexes	Present	Obtunded
Pathologic effects	Unlikely	Very likely

maximum force that can be applied to the teeth.[237] If 120 lb of force is applied (and some persons can easily reach 250 lb), the force-time activity reaches 57,600 lb/sec/day! It can easily be appreciated that force and duration of tooth contacts during parafunctional activity pose a much more serious consequence to the structures of the masticatory system than do those of functional activity.

Direction of Applied Forces. During chewing and swallowing, the mandible is moving primarily in a vertical direction.[238] As it closes and tooth contacts occur, the predominant forces applied to the teeth are also in a vertical direction. As discussed in Chapter 5, vertical forces are accepted well by the supportive structures of the teeth. During parafunctional activities, however (e.g., bruxism), heavy forces are applied to the teeth as the mandible shifts from side to side. This shifting causes horizontal forces, which are not well accepted and increase the likelihood of damage to the teeth and/or supportive structures.

Mandibular Position. Most functional activity occurs at or near the ICP. Although the ICP may not always be the most MS position for the condyles, it is stable for the occlusion because of the maximum number of tooth contacts it provides. Therefore the forces of functional activity are distributed to many teeth, minimizing potential damage to an individual tooth. Tooth wear patterns suggest that most parafunctional activity occurs in eccentric positions.[159] Few tooth contacts occur during this activity, and often the condyles are translated far from a stable position. Activity in this type of mandibular position places more strain on the masticatory system, rendering it more susceptible to breakdown. Such activity results in the application of heavy forces to a few teeth in an unstable joint position, and thus there is an increased likelihood of pathologic effects to the teeth and joints.

Type of Muscle Contraction. Most functional activity consists of well-controlled and rhythmic contraction and relaxation of the muscles involved during jaw function. This isotonic activity permits adequate blood flow to oxygenate the tissues and eliminate byproducts accumulated at the cellular level. Therefore functional activity is a

physiologic muscle activity. Parafunctional activity, by contrast, often results in sustained muscle contraction over long periods. This type of isometric activity inhibits normal blood flow within the muscle tissues. As a result, there is an increase in metabolic byproducts within the muscle tissues, creating the symptoms of fatigue, pain, and spasms.[227,241,242]

Influences of Protective Reflexes. Neuromuscular reflexes are present during functional activities, protecting the dental structures from damage. During parafunctional activities, however, the neuromuscular protecting mechanisms appear to be somewhat obtunded, resulting in less influence over muscle activity.[3,243,244] This allows parafunctional activity to increase and eventually reach levels high enough to create breakdown of the structures involved.

After considering these factors, it becomes apparent that parafunctional activity is more likely to be responsible for structural breakdown of the masticatory system and TMDs than functional activity. This is an important concept to remember because many patients come to the dental office complaining of functional disturbances such as difficulty in eating or pain during speaking. The clinician should remember that functional activities often bring to the patient's awareness the symptoms that have been created by parafunctional activities. In these instances treatment should be primarily directed toward controlling parafunctional activity. Altering the functional activity of which the patient is complaining can be helpful in reducing symptoms, but alone it is not sufficient treatment to resolve the disorder.

Another concept to remember is that parafunctional activities occur almost entirely subconsciously. Much of this damaging activity occurs during sleep in the form of bruxism and clenching. Often patients awake with no awareness of the activity that has occurred during sleep. They may even awake with TMD symptoms but not relate this discomfort to any causative factor. When they are questioned regarding bruxism, most will deny such activity.[207] Some studies suggest that 25% to 50% of the patients surveyed report bruxism.[55,245] Although these reports seem high, it is likely that the true percentage is even higher when one considers that many people surveyed are unaware of their parafunctional activity.

Etiology of Bruxing Events

Over the years, a great deal of controversy has surrounded the etiology of bruxism and clenching. Early on, the profession was quite convinced that bruxism was directly related to occlusal interferences.[3,132,246,247] Therefore treatments were directed toward correction of the occlusion condition. Later studies[130,161,248] did not support the concept that occlusal contacts cause bruxing events. Although it is clear that occlusal contacts influence function

of the masticatory system (see Chapter 2), they are not likely to contribute to bruxism (see previous discussion of the relationship between occlusal interferences and masticatory symptoms).

One factor that seems to influence bruxing activity is emotional stress.[249] Early studies that monitored levels of nocturnal bruxing activity demonstrated a strong temporal pattern associated with stressful events (Fig. 7-3).[135,136,231,248] This pattern can be seen clearly in Fig. 7-4 when a single subject is monitored over a long period of time. As the subject encountered a stressful event, the nocturnal masseter activity increased. Associated with this

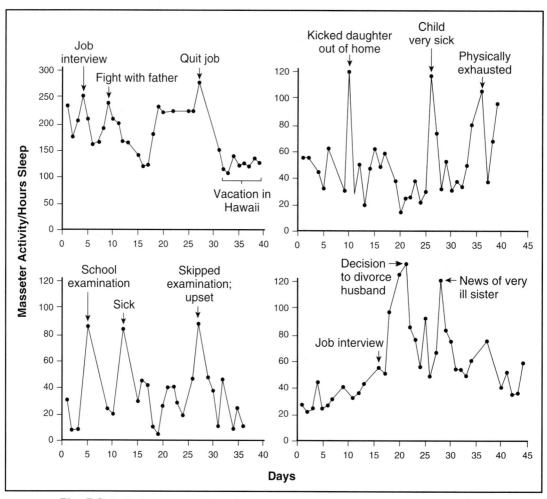

Fig. 7-3 Rugh demonstrated that daily stress is reflected in nocturnal masseter muscle activity. *(From Rugh JD, Solberg WK: In Zarb GA, Carlsson GE, editors:* Temporomandibular joint: function and dysfunction, *St Louis, 1979, Mosby.)*

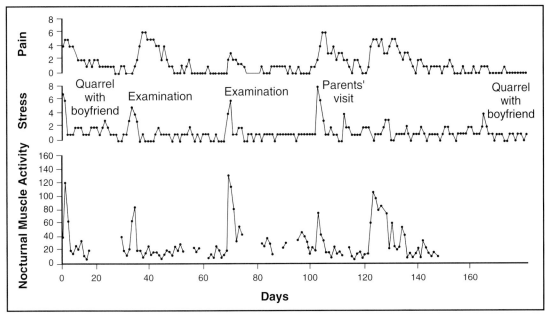

Fig. 7-4 Long-term relationship of stress, muscle activity, and pain. These three measurements have been obtained from a single subject for a 140-day period. Shortly after a stressful experience, the nocturnal muscle activity increases. Not long thereafter, the subject reports pain. *(From Rugh JD, Lemke RL: Significance of oral habits. In Matarazzo JD, Herd AJ, Weiss SM, editors:* Behavioral health: a handbook of health enhancement and disease prevention, *New York, 1984, John Wiley & Sons.)*

activity was a period of increased pain. Of note is that more recent studies found this relationship to be true in only a small percentage of the patients studied.[250,251]

Increase in emotional stress, however, is not the only factor that has been demonstrated to effect bruxism. Certain medications can increase bruxing events.[252-255] Some studies suggest a genetic predisposition to bruxism.[256,257] Other studies[258-260] report a relationship between bruxism and CNS disturbances.

At the writing of the first edition of this textbook (1983), a common and well-accepted concept was that parafunctional activity was a significant etiologic factor in TMDs. In fact, it was thought that if parafunctional activity could be controlled, TMD symptoms would be controlled. As the field has matured, new information has shed new light on the etiology of TMD. Presently it is still believed that parafunctional activity can be an etiologic factor, but it is far more complex than that. Clinicians also recognize that bruxing and clenching are common,

almost normal findings in the general population. Most individuals have some type of parafunctional activity that never results in any major consequence. However, on occasion parafunctional activity does precipitate problems, and therapy needs to be directed toward controlling it. In other instances it may not be the primary cause of the TMD symptoms but a perpetuating factor that maintains or accentuates symptoms. In this case both the major etiology and the parafunctional activity need to be addressed for complete resolution of symptoms. The effective clinician must be able to differentiate when parafunctional activity is important to the patient's symptoms and when it is only an accompanying condition. This is accomplished by carefully scrutinizing the patient's history and examination findings.

Bruxing in Children

Bruxing is a common finding in children. Often parents will hear their child bruxing during sleep and become concerned. They will show up in the dental office quite distressed about this finding and ask the dentist for advice or treatment. The dentist needs to properly respond to their concerns on the basis of sound data. Unfortunately, data in children are scarce. Experts generally accept that although bruxing in children is common, it is rarely associated with symptoms. A review of the pediatric literature on the subject of bruxing and TMDs fails to reveal any evidence of concern.[261] Although young children often wear their deciduous teeth, this is rarely associated with any difficulty in chewing or complaints of masticatory dysfunction. In one study[262] of 126 bruxing children (ages 6 to 9), only 17 were still bruxing 5 years later and none had symptoms. This study concluded that bruxing in children is a self-limiting phenomenon, not associated with significant symptoms and not related to an increased risk of bruxing as an adult. Concerned parents should be informed of the benign nature of this activity and asked to monitor any complaints of the child. If masticatory function is a problem, the child should be evaluated in the dental office. If the child complains of frequent and significant headaches, a TMD examination is also indicated to rule out masticatory dysfunction as a possible cause.

SUMMARY

This chapter has presented information regarding the epidemiology and etiology of TMDs. It has revealed that the signs and symptoms of TMD are common in the general population and are not always severe or debilitating. In fact, only a small percentage of the general population will seek advice for these complaints, with even fewer requiring treatment.[49] Nevertheless, individuals seeking care need to be managed effectively and, when possible, conservatively. To manage TMD effectively, the clinician must be able to recognize and understand its etiology. Unfortunately this is not always easy. Although for years the occlusal condition has been thought to be a major cause of TMD, this is not always the case. Certainly occlusion can be a factor, and when it is the clinician must address this effectively. However, occlusion represents only one of five etiologic considerations that have been

reviewed in this chapter. Before the clinician can begin treatment, a sound understanding of the precise cause of the TMD must be attained. This begins with a complete understanding of the different types of TMD patients. This information is presented in the next chapter.

In closing this chapter, it is important for the reader to remember that *the clinician who only evaluates the occlusion is likely missing as much as the clinician who never evaluates the occlusion.*

References

1. Costen JB: Syndrome of ear and sinus symptoms dependent upon functions of the temporomandibular joint, *Ann Otol Rhinol Laryngol* 3:1-4, 1934.
2. Shore NA: *Occlusal equilibration and temporomandibular joint dysfunction*, Philadelphia, 1959, JB Lippincott.
3. Ramfjord SP, Ash MM: *Occlusion*, Philadelphia, 1971, Saunders.
4. Gerber A: Kiefergelenk und zahnokklusion, *Dtsch Zahnaerztl* 26:119-123, 1971.
5. Graber G: Neurologische und psychosomatische aspekte der myoarthropathien des kauorgans, *Zwr* 80:997-1002, 1971.
6. Voss R: Behandlung von beschwerden des kiefergelenkes mit aufbissplatten, *Dtsch Zahanaerztl Z* 19:545-550, 1964.
7. Laskin DM: Etiology of the pain-dysfunction syndrome, *J Am Dent Assoc* 79:147-153, 1969.
8. Schwartz L: *Disorders of the temporomandibular joint*, Philadelphia, 1959, Saunders.
9. McNeill C, Danzig D, Farrar W, Gelb H, Lerman MD et al: Craniomandibular (TMJ) disorders—state of the art, *J Prosthet Dent* 44:434-437, 1980.
10. Bell WE: *Clinical management of temporomandibular disorders*, Chicago, 1982, Year Book Medical.
11. Griffiths RH: Report of the President's Conference on examination, diagnosis and management or temporomandibular disorders, *J Am Dent Assoc* 106:75-77, 1983.
12. Fowler EP: Deafness associated with dental occlusal disorders in contrast with deafness definitely not so associated, *N Y J Dent* 9:272-279, 1939.
13. Dingman RO: Diagnosis and treatment of lesions of the temporomandibular joint, *Am J Orthod Oral Surg* 26:374-379, 1940.
14. Junemann HR: Consequence of shortening the intermaxillary distance, *J Am Dent Assoc Dent Cosmos* 25:1427-1435, 1948.
15. Harvey W: Investigation and survey of malocclusion and ear symptoms, with particular reference to otitic barotrauma (pains in ears due to change in altitude), *Br Dent J* 85:219-223, 1940.
16. Bleiker RE: Ear disturbances of temporomandibular origin, *J Am Dent Assoc Dent Cosmos* 25:1390-1394, 1938.

17. Pippini BM: A method of repositioning the mandible in the treatment of lesions of the temporomandibular joint, *Wash U Dent J* 6:107-110, 1940.

18. Brussel IJ: Temporomandibular joint disease: differential diagnosis and treatment, *J Am Dent Assoc* 39:532-539, 1949.

19. Ramfjord SP: Diagnosis of traumatic temporomandibular joint arthritis, *J Calif Dent Assoc Nevada Dent Soc* 32:300-306, 1956.

20. Moyer RE: An electromyogram analysis of certain muscles involved in temporomandibular movement, *Am J Orthod* 36:481-489, 1950.

21. Perry HT, Harris SC: The role of the neuromuscular system in functional activity of the mandible, *J Am Dent Assoc* 48:665-673, 1954.

22. Jarabak JR: An electromyographic analysis of muscular and temporomandibular joint disturbances due to imbalance in occlusion, *J Am Dent Assoc* 26:170-179, 1956.

23. Sarnat BG: *The temporomandibular joint*, Springfield, Ill, 1951, Charles C. Thomas.

24. Farrar WB, McCarty WL Jr: The TMJ dilemma, *J Ala Dent Assoc* 63:19-26, 1979.

25. Okeson JP: *Bell's orofacial pains*, ed 6, Chicago, 2005, Quintessence.

26. *Dorland's illustrated medical dictionary*, ed 30, Philadelphia, 2003, Saunders, p 626.

27. Solberg WK, Woo MW, Houston JB: Prevalence of mandibular dysfunction in young adults, *J Am Dent Assoc* 98:25-34, 1979.

28. Osterberg T, Carlsson GE: Symptoms and signs of mandibular dysfunction in 70-year-old men and women in Gothenburg, Sweden, *Comm Dent Oral Epidemiol* 7:315-321, 1979.

29. Swanljung O, Rantanen T: Functional disorders of the masticatory system in southwest Finland, *Community Dent Oral Epidemiol* 7:177-182, 1979.

30. Ingervall B, Mohlin B, Thilander B: Prevalence of symptoms of functional disturbances of the masticatory system in Swedish men, *J Oral Rehabil* 7:185-197, 1980.

31. Nilner M, Lassing SA: Prevalence of functional disturbances and diseases of the stomatognathic system in 7-14 year olds, *Swed Dent J* 5:173-187, 1981.

32. Nilner M: Prevalence of functional disturbances and diseases of the stomatognathic system in 15-18 year olds, *Swed Dent J* 5:189-197, 1981.

33. Egermark-Eriksson I, Carlsson GE, Ingervall B: Prevalence of mandibular dysfunction and orofacial parafunction in 7-, 11- and 15-year-old Swedish children, *Eur J Orthod* 3:163-172, 1981.

34. Rieder CE, Martinoff JT, Wilcox SA: The prevalence of mandibular dysfunction. Part I: sex and age distribution of related signs and symptoms, *J Prosthet Dent* 50:81-88, 1983.

35. Gazit E, Lieberman M, Eini R, Hirsch N, Serfaty V et al: Prevalence of mandibular dysfunction in 10-18 year old Israeli schoolchildren, *J Oral Rehabil* 11:307-317, 1984.

36. Pullinger AG, Seligman DA, Solberg WK: Temporomandibular disorders. Part II: occlusal factors associated with temporomandibular joint tenderness and dysfunction, *J Prosthet Dent* 59:363-367, 1988.

37. Agerberg G, Inkapool I: Craniomandibular disorders in an urban Swedish population, *J Craniomandib Disord* 4:154-164, 1990.

38. De Kanter RJ, Truin GJ, Burgersdijk RC, Van 't Hof MA, Battistuzzi PG et al: Prevalence in the Dutch adult population and a meta-analysis of signs and symptoms of temporomandibular disorder, *J Dent Res* 72:1509-1518, 1993.

39. Magnusson T, Carlsson GE, Egermark I: Changes in subjective symptoms of craniomandibular disorders in children and adolescents during a 10-year period, *J Orofac Pain* 7:76-82, 1993.

40. Glass EG, McGlynn FD, Glaros AG, Melton K, Romans K: Prevalence of temporomandibular disorder symptoms in a major metropolitan area, *Cranio* 11:217-220, 1993.

41. Tanne K, Tanaka E, Sakuda M: Association between malocclusion and temporomandibular disorders in orthodontic patients before treatment, *J Orofac Pain* 7:156-162, 1993.

42. Nourallah H, Johansson A: Prevalence of signs and symptoms of temporomandibular disorders in a young male Saudi population, *J Oral Rehabil* 22:343-347, 1995.

43. Hiltunen K, Schmidt-Kaunisaho K, Nevalainen J, Narhi T, Ainamo A: Prevalence of signs of temporomandibular disorders among elderly inhabitants of Helsinki, Finland, *Acta Odontol Scand* 53:20-23, 1995.

44. Schiffman E: Mandibular dysfunction, occlusal dysfunction, and parafunctional habits in a non-clinical population, *J Dent Res* 65:306-314, 1986.

45. Rugh JD, Solberg WK: Oral health status in the United States: temporomandibular disorders. *J Dent Educ* 49:398-406, 1985.

46. Schiffman EL, Fricton JR, Haley DP, Shapiro BL: The prevalence and treatment needs of subjects with temporomandibular disorders, *J Am Dent Assoc* 120:295-303, 1990.

47. Magnusson T, Carlsson GE, Egermark-Eriksson I: An evaluation of the need and demand for treatment of craniomandibular disorders in a young Swedish population, *J Craniomandib Disord* 5:57-63, 1991.

48. Bibb CA: Jaw function status in an elderly non-population, *J Dent Res* 70:419-424, 1991.

49. De Kanter RJ, Kayser AF, Battistuzzi PG, Truin GJ, Van 't Hof MA: Demand and need for treatment of craniomandibular dysfunction in the Dutch adult population, *J Dent Res* 71:1607-1612, 1992.

50. Epker J, Gatchel RJ: Prediction of treatment-seeking behavior in acute TMD patients: practical application in clinical settings, *J Orofac Pain* 14:303-309, 2000.

51. Grossfeld O, Czarnecka B: Musculoarticular disorders of the stomatognathic system in school children examined according to clinical criteria, *J Oral Rehabil* 4:193-199, 1977.

52. Dibbets J: *Juvenile temporomandibular joint dysfunction and craniofacial growth*: thesis, Groningen, The Netherlands, 1977, University of Groningen.

53. Hansson T, Nilner M: A study of the occurrence of symptoms of diseases of the TMJ, masticatory musculature, and related structures, *J Oral Rehabil* 2:313-318, 1975.

54. Helkimo M: Studies on function and dysfunction of the masticatory system. IV. Age and sex distribution of symptoms

of dysfunction of the masticatory system in Lapps in the north of Finland, *Acta Odontol Scand* 32:255-267, 1974.

55. Agerberg G, Carlsson GE: Functional disorders of the masticatory system. I. Distribution of symptoms according to age and sex as judged from investigation by questionnaire, *Acta Odontol Scand* 30:597-613, 1972.

56. Ingervall B, Hedegard B: Subjective evaluation of functional disturbances of the masticatory system in young Swedish men, *Community Dent Oral Epidemiol* 2:149-152, 1974.

57. Agerberg G, Osterberg T: Maximal mandibular movements and symptoms of mandibular dysfunction in 70-year-old men and women, *Sven Tandlak Tidskr* 67:147-163, 1974.

58. Molin C, Carlsson GE, Friling B, Hedegard B: Frequency of symptoms of mandibular dysfunction in young Swedish men, *J Oral Rehabil* 3:9-18, 1976.

59. Posselt U: The temporomandibular joint syndrome and occlusion, *J Prosthet Dent* 25:432-438, 1971.

60. Mintz SS: Craniomandibular dysfunction in children and adolescents: a review, *J Craniomandib Pract* 11:224-231, 1993.

61. Osterberg T, Carlsson GE, Wedel A, Johansson U: A cross-sectional and longitudinal study of craniomandibular dysfunction in an elderly population, *J Craniomandib Disord* 6:237-245, 1992.

62. Von Korff M, Dworkin SF, Le Resche L, Kruger A: An epidemiologic comparison of pain complaints, *Pain* 32:173-183, 1988.

63. Ow RK, Loh T, Neo J, Khoo J: Symptoms of craniomandibular disorder among elderly people, *J Oral Rehabil* 22:413-419, 1995.

64. Greene CS: Temporomandibular disorders in the geriatric population, *J Prosthet Dent* 72:507-509, 1994.

65. Dworkin SF, Le Resche L, Von Korff MR: Diagnostic studies of temporomandibular disorders: challenges from an epidemiologic perspective, *Anesth Prog* 37:147-154, 1990.

66. Williamson EH, Simmons MD: Mandibular asymmetry and its relation to pain dysfunction, *Am J Orthod* 76:612-617, 1979.

67. De Boever JA, Adriaens PA: Occlusal relationship in patients with pain-dysfunction symptoms in the temporomandibular joint, *J Oral Rehabil* 10:1-7, 1983.

68. Egermark-Eriksson I, Ingervall B, Carlsson GE: The dependence of mandibular dysfunction in children on functional and morphologic malocclusion, *Am J Orthod* 83:187-194, 1983.

69. Brandt D: Temporomandibular disorders and their association with morphologic malocclusion in children. In Carlson DS, McNamara JA, Ribbens KA, editors: *Developmental aspects of temporomandibular joint disorders,* Ann Arbor, 1985, University of Michigan Press, pp 279-283.

70. Nesbitt BA, Moyers RE, TenHave T: Adult temporomandibular joint disorder symptomatology and its association with childhood occlusal relations: a preliminary report. In Carlson DS, McNamara JA, Ribbens KA, editors: *Developmental aspects of temporomandibular joint disorders,* Ann Arbor, 1985, University of Michigan Press, pp 183-189.

71. Thilander B: Temporomandibular joint problems in children. In Carlson DS, McNamara JA, Ribbens KA, editors: *Developmental aspects of temporomandibular joint disorders,* Ann Arbor, 1985, University of Michigan Press, p 89.

72. Budtz-Jorgensen E, Luan W, Holm-Pedersen P, Fejerskov O: Mandibular dysfunction related to dental, occlusal and prosthetic conditions in a selected elderly population, *Gerodontics* 1:28-33, 1985.

73. Bernal M, Tsamtsouris A: Signs and symptoms of temporomandibular joint dysfunction in 3- to 5-year-old children, *J Pedod* 10:127-140, 1986.

74. Nilner M: Functional disturbances and diseases of the stomatognathic system. A cross-sectional study, *J Pedod* 10:211-238, 1986.

75. Stringert HG, Worms FW: Variations in skeletal and dental patterns in patients with structural and functional alterations of the temporomandibular joint: a preliminary report, *Am J Orthod* 89:285-297, 1986.

76. Riolo ML, Brandt D, TenHave TR: Associations between occlusal characteristics and signs and symptoms of TMJ dysfunction in children and young adults, *Am J Orthod Dentofacial Orthop* 92:467-477, 1987.

77. Kampe T, Hannerz H: Differences in occlusion and some functional variable in adolescents with intact and restored dentitions, *Acta Odontol Scand* 45:31-39, 1987.

78. Kampe T, Carlsson GE, Hannerz H, Haraldson T: Three-year longitudinal study of mandibular dysfunction in young adults with intact and restored dentitions, *Acta Odontol Scand* 45:25-30, 1987.

79. Gunn SM, Woolfolk MW, Faja BW: Malocclusion and TMJ symptoms in migrant children, *J Craniomandib Disord* 2:196-200, 1988.

80. Seligman DA, Pullinger AG: Association of occlusal variables among refined TM patient diagnostic groups, *J Craniomandib Disord* 3:227-236, 1989.

81. Dworkin SF, Huggins KH, Le Resche L, Von KM, Howard J et al: Epidemiology of signs and symptoms in temporomandibular disorders: clinical signs in cases and controls, *J Am Dent Assoc* 120:273-281, 1990.

82. Linde C, Isacsson G: Clinical signs in patients with disk displacement versus patients with myogenic craniomandibular disorders, *J Craniomandib Disord* 4:197-204, 1990.

83. Kampe T, Hannerz H, Strom P: Five-year longitudinal recordings of functional variables of the masticatory system in adolescents with intact and restored dentitions: a comparative anamnestic and clinical study, *Acta Odontol Scand* 49:239-246, 1991.

84. Steele JG, Lamey PJ, Sharkey SW, Smith GM: Occlusal abnormalities, pericranial muscle and joint tenderness and tooth wear in a group of migraine patients, *J Oral Rehabil* 18:453-458, 1991.

85. Takenoshita Y, Ikebe T, Yamamoto M, Oka M: Occlusal contact area and temporomandibular joint symptoms, *Oral Surg Oral Med Oral Pathol* 72:388-394, 1991.

86. Pullinger AG, Seligman DA: Overbite and overjet characteristics of refined diagnostic groups of temporomandibular disorder patients, *Am J Orthod Dentofacial Orthop* 100:401-415, 1991.

87. Wanman A, Agerberg G: Etiology of craniomandibular disorders: evaluation of some occlusal and psychosocial factors in 19-year-olds, *J Craniomandib Disord* 5:35-44, 1991.

88. Cacchiotti DA, Plesh O, Bianchi P, McNeill C: Signs and symptoms in samples with and without temporomandibular disorders, *J Craniomandib Disord* 5:167-172, 1991.

89. Egermark I, Thilander B: Craniomandibular disorders with special reference to orthodontic treatment: an evaluation from childhood to adulthood, *Am J Orthod Dentofacial Orthop* 101:28-34, 1992.

90. Glaros AG, Brockman DL, Ackerman RJ: Impact of overbite on indicators of temporomandibular joint dysfunction, *Cranio* 10:277-281, 1992.

91. Huggare JA, Raustia AM: Head posture and cervicovertebral and craniofacial morphology in patients with craniomandibular dysfunction, *J Craniomandib Pract* 10:173-177, 1992.

92. Kirveskari P, Alanen P, Jamsa T: Association between craniomandibular disorders and occlusal interferences in children, *J Prosthet Dent* 67:692-696, 1992.

93. Kononen M: Signs and symptoms of craniomandibular disorders in men with Reiter's disease, *J Craniomandib Disord* 6:247-253, 1992.

94. Kononen M, Wenneberg B, Kallenberg A: Craniomandibular disorders in rheumatoid arthritis, psoriatic arthritis, and ankylosing spondylitis. A clinical study, *Acta Odontol Scand* 50:281-287, 1992.

95. List T, Helkimo M: Acupuncture and occlusal splint therapy in the treatment of craniomandibular disorders. II. A 1-year follow-up study, *Acta Odontol Scand* 50:375-385, 1992.

96. Shiau YY, Chang C: An epidemiological study of temporomandibular disorders in university students of Taiwan, *Community Dent Oral Epidemiol* 20:43-47, 1992.

97. Al Hadi LA: Prevalence of temporomandibular disorders in relation to some occlusal parameters, *J Prosthet Dent* 70:345-350, 1993.

98. Pullinger AG, Seligman DA: The degree to which attrition characterizes differentiated patient groups of temporomandibular disorders, *J Orofac Pain* 7:196-208, 1993.

99. Pullinger AG, Seligman DA, Gornbein JA: A multiple logistic regression analysis of the risk and relative odds of temporomandibular disorders as a function of common occlusal features, *J Dent Res* 72:968-979, 1993.

100. Scholte AM, Steenks MH, Bosman F: Characteristics and treatment outcome of diagnostic subgroups of CMD patients: retrospective study, *Community Dent Oral Epidemiol* 21:215-220, 1993.

101. Wadhwa L, Utreja A, Tewari A: A study of clinical signs and symptoms of temporomandibular dysfunction in subjects with normal occlusion, untreated, and treated malocclusions, *Am J Orthod Dentofacial Orthop* 103:54-61, 1993.

102. Keeling SD, McGorray S, Wheeler TT, King GJ: Risk factors associated with temporomandibular joint sounds in children 6 to 12 years of age, *Am J Orthod Dentofacial Orthop* 105:279-287, 1994.

103. Magnusson T, Carlsson GE, Egermark I: Changes in clinical signs of craniomandibular disorders from the age of 15 to 25 years, *J Orofac Pain* 8:207-215, 1994.

104. Tsolka P, Fenlon MR, McCullock AJ, Preiskel HW: A controlled clinical, electromyographic, and kinesiographic assessment of craniomandibular disorders in women, *J Orofac Pain* 8:80-89, 1994.

105. Vanderas AP: Relationship between craniomandibular dysfunction and malocclusion in white children with and without unpleasant life events, *J Oral Rehabil* 21:177-183, 1994.

106. Bibb CA, Atchison KA, Pullinger AG, Bittar GT: Jaw function status in an elderly community sample, *Community Dent Oral Epidemiol* 23:303-308, 1995.

107. Castro L: Importance of the occlusal status in the research diagnostic criteria of craniomandibular disorders, *J Orofac Pain* 9:98-102, 1995.

108. Hochman N, Ehrlich J, Yaffe A: Tooth contact during dynamic lateral excursion in young adults, *J Oral Rehabil* 22:221-224, 1995.

109. Lebbezoo-Scholte A, De Leeuw J, Steenks M, Bosman F, Buchner R et al: Diagnostic subgroups of craniomandibular disorders. Part 1: self-report data and clinical findings, *J Orofac Pain* 9:24-36, 1995.

110. Olsson M, Lindqvist B: Mandibular function before and after orthodontic treatment, *Eur J Orthod* 17:205-214, 1995.

111. Mauro G, Tagliaferro G, Bogini A, Fraccari F: A controlled clinical assessment and characterization of a group of patients with temporomandibular disorders, *J Orofac Pain* 9:101-105, 1995.

112. Tsolka P, Walter JD, Wilson RF, Preiskel HW: Occlusal variables, bruxism and temporomandibular disorders: a clinical and kinesiographic assessment, *J Oral Rehabil* 22:849-856, 1995.

113. Westling L: Occlusal interferences in retruded contact position and temporomandibular joint sounds, *J Oral Rehabil* 22:601-606, 1995.

114. Sato H, Osterberg T, Ahlqwist M, Carlsson G, Grondahl H-G et al: Temporomandibular disorders and radiographic findings of the mandibular condyle in an elderly population, *J Orofac Pain* 10:180-186, 1996.

115. Raustia AM, Pirttiniemi PM, Pyhtinen J: Correlation of occlusal factors and condyle position asymmetry with signs and symptoms of temporomandibular disorders in young adults, *Cranio* 13:152-156, 1995.

116. Seligman DA, Pullinger AG: A multiple stepwise logistic regression analysis of trauma history and 16 other history and dental cofactors in females with temporomandibular disorders, *J Orofac Pain* 10:351-361, 1996.

117. Conti PC, Ferreira PM, Pegoraro LF, Conti JV, Salvador MC: A cross-sectional study of prevalence and etiology of signs and symptoms of temporomandibular disorders in high school and university students, *J Orofac Pain* 10:254-262, 1996.

118. Ciancaglini R, Gherlone EF, Radaelli G: Association between loss of occlusal support and symptoms of functional disturbances of the masticatory system, *J Oral Rehabil* 26:248-253, 1999.

119. Seligman DA, Pullinger AG: Analysis of occlusal variables, dental attrition, and age for distinguishing healthy controls from female patients with intracapsular temporomandibular disorders, *J Prosthet Dent* 83:76-82, 2000.

120. McNamara JA Jr, Seligman DA, Okeson JP: Occlusion, orthodontic treatment, and temporomandibular disorders: a review, *J Orofac Pain* 9:73-90, 1995.

121. Clark GT, Tsukiyama Y, Baba K, Watanabe T: Sixty-eight years of experimental occlusal interference studies: what have we learned? *J Prosthet Dent* 82:704-713, 1999.

122. Okeson J: *Orofacial pain: guidelines for classification, assessment, and management*, Chicago, 1996, Quintessence.

123. Pullinger AG, Seligman DA: Quantification and validation of predictive values of occlusal variables in temporomandibular disorders using a multifactorial analysis, *J Prosthet Dent* 83:66-75, 2000.

124. Seligman DA, Pullinger AG: The role of intercuspal occlusal relationships in temporomandibular disorders: a review, *J Craniomandib Disord Facial Oral Pain* 5:96-106, 1991.

125. Miralles R, Manns A, Pasini C: Influence of different centric functions on electromyographic activity of elevator muscles, *Cranio* 6:26-33, 1988.

126. Miralles R, Bull R, Manns A, Roman E: Influence of balanced occlusion and canine guidance on electromyographic activity of elevator muscles in complete denture wearers, *J Prosthet Dent* 61:494-498, 1989.

127. Manns A, Miralles R, Valdivia J, Bull R: Influence of variation in anteroposterior occlusal contacts on electromyographic activity, *J Prosthet Dent* 61:617-623, 1989.

128. Williamson EH, Lundquist DO: Anterior guidance: its effect on electromyographic activity of the temporal and masseter muscles, *J Prosthet Dent* 49:816-823, 1983.

129. Sheikholeslam A, Holmgren K, Riise C: Therapeutic effects of the plane occlusal splint on signs and symptoms of craniomandibular disorders in patients with nocturnal bruxism, *J Oral Rehabil* 20:473-482, 1993.

130. Rugh JD, Barghi N, Drago CJ: Experimental occlusal discrepancies and nocturnal bruxism, *J Prosthet Dent* 51:548-553, 1984.

131. Ingervall B, Carlsson GE: Masticatory muscle activity before and after elimination of balancing side occlusal interference, *J Oral Rehabil* 9:183-192, 1982.

132. Ramfjord SP: Dysfunctional temporomandibular joint and muscle pain, *J Prosthet Dent* 11:353-362, 1961.

133. Krogh-Poulsen WG, Olsson A: Occlusal disharmonies and dysfunction of the stomatognathic system, *Dent Clin North Am* Nov:627-635, 1966.

134. Kloprogge MJ, van Griethuysen AM: Disturbances in the contraction and co-ordination pattern of the masticatory muscles due to dental restorations. An electromyographic study, *J Oral Rehabil* 3:207-216, 1976.

135. Rugh JD, Solberg WK: Electromyographic studies of bruxist behavior before and during treatment, *J Calif Dent Assoc* 3:56-59, 1975.

136. Solberg WK, Clark GT, Rugh JD: Nocturnal electromyographic evaluation of bruxism patients undergoing short term splint therapy, *J Oral Rehabil* 2:215-223, 1975.

137. Lavigne GI, Montplaisir JY: Bruxism: epidemiology, diagnosis, pathophysiology, and pharmacology. In Fricton JR, Dubner RB, editors: *Orofacial pain and temporomandibular disorders*, New York, 1995, Raven, pp 387-404.

138. Lavigne GJ, Velly-Miguel AM, Montplaisir J: Muscle pain, dyskinesia, and sleep, *Can J Physiol Pharmacol* 69:678-682, 1991.

139. Miguel AV, Montplaisir J, Rompre PH, Lund JP, Lavigne GJ: Bruxism and other orofacial movements during sleep, *J Craniomandib Disord* 6:71-81, 1992.

140. Maruyama T, Miyauchi S, Umekoji E: Analysis of the mandibular relationship of TMJ dysfunction patients using the mandibular kinesiograph, *J Oral Rehabil* 9:217-223, 1982.

141. Graham MM, Buxbaum J, Staling LM: A study of occlusal relationships and the incidence of myofascial pain, *J Prosthet Dent* 47:549-555, 1982.

142. Mohlin B, Ingervall B, Thilander B: Relation between malocclusion and mandibular dysfunction in Swedish men, *Eur J Orthod* 2:229-238, 1980.

143. Kirveskari P, Alanen P: Association between tooth loss and TMJ dysfunction, *J Oral Rehabil* 12:189-194, 1985.

144. Lieberman MA, Gazit E, Fuchs C, Lilos P: Mandibular dysfunction in 10-18 year old school children as related to morphological malocclusion, *J Oral Rehabil* 12:209-214, 1985.

145. Kirveskari P, Alanen P, Jamsa T: Association between craniomandibular disorders and occlusal interferences, *J Prosthet Dent* 62:66-69, 1989.

146. Harriman LP, Snowdon DA, Messer LB, Rysavy DM, Ostwald SK et al: Temporomandibular joint dysfunction and selected health parameters in the elderly, *Oral Surg Oral Med Oral Pathol* 70:406-413, 1990.

147. Egermark-Eriksson I, Carlsson GE, Magnusson T: A long-term epidemiologic study of the relationship between occlusal factors and mandibular dysfunction in children and adolescents, *J Dent Res* 66:67-71, 1987.

148. Mohlin B, Kopp S: A clinical study on the relationship between malocclusions, occlusal interferences and mandibular pain and dysfunction, *Swed Dent J* 2:105-112, 1978.

149. Droukas B, Lindee C, Carlsson GE: Occlusion and mandibular dysfunction: a clinical study of patients referred for functional disturbances of the masticatory system, *J Prosthet Dent* 53:402-406, 1985.

150. Bush FM: Malocclusion, masticatory muscle, and temporomandibular joint tenderness, *J Dent Res* 64:129-133, 1985.

151. Huber MA, Hall EH: A comparison of the signs of temporomandibular joint dysfunction and occlusal discrepancies in a symptom-free population of men and women, *Oral Surg Oral Med Oral Pathol* 70:180-183, 1990.

152. Vanderas AP: The relationship between craniomandibular dysfunction and malocclusion in white children with unilateral cleft lip and cleft lip and palate, *Cranio* 7:200-204, 1989.

153. Helm S, Petersen PE: Mandibular dysfunction in adulthood in relation to morphologic malocclusion at adolescence, *Acta Odontol Scand* 47:307-314, 1989.

154. Witter DJ, Van EP, Kayser AF, Van RGM: Oral comfort in shortened dental arches, *J Oral Rehabil* 17:137-143, 1990.

155. Seligman DA, Pullinger AG: The role of functional occlusal relationships in temporomandibular disorders: a review, *J Craniomandib Disord* 5:265-279, 1991.

156. Belser UC, Hannan AG: The influence of altered working-side guidance, *J Prosthet Dent* 53:406-411, 1985.

157. Riise C, Sheikholeslam A: Influence of experimental interfering occlusal contacts on the activity of the anterior temporal and masseter muscles during mastication, *J Oral Rehabil* 11:325-333, 1984.

158. Shupe RJ, Mohamed SE, Christensen LV, Finger IM, Weinberg R: Effects of occlusal guidance on jaw muscle activity, *J Prosthet Dent* 51:811-818, 1989.

159. Seligman DA, Pullinger AG, Solberg WK: The prevalence of dental attrition and its association with factors of age, gender, occlusion, and TMJ symptomatology, *J Dent Res* 67:1323-1333, 1988.

160. Bailey JO, Rugh JD: Effects of occlusal adjustment on bruxism as monitored by nocturnal EMG recordings, *J Dent Res* 59(special issue):317, 1980.

161. Kardachi BJ, Bailey JO, Ash MM: A comparison of biofeedback and occlusal adjustment on bruxism, *J Periodontol* 49:367-372, 1978.

162. Rugh JD, Graham GS, Smith JC, Ohrbach RK: Effects of canine versus molar occlusal splint guidance on nocturnal bruxism and craniomandibular symptomatology, *J Craniomandib Disord* 3:203-210, 1989.

163. Sheikholeslam A, Riise C: Influence of experimental interfering occlusal contacts on the activity of the anterior temporal and masseter muscles during submaximal and maximal bite in the intercuspal position, *J Oral Rehabil* 10:207-214, 1983.

164. Randow K, Carlsson K, Edlund J, Oberg T: The effect of an occlusal interference on the masticatory system. An experimental investigation, *Odontol Rev* 27:245-256, 1976.

165. Magnusson T, Enbom L: Signs and symptoms of mandibular dysfunction after introduction of experimental balancing-side interferences, *Acta Odontol Scand* 42:129-135, 1984.

166. Karlsson S, Cho SA, Carlsson GE: Changes in mandibular masticatory movements after insertion of nonworking-side interference, *J Craniomandib Disord* 6:177-183, 1992.

167. Tsolka P, Morris RW, Preiskel HW: Occlusal adjustment therapy for craniomandibular disorders: a clinical assessment by a double-blind method [see comments], *J Prosthet Dent* 68:957-964, 1992.

168. Goodman P, Greene CS, Laskin DM: Response of patients with myofascial pain-dysfunction syndrome to mock equilibration, *J Am Dent Assoc* 92:755-758, 1976.

169. Forssell H, Kirveskari P, Kangasniemi P: Effect of occlusal adjustment on mandibular dysfunction. A double-blind study, *Acta Odontol Scand* 44:63-69, 1986.

170. Kirveskari P, Le Bell Y, Salonen M, Forssell H, Grans L: Effect of elimination of occlusal interferences on signs and symptoms of craniomandibular disorder in young adults, *J Oral Rehabil* 16:21-26, 1989.

171. Kirveskari P: The role of occlusal adjustment in the management of temporomandibular disorders, *Oral Surg Oral Med Oral Pathol Oral Radiol Endod* 83:87-90, 1997.

172. Kirveskari P, Jamsa T, Alanen P: Occlusal adjustment and the incidence of demand for temporomandibular disorder treatment, *J Prosthet Dent* 79:433-438, 1998.

173. Stohler CS, Ash MM: Excitatory response of jaw elevators associated with sudden discomfort during chewing, *J Oral Rehabil* 13:225-233, 1986.

174. Yemm R: Neurophysiologic studies of temporomandibular joint dysfunction. In Zarb GA, Carlsson GE, editors: *Temporomandibular joint: function and dysfunction*, St Louis, 1979, Mosby, pp 215-237.

175. Williamson EH: The role of craniomandibular dysfunction in orthodontic diagnosis and treatment planning, *Dent Clin North Am* 27:541-560, 1983.

176. Manns A: Influence of group function and canine guidance on electromyographic activity of elevator muscles, *J Prosthet Dent* 57:494-501, 1987.

177. Egermark I, Ronnerman A: Temporomandibular disorders in the active phase of orthodontic treatment, *J Oral Rehabil* 22:613-618, 1995.

178. Smith BR: Effects of orthodontic archwire changes on masseter muscle activity, *J Dent Res* 63(special issue) abst# 784:258, 1984.

179. Goldreich H, Rugh JD, Gazit E, Lieberman A: The effects of orthodontic archwire adjustment on masseter muscle EMG activity, *J Dent Res* 70 (special issue) abst# 1976:513, 1991.

180. Choi JK: A study on the effects of maximum voluntary clenching on the tooth contact points and masticatory muscle activities in patients with temporomandibular disorders, *J Craniomandib Disord* 6:41-49, 1992.

181. Kampe T, Hannerz H: Five-year longitudinal study of adolescents with intact and restored dentitions: signs and symptoms of temporomandibular dysfunction and functional recordings, *J Oral Rehabil* 18:387-398, 1991.

182. Silvennoinen U, Raustia AM, Lindqvist C, Oikarinen K: Occlusal and temporomandibular joint disorders in patients with unilateral condylar fracture. A prospective one-year study, *Int J Oral Maxillofac Surg* 27:280-285, 1998.

183. Melugin MB, Indresano AT, Clemens SP: Glenoid fossa fracture and condylar penetration into the middle cranial fossa: report of a case and review of the literature, *J Oral Maxillofac Surg* 55:1342-1347, 1997.

184. Brooke RI, Stenn PG: Postinjury myofascial pain dysfunction syndrome: its etiology and prognosis, *Oral Surg Oral Med Oral Pathol* 45:846-850, 1978.

185. Brown CR: TMJ injuries from direct trauma, *Pract Periodontics Aesthet Dent* 9:581-582, 1997.

186. Burgess JA, Kolbinson DA, Lee PT, Epstein JB: Motor vehicle accidents and TMDs: assessing the relationship, *J Am Dent Assoc* 127:1767-1772, 1996.

187. DeVita CL, Friedman JM, Meyer S, Breiman A: An unusual case of condylar dislocation, *Ann Emerg Med* 17:534-536, 1988.

188. Ferrari R, Leonard MS: Whiplash and temporomandibular disorders: a critical review [see comments], *J Am Dent Assoc* 129:1739-1745, 1998.

189. Howard RP, Hatsell CP, Guzman HM: Temporomandibular joint injury potential imposed by the low-velocity extension-flexion maneuver, *J Oral Maxillofac Surg* 53:256-262, 1995.

190. Kolbinson DA, Epstein JB, Burgess JA: Temporomandibular disorders, headaches, and neck pain following motor vehicle accidents and the effect of litigation: review of the literature, *J Orofac Pain* 10:101-25, 1996.

191. Levy Y, Hasson O, Zeltser R, Nahlieli O: Temporomandibular joint derangement after air bag deployment: report of two cases, *J Oral Maxillofac Surg* 56:1000-1003, 1998.

192. Probert TCS, Wiesenfeld PC, Reade PC: Temporomandibular pain dysfunction disorder resulting from road traffic accidents—an Australian study, *Int J Oral Maxillofac Surg* 23:338-341, 1994.

193. Pullinger AG, Seligman DA: Trauma history in diagnostic groups of temporomandibular disorders, *Oral Surg Oral Med Oral Pathol* 71:529-534, 1991.

194. Reynolds MD: Myofascial trigger points in persistent posttraumatic shoulder pain, *South Med J* 77:1277-1280, 1984.

195. Thoren H, Iizuka T, Hallikainen D, Nurminen M, Lindqvist C: An epidemiological study of patterns of condylar fractures in children, *Br J Oral Maxillofac Surg* 35:306-311, 1997.

196. De Boever JA, Keersmaekers K: Trauma in patients with temporomandibular disorders: frequency and treatment outcome, *J Oral Rehabil* 23:91-96, 1996.

197. Zhang ZK, Ma XC, Gao S, Gu ZY, Fu KY: Studies on contributing factors in temporomandibular disorders, *Chin J Dent Res* 2:7-20, 1999.

198. Carlson CR, Okeson JP, Falace DA, Nitz AJ, Curran SL et al: Comparison of psychologic and physiologic functioning between patients with masticatory muscle pain and matched controls, *J Orofac Pain* 7:15-22, 1993.

199. Selye H: *Stress without distress*, Philadelphia, 1974, JB Lippincott, pp 32-34.

200. Grassi C, Passatore M: Action of the sympathetic system on skeletal muscle, *Ital J Neurol Sci* 9:23-28, 1988.

201. Passatore M, Grassi C, Filippi GM: Sympathetically-induced development of tension in jaw muscles: the possible contraction of intrafusal muscle fibres, *Pflugers Arch* 405:297-304, 1985.

202. Carlson CR, Okeson JP, Falace DA, Nitz AJ, Lindroth JE: Reduction of pain and EMG activity in the masseter region by trapezius trigger point injection, *Pain* 55:397-400, 1993.

203. Gavish A, Halachmi M, Winocur E, Gazit E: Oral habits and their association with signs and symptoms of temporomandibular disorders in adolescent girls, *J Oral Rehabil* 27:22-32, 2000.

204. Rugh JD, Robbins JW: Oral habits disorders. In Ingersoll B, editor: *Behavioral aspects in dentistry*, New York, 1982, Appleton-Century-Crofts, pp 179-202.

205. Howard JA: Temporomandibular joint disorders, facial pain and dental problems of performing artists. In Sataloff R, Brandfonbrener A, Lederman R, editors: *Textbook of performing arts medicine*, New York, 1991, Raven, pp 111-169.

206. Taddy JJ: Musicians and temporomandibular disorders: prevalence and occupational etiologic considerations, *J Craniomandib Pract* 10:241-246, 1992.

207. Marbach JJ, Raphael KG, Dohrenwend BP, Lennon MC: The validity of tooth grinding measures: etiology of pain dysfunction syndrome revisited, *J Am Dent Assoc* 120:327-333, 1990.

208. Hauri P: *Current concepts: the sleep disorders*, Kalamazoo, Mich, 1982, Upjohn.

209. Synder F: Psychophysiology of human sleep, *Clin Neurosurg* 18:503-510, 1971.

210. Fuchs P: The muscular activity of the chewing apparatus during night sleep. An examination of healthy subjects and patients with functional disturbances, *J Oral Rehabil* 2:35-48, 1975.

211. Dement W: The effect of sleep deprivation, *Science* 131:1705-1713, 1960.

212. Moldofsky H, Scarisbrick P: Induction of neurasthenic musculoskeletal pain syndrome by selective sleep stage deprivation, *Psychosom Med* 38:35-44, 1976.

213. Clarke NG, Townsend GC, Carey SE: Bruxing patterns in man during sleep, *J Oral Rehabil* 11:123-127, 1983.

214. Reding GR: Sleep patterns of tooth grinding: its relationship to dreaming, *Science* 145:725-730, 1964.

215. Satoh T, Harada Y: Electrophysiological study on tooth-grinding during sleep. *Electroencephalogr Clin Neurophysiol* 35:267-275, 1973.

216. Satoh T, Harada Y: Tooth-grinding during sleep as an arousal reaction, *Experientia* 27:785-791, 1971.

217. Tani K et al: Electroencephalogram study of parasomnia, *Physiol Animal Behav* 1:241-248, 1966.

218. Reding GR, Zepelin H, Robinson JE Jr, Zimmerman SO, Smith VH: Nocturnal teeth-grinding: all-night psychophysiologic studies, *J Dent Res* 47:786-797, 1968.

219. Okeson JP, Phillips BA, Berry DT, Cook Y, Paesani D et al: Nocturnal bruxing events in healthy geriatric subjects, *J Oral Rehabil* 17:411-418, 1990.

220. Okeson JP, Phillips BA, Berry DT, Cook YR, Cabelka JF: Nocturnal bruxing events in subjects with sleep-disordered breathing and control subjects, *J Craniomandib Disord* 5:258-264, 1991.

221. Okeson JP, Phillips BA, Berry DT, Baldwin RM: Nocturnal bruxing events: a report of normative data and cardiovascular response, *J Oral Rehabil* 21:623-630, 1994.

222. Ware JC, Rugh JD: Destructive bruxism: sleep stage relationship, *Sleep* 11:172-181, 1988.

223. Kydd WL, Daly C: Duration of nocturnal tooth contacts during bruxing, *J Prosthet Dent* 53:717-721, 1985.

224. Clarke NG, Townsend GC: Distribution of nocturnal bruxing patterns in man, *J Oral Rehabil* 11:529-534, 1984.

225. Trenouth MJ: The relationship between bruxism and temporomandibular joint dysfunction as shown by computer analysis of nocturnal tooth contact patterns, *J Oral Rehabil* 6:81-87, 1979.

226. Christensen LV: Facial pain from experimental tooth clenching, *Tandlaegebladet* 74:175-182, 1970.

227. Christensen LV, Mohamed SE: Contractile activity of the masseter muscle in experimental clenching and grinding of the teeth in man, *J Oral Rehabil* 11:191-199, 1984.

228. Christensen LV: Some subjective-experiential parameters in experimental tooth clenching in man, *J Oral Rehabil* 6:119-136, 1979.

229. Clarke NG, Townsend GC, Carey SE: Bruxing patterns in man during sleep, *J Oral Rehabil* 11:123-127, 1984.

230. Rugh JD: Feasibility of a laboratory model of nocturnal bruxism, *J Dent Res* 70:554-561, 1991.

231. Clark GT, Beemsterboer PL, Solberg WK, Rugh JD: Nocturnal electromyographic evaluation of myofascial pain dysfunction in patients undergoing occlusal splint therapy, *J Am Dent Assoc* 99:607-611, 1979.

232. Colquitt T: The sleep-wear syndrome, *J Prosthet Dent* 57:33-41, 1987.

233. Phillips BA, Okeson J, Paesani D, Gilmore R: Effect of sleep position on sleep apnea and parafunctional activity, *Chest* 90:424-429, 1986.

234. Sjoholm TT, Polo OJ, Alihanka JM: Sleep movements in teethgrinders, *J Craniomandib Disord* 6:184-191, 1992.

235. Ware JC: Sleep related bruxism: differences in patients with dental and sleep complaints, *Sleep Res* 11:182-189, 1982.

236. Dao TT, Lund JP, Lavigne GJ: Comparison of pain and quality of life in bruxers and patients with myofascial pain of the masticatory muscles, *J Orofac Pain* 8:350-356, 1994.

237. Gibbs CH, Mahan PE, Lundeen HC, Brehnan K, Walsh EK et al: Occlusal forces during chewing and swallowing as measured by sound transmission, *J Prosthet Dent* 46:443-449, 1981.

238. Lundeen HC, Gibbs CH: *Advances in occlusion*, Boston, 1982, John Wright PSC.

239. Graf H: Bruxism, *Dent Clin North Am* 13:659-665, 1969.

240. Flanagan JB: The 24-hour pattern of swallowing in man, *J Dent Res* 42(abstr # 165):1072, 1963.

241. Christensen LV: Facial pain and internal pressure of masseter muscle in experimental bruxism in man, *Arch Oral Biol* 16:1021-1031, 1971.

242. Christensen LV, Mohamed SE, Harrison JD: Delayed onset of masseter muscle pain in experimental tooth clenching, *J Prosthet Dent* 48:579-584, 1982.

243. Guyton AC: *Textbook of medical physiology*, Philadelphia, 1991, Saunders, p 1013.

244. Manns AE, Garcia C, Miralles R, Bull R, Rocabado M: Blocking of periodontal afferents with anesthesia and its influence on elevator EMG activity, *Cranio* 9:212-219, 1991.

245. Agerberg G, Carlsson GE: Functional disorders of the masticatory system. II. Symptoms in relation to impaired mobility of the mandible as judged from investigation by questionnaire, *Acta Odontol Scand* 31:337-347, 1973.

246. Guichet NE: *Occlusion: a teaching manual*, Anaheim, Calif, 1977, Denar Corporation.

247. Ramfjord S: Bruxism: a clinical and electromyographic study, *J Am Dent Assoc* 62:21-28, 1961.

248. Yemm R: Cause and effect of hyperactivity of the jaw muscles. In Bayant E, editor: *NIH Publication 79-1845*, Bethesda, Md, 1979, National Institutes of Health.

249. Schiffman EL, Fricton JR, Haley D: The relationship of occlusion, parafunctional habits and recent life events to mandibular dysfunction in a non-patient population, *J Oral Rehabil* 19:201-223, 1992.

250. Pierce CJ, Chrisman K, Bennett ME, Close JM: Stress, anticipatory stress, and psychologic measures related to sleep bruxism, *J Orofac Pain* 9:51-56, 1995.

251. Dao TT, Lavigne GJ, Charbonneau A, Feine JS, Lund JP: The efficacy of oral splints in the treatment of myofascial pain of the jaw muscles: a controlled clinical trial, *Pain* 56:85-94, 1994.

252. Ashcroft GW: Recognition of amphetamine addicts, *Br Med J* 1:57-61, 1965.

253. Magee KR: Bruxism related to levodopa therapy, *JAMA* 214:147, 1970.

254. Brandon S: Unusual effect of fenfluramine, *Br Med J* 4:557-558, 1969.

255. Hartman E: Alcohol and bruxism, *N Engl J Med* 301:333-335, 1979.

256. Abe K, Shimakawa M: Genetic and developmental aspects of sleeptalking and teeth-grinding, *Acta Paedopsychiatr* 33:339-344, 1966.

257. Reding GR, Rubright WC, Zimmerman SO: Incidence of bruxism, *J Dent Res* 45:1198-1204, 1966.

258. Lindqvist B, Heijbel J: Bruxism in children with brain damage, *Acta Odontol Scand* 32:313-319, 1974.

259. Rosenbaum CH, McDonald RE, Levitt EE: Occlusion of cerebral-palsied children, *J Dent Res* 45:1696-1700, 1966.

260. Richmond G, Rugh JD, Dolfi R, Wasilewsky JW: Survey of bruxism in an institutionalized mentally retarded population, *Am J Ment Defic* 88:418-421, 1984.

261. Okeson JP: Temporomandibular disorders in children, *Pediatr Dent* 11:325-329, 1989.

262. Kieser JA, Groeneveld HT: Relationship between juvenile bruxing and craniomandibular dysfunction, *J Oral Rehabil* 25:662-665, 1998.

Signs and Symptoms of Temporomandibular Disorders

8

CHAPTER

"You can never diagnose something you have never heard about."

—JPO

The previous chapter described certain events and conditions that can lead to alteration of the normal function of the masticatory system. Etiologic factors such as trauma, emotional stress, orthopedic instability, and sources of deep pain and muscle hyperactivity were implicated as significant components. In this chapter the common signs and symptoms of masticatory dysfunction are discussed. The clinical signs and symptoms of masticatory dysfunction can be grouped into categories according to structures that are affected: (1) the muscles, (2) the temporomandibular joints (TMJs), and (3) the dentition. Muscle and TMJ disorders make up the group of conditions known as *temporomandibular disorders* (TMDs). Included with the signs and symptoms of each are the etiologic factors that either cause or contribute to the disorder.

When evaluating a patient, it is important to identify both signs and symptoms clearly. A *sign* is an objective clinical finding that the clinician uncovers during a clinical examination. A *symptom* is a description or complaint reported by the patient. Patients are acutely aware of their symptoms, yet they may not be aware of their clinical signs. For example, a person reports muscle tenderness during mandibular opening yet is totally unaware of the joint sounds that are also present. Both the muscle tenderness and the joint sounds are clinical signs, but only the muscle tenderness is considered a symptom. To avoid overlooking subclinical signs, the examiner must be acutely aware of the common signs and symptoms for each specific disorder.

FUNCTIONAL DISORDERS OF THE MUSCLES

Functional disorders of masticatory muscles are probably the most common TMD complaint of patients seeking treatment in the dental office.[1,2] With regard to pain, they are second only to odontalgia (i.e., tooth or periodontal pain) in terms of frequency. They are generally grouped in a large category known as *masticatory muscle disorders*.[3] As with any pathologic state, two major symptoms can be observed: (1) pain and (2) dysfunction.

PAIN

Certainly the most common complaint of patients with masticatory muscle disorders is muscle pain, which may range from slight tenderness to extreme discomfort. Pain felt in muscle tissue is called *myalgia*. Myalgia can arise from increased levels of muscular use. The symptoms are often associated with a feeling of muscle fatigue and tightness. Although the exact origin of this type of muscle pain is debatable, some authors suggest it is related to vasoconstriction of the relevant nutrient arteries and the accumulation of metabolic waste products in the muscle tissues. Within the ischemic area of the muscle, certain algogenic substances (e.g., bradykinins, prostaglandins) are released, causing muscle pain.[3-7]

Muscle pain, however, is far more complex than simple overuse and fatigue. In fact, muscle pain associated with most TMD does not seem to be strongly correlated with increased activity such as spasm.[8-12] It is now appreciated that muscle pain can be greatly influenced by central mechanisms[7,13,14] (discussed later in this chapter).

The severity of muscle pain is directly related to the functional activity of the muscle involved. Therefore patients often report that the pain affects their functional activity. Remember, when a patient reports pain during chewing or speaking, these functional activities are not usually the cause of the disorder. Instead they heighten the patient's awareness of it. More likely some type of activity or central nervous system (CNS) effect has led to the muscle pain, and thus treatment directed toward the functional activity will not be appropriate or successful; rather, treatment needs to be directed toward diminishing the CNS effects or possibly muscle hyperactivity.

The clinician must also remember that myogenous pain (pain originating in muscle tissue) is a type of deep pain and, if it becomes constant, can produce central excitatory effects. As described in Chapter 2, these effects may present as sensory effects (i.e., referred pain or secondary hyperalgesia), efferent effects (i.e., muscle effects), or even autonomic effects. In particular, remember that muscle pain can therefore reinitiate more muscle pain (i.e., the cyclic effect discussed in Chapter 2). This clinical phenomenon was first described[15] in 1942 as *cyclic muscle spasm* and later related to the masticatory muscles by Schwartz.[16] More recently with the findings that the painful muscles are not truly in spasm, the term *cyclic muscle pain* was coined for this text. The importance of cyclic muscle pain is discussed later in this chapter.

Another common symptom associated with masticatory muscle pain is headache. Because there are numerous types of headaches, this symptom is discussed in a separate section later in this chapter.

DYSFUNCTION

Dysfunction is a common clinical symptom associated with masticatory muscle disorders. Usually it is seen as a decrease in the range of mandibular movement. When muscle tissues have been compromised by overuse, any contraction or stretching increases the pain. Therefore to maintain comfort, the patient restricts movement within a range that does not increase pain levels. Clinically this is seen as an inability to open widely. The restriction may be at any degree of opening depending on where discomfort is felt. In some myalgic disorders the patient can slowly open wider, but the pain is still present and may even become worse.

Acute malocclusion is another type of dysfunction. *Acute malocclusion* refers to any sudden change in the occlusal condition that has been created by a disorder. An acute malocclusion may result from a sudden change in the resting length of a muscle that controls jaw position. When this occurs the patient describes a change in the occlusal contact of the teeth. The mandibular position and resultant alteration in occlusal relationships depend on the muscles involved. For example, with slight functional shortening of the inferior lateral pterygoid, disocclusion of the posterior teeth will occur on the ipsilateral side and premature contact of the anterior teeth (especially the canines) on the contralateral side. With functional shortening of the elevator muscles (clinically a less detectable acute malocclusion), the patient will generally complain of an inability to occlude normally. The clinician should remember that an acute malocclusion is the *result* of the muscle disorder and not the *cause*. Therefore treatment should never be directed toward correcting the malocclusion. Rather, it should be aimed at eliminating the muscle disorder. When this condition is reduced, the occlusal condition will return to normal. As discussed later, certain intracapsular disorders can also lead to acute malocclusion.

All masticatory muscle disorders are not the same clinically. At least five different types exist, and being able to distinguish among them is important because the treatment of each is quite different. The five types are protective co-contraction (muscle splinting), local muscle soreness, myofascial (trigger point) pain, myospasm, and chronic centrally mediated myalgia. A sixth condition known as *fibromyalgia* also needs to be discussed. The first three conditions (protective co-contraction, local muscle soreness, and myofascial pain) are commonly seen in the dental office. Myospasm and chronic centrally mediated myalgia are less frequently seen. Many of these muscle disorders occur and resolve in a relatively short time. When these conditions are not resolved, more chronic pain disorders may result. Chronic masticatory muscle disorders become more complicated and treatment is generally oriented differently than for acute problems. Therefore the clinician must be able to distinguish acute muscle disorders from chronic disorders so that proper therapy can be applied. Fibromyalgia is a chronic myalgic disorder, which presents as a systemic musculoskeletal pain problem that needs to be recognized by the dentist and is best managed by referral to appropriate medical personnel.

CLINICAL MASTICATORY MUSCLE PAIN MODEL

To understand the relationships among different muscle pain disorders, a masticatory muscle pain model is presented (Fig. 8-1). The model begins with the assumption that the muscles of mastication are healthy and functioning normally (as depicted in Chapter 2). Normal muscle function can be interrupted by certain types of events. If an event is significant, a muscle response known as *protective co-contraction* (muscle splinting) occurs. In many instances the consequence of the event is minor and co-contraction resolves quickly, allowing muscle function to return to normal. If, however, protective co-contraction is prolonged, local biochemical and later structural changes can occur, creating a condition known as *local muscle soreness*. This condition may resolve spontaneously with rest or may need the assistance of treatment.

If local muscle soreness does not resolve, changes in the muscle tissues may develop, resulting in prolonged pain input. This constant deep pain input can affect the CNS, leading to certain

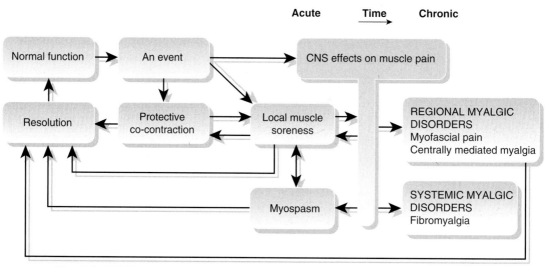

Fig. 8-1 MASTICATORY MUSCLE MODEL. This model depicts the relationship among various clinically identifiable muscle pain disorders along with some etiologic considerations. A thorough explanation of the model is given in the text. *(Modified from the original model developed by J.P. Okeson, D.A. Falace, C.R. Carlson, A. Nitz, and D.T. Anderson, Orofacial Pain Center, University of Kentucky, 1991.)*

muscle responses (see Chapter 2). Two examples of CNS-influenced muscle pain disorders are *myofascial pain* and *myospasm*. In some instances the CNS responds to certain events or local conditions by inducing an involuntary contraction seen clinically as a muscle spasm. Myospasms are not chronic but instead represent a condition of relatively short duration. At one time myospasm was thought to be the primary condition responsible for myalgia. Recent studies[11,12,17-19] suggest that true myospasms are not common in patients suffering from masticatory muscle pain.

These masticatory muscle disorders usually present as relatively acute problems and, once identified and treated, the muscle returns to normal function.[20] If, however, these acute myalgic disorders are not recognized or appropriately managed, certain perpetuating conditions can advance the problem into a more chronic myalgic disorder. As the myalgic disorder becomes more chronic, the CNS contributes more to maintaining the condition. Because the CNS is an important factor in this condition, it is referred to as *centrally mediated myalgia*. Chronic centrally mediated myalgia is often very difficult to resolve, and treatment strategies must be changed from those used with the acute myalgic disorders.

Another example of a chronic musculoskeletal pain disorder is *fibromyalgia*. Although this is not primarily a masticatory pain disorder, the dentist needs to recognize this condition so as to avoid unnecessary dental therapy. Unlike the other muscle pain disorders that are regional, fibromyalgia is a widespread, global, musculoskeletal pain condition. The dentist needs to be aware that the management of these chronic pain disorders is quite different than that of an acute muscle disorder.

To better understand the masticatory muscle pain model, each component of the model is discussed in detail.

EVENTS

Normal muscle function can be interrupted by various types of events. These events can arise from either local or systemic factors. Local factors represent any events that acutely alter sensory or proprioceptive input in the masticatory structures (e.g., the fracture of a tooth or the placement of a restoration in supraocclusion). Trauma to local structures such as tissue damage caused by a dental injection represents another type of local event. Trauma might also arise from excessive or unaccustomed use of masticatory structures, such as chewing unusually hard food or chewing for a long period of time (i.e., gum chewing). Opening too wide may produce a strain to ligaments supporting the joint and/or muscles. This may occur as a result of a long dental procedure or even by simply opening too wide (i.e., yawning).

Any source of constant deep pain input may also represent a local factor that alters muscle function. This pain input may have its source in local structures such as the teeth, joints, or even the muscles themselves. The source of the pain, however, is not significant because any constant deep pain, even idiopathic pain, may create a muscle response.[21]

Systemic factors may also represent events that can interrupt normal muscle function. One of the most commonly recognized systemic factors is emotional stress.[2,22-24] Stress seems to alter muscle function through either the gamma efferent system to the muscle spindle or by means of sympathetic activity to the muscle tissues and related structures.[25-27] Of course, responses to emotional stress are quite individualized. Therefore the patient's emotional reaction and psychophysiologic response to stressors may vary greatly. It has been demonstrated that exposing a subject to an experimental stressor can immediately increase the resting electromyographic (EMG) activity of masticatory muscles.[11,12] This physiologic response provides direct insight into how emotional stress directly influences muscle activity and muscle pain.

Other systemic factors can influence muscle function and are less understood, such as acute illness or viral infections. Likewise, a broad category of poorly understood constitutional factors that are unique to each patient exists. Such factors include immunologic resistance and autonomic balance of the patient. These factors seem to reduce the individual's ability to resist or combat the challenge or demand created by the event. Constitutional factors are likely to be influenced by age, gender, diet, and perhaps even genetic predisposition.

Clinicians realize that individual patients often respond quite differently to similar events. Therefore it is assumed that certain constitutional factors do exist and can influence the individual's response. At this time these factors are poorly understood and not well defined as they relate to muscle pain disorders.

PROTECTIVE CO-CONTRACTION (MUSCLE SPLINTING)

The first response of the masticatory muscles to one of the previously described events is protective co-contraction. Protective co-contraction is a CNS response to injury or threat of injury. This response has also been called *protective muscle splinting*.[28] It has been described for many years but only recently documented.[29-33] In the presence of an injury or threat of injury, normal sequencing of muscle activity seems to be altered so as to protect the threatened part from further injury. Protective co-contraction can be likened to the co-contraction[34] observed during many normal functional activities, such as bracing the arm when attempting a task with the fingers. In the presence of altered sensory input or pain, antagonistic muscle groups seem to fire during movement in an attempt to protect the injured part. In the masticatory system, for example, a patient experiencing co-contraction will demonstrate an increase in muscle activity of the elevator muscles during mouth opening.[29,35,36] During closing of the mouth an increased activity is noted in the depressing muscles. This coactivation of antagonistic muscles is thought to be a normal protective or guarding mechanism and needs to be recognized by the clinician. Protective co-contraction is not a pathologic condition, although when prolonged it may lead to muscle symptoms.

The etiology of protective co-contraction can be any change in sensory or proprioceptive input from associated structures. An example of such an event in the masticatory system is the placement of a high crown. Protective co-contraction can also be caused by any source of deep pain input or an increase in emotional stress.

Co-contraction is reported clinically as a feeling of muscle weakness directly following an event.

No pain occurs when the muscle is at rest, but use of the muscle usually increases the pain. The patient often presents with limited mouth opening, but when asked to open slowly, full opening can be achieved. The key to identifying co-contraction is that it immediately follows an event, and therefore the history is important. If protective co-contraction continues for several hours or days, the muscle tissue can become compromised and a local muscle problem may develop.

LOCAL MUSCLE SORENESS (NONINFLAMMATORY MYALGIA)

Local muscle soreness is a primary, noninflammatory, myogenous pain disorder. It is often the first response of the muscle tissue to prolonged co-contraction. Whereas co-contraction represents a CNS-induced muscle response, local muscle soreness represents a condition that is characterized by changes in the local environment of the muscle tissues. These changes are characterized by the release of certain algogenic substances (i.e., bradykinin, substance P, even histamine[37]) that produce pain. These initial changes may represent nothing more than fatigue. Along with protracted co-contraction, other causes of local muscle soreness are local trauma or excessive use of the muscle. When excessive use is the etiology, a delay in the onset of muscle soreness can occur.[38] This type of local muscle soreness is often referred to as *delayed onset muscle soreness* or *postexercise muscle soreness*.[39,40-43]

Because local muscle soreness itself is a source of deep pain, an important clinical event can occur. Deep pain produced by muscle soreness can, in fact, produce protective co-contraction. This additional co-contraction can, in turn, produce more muscle soreness. Therefore a cycle can be created whereby muscle soreness produces more co-contraction and so on. This cyclic muscle pain has already been discussed in earlier chapters.

The clinician needs to be aware of the complications this might pose with diagnosis. For example, the medial pterygoid muscle is injured by an inferior alveolar nerve block. This trauma causes local muscle soreness. The pain associated with the soreness in turn produces protective co-contraction. Because protective co-contraction can lead to muscle soreness, a cycle begins. During this cycling, the original tissue damage produced by the injections resolves. When tissue repair is complete, the original source of pain is eliminated; however, the patient may continue to suffer with a cyclic muscle pain disorder. Because the original cause of the pain is no longer part of the clinical picture, the clinician can easily be confused during the examination. The clinician needs to recognize that even though the original cause has resolved, a cyclic muscle pain condition exists and needs to be treated. This condition is an extremely common clinical finding and, if not recognized, often leads to mismanagement of the patient.

Local muscle soreness presents clinically with muscles that are tender to palpation and reveal increased pain with function. Structural dysfunction is common, and when the elevator muscles are involved, limited mouth opening results. Unlike protective co-contraction, the patient has great difficulty opening any wider. With local muscle soreness there is an actual muscle weakness.[44-46] Muscle strength is returned to normal when the muscle soreness is resolved.[45-47]

CENTRAL NERVOUS SYSTEM EFFECTS ON MUSCLE PAIN

The muscle pain conditions described to this point are relatively simple, having their origins predominately in the local muscle tissues. Unfortunately muscle pain can become much more complex. In many instances, activity within the CNS can either influence or actually *be* the origin of the muscle pain. This may occur either secondary to ongoing deep pain input or altered sensory input or arise from central influences such as upregulation of the autonomic nervous system (i.e., emotional stress). This occurs when conditions within the CNS excite peripheral sensory neurons (primary afferents) creating the antidromic release algogenic substances into the peripheral tissues, resulting in muscle pain (i.e., neurogenic inflammation).[14,48-50] These central excitatory effects can also lead to motor effects (primary efferents), resulting in an increase in muscle tonicity (co-contraction).[12,51]

Therapeutically, it is important that the clinician appreciates that the muscle pain now has a central origin. The CNS responds in this manner secondary to one of three factors: (1) the presence of ongoing deep pain input; (2) increased levels of emotional stress (i.e., an upregulation of the autonomic nervous system); or (3) changes in the descending inhibitory system that lead to a decrease in the ability to counter the afferent input, whether nociceptive or not.

Centrally influenced muscle pain disorders are therapeutically divided into *acute myalgic disorders* such as *myospasm* or *chronic myalgic disorders*, which are further divided into *regional myalgic disorders* or *systemic myalgic disorders*. Regional myalgic disorders are subdivided into *myofascial pain* and *chronic centrally mediated myalgia*. An example of a systemic myalgic disorder is fibromyalgia. Each of these conditions is discussed as follows.

MYOSPASM (TONIC CONTRACTION MYALGIA)

Myospasm is a CNS-induced tonic muscle contraction. For many years the dental profession believed that myospasms were the most common source of myogenous pain. More recent studies, however, shed new light on muscle pain and myospasms.

It is reasonable to expect that a muscle in spasm or tonic contraction would reveal a relatively high level of EMG activity. Studies, however, do not support the assumption that painful muscles have a significant increase in their EMG output.[8,12,17,30,51] These studies have forced us to rethink the classification of muscle pain and differentiate myospasms from other muscle pain disorders. Although myospasms of the muscles of mastication do occur, this condition is not common and when present is usually easily identified by clinical characteristics.

The etiology of myospasms has not been well documented. Several factors are likely to combine to promote myospasms. Local muscle conditions certainly seem to foster myospasms. These conditions involve muscle fatigue and changes in local electrolyte balances. Deep pain input may also precipitate myospasms.

Myospasms are easily recognized by the structural dysfunction that is produced. Because a muscle in spasm is contracted, major jaw positional changes result according to the muscle or muscles in spasm. These positional changes create certain acute malocclusions (discussed in detail in later chapters). Myospasms are also characterized by firm muscles as noted by palpation.

Myospasms are usually short lived, lasting for only minutes at a time. They are the same as one would feel from an acute cramp in a leg muscle. On occasion these uncontrolled muscle contractions can become repeated over time. When they are repeated, the condition may be classified as a dystonia. Dystonic conditions are thought to be related to CNS mechanisms and need to be managed differently than true myospasm. Certain, well-described oromandibular dystonias predominately affect the muscle of mastication. During these dystonic episodes the mouth may be forced open (opening dystonia) or closed (closing dystonia) or even off to one side. The precise jaw position is determined by the muscles involved.

REGIONAL MYALGIC DISORDERS

Myofascial Pain (Trigger Point Myalgia)

Myofascial pain is a regional myogenous pain condition characterized by local areas of firm, hypersensitive bands of muscle tissue known as *trigger points*. This condition is sometimes referred to as *myofascial trigger point pain*. It is a type of muscle disorder that is not widely appreciated or completely understood, yet it commonly occurs in patients with myalgic complaints. In one study[52] more than 50% of the patients reporting to a university pain center were diagnosed as having this type of pain.

Myofascial pain was first described by Travell and Rinzler[53] in 1952, yet the dental and medical communities have been slow to appreciate its significance. In 1969 Laskin[54] described the myofascial pain dysfunction (MPD) syndrome as having certain clinical characteristics. Although Laskin borrowed the term *myofascial*, he was not describing myofascial trigger point pain. Instead MPD syndrome has been used in dentistry as a general term to denote any muscle disorder (not an intracapsular disorder). Because the term is so broad and general, it is not useful in the specific diagnosis and management of masticatory muscle disorders. MPD syndrome should not be confused with Travell and Rinzler's description, which will be used in this textbook. The term *masticatory muscle pain* should be used as a generic term for all the types of masticatory muscle pain. *Myofascial pain* should be used only if the condition meets the original description in the medical literature (discussed in the following section).

Myofascial pain arises from hypersensitive areas in muscles called *trigger points*. These localized areas in muscle tissues, tendinous attachments, or both are often felt as taut bands when palpated, which elicits pain. The exact nature of a trigger point is not known. It has been suggested[4,55] that certain nerve endings in the muscle tissues may become sensitized by algogenic substances that create a localized zone of hypersensitivity.[56] A local temperature rise may occur at the site of the trigger point, suggesting an increase in metabolic demand, reduction of blood flow, or both to these tissues.[57,58] A trigger point is a circumscribed region in which just a relatively few motor units seem to be contracting.[59] If all the motor units of a muscle contract, the muscle will of course shorten in length (see Chapter 2). This condition is called *myospasm* and is discussed earlier in this chapter. Because a trigger point has only a select group of motor unit contracting, no overall shortening of the muscle results (as occurs with myospasm).

The unique characteristic of trigger points is that they are a source of constant deep pain and therefore can produce central excitatory effects (see Chapter 2). If a trigger point centrally excites a group of converging afferent interneurons, referred pain will often result, generally in a predictable pattern according to the location of the involved trigger point (Figs. 8-2 to 8-4). The pain is often reported by the patient as headache pain.

The etiology of myofascial pain is complex. Unfortunately, we lack a complete understanding of this myogenous pain condition. Therefore it is difficult to be specific concerning all etiologic factors. Travell and Simons[60] have described certain local and systemic factors that seem to be associated, such as trauma, hypovitaminosis, poor

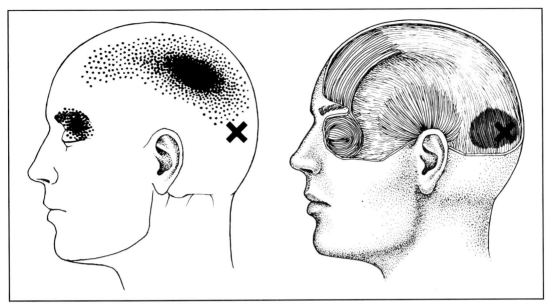

Fig. 8-2 A trigger point (marked with *x*) in the occipital belly of the occipitofrontalis muscle produces referred headache pain behind the eye. *(From Travell JG, Simons DG:* Myofascial pain and dysfunction. The trigger point manual, *Baltimore, 1983, Williams & Wilkins, p 291.)*

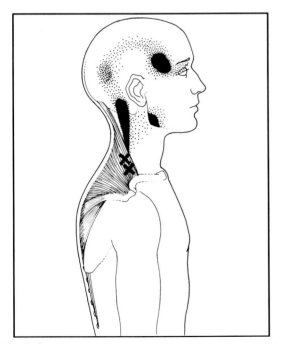

Fig. 8-3 The trigger points located in the trapezius muscle (marked with *x*) refer pain to behind the ear, the temple, and the angle of the jaw. *(From Travell JG, Simons DG:* Myofascial pain and dysfunction. The trigger point manual, *Baltimore, 1983, Williams & Wilkins, p 184.)*

physical conditioning, fatigue, and viral infections. Other important factors are likely to be emotional stress and deep pain input.

The most common clinical feature of myofascial pain is the presence of local areas of firm, hypersensitive bands of muscle tissue (i.e., trigger points). Although palpation of trigger points produces pain, local muscle sensitivity is not the most common complaint of patients suffering from myofascial trigger point pain. The most common symptom is usually associated with the central excitatory effects created by the trigger points. In many instances patients may be aware only of the referred pain and not even acknowledge the trigger points. A perfect example is the patient suffering from myofascial trigger point pain in the trapezius muscle that creates referred pain to the temple region (see Fig. 8-3).[61,62] The chief complaint is temporal headache, with little acknowledgment of the trigger point in the shoulder. This clinical presentation can easily distract the clinician from the source of the problem. The patient will draw the clinician's attention to the site of the pain (the temporal headache) and not the source. The clinician must

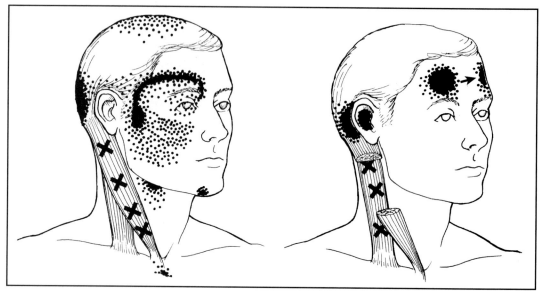

Fig. 8-4 Trigger points located in the sternocleidomastoideus refer pain to the temple area (i.e., typical temporal headache). *(From Travell JG, Simons DG: Myofascial pain and dysfunction. The trigger point manual, Baltimore, 1983, Williams & Wilkins, p 203.)*

always remember that for treatment to be effective, it must be directed toward the source of the pain, not the site. Therefore a clinician must always search for the true source of the pain.

Because trigger points can create central excitatory effects,[63-65] it is also important to be aware of all the possible clinical manifestations. As stated in Chapter 2, central excitatory effects can appear as referred pain, secondary hyperalgesia, protective co-contraction, or even autonomic responses. These conditions must be considered when evaluating the patient.

An interesting clinical feature of a trigger point is that it may present in either an active or a latent state. In the active state it produces central excitatory effects. Therefore when a trigger point is active, a headache is commonly felt. Because referred pain is wholly dependent on its original source, palpation of an active trigger point (local provocation) often increases such pain. Although not always present, when this characteristic appears it is an extremely helpful diagnostic aid. In the latent state a trigger point is no longer sensitive to palpation and therefore does not produce referred pain. When trigger points are latent, they cannot be

found by palpation and the patient does not complain of headache pain. In this case the history is the only datum that leads the clinician to make the diagnosis of myofascial pain. In some instances the clinician should consider asking the patient to return to the office when the headache is present so that confirmation of the pattern of pain referral can be verified and the diagnosis confirmed.

Experts believe that trigger points do not resolve without treatment. Trigger points may in fact become latent or dormant, creating a temporary relief of the referred pain. Trigger points may be activated by various factors[66] such as increased use of a muscle, strain on the muscle, emotional stress, or even an upper respiratory infection. When trigger points are activated, the headache returns. This is a common finding with patients who complain of regular late-afternoon headaches following a trying and stressful day.

Along with referred pain, other central excitatory effects may be felt. When secondary hyperalgesia is present, it is commonly felt as an increased sensitivity to touching of the scalp. Some patients will even report that their "hair hurts" or that it is painful to brush their hair. Co-contraction is another common condition associated with myofascial pain. Trigger points in the shoulder or cervical muscles can produce co-contraction in the muscles of mastication.[51] If this continues, local muscle soreness in the masticatory muscles can develop. Treatment of the masticatory muscles will not resolve the condition because its source is the trigger points of the cervicospinal and shoulder muscles. However, treatment of the trigger points in the shoulder muscles will resolve the masticatory muscle disorder. Management may become difficult when muscle soreness has been present for a long time because it can initiate cyclic muscle pain (see Chapter 2). In these cases extending treatment to both the muscles of mastication and the trigger points in the cervicospinal and shoulder muscles will usually resolve the problem.

On occasion, autonomic effects are produced by deep pain input from trigger points. These may result in such clinical findings as tearing or drying of the eye, or vascular changes (e.g., blanching, reddening of tissue, or both) may occur. Sometimes the conjunctiva will become red. Mucosal changes may even produce nasal discharge similar to an allergic response. The key to determining whether the autonomic effects are related to central excitatory effects or to a local reaction such as allergies is the unilateral appearance. Central excitatory effects in the trigeminal area rarely cross the midline. Therefore if the deep pain is unilateral, the autonomic effects will be on the same side as the pain. In other words, one eye will be red and the other normal, one nostril draining mucus and the other not. With allergic responses, both eyes or both nostrils will be involved.

By way of summary, the clinical symptoms reported with myofascial pain are most commonly associated with the *central excitatory effects* created by the trigger points and not the trigger points themselves. The clinician must be aware of this and find the involved trigger points. When these are palpated, they appear as hypersensitive areas often felt as taut bands within the muscle. Usually no local pain occurs when the muscle is at rest, but some pain is felt when the muscle is used. Often slight structural dysfunction will be seen in the muscle harboring the trigger points. This is commonly reported as a "stiff neck."

CONSIDERATIONS OF CHRONIC MUSCLE PAIN

The myalgic disorders that have been described are commonly seen in the general practice of dentistry and usually represent problems of short duration. With proper therapy, these disorders can be completely resolved. However, when myogenous pain persists, more chronic and often complex muscle pain disorders can develop. With chronicity, myogenous pain disorders become even more influenced by the CNS, resulting in a more regional or even occasionally global pain condition. Often cyclic muscle pain also becomes an important feature that perpetuates the condition.

As a general rule, chronic pain is considered to be pain that has been present for 6 months or longer. However, the duration of pain may not be the most important factor in determining chronicity. Some pains are experienced for years but never become chronic pain conditions. Likewise, some pain conditions become clinically chronic in a matter of months. The additional factor that must be considered is the continuity of the pain. When a pain experience is constant, with no periods of relief, the clinical manifestations of chronicity develop quickly. On the other hand, if the pain is interrupted with periods of remission (no pain), the condition may never become a chronic pain disorder. For example, cluster headache is an extremely painful neurovascular pain condition that may last for years and never become a chronic pain disorder. The reason for this is because significant periods of relief occur between episodes of pain. Conversely, the constant pain associated with centrally mediated myalgia, when left untreated, can develop the clinical manifestations of chronicity within several months.

The dentist must recognize that as myalgic complaints progress from an acute to a chronic disorder, the effectiveness of local treatment is greatly reduced. Chronic pain disorders most often need to be managed by a multidisciplinary approach. In many instances the dentist alone is not equipped to manage these disorders. Therefore it is important for the dentist to recognize chronic pain disorders and consider referring the patient to a team of appropriate therapists who are better able to manage the pain condition.

Perpetuating Factors

Certain conditions or factors, when present, may prolong the muscle pain condition. These factors are known as *perpetuating factors* and can be divided into those of a local source and those of a systemic source.

Local Perpetuating Factors. The following conditions represent local factors that can be responsible for the progression of a relatively simple acute muscle disorder into a more complex chronic pain condition:

1. *Protracted cause.* If the clinician fails to eliminate the cause of an acute myalgic disorder, a more chronic condition is likely to develop.
2. *Recurrent cause.* If the patient experiences recurrent episodes of the same etiology that produced an acute myalgic disorder, it is likely that the disorder will progress to a more chronic condition (e.g., bruxism, repeated trauma).
3. *Therapeutic mismanagement.* When a patient is improperly treated for an acute myalgic disorder, symptoms do not readily resolve. This can lead to a more chronic condition. This type of perpetuating factor emphasizes the importance of establishing the proper diagnosis and initiating effective therapy.

Systemic Perpetuating Factors. The following conditions represent systemic factors that can be responsible for the progression of an acute muscle disorder into a chronic pain condition:

1. *Continued emotional stress.* Because increased emotional stress can be an etiologic factor in the development of an acute muscle disorder, continued experience of significant levels of emotional stress can represent a perpetuating factor that may advance the condition to a more chronic pain disorder.
2. *Downregulation of the descending inhibitory system.* As mentioned in Chapter 2, the descending inhibitory system represents a group of brainstem structures that regulates ascending neural activity. An effective descending inhibitory system minimizes nociceptive input as it ascends to the cortex. If this system becomes less efficient, increased nociception can reach the cortex, resulting in a greater pain experience. The factors that lead to a downregulation

of the system are unclear, but this concept may in part help explain the marked differences in individuals' responses to various events. Perhaps factors such as nutritional deficiency and physical fitness play a role. Although a decrease in the function of the descending inhibitory system seems to fit the clinical presentation of continued pain problems, these factors have yet to be documented adequately.

3. *Sleep disturbances.* Sleep disturbances appear to be commonly associated with many chronic myalgic pain disorders.[67-72] Whether the chronic pain condition produces a sleep disturbance or whether a sleep disturbance is a significant factor in the initiation of the chronic pain condition is unknown. Regardless of this cause-and-effect question, the relationship between sleep disturbances and chronic pain disorders must be recognized because it may need to be addressed during therapy.
4. *Learned behavior.* Patients who experience prolonged suffering can develop an illness behavior that seems to perpetuate the pain disorder. In other words, people learn to be sick instead of well. Patients who present with illness behavior need to receive therapy to promote wellness behavior before complete recovery can be accomplished.
5. *Secondary gain.* Chronic pain disorders can produce certain secondary gains for the suffering patient.[73-75] When a patient learns that chronic pain can be used to alter normal life events, the patient may have difficulty giving up the pain and going back to normal responsibilities. For example, if chronic pain becomes an excuse to avoid work, it will be difficult for the clinician to resolve the pain problem unless the patient wants to return to work. Importantly, the therapist must recognize the presence of secondary gains so that they can be properly addressed. Failure to eliminate secondary gains will lead to failure in resolving the chronic pain disorder.
6. *Depression.* Psychologic depression is a common finding in chronic pain patients.[76-84] Patients who suffer for long periods of time will frequently become depressed.[85-88] Because

depression can result in an independent psychologic problem, it must be properly addressed in order to manage the patient completely.[89,90] Elimination of the pain problem alone will not necessarily eliminate depression.

Centrally Mediated Myalgia (Chronic Myositis)

Centrally mediated myalgia is a chronic, continuous muscle pain disorder originating predominantly from CNS effects that are felt peripherally in the muscle tissues. This disorder clinically presents with symptoms similar to an inflammatory condition of the muscle tissue and therefore is sometimes referred to as *myositis*. This condition, however, is not characterized by the classic clinical signs associated with inflammation (e.g., reddening, swelling), and therefore myositis is not an accurate term. A more accurate term is neurogenic inflammation. Experts now know that when the CNS becomes exposed to prolonged nociceptive input, brainstem pathways can functionally change. This can result in an antidromic effect on afferent peripheral neurons. In other words, neurons that normally only carry information from the periphery into the CNS can now be reversed to carry information from the CNS out to the peripheral tissues. This is likely to occur through the axon transport system.[21] When this occurs, the afferent neurons in the periphery can release nociceptive neurotransmitters (e.g., substance P, bradykinin), which in turn cause peripheral tissue pain. This process is called *neurogenic inflammation*.[91-95]

The important concept to remember is that the muscle pain expressed by the patient with chronic centrally mediated myalgia cannot be treated by manipulating the painful muscle tissue itself. Management must be directed to the central mechanisms, a thought process that can be foreign to dentists.

Chronic centrally mediated myalgia may be caused by the prolonged input of muscle pain associated with local muscle soreness or myofascial pain. In other words, the longer the patient complains of myogenous pain, the greater the likelihood of chronic centrally mediated myalgia. However, other central mechanisms may play a significant role in the etiology of centrally mediated myalgia, such as chronic upregulation of the autonomic nervous system, chronic exposure to emotional stress, or other sources of deep pain input.

The clinician should note that chronic centrally mediated myalgia is more closely associated with continuity of muscle pain rather than actual duration. Many muscle pain disorders are episodic, leaving intermittent times of no muscle pain. Periodic episodes of muscle pain do not produce chronic centrally mediated myalgia. A prolonged and constant period of muscle pain, however, is likely to lead to chronic centrally mediated myalgia.

On occasion, a bacterial or viral infection can spread to a muscle, producing a true infectious myositis. This condition is not common but when present needs to be identified and properly treated.

A clinical characteristic of chronic centrally mediated myalgia is the presence of constant, aching myogenous pain. The pain is present during rest and increases with function. The muscles are tender to palpate, and structural dysfunction is common. The most common clinical feature is the extended duration of the symptoms.

Chronic Systemic Myalgic Disorders (Fibromyalgia)

Chronic systemic myalgic disorders need to be recognized as such because therapy demands it. The word *systemic* is used because the symptoms are reported by the patient to be widespread or global, and the etiology appears to be associated with a central mechanism. The treatment of these conditions becomes more complicated because perpetuating factors and cyclic muscle pain also need to be addressed. A chronic systemic myalgic disorder that the dentist needs to be aware of is fibromyalgia. This condition represents a global musculoskeletal pain disorder that can often be confused with an acute masticatory muscle disorder. In the past, fibromyalgia was referred to in the medical literature as *fibrositis*. According to a major consensus report,[96] fibromyalgia is a widespread musculoskeletal pain disorder in which tenderness is found in 11 or more of 18 specific tender point sites throughout the body. Fibromyalgia is not a masticatory pain disorder, yet many patients with fibromyalgia often report similar clinical complaints as TMDs.[97-102] This similar presentation may lead to some fibromyalgia patients being mistreated with TMD therapies.[103] This occurs because 42% of patients with fibromyalgia also report TMD-like symptoms.[103] Because several chronic systemic muscle pain conditions can coexist,[104] the clinician needs to recognize them and refer the patient to the appropriate medical personnel. This chronic systemic myalgic disorder is discussed more completely in Chapter 12 so that it may be properly identified and distinguished from a masticatory muscle disorder.

FUNCTIONAL DISORDERS OF THE TEMPOROMANDIBULAR JOINTS

Functional disorders of the TMJs are probably the most common findings one sees when examining a patient for masticatory dysfunction. The reason for this is the high prevalence of signs (not necessarily the symptoms). Many of the signs, such as joint sounds, are not painful and therefore the patient may not seek treatment. When present, however, they generally fall into three broad categories: *derangements of the condyle-disc complex, structural incompatibility of the articular surfaces,* and *inflammatory joint disorders.* The first two categories have been collectively referred to as disc-interference disorders. The term *disc-interference disorder* was first introduced by Welden Bell[105] to describe a category of functional disorders that arises from problems with the condyle-disc complex. Some of these problems are caused by a derangement or alteration of the attachment of the disc to the condyle; others to an incompatibility among the articular surfaces of the condyle, disc, and fossa; and still others to the fact that relatively normal structures have been extended beyond their normal range of movement. Although these broad categories have similar clinical presentations, they are treated quite differently. Therefore it is important that they be clinically differentiated.

Inflammatory disorders arise from any localized response of the tissues that make up the TMJ. They are often the result of chronic or progressive disc derangement disorders. The two major symptoms of functional TMJ problems are pain and dysfunction.

PAIN

Pain in any joint structure (including the TMJs) is called *arthralgia*. It would seem logical that such pain should originate from the articular surfaces when the joint is loaded by the muscles. This is impossible, however, in a healthy joint because there is no innervation of the articular surfaces. Arthralgia therefore can originate only from nociceptors located in the soft tissues surrounding a joint.

Three periarticular tissues contain such nociceptors: discal ligaments, capsular ligaments, and retrodiscal tissues. When these ligaments are elongated or the retrodiscal tissues compressed, the nociceptors send out signals and pain is perceived. The person cannot differentiate among the three structures, so any nociceptors that are stimulated in any of these structures radiate signals that are perceived as joint pain. Stimulation of the nociceptors creates inhibitory action in the muscles that move the mandible. Therefore when pain is suddenly and unexpectedly felt, mandibular movement immediately ceases (nociceptive reflex). When chronic pain is felt, movement becomes limited and deliberate (protective co-contraction).

Arthralgia from normal healthy structures of the joint is a sharp, sudden, and intense pain that is closely associated with joint movement. When the joint is rested, the pain resolves quickly. If the joint structures break down, inflammation can produce a constant pain that is accentuated by joint movement. As discussed later, a breakdown of joint tissues results in a loss of normal articular surfaces, creating pain that can actually originate in the subarticular bone.

DYSFUNCTION

Dysfunction is common with functional disorders of the TMJ. Usually it presents as a disruption of the normal condyle-disc movement, with the production of joint sounds.[106-108] The joint sounds may be a single event of short duration known as a *click.* If this is loud, it may be referred to as a *pop.* *Crepitation* is a multiple, rough, gravel-like sound described as grating and complicated. Dysfunction of the TMJ may also present as catching sensations when the patient opens his or her mouth. Sometimes the jaw can actually lock. Dysfunction of the TMJ is always directly related to jaw movement.

CONTINUUM OF FUNCTIONAL DISORDERS OF THE TEMPOROMANDIBULAR JOINT

As with muscle disorders, all functional disorders of the TMJ are not the same. Therefore proper identification of symptoms and the establishment of an accurate diagnosis are essential for successful treatment. The three major categories of disorders of the TMJ are discussed, along with their various subcategories. The clinical presentation of each is identified, and the more common etiologic factors are enumerated.

Derangements of the Condyle-Disc Complex

These disorders present as a range of conditions, most of which can be viewed as a continuum of progressive events. They occur because the relationship between the articular disc and the condyle changes. To understand the relationships, it is appropriate to review briefly a description of normal joint function (see Chapter 1).

Remember that the disc is laterally and medially bound to the condyle by the discal collateral ligaments; thus translatory movement in the joint can occur only between the condyle-disc complex and the articular fossa. The only physiologic movement that can occur between the condyle and the articular disc is rotation. The disc can rotate on the condyle around the attachments of the discal collateral ligaments to the poles of the condyle. The extent of rotational movement is limited by the length of the discal collateral ligaments, as well as by the inferior retrodiscal lamina posteriorly and the anterior capsular ligament anteriorly. The amount of rotation of the disc on the condyle is also determined by the morphology of the disc, the degree of interarticular pressure, and the superior lateral pterygoid muscle and superior retrodiscal lamina.

When the mouth opens, the condyle moves forward and the disc rotates posteriorly on the condyle. The superior retrodiscal lamina becomes elongated, allowing the condyle-disc complex to translate out of the fossa. Interarticular pressure provided by the elevator muscles maintains the condyle on the thinner intermediate zone of the articular disc and prevents the thicker anterior border from passing posteriorly through the discal space between the condyle and the articular surface of the eminence. When a person bites on firm food, the interarticular pressure decreases in the ipsilateral (biting side) joint. To stabilize the joint during this power stroke, the superior lateral pterygoid pulls the condyle-disc complex forward. The fibers of the superior lateral pterygoid that are attached to the disc produce a forward rotation of the disc, allowing the thicker posterior border to maintain intimate contact between the two articular surfaces. The fibers of the superior lateral pterygoid that are attached to the neck of the condyle pull the condyle forward, bracing it against the posterior slope of the eminence.

Remember that the superior retrodiscal lamina is the only structure that can retract the disc posteriorly. This force, however, can be applied only when the condyle is translated forward, unfolding and stretching the superior retrodiscal lamina. (In the closed joint position there is no tension in the superior retrodiscal lamina.) The disc can be rotated forward by action of the superior lateral pterygoid, to which it is attached. In the healthy joint the surfaces of the condyle, disc, and articular fossa are smooth and slippery and allow easy frictionless movement.

The disc therefore maintains its position on the condyle during movement because of its morphology and interarticular pressure. Its morphology (i.e., the thicker anterior and posterior borders) provides a self-positioning feature that, in conjunction with the interarticular pressure, centers it on the condyle. Backing up this self-positioning feature are the medial and lateral discal collateral ligaments, which do not permit sliding movements of the disc on the condyle.

If the morphology of the disc is altered and the discal ligaments become elongated, the disc is then permitted to slide (translate) across the articular surface of the condyle. This type of movement is not present in the healthy joint. Its degree is determined by changes that have occurred in the morphology of the disc and the degree of elongation of the discal ligaments.

For discussion purposes, the clinician can assume that the discal ligaments become elongated. (Ligaments can only be elongated, not stretched. *Stretch* implies extension followed by a return to the original length. Ligaments do not have elasticity and therefore, once elongated, generally remain at that length; see Chapter 1.) In the normal closed joint position and during function, interarticular pressure still allows the disc to position itself on the condyle and no unusual symptoms are noted. Alteration in the morphology of the disc accompanied by elongation of the discal ligaments can change this normal functioning relationship. In the resting closed joint position, the interarticular pressure is low. If the discal ligaments become elongated, the disc is free to move on the articular surface of the condyle. Because in the closed joint position the superior retrodiscal lamina does not provide much influence on disc position, tonicity of the superior lateral pterygoid muscle will encourage the disc to assume a more forward position on the condyle.

The forward movement of the disc will be limited by the length of the discal ligaments and the thickness of the posterior border of the disc. Actually, the attachment of the superior lateral pterygoid pulls the disc not only forward but also medially on the condyle (Fig. 8-5). If the pull of this muscle is protracted, over time the posterior border of the disc can become more thinned. As this area is thinned, the disc may be displaced more in the anteromedial direction. Because the superior retrodiscal lamina provides little resistance in the closed joint position, the medial and anterior positions of the disc are maintained. As the posterior border of the disc becomes thinned, it can be displaced further into the discal space so that the condyle becomes positioned on the posterior border of the disc. This condition is known as *functional disc displacement* (Fig. 8-6). Most persons report functional displacements of the disc initially as a momentary altered sensation during movement but not usually pain. Pain may occasionally be experienced when the person bites (a power stroke) and activates the superior lateral pterygoid. As this muscle pulls, the disc is displaced further and tightness in the already elongated discal ligament can produce joint pain.

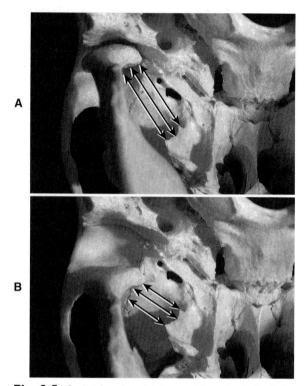

Fig. 8-5 A, In the closed joint position, the pull of the superior lateral pterygoid muscle is in an anteromedial direction *(arrows)*. **B,** When the mandible translates forward into a protrusive position, the pull of the superior head is even more medially directed *(arrows)*. In this protruded position, the major directional pull of the muscle is medial and not anterior.

When the disc is in this more forward and medial position, function of the joint can be somewhat compromised. As the mouth opens and the condyle moves forward, a short distance of translatory movement can occur between the condyle and the disc until the condyle once again assumes its normal position on the thinnest area of the disc (intermediate zone). Once it has translated over the posterior surface of the disc to the intermediate zone, interarticular pressure maintains this relationship and the disc is again carried forward with the condyle through the remaining portion of the translatory movement. After the full forward movement is completed, the condyle begins to return and the stretched fibers of the superior retrodiscal lamina actively assist in returning the

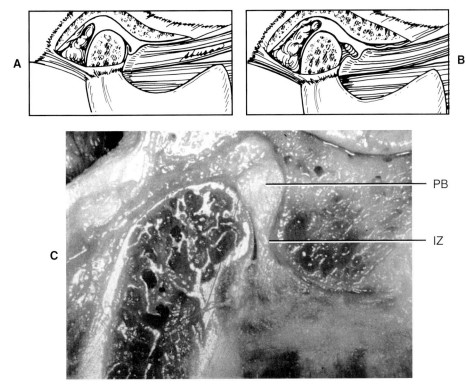

Fig. 8-6 **A,** Normal position of the disc on the condyle in the closed joint position. **B,** Functional displacement of the disc. Its posterior border has been thinned, and the discal and inferior retrodiscal ligaments are elongated, allowing activity of the superior lateral pterygoid to displace the disc anteriorly (and medially). **C,** In this specimen the condyle is articulating on the posterior band of the disc *(PB)* and not on the intermediate zone *(IZ).* This depicts an anterior displacement of the disc. *(Courtesy Dr. Julio Turell, University of Montevideo, Uruguay.)*

disc with the condyle to the closed joint position. Again, the interarticular pressure maintains the articular surface of the condyle on the intermediate zone of the disc by not allowing the thicker anterior border to pass between the condyle and the articular eminence.

Once in the closed joint position, the disc is again free to move according to the demands of its functional attachments. The presence of muscle tonicity will again encourage the disc to assume the most anteromedial position allowed by the discal attachments and its own morphology. One can imagine that if muscle hyperactivity were present, the superior lateral pterygoid muscle would have an even greater influence on the disc position.

The important feature of this functional relationship is that the condyle translates across

the disc to some degree when movement begins. This type of movement does not occur in the normal joint. During such movement the increased interarticular pressure may prevent the articular surfaces from sliding across each other smoothly. The disc can stick or be bunched slightly, causing an abrupt movement of the condyle over it into the normal condyle-disc relationship. A clicking sound often accompanies this abrupt movement. Once the joint has clicked, the normal relationship of the disc and condyle is reestablished and this relationship is maintained during the rest of the opening movement. During closing of the mouth the normal relationship of the disc and condyle is maintained because of interarticular pressure. However, once the mouth is closed and the interarticular pressure is lower, the disc can once again be displaced forward by tonicity of the superior lateral pterygoid muscle. In many instances if the displacement is slight and the interarticular pressure is low, no click is noted during this redisplacement (Fig. 8-7). This single click observed during opening movement represents the early stages of disc derangement disorder, also called *internal derangement*.

If this condition persists, a second stage of derangement is noted. As the disc is more chronically repositioned forward and medially by muscle action of the superior lateral pterygoid, the discal ligaments are further elongated. Continued forward positioning of the disc also causes elongation of the inferior retrodiscal lamina. Accompanying this breakdown is a continued thinning of the

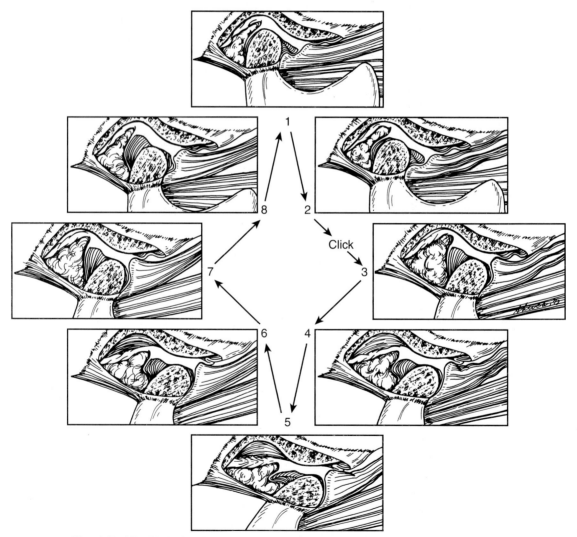

Fig. 8-7 SINGLE CLICK. Between positions 2 and 3 a click is felt as the condyle moves across the posterior border into the intermediate zone of the disc. Normal condyle-disc function occurs during the remaining opening and closing movement. In the closed joint position (*1*) the disc is again displaced forward (and medially) by activity of the superior lateral pterygoid.

posterior border of the disc, which permits the disc to be repositioned more anteriorly, resulting in the condyle being positioned more posteriorly on the posterior border.[107-109] The morphologic changes of the disc at the area where the condyle rests can create a second click during the later stages of condylar return just before the closed

joint position. This stage of derangement is called the *reciprocal click*.[110]

Reciprocal clicking (Fig. 8-8) is characterized as follows:

1. During mandibular opening, a sound is heard that represents the condyle moving across the posterior border of the disc to its normal

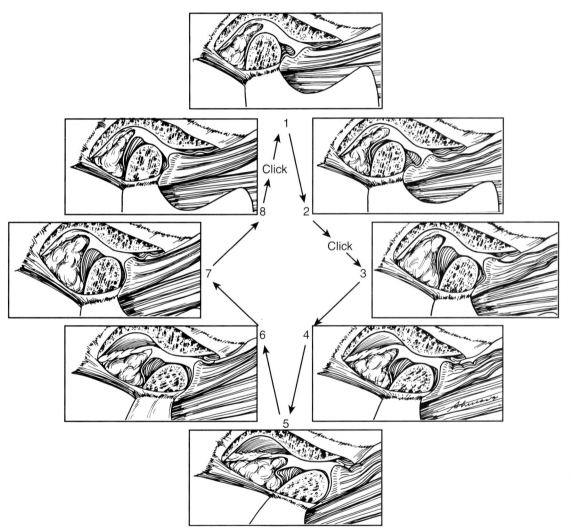

Fig. 8-8 RECIPROCAL CLICK. Between positions 2 and 3 a click is felt as the condyle moves across the posterior border of the disc. Normal condyle-disc function occurs during the remaining opening and closing movement until the closed joint position is approached. Then a second click is heard as the condyle once again moves from the intermediate zone to the posterior border of the disc (between *8* and *1*).

position on the intermediate zone. The normal disc-condyle relationship is maintained through the remaining opening movement.

2. During closing, the normal disc position is maintained until the condyle returns to near the closed joint position.

3. As the closed joint position is approached, the posterior pull of the superior retrodiscal lamina is decreased.

4. The combination of disc morphology and pull of the superior lateral pterygoid allows the disc to slip back into the more anterior position, where movement began. This final movement of the condyle across the posterior border of the disc creates a second clicking sound, and thus the reciprocal click.

The opening click can occur at any time during that movement depending on disc-condyle morphology, muscle pull, and the pull of the superior retrodiscal lamina. The closing click almost always occurs near the closed or intercuspal position (ICP).

The clinician should remember that when the disc is anteriorly displaced by the muscles, the superior retrodiscal lamina is being slightly elongated. If this condition is maintained for a prolonged period, the elasticity of the superior retrodiscal lamina can

break down and be lost. Importantly, this area is the only structure that can apply retractive force on the disc. Once this force is lost, no mechanism can retract the disc posteriorly.

Some authors[111] suggested that the superior lateral pterygoid muscle is not the major influencing factor on the anterior medial displacement of the disc. Although this would appear to be the obvious influencing factor, other features certainly need to be considered. Tanaka[112,113] has identified the presence of a ligamentous attachment of the medial portion of the condyle-disc complex to the medial wall of the fossa (Fig. 8-9). If this ligament were tightly bound, forward movement of the condyle might create a tethering of the disc to the medial. Tanaka[112] has also identified the retrodiscal tissues as being tightly attached in the medial aspect of the posterior fossa but not in the lateral aspect. This would suggest that the lateral aspect of the disc can be more easily displaced than the medial, allowing the direction of the disc displacement to be more anteromedial. Additional factors that have not yet been described are likely to exist. Further investigation in this area is necessary.

With this in mind the next stage of disc derangement can be discussed. The clinician

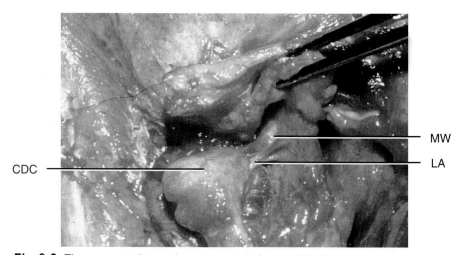

Fig. 8-9 This specimen shows a ligamentous attachment *(LA)* of the condyle-disc complex *(CDC)* to the medial wall of the fossa *(MW)*. During forward movement of the condyle, this attachment may tether the disc in an anteromedial direction. This attachment has been demonstrated by Tanaka and may help explain the anteromedial directional displacement of some discs. *(Courtesy Dr. Terry Tanaka, Chula Vista, Calif.)*

should remember that the longer the disc is displaced anteriorly and medially, the greater the thinning of its posterior border and the more the lateral discal ligament and inferior retrodiscal lamina will be elongated.[114] Also, protracted anterior displacement of the disc leads to a greater loss of elasticity in the superior retrodiscal lamina. As the disc becomes flatter, it further loses its ability to self-position on the condyle, allowing more translatory movement between condyle and disc. The more freedom of the disc to move, the more positional influence from the attachment of the superior lateral pterygoid muscle. Eventually the disc can be forced through the discal space, collapsing the joint space behind. In other words,

if the posterior border of the disc becomes thin, the functional attachment of the superior lateral pterygoid can encourage an anterior migration of the disc completely through the discal space. When this occurs, interarticular pressure will collapse the discal space, trapping the disc in the forward position. Then the next full translation of the condyle is inhibited by the anterior and medial position of the disc. The person feels the joint being locked in a limited closed position. Because the articular surfaces have actually been separated, this condition is referred to as a *functional dislocation of the disc* (Fig. 8-10).

As already described, a functionally displaced disc can create joint sounds as the condyle skids

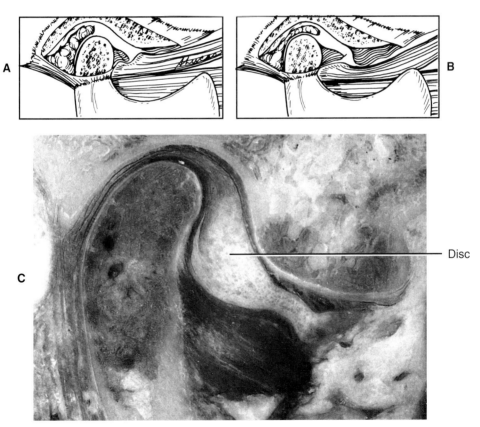

Fig. 8-10 A, Functionally displaced discs. **B,** Functionally dislocated discs. In the functionally dislocated disc, the joint space has narrowed and the disc is trapped anteriorly (and medially). **C,** In this specimen the disc is functionally dislocated anterior to the condyle. *(Courtesy Dr. Per-Lennart Westesson, University of Rochester, NY.)*

across the disc during normal translation of the mandible. If the disc becomes functionally dislocated, the joint sounds are eliminated because no skidding can occur. This can be helpful information in distinguishing a functional displacement from a functional dislocation.

Some persons with a functional dislocation of the disc can move the mandible in various lateral or protrusive directions to accommodate the movement of the condyle over the posterior border

of the disc, and the locked condition is resolved. If the lock occurs only occasionally and the person can resolve it with no assistance, it is referred to as a *functional dislocation with reduction*. The patient will often report that the jaw "catches" when opening wide (Fig. 8-11). This condition may or may not be painful depending on the severity and duration of the lock and the integrity of the structures in the joint. If it is acute, having a short history and duration, joint pain may only be associated with

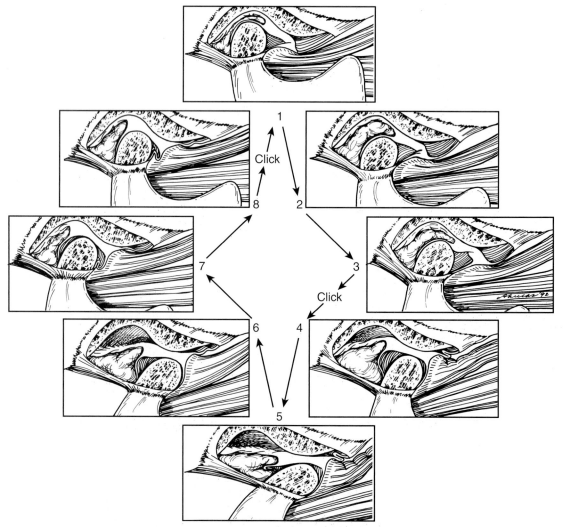

Fig. 8-11 FUNCTIONAL DISLOCATION OF THE DISC WITH REDUCTION. During opening, the condyle passes over the posterior border of the disc onto the intermediate area of the disc, thus reducing the dislocated disc (between positions *3* and *4*). A second click is heard as the condyle moves off the posterior portion of the disc as the disc is once again dislocated (between positions *8* and *1*).

elongation of the joint ligaments (such as trying to force the jaw open). As episodes of catching or locking become more frequent and chronic, ligaments break down and innervation is lost. Pain becomes less associated with ligaments and more related to forces placed on the retrodiscal tissues.

The next stage of disc derangement is known as *functional disc dislocation without reduction*. This condition occurs when the person is unable to return the dislocated disc to its normal position on the condyle.

The mouth cannot be opened maximally because the position of the disc does not allow full translation of the condyle (Fig. 8-12). Typically the initial opening will be only 25 to 30 mm interincisally, which represents the maximum rotation of the joint. The person is usually aware of which joint is involved and can remember the occasion that led to the locked feeling. Because only one joint usually becomes locked, a distinct pattern of mandibular movement is observed clinically.

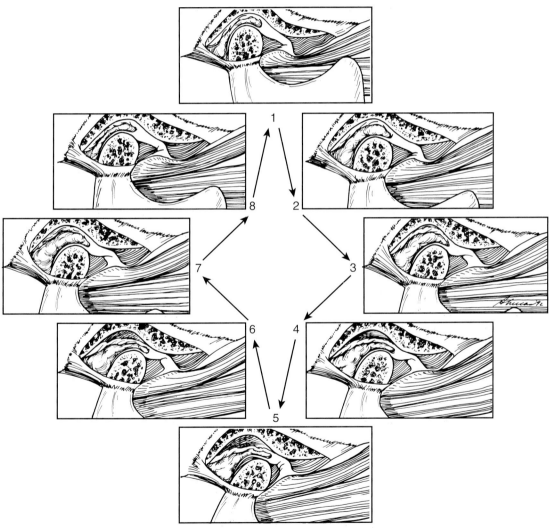

Fig. 8-12 CLOSED LOCK. The condyle never assumes a normal relationship on the disc but instead causes the disc to move forward ahead of it. This condition limits the distance it can translate forward.

The joint with the functionally dislocated disc without reduction does not allow complete translation of its condyle, whereas the other joint functions normally. Therefore when the patient opens wide, the midline of the mandible is deflected to the affected side. Also, the patient is able to perform a normal lateral movement to the affected side (the condyle on the affected side only rotates). However, when movement is attempted to the unaffected side, a restriction develops (the condyle on the affected side cannot translate past the anterior functionally dislocated disc). The dislocation without reduction has also been termed a *closed lock*[110] because the patient feels he or she is locked near the closed mouth position. Patients may report pain when the mandible is moved to the point of limitation, but pain does not necessarily accompany this condition.[115-118]

If the closed lock continues, the condyle will be chronically positioned on the retrodiscal tissues. These tissues are not anatomically structured to accept force. Therefore as force is applied, a great likelihood arises that the tissues may break down.[108,119,120] With this breakdown comes tissue inflammation (which is discussed as another category of TMJ disorders).

Any condition or event that leads to elongation of the discal ligaments or thinning of the disc can cause these derangements of the condyle-disc complex disorders. Certainly one of the most common factors is trauma. Two general types of trauma need to be considered: *macrotrauma* and *microtrauma*.

Macrotrauma. Macrotrauma is considered any sudden force to the joint that can result in structural alterations. The most common structural alteration affecting the TMJ is elongation of the discal ligaments. Macrotrauma can be subdivided into two types: direct trauma or indirect trauma.

Direct trauma. Significant direct trauma to the mandible, such as a blow to the chin, can instantly create an intracapsular disorder. If this trauma occurs when the teeth are separated (open mouth trauma) the condyle can be suddenly displaced from the fossa. This sudden movement of the condyle is resisted by the ligaments. If the force is great, the ligaments can become elongated, which may compromise normal condyle-disc mechanics. The resulting increased looseness can lead to

discal displacement and to the symptoms of clicking and catching. Unexpected macrotrauma to the jaw (as might be sustained during a fall or in a motor vehicle accident) may lead to discal displacement and/or dislocation.[121-132]

Of note is that with open mouth trauma, often the joint opposite the site of the trauma receives the most injury. For example, if an individual receives a blow to the right side of the mandible, the mandible is quickly shifted to the left. The right condyle is well supported by the medial wall of the fossae. Therefore this condyle is not displaced and ligaments are not injured. However, when a blow comes to the right side, the left condyle can be quickly forced laterally where there is no bony support, only ligaments. These ligaments can be suddenly elongated, resulting in a left TMJ disc displacement.

Macrotrauma can also occur when the teeth are together (closed mouth trauma). If trauma occurs to the mandible when the teeth are together, the intercuspation of the teeth maintains the jaw position, resisting joint displacement. Closed mouth trauma is therefore less injurious to the condyle-disc complex. This reduction of potential injury becomes obvious when one examines the incidence of injury associated with athletic activity. Athletes who wear soft protective mouth appliances have significantly fewer jaw-related injuries than those that do not.[133,134] It would be wise, therefore, if facial trauma were expected, to have a soft appliance in place or at least hold the teeth tightly in the ICP. Unfortunately, most direct macrotrauma is unexpected (i.e., motor vehicle accident) and therefore the teeth are separated, commonly resulting in injury to the joint structures.

Closed mouth trauma is not likely to be without some consequence. Although ligaments may not be elongated, articular surfaces can certainly receive sudden traumatic loading.[135] This type of impact loading may disrupt the articular surface of the condyle, fossa, or disc, which may lead to alterations in the smooth sliding surfaces of the joint, causing roughness and even sticking during movement. Therefore this type of trauma may result in adhesions, which are addressed later in this chapter.

Direct trauma may also be iatrogenic. Anytime the jaw is overextended, elongation of the ligaments can occur. Patients are more at risk for this type of injury if they have been sedated, reducing normal joint stabilization by the muscles. A few common examples of iatrogenic trauma are intubation procedures,[136-139] third molar extraction procedures, and a long dental appointment. In fact, any extended wide opening of the mouth (e.g., a yawn) has the potential to elongate the discal ligaments.[121] The medical and dental professions need to be acutely aware of these conditions so as not to create a disc derangement problem that might last the patient's lifetime.

Indirect trauma. Indirect trauma refers to injury that may occur to the TMJ secondary to a sudden force, but not one that occurs directly to the mandible. The most common type of indirect trauma reported is associated with a cervical extension/flexion injury (whiplash injury).[123,129,140,141] Although the literature reflects an association between whiplash injury and TMD symptoms, the data are still lacking regarding the precise nature of this relationship.[142-145]

Computer modeling suggests that certain motor vehicle injuries do not produce a TMJ flexion-extension event similar to that seen in the neck.[146,147] In support, human volunteers in motor vehicle crash tests fail to show jaw movement during a rear-end impact.[148] Therefore there is little compelling evidence at this time to support the concept that indirect trauma commonly results in the condyle being quickly moved within the fossa, creating a soft tissue injury similar to that seen in the cervical spine.[149,150] This is not to say that this type of injury could never occur, only that it is likely rare.

If this statement is true, why are TMD symptoms so commonly associated with cervical spine injuries?[123,129,141,144,145] The answer to this question lies in the understanding of heterotopic symptoms (see Chapter 2). The clinician always needs to be mindful that constant deep pain input originating in the cervical spine commonly creates heterotopic symptoms in the face.[48] These heterotopic symptoms may be referred pain (sensory) and/or co-contraction of masticatory muscles (motor). Kronn[141] reported that patients who experienced recent whiplash injuries have a greater incidence of TMJ pain, limited mouth opening, and masticatory muscle pain to palpation than a matched group of controls. All of these symptoms can be explained as heterotopic symptoms associated with deep pain input from the cervical spine. The clinical significance of understanding this concept is enormous because it dictates therapy. As discussed in future chapters, when these circumstances occur, therapy extended to the masticatory structures will have little effect on resolving the cervical deep pain input. Primary emphasis needs to be directed to the cervical injury (the origin of the pain).

Microtrauma. *Microtrauma* refers to any small force that is repeatedly applied to the joint structures over a long period of time. As discussed in Chapter 1, the dense fibrous connective tissues that cover the articular surfaces of the joints can well tolerate loading forces. In fact, these tissues need a certain amount of loading to survive because loading forces drive synovial fluid in and out of the articular surfaces, passing with it nutrients coming in and waste products going out. If, however, loading exceeds the functional limit of the tissue, irreversible changes or damage can result. When the functional limitation has been exceeded, the collagen fibrils become fragmented, resulting in a decrease in the stiffness of the collagen network. This allows the proteoglycan-water gel to swell and flow out into the joint space, leading to a softening of the articular surface. This softening is called *chondromalacia*.[151] This early stage of chondromalacia is reversible if the excessive loading is reduced. If, however, the loading continues to exceed the capacity of the articular tissues, irreversible changes can occur. Regions of fibrillation can begin to develop, resulting in focal roughening of the articular surfaces.[152] This alters the frictional characteristics of the surface and may lead to sticking of the articular surfaces, causing changes in the mechanics of condyle-disc movement. Continued sticking and/or roughening leads to strains on the discal ligaments during movements and eventually disc displacements[151] (discussed later in this section).

Another consideration regarding loading is the hypoxia/reperfusion theory. As previously stated, loading of the articular surfaces is normal and necessary for health. However, on occasion the forces applied to the articular surfaces can exceed the capillary pressure of the supplying vessels. If this pressure is maintained, hypoxia can develop in the structures supplied by the vessels. When the interarticular pressure is returned to normal, there is a reperfusion phase. Experts believe that during this reperfusion phase, free radicals are released into the synovial fluid. These free radicals can rapidly break down the hyaluronic acid, which protects the phospholipids that line the joint surfaces and provide important lubrication.[153-159] When the phospholipids are lost,[160] the articular surfaces joint no longer slides frictionless, leading to breakdown. The resulting "sticking" can also lead to disc displacement. Free radicals are also associated with hyperalgesic states and can therefore produce a painful joint.[161-164]

Microtrauma can result from joint loading associated with muscle hyperactivity such as bruxism or clenching.[165,166] This may be especially true if the bruxing activity is intermittent and the tissues have not had an opportunity to adapt. It is likely that if the bruxing is long-standing, the articular tissues have adapted to the loading forces and changes will not be seen. In fact, in most patients gradual loading of the articular surfaces leads to a thicker, more tolerant articular tissue.[167-169]

Another type of microtrauma results from mandibular orthopedic instability. As previously described, orthopedic stability exists when the stable ICP of the teeth is in harmony with the musculoskeletally stable position of the condyles. When this condition does not exist, microtrauma can result. This trauma occurs not when the teeth are initially brought into contact but only during loading of the masticatory system by the elevator muscles. Once the teeth are in the ICP, elevator muscle activity loads the teeth and the joints. Because the ICP represents the most stable position for the teeth, loading is accepted by the teeth without consequence. If the condyles are also in a stable relationship in the fossae, loading occurs with no adverse effect to the joint structures. If, however, loading occurs when a joint is not in a stable relationship with the disc and fossa, unusual movement can occur in an attempt to gain stability. This movement is often a translatory shift between disc and condyle. This movement can lead to elongation of the discal ligaments and thinning of the disc. Remember that the amount and intensity of the loading greatly influence whether the orthopedic instability will lead to a disc derangement disorder. Bruxing patients with orthopedic instability, therefore, are more likely to create problems than nonbruxers with the same occlusion.

An important question that arises in dentistry is, "What occlusal conditions are commonly associated with disc derangements?" It has been demonstrated that when an occlusal condition causes a condyle to be positioned posterior to the musculoskeletally stable position, the posterior border of the disc can be thinned.[170] A common occlusal condition that has been suggested to provide this environment is the skeletal Class II deep bite, which may be further aggravated when a division 2 anterior relationship also exists.[171-175] One needs to be aware, however, that not all patients with Class II malocclusions present with disc derangement disorders. Some studies show no relationship between Class II malocclusion and these disorders.[176-185] Other studies show no association between the horizontal and vertical relationship of the anterior teeth and disc derangement disorders.[186-190] The important feature of an occlusal condition that leads to disc derangement disorders is the lack of joint stability when the teeth are tightly occluded. Some Class II malocclusions likely provide joint stability, whereas others do not. Another factor that must be considered is the amount and duration of joint loading. Perhaps joint loading is more damaging with certain Class II malocclusions.

Another consideration regarding orthopedic stability and intracapsular disorders relates to tooth contacts associated with eccentric mandibular movements. Most studies to date have looked at the static relationship of the teeth and TMD symptoms. Perhaps studying tooth contacts during mandibular movements would reveal new insights. In one study a positive relationship was found between disc dislocation and nonworking tooth contacts.[191] Evidence suggests that if a nonworking contact was the predominant tooth contact during an eccentric movement, the ipsilateral condyle will experience significant reduction in loading force. If this occlusion is coupled with heavy loading such as bruxism, joint stability may result. Future studies need to be directed to the relationship of orthopedic instability and loading.

Obviously, no simple relationship exists among occlusion, orthopedic instability, and intracapsular disorders. However, it is vitally important that when orthopedic instability exists it be identified as a potential etiologic factor. The relationship between these findings and the TMD symptoms need to be evaluated in a manner that will be presented later in this text.

Orthodontics and Disc Derangement Disorders. In recent years concern has arisen regarding the effect of orthodontic treatment on disc derangement disorders. Some authors have suggested that certain orthodontic treatments can lead to disc derangement disorders.[192-195] Long-term studies of orthodontically treated populations, however, do not support these concerns.[196-207] These studies report that the incidence of TMD symptoms in a population of orthodontically treated patients is no greater than that of the untreated general population.

Furthermore, studies that looked at the specific type of orthodontic mechanisms used, such as Begg technique versus various functional techniques, also failed to show a relationship between intracapsular disorders (or any TMD symptoms) and orthodontic treatment.[199,208-211] Even the extraction of teeth for orthodontic purposes did not reveal a greater incident of TMD symptoms posttreatment.[212-216]

Although these studies are comforting to the orthodontist, one should also note that the incidence of TMD symptoms in the orthodontically treated populations was generally no lower than that of the untreated population. Therefore these findings suggest that orthodontic treatment is not effective in preventing TMDs.

Although these studies do not reveal a relationship between orthodontic therapy and TMDs, it would be naive to suggest that orthodontic therapy has no potential to predispose a patient to disc derangement disorders. Any dental procedure that produces an occlusal condition that is not in harmony with the musculoskeletally stable position of the joint can predispose the patient to these problems. This may occur secondary to orthodontic or prosthodontic or even surgical therapies.

These studies merely suggest that patients who receive conventional orthodontic therapy are no more at risk of developing TMD than those who do not.

Structural Incompatibility of the Articular Surfaces

Some disc derangement disorders result from problems between the articular surfaces of the joints. In a healthy joint the articular surfaces are firm and smooth and, when lubricated with synovial fluid, move almost without friction against each other. However, if these surfaces become altered by the microtrauma that has been described, movement is impaired. Alterations can occur because of insufficient lubrication or because of the development of adherences between the surfaces.

As described in Chapter 1, smooth articulation of the TMJs is ensured by two mechanisms: boundary lubrication and weeping lubrication. If, for any reason, the amount or quality of the synovial fluid is decreased, friction increases between the articular surfaces, which can abrade the surfaces and lead to breakdown or sticking.

Adherences are considered to be a temporary sticking of the articular surfaces, whereas adhesions are more permanent. Sometimes adherences may develop between articular surfaces even in the presence of sufficient fluid. When a joint is statically loaded, a small amount of previously absorbed synovial fluid is expressed from the articular surfaces and lubricates them (weeping lubrication). As soon as the joint moves, the reservoir of fluid in the peripheral area of the joint relubricates the surfaces, preparing them for future loading (boundary lubrication). If static loading continues for a prolonged time, however, weeping lubrication can become exhausted and sticking of the articular surfaces can result. When the static loading is finally discontinued and movement begins, a sense of stiffness is felt in the joint until enough energy is exerted to break apart the adhering surfaces.

This breaking apart of adherences can be felt as a click, and it denotes the instant return to normal range of mandibular movement (Fig. 8-13). Static loading of the joint may occur as a result of muscle hyperactivity such as clenching. For example, a patient may wake up in the morning after a night of

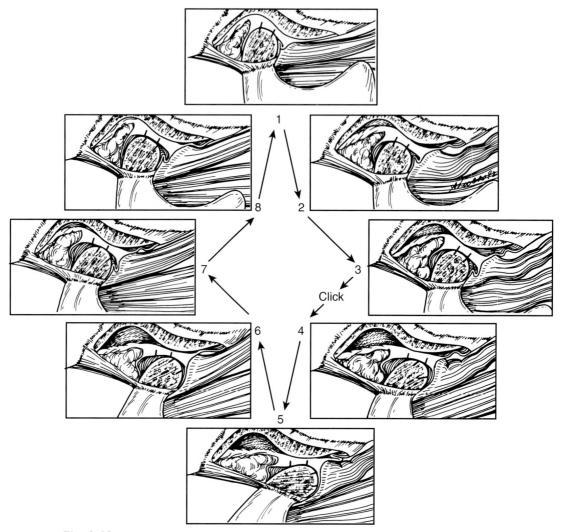

Fig. 8-13 In position 1 the adhesion is demonstrated between condyle and disc. During opening, no discal rotation occurs. In position 3 the adhesion is broken, resulting in a click and normal function from that point on. No reciprocal or additional clicking occurs unless followed by a period of static loading of the joint.

clenching and have the sensation of restricted jaw movement. As the patient tries to open his or her mouth, resistance is felt until suddenly there is a click and normal function returns. This sound represents the breaking apart of sticking surfaces. Clicks caused by temporary adherences can be differentiated from clicks associated with disc displacements by the fact that they occur only once following a period of static loading. After the single click, the joint becomes lubricated with boundary lubrication and it is silent during subsequent opening and closing. With a disc displacement, the clicking is repeated during each opening and closing cycle.

Adherences can occur between the disc and the condyle, as well as between the disc and the fossa. When they occur in the inferior joint space, the condyle and disc stick together, inhibiting normal rotational movement between them. Although the patient can translate the condyle forward to a relatively normal mouth opening, the movement is felt as rough and jumpy. Often there is also joint stiffness. When adherences occur in the superior joint space, the disc and fossa stick together, inhibiting normal translatory movement between them.[217,218] The patient can usually separate the teeth only 25 to 30 mm. This condition is similar to a closed lock. An accurate diagnosis is made by taking a careful history.

The clinician should remember that the term *adherence* implies that the articular structures have become temporarily stuck together but there have not been any changes to physically bind the tissues together. Once enough force is generated to break the adherence, normal function returns. If, however, the adherence remains for a significant period of time, fibrous tissue can develop between the articular structures and a true adhesion can develop. This condition represents a mechanical connection that limits normal condyle/disc/fossa function on a more permanent base.[219]

Both macrotrauma and microtrauma can be significant etiologic factors in TMJ adhesion problems. When trauma alters the articular surfaces, they can be abraded, leading to sticking problems. Generally, closed mouth trauma is the specific type of injury that leads to adhesions. When the jaw sustains a blow with the teeth in occlusion, the major structures receiving the force of impact are the articular surfaces of the joints and the teeth. This type of injury can alter the smooth frictionless surfaces of the joint. Another etiologic factor of adhesions is hemarthrosis (bleeding within the joint). The presence of blood byproducts seems to provide a matrix for the fibrous unions found within adhesions.[156] Hemarthrosis can occur when the retrodiscal tissues are disrupted by either external jaw trauma or surgical intervention.

As with any mobile joint, the articular surfaces of the TMJs are maintained in constant close contact. Because of this, the morphologic characteristics of the surfaces usually conform to each other closely. If the morphology of the disc, condyle, or fossa is altered, joint function can be impaired. For example, a bony protuberance on the condyle or fossa may catch the disc at certain degrees of opening, causing alterations in function. The disc itself may become thinned (as with disc displacement) or even perforated, causing significant changes in function. These alterations in form can create clicking and catching of the jaw similar to that seen with functional disc displacements.

The main clinical characteristic differentiating this type of problem from disc displacements is the consistent presence and location of symptoms during jaw movement. Because the disorder is associated with altered form, the symptoms always occur at the degree of mandibular opening at which normal function is disrupted (Fig. 8-14). During mandibular closure the symptoms likewise occur at the same interincisal opening, even when the speed and force of opening and closing change. As previously stated, with disc displacements the opening and closing clicks are usually at different interincisal distances. Also, with disc displacements, changing the speed and force of opening can often alter the associated symptoms associated.

Alterations in form may be caused by developmental conditions or direct trauma. Some of the inflammatory conditions discussed in the next section may also lead to alterations in articular surface form.

Subluxation. The term *subluxation* (sometimes referred to as *hypermobility*) is used to describe certain clinically observed movements of the TMJ during wide opening. Normal joint anatomy permits a relatively smooth movement of the condyle as it translates down and over the articular eminence. This movement is assisted by the posterior rotation of the disc on the condyle during translation. The anatomy of some joints, however, does not lend itself to this smooth movement. Clinical observations of some joints reveal that as the mouth opens to its fullest extent, a momentary pause occurs, followed by a sudden jump or leap to the maximally open position. This jump does not produce a clicking sound but instead is accompanied by more of a thud. The examiner can readily see it by watching the side of the patient's face. During maximum opening the lateral poles of the condyles will jump forward, causing a noticeable preauricular depression. This condition is called *subluxation* or *hypermobility*.[220]

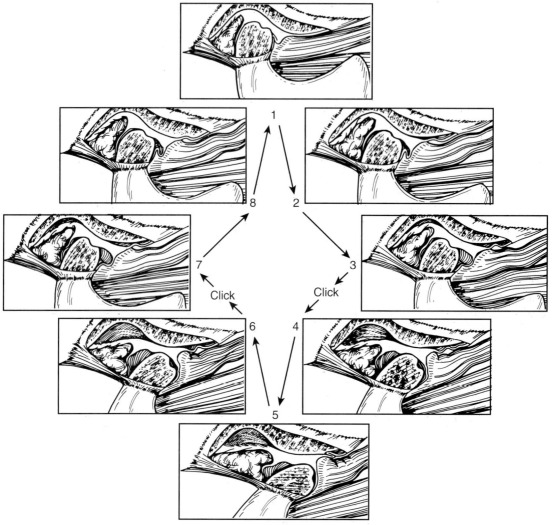

Fig. 8-14 In position 1 the structural defect (alteration in form) occurs in the condyle and disc. Between positions 3 and 4 the condyle moves out of the defect, creating a click. The condyle returns to this defect between positions 6 and 7. The opening and closing clicks occur at the same degree of opening.

The cause of subluxation is usually not pathologic. Subluxation is more likely to occur in a TMJ whose articular eminence has a short steep posterior slope followed by a longer, flatter anterior slope. The anterior slope is often more superior than the crest of the eminence. During opening the steep eminence requires a significant amount of discal rotation to occur before the condyle reaches the crest. As the condyle reaches the crest, the disc rotates posteriorly on the condyle to the maximum degree allowed by the anterior capsular ligament. In the normal joint, maximum posterior rotation of the disc and maximum translation of the condyle are reached at the same point of movement. In the subluxating joint, maximum rotational movement of the disc is reached before maximum translation of the condyle. Therefore as the mouth opens wider, the last portion of the translatory movement occurs with a bodily shift of the condyle and disc as a unit. This is abnormal, and it creates a quick forward leap and thud of the condyle-disc complex. The actual relationship between subluxation and TMD is not well established.[221] Subluxation is an anatomic feature of some joints and not pathology. However, if an individual repeatedly subluxates the mandible, elongation of ligaments could occur, potentially leading to some to the disc interference disorders described in this chapter.

Spontaneous Dislocation. On occasion the mouth is opened beyond its normal limit, and the mandible locks. This is called *spontaneous dislocation* or an *open lock*. Most dentists will eventually experience this condition in a patient following a wide opening dental procedure. It should not be confused with the closed lock, which occurs with a functionally dislocated disc without reduction. With spontaneous dislocation, the patient cannot close the mouth. This condition is almost always produced by wide opening (e.g., an extended yawn or a long dental procedure).

Spontaneous dislocation typically occurs in a patient who has the fossa anatomy that permits subluxation. As with subluxation, the disc becomes maximally rotated on the condyle before full translation of the condyle occurs. The end of translation therefore represents a sudden movement of the condyle-disc complex as a unit. If, in the maximally open position of the mouth, pressure is applied to force it open wider, the tight attachment of the anterior capsular ligament can cause a bodily rotation of the condyle and disc, moving the disc farther anteriorly through the discal space (Fig. 8-15). The discal space collapses as the condyle rides up on the retrodiscal tissues, and this traps the disc forward. This concept was proposed by Bell,[222] but other authors[223,224] have found that in some individuals the condyle actually moves in front of the disc, trapping it behind (Fig. 8-16). Although there is some debate on the precise position of the disc during an open lock, in both concepts the disc and condyle are trapped anterior to the crest of the eminence.

When this occurs the patient often becomes panicked and will react by attempting to close the mouth, which activates the elevator muscles and collapses the discal space even more. Therefore the patient's efforts can actually prolong the dislocation. In these joints the anterior slope is commonly more superior to the crest of the eminence, and therefore a mechanical locking exists in the open mouth position.

Importantly, the clinician should note that spontaneous dislocation can occur in any TMJ that is forced beyond the maximum limit of opening. However, it

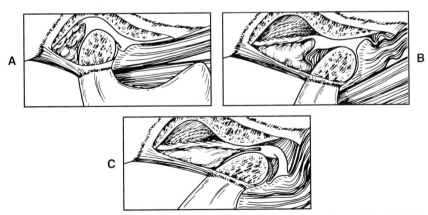

Fig. 8-15 SPONTANEOUS DISLOCATION (WITH DISC ANTERIORLY DISLOCATED). A, Normal condyle-disc relationship in the resting closed joint position. **B,** In the maximum translated position, the disc has rotated posteriorly on the condyle as far as permitted by the anterior capsular ligament. **C,** If the mouth is forced open wider, the disc is pulled forward by the anterior capsular ligament through the disc space. As the condyle moves superiorly, the disc space collapses, trapping the disc forward.

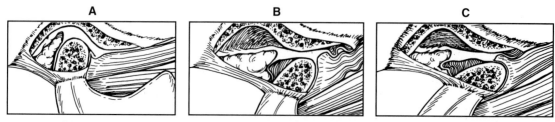

Fig. 8-16 SPONTANEOUS DISLOCATION (WITH DISC POSTERIORLY DISLOCATED). A, Normal condyle-disc relationship in the resting closed joint position. **B,** In the maximum translated position, the disc has rotated posteriorly on the condyle as far as permitted by the anterior capsular ligament. **C,** If the mouth is forced open wider, the condyle is forced over the disc, dislocating it posterior to the condyle. As the condyle moves superiorly, the disc space collapses, trapping the disc posteriorly.

usually presents in a joint that shows subluxation tendencies. Spontaneous dislocation is not the result of a pathologic condition. It is a normal joint that has been moved beyond normal border limits.

Factors That Predispose to Disc Derangement Disorders

Several anatomic features of a joint may predispose a patient to disc derangement disorders. Although they may not be changeable features, knowledge of them can explain why some joints seem to be more susceptible than others to these disorders.

Steepness of the Articular Eminence. As discussed in Chapter 6, the steepness of the posterior slope of the articular eminence varies from patient to patient. The degree of steepness of the posterior slope greatly influences condyle-disc function. In a patient with a flat eminence, there is a minimum amount of posterior rotation of the disc on the condyle during opening. As the steepness increases, more rotational movement is required between the disc and condyle during forward translation of the condyle (Fig. 8-17).[225] Therefore patients with steep eminences are more likely

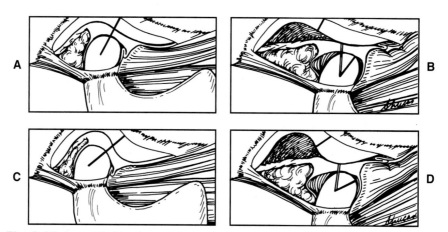

Fig. 8-17 A and **B,** Translation of a joint with a shallow articular eminence. Note the degree of rotational movement that occurs between the condyle and the articular disc. **C** and **D,** Steep articular eminence. The degree of rotational movement between the condyle and the disc is much greater in the joint with a steeper articular eminence. *(Modified from Bell WE: Temporomandibular disorders, ed 2, Chicago, 1986, Year Book Medical.)*

to demonstrate greater condyle-disc movement during function. This exaggerated condyle-disc movement may increase the risk of ligament elongation that leads to disc derangement disorders. Although some studies have found this relationship to be true,[226,227] others have not.[228-230] Perhaps this predisposing factor is only significant when combined with other factors that relate to the amount of joint function and loading.

Morphology of the Condyle and Fossa. Evidence from autopsy studies[231] suggests that the anatomic form of the condyle and fossa may predispose the disc to displacement. Flat or gablelike condyles that articulate against inverted V-shaped temporal components seem to have an increased incidence of disc derangement disorders and degenerative joint disease. It would appear that flatter, broader condyles distribute forces better, leading to fewer loading problems.[232]

Joint Laxity. As stated in Chapter 1, ligaments act as guide wires to restrict certain movements of the joint. Although the purpose of ligaments is to restrict movement, the quality and integrity of these collagenous fibers vary from patient to patient. As a result, some joints will show slightly more freedom or laxity than others. Some generalized laxity may be caused by increased levels of estrogen.[233-235] For example, women's joints are generally more flexible and lax than men's.[236] Some studies demonstrate[125,237-246] that women with general joint laxity have a higher incidence of TMJ clicking than do women without this trait. Still other studies find no relationship.[247-254] Although this relationship is not clear, it likely represents one of many factors that may help explain the higher incidence of females than males with TMDs.

Hormonal Factors. Another such factor may relate to hormonal changes associated with menstruation. It has been demonstrated that the premenstrual phase is associated with increases in EMG activity that may be related to pain.[255] The premenstrual phase seems to be associated with an increase of TMD symptoms.[256-258] The use of oral contraceptives has also been associated with TMD pain.[259] Estrogen has been found to be an important factor in certain pain pathways,[260,261] suggesting that shifting levels of estrogen may alter some nociceptive transmission.

Another interesting finding regarding sex differences is that female muscles appear to have a lower endurance time than male muscles.[262] Whether this factor has any effect on clinical pain in unknown.

Attachment of the Superior Lateral Pterygoid Muscle. Chapter 1 stated that the superior lateral pterygoid muscle originates at the infratemporal surface of the greater sphenoid wing and attaches to the articular disc and neck of the condyle. The exact percentage of attachment to the disc and condyle has been debated and is apparently variable. However, it would be reasonable to assume that if the attachment of the muscle is greater to the neck of the condyle (and less to the disc), muscle function will have correspondingly less influence on disc position. Conversely, if the attachment is greater to the disc (and less to the condylar neck), muscle function will correspondingly influence disc position more. This anatomic variation may help explain why in some patients the discs seem to be displaced quickly, even dislocated, without particularly remarkable histories or other clinical findings.[263]

Inflammatory Joint Disorders

Inflammatory joint disorders are a group of disorders in which various tissues that make up the joint structure become inflamed as a result of insult or breakdown. Any or all of the joint structures may be involved. Disorders that fit into this category are synovitis, capsulitis, retrodiscitis, and the arthritides. A few inflammatory disorders are also related to structures associated with the TMJ.

Unlike disc derangement disorders, in which pain is often momentary and associated with joint movement, inflammatory disorders are characterized by constant, dull, aching pain that is accentuated by joint movement.

Synovitis. When the synovial tissues that line the recess areas of the joint become inflamed, the condition is called *synovitis*.[264,265] This type of pain is characterized by constant intracapsular pain that is enhanced with joint movement. Synovitis is commonly caused by any irritating condition within the joint. It may result in unusual function or trauma. It is usually difficult to clinically differentiate the inflammatory disorders from each other because the clinical presentations are similar.[265,266] For example, synovitis and capsulitis are nearly impossible to clinically separate. Often, differential diagnosis is only important if treatment is different, as discussed in later chapters.

Capsulitis. When the capsular ligament becomes inflamed, the condition is called *capsulitis*. It usually presents clinically as tenderness when the lateral pole of the condyle is palpated. Capsulitis produces pain even in the static joint position, but joint movement generally increases the pain. Although a number of etiologic factors can contribute to capsulitis, the most common is macrotrauma (especially an open mouth injury). Thus whenever the capsular ligament is abruptly elongated and an inflammatory response is detected, it is likely that trauma will be found in the patient's history. Capsulitis can also develop secondary to adjacent tissue breakdown and inflammation.

Retrodiscitis. The retrodiscal tissues are highly vascularized and innervated. Thus they are unable to tolerate much loading force. If the condyle encroaches on these tissues, breakdown and inflammation are likely.[267] As with other inflammatory disorders, inflammation of the retrodiscal tissues *(retrodiscitis)* is characterized by constant, dull, aching pain that is often increased by clenching. If the inflammation becomes great, swelling may occur and force the condyle slightly forward down the posterior slope of the articular eminence. This shift can cause an acute malocclusion. Clinically such an acute malocclusion is seen as disengagement of the ipsilateral posterior teeth and heavy contact of the contralateral canines.

As with capsulitis, trauma is the major etiologic factor with retrodiscitis. Open mouth macrotrauma (a blow to the chin) can suddenly force the condyle onto the retrodiscal tissues. Microtrauma can also be a factor and is usually associated with discal displacement. As the disc is thinned and the ligaments become elongated, the condyle begins to encroach on the retrodiscal tissues. The first area of breakdown is the inferior retrodiscal lamina,[268] which allows even more discal displacement. With continued breakdown, disc dislocation occurs and forces the entire condyle to articulate on the retrodiscal tissues. If the loading is too great for

the retrodiscal tissue, breakdown continues and perforation can occur. With perforation of the retrodiscal tissues, the condyle may eventually move through these tissues and articulate with the fossa.

Arthritides. Joint *arthritides* represent a group of disorders in which destructive bony changes are seen. One of the most common types of TMJ arthritides is called *osteoarthritis* (sometimes called *degenerative joint disease*). Osteoarthritis represents a destructive process by which the bony articular surfaces of the condyle and fossa become altered. It is generally considered to be the body's response to increased loading of a joint.[269] As loading forces continue, the articular surface becomes softened (chondromalacia) and the subarticular bone begins to resorb. Progressive degeneration eventually results in loss of the subchondral cortical layer, bone erosion, and subsequent radiographic evidence of osteoarthritis.[264] Importantly, the clinician should note that radiographic changes are only seen in later stages of osteoarthritis and may not reflect the disease accurately (see Chapter 9).

Osteoarthritis is often painful, and jaw movement accentuates the symptoms. Crepitation (grating joint sounds) is a common finding with this disorder. Osteoarthritis can occur any time the joint is overloaded but is most commonly associated with disc dislocation[270,271] or perforation.[272] Once the disc is dislocated and the retrodiscal tissues break down, the condyle begins to articulate directly with the fossa, accelerating the destructive process. In time the dense fibrous articular surfaces are destroyed, and bony changes occur. Radiographically, the surfaces seem to be eroded and flattened. Any movement of these surfaces creates pain, so jaw function usually becomes restricted. Although osteoarthritis is in the category of inflammatory disorders, it is not a true inflammatory condition. Often once loading is decreased, the arthritic condition can become adaptive. The adaptive stage has been referred to as *osteoarthrosis*.[269,273] (A more detailed description of osteoarthritis/osteoarthrosis is provided in Chapter 13.)

Other types of arthritides certainly affect the TMJ. These conditions are discussed in later chapters.

SUMMARY OF THE CONTINUUM

Disorders of the TMJs may follow a path of progressive events, a continuum, from the initial signs of dysfunction to osteoarthritis. They are summarized in Fig. 8-18 and as follows:

1. Normal healthy joint
2. Loss of normal condyle/disc function caused by one of the following:
   a. Macrotrauma that resulted in elongation of the discal ligaments

   or

   b. Microtrauma that created changes in the articular surface, reducing the frictionless movement between the articular surfaces
3. Abnormal translatory movement begins between the disc and condyle.
4. Posterior border of the disc becomes thinned.
5. Further elongation of the discal and inferior retrodiscal ligaments

6. Disc becomes functionally displaced.
   a. Single click
   b. Reciprocal click
7. Disc becomes functionally displaced.
   a. Dislocation with reduction (catching)
   b. Dislocation without reduction (closed lock)
8. Retrodiscitis
9. Osteoarthritis

Although this continuum is logical, the question must be asked whether these events are always progressive. This question is of great significance because if all patients continue to progress in this manner, steps must be taken to resolve any joint symptoms as soon as they first appear. The sequence of breakdown is logical and has clinical support.[274-277] Factors such as trauma, however, may alter it. The question of real significance is whether the sequence is a continuing progression for each patient. Clinically it appears that some

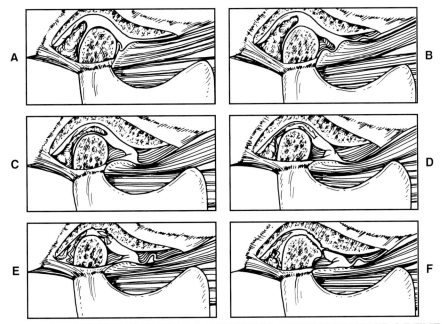

Fig. 8-18 VARIOUS STATES OF INTERNAL DERANGEMENT OF THE TEMPOROMANDIBULAR JOINT. A, Normal joint. **B,** Functional displacement of the disc. **C,** Functional dislocation of the disc. **D,** Impingement of retrodiscal tissues. **E,** Retrodiscitis and tissue breakdown. **F,** Osteoarthritis. *(Modified from Farrar WB, McCarty WL: A clinical outline of temporomandibular joint diagnosis and treatment, ed 7, Montgomery, Ala, 1983, Normandie Publications, p 72.)*

patients will present in one stage but may not necessarily progress to the next. At a given stage of disc derangement the patient may reach a level of adaptability, and no further breakdown will occur.[278,279] This can be supported by histories of asymptomatic single and reciprocal clicks over many years. It also implies that not all patients with joint sounds need treatment. Perhaps the key to treatment lies in the obvious progression from one stage to the next. Also, the presence of pain is important because it implies continuous breakdown. (Later chapters discuss treatment considerations for these disorders.)

FUNCTIONAL DISORDERS OF THE DENTITION

Like the muscles and joints, the dentition can show signs and symptoms of functional disorders. These are normally associated with breakdown created by heavy occlusal forces to the teeth and their supportive structures. Signs of breakdown in the dentition are common, yet only on occasion do patients complain of these symptoms.

MOBILITY

One site of dental breakdown is the supportive structures of the teeth. When this occurs, the clinical sign is tooth mobility, observed clinically as an unusual degree of movement of a tooth within its bony socket.

Two factors can lead to tooth mobility: loss of bony support and unusually heavy occlusal forces.

As chronic periodontal disease reduces the bony support of a tooth, mobility occurs. This type of mobility is apparent regardless of the occlusal forces placed on the teeth (although heavy forces may enhance the degree). The loss of bony support is primarily a result of periodontal disease (Fig. 8-19, *A*).

The second factor that can cause tooth mobility is unusually heavy occlusal forces. This type of mobility is closely related to muscle hyperactivity and thus becomes a sign of a functional disturbance of the masticatory system. As unusually heavy forces (especially those directed horizontally) are

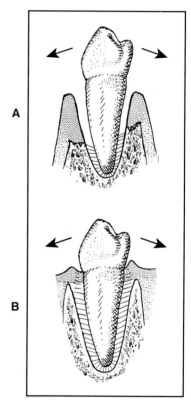

Fig. 8-19 TOOTH MOBILITY. Tooth mobility can be caused by loss of periodontal supportive structures (secondary traumatic occlusion) **(A)** or unusually heavy occlusal forces (primary traumatic occlusion) **(B).** (The width of the periodontal ligament has been exaggerated for illustrative purposes.)

placed on the teeth, the periodontal ligament cannot successfully distribute them to the bone. When heavy horizontal forces are applied to the bone, the pressure side of the root shows signs of cellular breakdown, whereas the opposite side (tension side) shows signs of vascular dilation and elongation of the periodontal ligament.[280,281] This increases the width of the periodontal space on both sides of the tooth; the space is initially filled with soft granulation tissue, but as the condition becomes chronic, the granulation tissue changes to collagenous and fibrous connective tissue, still leaving the increased periodontal space.[282] This increased width creates increased mobility of the tooth (Fig. 8-19, *B*).

The amount of clinical mobility depends on the duration and degree of force applied to the tooth or teeth. Sometimes a tooth can become so mobile that it will move out of the way, allowing the heavy forces to be placed on other teeth. For example, during a laterotrusive movement, heavy contact occurs on a lower first premolar, which disoccludes the canine. If this force is too extreme for the tooth, mobility results. As the mobility increases, continued laterotrusive movement displaces the first premolar, resulting in contact with the canine. The canine is usually a structurally sound tooth and able to tolerate this force. Therefore the amount of mobility of the premolar is limited to the degree and direction of contact before it is disoccluded by the canine.

Because two independent factors cause tooth mobility (periodontal disease and occlusal forces), the question arises: How, if at all, can they interact? More specifically, can occlusal force cause periodontal disease? This question has been researched and debated for some time and is still not completely resolved. It has been widely accepted that occlusal forces can create resorption of the lateral bony support of the tooth but do not create breakdown of the supracrestal fibers of the periodontal ligament. In other words, heavy occlusal force does not create apical migration of the epithelial attachment of the gingiva.[283,284] With the attachment remaining healthy, pathologic changes occur only at the level of the bone. Once the heavy occlusal forces are removed, the bony tissue resolves and the mobility decreases to a normal level. Therefore no permanent alteration in the gingival attachment or supportive structures of the tooth has occurred.

However, a different sequence of destruction appears to occur when an inflammatory reaction to plaque (gingivitis) is also present. The presence of gingivitis causes a loss of the epithelial attachment of the gingiva. This marks the beginning of periodontal disease, regardless of the occlusal forces. Once the attachment is lost and inflammation nears the bone, it appears that heavy occlusal forces can play a significant role in the destructive loss of supportive tissue. In other words, periodontal disease coupled with heavy occlusal forces tends to result in a more rapid loss of bony tissue.[281,285,286]

Unlike mobility without inflammation, mobility with associated bone loss is irreversible. Although evidence tends to support this concept, some research nevertheless does not substantiate it.[287]

Specific terminology is used to describe tooth mobility that relates to inflammation and heavy occlusal stress. *Primary traumatic occlusion* is mobility resulting from unusually heavy occlusal forces applied to a tooth with basically normal periodontal supportive structure. This type is usually reversible when the heavy occlusal forces are eliminated. *Secondary traumatic occlusion* results from occlusal forces, which may be either normal or unusually heavy, acting on already weakened periodontal supportive structures. With this type, periodontal disease is present and needs to be addressed.

Another interesting phenomenon originally thought to be associated with heavy loading of the teeth is the development of mandibular tori. Studies[288,289] have found a significant association between the presence of mandibular tori in a TMD population, as compared with a control group. However, no findings could help explain the relationship. A more common thought today is that the etiology of mandibular tori relates to an interplay between genetic factors and environmental conditions.[290]

PULPITIS

Another symptom that is sometimes associated with functional disturbances of the dentition is pulpitis. The heavy forces of parafunctional activity, especially when placed on a few teeth, can create the symptoms of pulpitis.[291] Typically the patient complains of hot or cold sensitivity. The pain is usually of short duration and characterized as a reversible pulpitis. In extreme cases the trauma can be great enough that the pulpal tissues reach a point of irreversibility, and pulpal necrosis ensues.

Some experts have suggested that an etiology of pulpitis is the chronic application of heavy forces to the tooth. This overloading can alter the blood flow through the apical foramen.[292] This alteration in the blood supply to the pulp gives rise to the symptoms of pulpitis. If the blood supply is

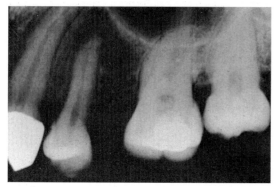

Fig. 8-20 The maxillary first premolar is nonvital because of heavy occlusal forces. This condition began when a crown was placed on the maxillary canine. The original laterotrusive guidance was not reestablished on the crown, resulting in heavy laterotrusive contact on the premolar (traumatic occlusion). The canine root is of a much more favorable size for accepting lateral (horizontal) forces than is the smaller premolar root.

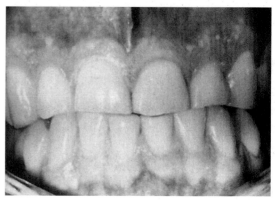

Fig. 8-21 Tooth wear during a protrusive movement.

severely altered or if lateral forces are great enough to completely block or sever the tiny artery passing into the apical foramen, pulpal necrosis may occur (Fig. 8-20).

Pulpitis can also result from other etiologic factors, such as caries or a recent dental procedure. Clinical and radiographic examination procedures are helpful in ruling out these other factors. When more obvious factors have been ruled out, occlusal trauma should be considered. Often a thorough history assists in identifying this frequently missed diagnosis.

TOOTH WEAR

By far the most common sign associated with functional disturbances of the dentition is tooth wear. This is observed as shiny flat areas of the teeth that do not match the natural occlusal form of the tooth. An area of wear is called a *wear facet.* Although wear facets are an extremely common finding in patients, symptoms are rarely reported. Those that are reported usually center around aesthetic concerns and not discomfort.

The etiology of tooth wear stems predominantly from parafunctional activity. This can be verified by merely observing the location of most wear facets.

If tooth wear were associated with functional activities, it would logically be found on the functional tooth surfaces (i.e., maxillary lingual cusps and mandibular buccal cusps). After examining patients it becomes evident that most tooth wear results from eccentric tooth contacts created by bruxing types of movement (Fig. 8-21). The position of the mandible that allows the facets to match up clearly falls outside the normal range of functional (Fig. 8-22). The only way to explain the presence of these facets is through the eccentric positions assumed during nocturnal bruxism.

In a careful examination of 168 general dental patients,[293] 95% were observed to have some form of tooth wear. This finding suggests that nearly all

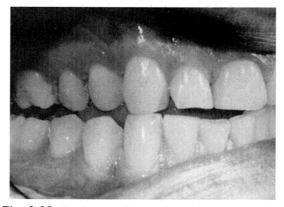

Fig. 8-22 Tooth wear during a laterotrusive movement. When the wear facets are positioned to oppose each other, the posterior teeth are beyond any functional range.

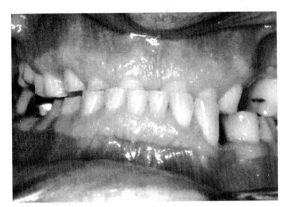

Fig. 8-23 Severe tooth wear secondary to bruxism, which compromises functional activities of the masticatory system.

patients experience some level of parafunctional activity at some time during their lives. It further suggests that parafunctional activity is a normal process, but certainly not without complications in some patients. Tooth wear can be a destructive process and may eventually lead to functional problems (Fig. 8-23). For the most part, however, tooth wear is normally asymptomatic and therefore perhaps the most tolerated form of breakdown in the masticatory system. Tooth wear has not been found to be strongly associated with TMD symptoms.[294]

Some wear facets are found near the centric occlusal stops of opposing teeth. This is especially common in the anterior region. Although these may be the result of parafunctional activity, some clinicians[295] have suggested that this type of tooth wear results when tooth structure infringes on the functional envelope of motion. In other words, this may result more often in patients who have their anterior teeth contacting heavier than the posterior teeth in the alert feeding position. When this condition exists, the functional activity of chewing results in heavy anterior tooth contact. If this continues, wear may be produced.

The difference between these two types of tooth wear is important because the etiology is quite different. Tooth wear secondary to nocturnal bruxism is centrally induced (see Chapter 7) and needs to be managed by attempting to control central mechanisms (e.g., stress management) and/or protecting the teeth with an occlusal appliance. On the other hand, tooth wear secondary to tooth structure that is infringing on the functional envelope of motion may be treated by adjusting the teeth to produce more freedom during functional movements. At this time the data on this subject are still weak. Whether these differences actually exist and how one can differentiate them for the proper selection of treatment has yet to be determined.

OTHER SIGNS AND SYMPTOMS ASSOCIATED WITH TEMPOROMANDIBULAR DISORDERS

HEADACHE

Headache is one of the most common pain problems related to human suffering.[296] The Nuprin report[297] revealed that 73% of the adult population experienced at least one headache in the previous 12 months. These same studies reported that 5% to 10% of the general population seeks medical advice for severe headache pain. The clinician should recognize that headache is not a disorder but instead a symptom created by a disorder. The therapist must therefore be able to identify the actual disorder causing the headache before effective treatment can be instituted.

When headache pain arises from masticatory structures, the dentist can play an important role in managing the pain. Many studies reveal that headache is a common symptom associated with TMDs.[298-311] Other studies demonstrated that various TMD treatments can significantly decrease headache pain.[307,312-321] If, however, the headache arises from nonmasticatory structures, the dentist may have little to offer the patient. The dentist, therefore, needs to be able to differentiate headaches that are likely to respond to dental therapies from those that are not. A knowledgeable practitioner should be able to determine this relationship before treatment begins so as to avoid unnecessary procedures.

Many different types of headaches originate from a variety of different etiologic considerations. The International Headache Society has offered a classification for headache that includes more than 230 types in 13 broad categories.[322] Headache is certainly a complex and significant problem for many people. Some headaches are the result of problems in the cranial structures, such as a brain tumor or increased intracranial pressure. Because these types of headaches can represent a serious problem, they must be identified quickly and referred for proper treatment. Usually these types of headaches are accompanied by other systemic symptoms that help the clinician identify the condition. These other symptoms may be muscle weakness, paralysis, paresthesia, seizure activity, or even loss of consciousness. When these symptoms accompany a headache, the patient should be immediately referred to the appropriate medical specialist.[323,324]

Fortunately, headaches produced by disorders of intracranial structures represent only a small percentage of all headache pain. Most headaches present as heterotopic pain produced by associated or even remote structures. Two of the most common structures that produce this heterotopic pain are vascular tissues and muscle tissues. Headache pain that has its origin in vascular structures is called a *migraine*. Studies have demonstrated that migraine is the result of neurologic activity on intracranial vascular structures. Therefore *migraine* is better classified as *neurovascular pain*.

Headache pain that has its origin in muscle tissue was previously referred to as *muscle tension headache* or *muscle contraction headache*. Both terms, however, are inappropriate because there is actually no significant increase in the EMG activity associated with the muscles.[325-328] The type of headache pain that originates from muscle structures fits into the category of *tension-type headache*.[322] Of note is that not all tension-type headaches originate from muscle sources. Numerous other sources can produce tension-type headaches. In this text, however, the term *tension-type headache* is used to describe headache pain with its origin in muscle tissues.

Certainly migraine and tension-type headache account for the vast majority of headache pain experienced by the general population. Between these two types, it is estimated that tension-type headache is the most common, representing 80% of all headaches.[329] Because neurovascular

headache and tension-type headache present with different clinical symptoms, it was originally believed that the mechanisms by which they produce headaches were quite different. Although this may be basically true, some suggest a common mechanism.[330] Because the management of neurovascular headache and tension-type headache are quite different, they need to be clinically differentiated.

Neurovascular Headache (Migraine)

Neurovascular headache usually presents as severe, pulsating, unilateral pain that is quite debilitating.[331] Often accompanying the pain is nausea, photophobia, and phonophobia. Two thirds of the patients who experience migraine pain will report the pain as unilateral. Typically a migraine episode will last from 4 to 72 hours and often be relieved by sleep. Some patients report an aura about 5 to 15 minutes before the pain begins. The aura commonly produces temporary neurologic symptoms such as paresthesias, visual impairment, or sensations of luminous appearances such as flashes, sparks, or zigzags before the eyes (teichopsia). In the past, migraines with aura have been called *classic migraines*, whereas migraines with no aura have been called *common migraines*.

The etiology of neurovascular headache is still not well understood. Earlier work suggested a cerebrovascular spasm,[332] whereas others proposed a disorder of blood platelets.[333] Another theory suggests some type of biochemical dysnociception.[334] Alterations in the regional cerebral blood flow have been demonstrated during the onset of a migraine,[335] which certainly suggests a vascular relationship to the pain. More recently the concept of neurogenic inflammation of the cerebral vessels has gained favor.[331,336] A genetic factor is apparent in migraine, with more women being affected than men.[337-339]

Often migraines are associated with certain factors that seem to trigger the onset of the headache. These initiating factors may be as simple as an exposure to different foods, such as chocolate, red wine, or certain cheeses. Some migraine sufferers will experience an attack following exposure to certain odors such as cigarette smoke or perfume. The presence of parafunctional activity, such as nocturnal bruxism, has been linked to early morning migraines,[340] perhaps as a triggering mechanism. Once these triggering mechanisms are learned, the patient may be able to control the frequency of the attacks by avoiding the triggers. Unfortunately for other patients, these trigger mechanisms are not as easily controlled. For some sufferers, migraine may be precipitated by factors such as fatigue, alterations in sleep patterns, emotional stress, deep pain, menstruation, or even sunlight. Patients with these types of triggering mechanisms often find it difficult to control their attacks.

Because neurovascular pain is not a TMD, its treatment is not discussed in this text. The only relationship that may exist between TMD and migraine is by way of a triggering mechanism. When a migraine sufferer experiences musculoskeletal pain associated with a TMD, the pain may represent a trigger for a migraine attack. This trigger is likely related to the fact that the nociceptive input associated with migraine is carried on the trigeminal nerve (predominately the ophthalmic division), just like TMD nociception. Perhaps this explains why some migraine patients who also have TMD pains may find that the TMD pain precipitates a migraine attack. When this occurs, successful treatment for the TMD is likely to reduce the number of migraine attacks. One must always remember that the TMD treatment does not cure the patient of migraine headaches. At best it merely reduces the number of attacks. Although this may be helpful, the patient should be educated regarding the actual reason for the headache reduction and not be denied more traditional migraine treatment when indicated. Patients with neurovascular headache should be referred to appropriate medical personnel for evaluation and treatment.[331]

Tension-Type Headache

Tension-type headache presents as a constant, steady, aching pain. It is commonly described as the feeling of wearing a tight headband. Tension-type headaches are not usually debilitating. In other words, patients will report carrying out their daily activities even though they are experiencing the headache. Most tension-type headaches are bilateral and can last for days or even weeks. Tension-type headaches are not accompanied by auras, and nausea is not common unless the pain becomes severe.

Numerous etiologic factors likely produce tension-type headache. One of the more common sources of this headache, however, is myofascial pain. When trigger points develop in muscles, the deep pain felt commonly produces heterotopic pain expressed as headache[341] (see the discussion on myofascial pain). Because this type of headache may relate to masticatory structures, the dentist needs to be able to differentiate it from migraine so that proper treatment may be instituted. The diagnosis and management of tension-type headache is discussed in later chapters in the sections on myofascial pain.

OTOLOGIC SYMPTOMS

The most common signs and symptoms of TMDs have been reviewed. However, other signs appear less often but may also relate to functional disturbances of the masticatory system. Some of these are ear complaints, such as pain.[342] Ear pain can actually be TMJ pain perceived more posteriorly.[48,343] Only one thin area of the temporal bone separates the TMJ from the external auditory meatus and middle ear. This anatomic proximity, along with similar phylogenetic heritage and nerve innervation, can confuse the patient's ability to locate the pain.

Persons also frequently complain of a sensation of fullness in the ear or ear stuffiness.[344,345] These symptoms can be explained by reviewing the anatomy. The eustachian tube connects the cavity of the middle ear with the nasopharynx (posterior aspect of the throat). During swallowing the palate is elevated, closing off the nasopharynx. As the palate is elevated, the tensor palati muscle contracts. This straightens the eustachian tube, equalizing the air pressure between the middle ear and the throat.[346] When the tensor palati muscle fails to elevate and straighten the eustachian tube, a stuffy feeling is felt in the ear.

The tensor tympani muscle, which is attached to the tympanic membrane, is another muscle that can affect ear symptoms. When oxygen is absorbed from the air by the mucosal membranes in the middle ear cavity, a negative pressure is created in that cavity. This decrease in pressure pulls the tympanic membrane inward (retraction), which diminishes the tension on the tensor tympani. The decrease in tonus of this muscle reflexly causes it and the tensor palati to increase their tonuses, which then causes the eustachian tube to open during the next swallow.[347]

Tinnitus (ear ringing) and vertigo (dizziness) have also been reported by patients suffering from a TMD.[348-359] Some patients complain of altered hearing as a result of protective co-contraction of the tensor tympani. When this muscle contracts, the eardrum is flexed and tightened. The tensor tympani, like the tensor palati, is innervated by the fifth cranial nerve (trigeminal). Therefore deep pain in any structure served by the trigeminal nerve may be able to affect ear function and create sensations. This alteration is more likely to result from central excitatory effects and not a reflex contraction of the muscle.[360] Some studies[348,361-368] have demonstrated that TMD therapy may reduce otologic symptoms, whereas another study[369] failed to show any relationship. The correlation between ear symptoms and TMDs is not well documented and remains an area of considerable controversy.[356,370-372]

References

1. Schiffman EL, Fricton JR, Haley DP, Shapiro BL: The prevalence and treatment needs of subjects with temporomandibular disorders, *J Am Dental Assoc* 120:295-303, 1990.
2. McCreary CP, Clark GT, Merril RL et al: Psychological distress and diagnostic subgroups of temporomandibular disorder patients, *Pain* 44:29-34, 1991.
3. Okeson JP: *Bell's orofacial pains*, ed 6, Chicago, 2005, Quintessence, pp 287-328.
4. Mense S, Meyer H: Bradykinin-induced sensitization of high-threshold muscle receptors with slowly conducting afferent fibers, *Pain* (Suppl):S204, 1981.
5. Keele KD: A physician looks at pain. In Weisenberg M, editor: *Pain: clinical and experimental perspectives*, St Louis, 1975, Mosby, pp 45-52.
6. Layzer RB: Muscle pain, cramps and fatigue. In Engel AG, Franzini-Armstrong C, editors: *Myology*, New York, 1994, McGraw-Hill, pp 1754-1786.
7. Svensson P, Graven-Nielsen T: Craniofacial muscle pain: review of mechanisms and clinical manifestations, *J Orofac Pain* 15:117-145, 2001.
8. Lund JP, Widmer CG: Evaluation of the use of surface electromyography in the diagnosis, documentation, and treatment of dental patients, *J Craniomandib Disord* 3:125-137, 1989.
9. Lund JP, Widmer CG, Feine JS: Validity of diagnostic and monitoring tests used for temporomandibular disorders, *J Dent Res* 74:1133-1143, 1995.
10. Paesani DA, Tallents RH, Murphy WC, Hatala MP, Proskin HM: Evaluation of the reproducibility of rest activity of the anterior temporal and masseter muscles in asymptomatic and symptomatic temporomandibular subjects, *J Orofac Pain* 8:402-406, 1994.
11. Carlson CR, Okeson JP, Falace DA et al: Comparison of psychological and physiological functioning between patients with masticatory muscle pain and matched controls, *J Orofac Pain* 7:15-22, 1993.
12. Curran SL, Carlson CR, Okeson JP: Emotional and physiologic responses to laboratory challenges: patients with temporomandibular disorders versus matched control subjects, *J Orofac Pain* 10:141-150, 1996.
13. Mense S: Considerations concerning the neurobiological basis of muscle pain, *Can J Physiol Pharmacol* 69:610-616, 1991.
14. Mense S: Nociception from skeletal muscle in relation to clinical muscle pain, *Pain* 54:241-289, 1993.
15. Travell JG, Rinzler S, Herman M: Pain and disability of the shoulder and arm, *JAMA* 120:417, 1942.
16. Schwartz LL: A temporomandibular joint pain-dysfunction syndrome, *J Chron Dis* 3:284-292, 1956.
17. Yemm R: A neurophysiological approach to the pathology and aetiology of temporomandibular dysfunction, *J Oral Rehabil* 12:343-353, 1985.
18. Schroeder H, Siegmund H, Santibanez G, Kluge A: Causes and signs of temporomandibular joint pain and dysfunction: an electromyographical investigation, *J Oral Rehabil* 18:301-310, 1991.
19. Flor H, Birbaumer N, Schulte W, Roos R: Stress-related electromyographic responses in patients with chronic temporomandibular pain, *Pain* 46:145-152, 1991.
20. Linton SJ, Hellsing AL, Andersson D: A controlled study of the effects of an early intervention on acute musculoskeletal pain problems, *Pain* 54:353-359, 1993.
21. Okeson JP: *Bell's orofacial pains*, ed 6, Chicago, 2005, Quintessence, pp 45-62.
22. Sternbach RA: Pain and 'hassles' in the United States: findings of the Nuprin pain report, *Pain* 27:69-80, 1986.
23. Selye H: *Stress without distress*, Philadelphia, 1974, JB Lippincott, p 32.
24. Schiffman EL, Fricton JR, Haley D: The relationship of occlusion, parafunctional habits and recent life events to mandibular dysfunction in a non-patient population, *J Oral Rehabil* 19:201-223, 1992.
25. Grassi C, Passatore M: Action of the sympathetic system on skeletal muscle, *Ital J Neurol Sci* 9:23-28, 1988.
26. Passatore M, Grassi C, Filippi GM: Sympathetically-induced development of tension in jaw muscles: the possible contraction of intrafusal muscle fibres, *Pflugers Arch* 405:297-304, 1985.

27. McNulty WH, Gevirtz RN, Hubbard DR, Berkoff GM: Needle electromyographic evaluation of trigger point response to a psychological stressor, *Psychophysiology* 31:313-316, 1994.

28. Bell WE: *Temporomandibular disorders: classification, diagnosis, management,* ed 3, Chicago, 1990, Year Book Medical, pp 60-61.

29. Ashton-Miller JA, McGlashen KM, Herzenberg JE, Stohler CS: Cervical muscle myoelectric response to acute experimental sternocleidomastoid pain, *Spine* 15:1006-1012, 1990.

30. Lund JP, Donga R, Widmer CG, Stohler CS: The pain-adaptation model: a discussion of the relationship between chronic musculoskeletal pain and motor activity, *Can J Physiol Pharmacol* 69:683-694, 1991.

31. Lund JP, Olsson KA: The importance of reflexes and their control during jaw movements, *Trends Neurosci* 6:458-463, 1983.

32. Stohler CS, Ash MM Jr: Demonstration of chewing motor disorder by recording peripheral correlates of mastication, *J Oral Rehabil* 12:49-57, 1985.

33. Stohler CS, Ash MM: Excitatory response of jaw elevators associated with sudden discomfort during chewing, *J Oral Rehabil* 13:225-233, 1986.

34. Smith AM: The coactivation of antagonist muscles, *Can J Physiol Pharmacol* 59:733-741, 1981.

35. Stohler CS: Clinical perspectives on masticatory and related muscle disorders. In Sessle BJ, Bryant PS, Dionne RA, editors: *Temporomandibular disorders and related pain conditions,* Seattle, 1995, IASP Press, pp 3, 29, 43.

36. Stohler CS, Ashton-Miller JA, Carlson DS: The effects of pain from the mandibular joint and muscles on masticatory motor behavior in man, *Arch Oral Biol* 33:175-182, 1988.

37. Watanabe M, Tabata T, Huh JI, Inai T, Tsuboi A et al: Possible involvement of histamine in muscular fatigue in temporomandibular disorders: animal and human studies, *J Dent Res* 78:769-775, 1999.

38. Christensen LV, Mohamed SE, Harrison JD: Delayed onset of masseter muscle pain in experimental tooth clenching, *J Prosthet Dent* 48:579-584, 1982.

39. Abraham WM: Factors in delayed muscle soreness, *Med Sci Sports* 9:11-20, 1977.

40. Tegeder L, Zimmermann J, Meller ST, Geisslinger G: Release of algesic substances in human experimental muscle pain, *Inflamm Res* 51:393-402, 2002.

41. Evans WJ, Cannon JG: The metabolic effects of exercise-induced muscle damage, *Exerc Sport Sci Rev* 19:99-125, 1991.

42. Byrnes WC, Clarkson PM: Delayed onset muscle soreness and training, *Clin Sports Med* 5:605-614, 1986.

43. Bobbert MF, Hollander AP, Huijing PA: Factors in delayed onset muscular soreness of man, *Med Sci Sports Exerc* 18:75-81, 1986.

44. Bakke M, Michler L: Temporalis and masseter muscle activity in patients with anterior open bite and craniomandibular disorders, *Scand J Dent Res* 99:219-228, 1991.

45. Tzakis MG, Dahlstrom L, Haraldson T: Evaluation of masticatory function before and after treatment in patients with craniomandibular disorders, *J Craniomandib Disord* 6:267-272, 1992.

46. Sinn DP, de Assis EA, Throckmorton GS: Mandibular excursions and maximum bite forces in patients with temporomandibular joint disorders, *J Oral Maxillofac Surg* 54:671-679, 1996.

47. High AS, MacGregor AJ, Tomlinson GE: A gnathodynanometer as an objective means of pain assessment following wisdom tooth removal, *Br J Maxillofac Surg* 26:284-290, 1988.

48. Okeson JP: *Bell's orofacial pains,* ed 6, Chicago, 2005, Quintessence, pp 63-94.

49. Gonzales R, Coderre TJ, Sherbourne CD, Levine JD: Postnatal development of neurogenic inflammation in the rat, *Neurosci Lett* 127:25-27, 1991.

50. Levine JD, Dardick SJ, Basbaum AI, Scipio E: Reflex neurogenic inflammation. I. Contribution of the peripheral nervous system to spatially remote inflammatory responses that follow injury, *J Neurosci* 5:1380-1386, 1985.

51. Carlson CR, Okeson JP, Falace DA, Nitz AJ, Lindroth JE: Reduction of pain and EMG activity in the masseter region by trapezius trigger point injection, *Pain* 55:397-400, 1993.

52. Fricton JR, Kroening R, Haley D, Siegert R: Myofascial pain syndrome of the head and neck: a review of clinical characteristics of 164 patients, *Oral Surg Oral Med Oral Pathol* 60:615-623, 1985.

53. Travell JG, Rinzler SH: The myofascial genesis of pain, *Postgrad Med* 11:425-434, 1952.

54. Laskin DM: Etiology of the pain-dysfunction syndrome, *J Am Dent Assoc* 79:147-153, 1969.

55. Simons DG, Travell J: Myofascial trigger points, a possible explanation [letter], *Pain* 10:106-109, 1981.

56. McMillan AS, Blasberg B: Pain-pressure threshold in painful jaw muscles following trigger point injection, *J Orofac Pain* 8:384-390, 1994.

57. Travell J: Introductory comments. In Ragan C, editor: *Connective tissues. Transactions of the fifth conference,* New York, 1954, Josiah Macy Jr, pp 12-22.

58. Simons DG, Travell JG, Simons LS: *Travell & Simons' myofascial pain and dysfunction: the trigger point manual,* ed 2, Baltimore, 1999, Lippincott Williams & Wilkins, pp 67-78.

59. Hubbard DR, Berkoff GM: Myofascial trigger points show spontaneous needle EMG activity, *Spine* 18:1803-1807, 1993.

60. Simons DG, Travell JG, Simons LS: *Travell & Simons' myofascial pain and dysfunction: the trigger point manual,* ed 2, Baltimore, 1999, Lippincott Williams & Wilkins, pp 178-235.

61. Giunta JL, Kronman JH: Orofacial involvement secondary to trapezius muscle trauma, *Oral Surg Oral Med Oral Pathol* 60:368-369, 1985.

62. Wright EF: Referred craniofacial pain patterns in patients with temporomandibular disorder, *J Am Dent Assoc* 131:1307-1315, 2000.

63. Simons DG: The nature of myofascial trigger points, *Clin J Pain* 11:83-84, 1995.

64. Hoheisel U, Mense S, Simons DG, Yu XM: Appearance of new receptive fields in rat dorsal horn neurons following noxious stimulation of skeletal muscle: a model for referral of muscle pain? *Neurosci Lett* 153:9-12, 1993.

65. Hong CZ, Simons DG: Pathophysiologic and electrophysiologic mechanisms of myofascial trigger points, *Arch Phys Med Rehabil* 79:863-872, 1998.

66. Simons DG, Travell JG, Simons LS: *Travell & Simons' myofascial pain and dysfunction: the trigger point manual*, ed 2, Baltimore, 1999, Lippincott Williams & Wilkins, pp 110-112.

67. Moldofsky H, Scarisbrick P: Induction of neurasthenic musculoskeletal pain syndrome by selective sleep stage deprivation, *Psychosom Med* 38:35-44, 1976.

68. Moldofsky H, Scarisbrick P, England R, Smythe H: Musculoskeletal symptoms and non-REM sleep disturbance in patients with "fibrositis" and healthy subjects, *Psychosom Med* 37:341-349, 1986.

69. Moldofsky H, Tullis C, Lue FA: Sleep related myoclonus in rheumatic pain modulation disorder (fibrositis syndrome), *J Rheumatol* 13:614-617, 1986.

70. Molony RR, MacPeek DM, Schiffman PL, Frank M, Neubauer JA et al: Sleep, sleep apnea and the fibromyalgia syndrome, *J Rheumatol* 13:797-800, 1986.

71. Moldofsky H: Sleep and pain, *Sleep Med Rev* 5:385-396, 2001.

72. Mease P: Fibromyalgia syndrome: review of clinical presentation, pathogenesis, outcome measures, and treatment, *J Rheumatol Suppl* 75:6-21, 2005.

73. Marbach JJ, Lennon MC, Dohrenwend BP: Candidate risk factors for temporomandibular pain and dysfunction syndrome: psychosocial, health behavior, physical illness and injury, *Pain* 34:139-151, 1988.

74. Burgess JA, Dworkin SF: Litigation and post-traumatic TMD: how patients report treatment outcome, *J Am Dent Assoc* 124:105-110, 1993.

75. Hopwood MB, Abram SE: Factors associated with failure of trigger point injections, *Clin J Pain* 10:227-234, 1994.

76. Tauschke E, Merskey H, Helmes E: Psychological defense mechanisms in patients with pain, *Pain* 40:161-170, 1990.

77. Marbach JJ, Lund P: Depression, anhedonia and anxiety in temporomandibular joint and other facial pain syndromes, *Pain* 11:73-84, 1981.

78. Magni G, Marchetti M, Moreschi C, Merskey H, Luchini SR: Chronic musculoskeletal pain and depressive symptoms in the National Health and Nutrition Examination I. Epidemiologic follow-up study, *Pain* 53:163-168, 1993.

79. Auerbach SM, Laskin DM, Frantsve LM, Orr T: Depression, pain, exposure to stressful life events, and long-term outcomes in temporomandibular disorder patients, *J Oral Maxillofac Surg* 59:628-633, 2001.

80. Dworkin SF: Perspectives on the interaction of biological, psychological and social factors in TMD, *J Am Dent Assoc* 125:856-863, 1994.

81. Gallagher RM, Marbach JJ, Raphael KG, Dohrenwend BP, Cloitre M: Is major depression comorbid with temporomandibular pain and dysfunction syndrome? A pilot study, *Clin J Pain* 7:219-225, 1991.

82. Glaros AG: Emotional factors in temporomandibular joint disorders, *J Indiana Dent Assoc* 79:20-23, 2000.

83. Parker MW, Holmes EK, Terezhalmy GT: Personality characteristics of patients with temporomandibular disorders: diagnostic and therapeutic implications, *J Orofac Pain* 7:337-344, 1993.

84. Vickers ER, Boocock H: Chronic orofacial pain is associated with psychological morbidity and negative personality changes: a comparison to the general population, *Aust Dent J* 50:21-30, 2005.

85. Fine EW: Psychological factors associated with non-organic temporomandibular joint pain dysfunction syndrome, *Br Dent J* 131:402-404, 1971.

86. Haley WE, Turner JA, Romano JM: Depression in chronic pain patients: relation to pain, activity, and sex differences, *Pain* 23:337-343, 1985.

87. Hendler N: Depression caused by chronic pain, *J Clin Psychiatry* 45:30-38, 1984.

88. Faucett JA: Depression in painful chronic disorders: the role of pain and conflict about pain, *J Pain Symptom Manage* 9:520-526, 1994.

89. Dworkin RH, Richlin DM, Handlin DS, Brand L: Predicting treatment response in depressed and non-depressed chronic pain patients, *Pain* 24:343-353, 1986.

90. Fricton JR, Olsen T: Predictors of outcome for treatment of temporomandibular disorders, *J Orofac Pain* 10:54-65, 1996.

91. Bowsher D: Neurogenic pain syndromes and their management, *Br Med Bull* 47:644-666, 1991.

92. LaMotte RH, Shain CN, Simone DA, Tsai EF: Neurogenic hyperalgesia: psychophysical studies of underlying mechanisms, *J Neurophysiol* 66:190-211, 1991.

93. Sessle BJ: The neural basis of temporomandibular joint and masticatory muscle pain, *J Orofac Pain* 13:238-245, 1999.

94. Simone DA, Sorkin LS, Oh U, Chung JM, Owens C et al: Neurogenic hyperalgesia: central neural correlates in responses of spinothalamic tract neurons, *J Neurophysiol* 66:228-246, 1991.

95. Wong JK, Haas DA, Hu JW: Local anesthesia does not block mustard-oil-induced temporomandibular inflammation, *Anesth Analg* 92:1035-1040, 2001.

96. Wolfe F, Smythe HA, Yunus MB, Bennett RM, Bombardier C et al: The American College of Rheumatology 1990 Criteria for the Classification of Fibromyalgia. Report of the Multicenter Criteria Committee, *Arthritis Rheum* 33:160-172, 1990.

97. Fricton JR: The relationship of temporomandibular disorders and fibromyalgia: implications for diagnosis and treatment, *Curr Pain Headache Rep* 8:355-363, 2004.

98. Rhodus NL, Fricton J, Carlson P, Messner R: Oral symptoms associated with fibromyalgia syndrome, *J Rheumatol* 30:1841-1845, 2003.

99. Hedenberg-Magnusson B, Ernberg M, Kopp S: Presence of orofacial pain and temporomandibular disorder in fibromyalgia. A study by questionnaire, *Swed Dent J* 23:185-192, 1999.

100. Aaron LA, Burke MM, Buchwald D: Overlapping conditions among patients with chronic fatigue syndrome, fibromyalgia, and temporomandibular disorder, *Arch Intern Med* 160:221-227, 2000.

101. Hedenberg-Magnusson B, Ernberg M, Kopp S: Symptoms and signs of temporomandibular disorders in patients with fibromyalgia and local myalgia of the

temporomandibular system. A comparative study, *Acta Odontol Scand* 55:344-349, 1997.

102. Plesh O, Wolfe F, Lane N: The relationship between fibromyalgia and temporomandibular disorders: prevalence and symptom severity, *J Rheumatol* 23:1948-1952, 1996.

103. Korszun A, Papadopoulos E, Demitrack M, Engleberg C, Crofford L: The relationship between temporomandibular disorders and stress-associated syndromes, *Oral Surg Oral Med Oral Pathol Oral Radiol Endod* 86:416-420, 1998.

104. Aaron LA, Burke MM, Buchwald D: Overlapping conditions among patients with chronic fatigue syndrome, fibromyalgia, and temporomandibular disorder [see comments], *Arch Intern Med* 160:221-227, 2000.

105. Bell WE: Management of temporomandibular joint problems. In Goldman HM et al, editors: *Current therapy in dentistry*, St Louis, 1970, Mosby, pp 398-415.

106. Eriksson L, Westesson PL, Rohlin M: Temporomandibular joint sounds in patients with disc displacement, *Int J Oral Surg* 14:428-436, 1985.

107. Guler N, Yatmaz PI, Ataoglu H, Emlik D, Uckan S: Temporomandibular internal derangement: correlation of MRI findings with clinical symptoms of pain and joint sounds in patients with bruxing behavior, *Dentomaxillofac Radiol* 32:304-310, 2003.

108. Taskaya-Yylmaz N, Ogutcen-Toller M: Clinical correlation of MRI findings of internal derangements of the temporomandibular joints, *Br J Oral Maxillofac Surg* 40:317-321, 2002.

109. Westesson PL, Bronstein SL, Liedberg J: Internal derangement of the temporomandibular joint: morphologic description with correlation to joint function, *Oral Surg Oral Med Oral Pathol* 59:323-331, 1985.

110. Farrar WB, McCarty WL Jr: The TMJ dilemma, *J Ala Dent Assoc* 63:19-26, 1979.

111. Wilkinson TM: The relationship between the disk and the lateral pterygoid muscle in the human temporomandibular joint, *J Prosthet Dent* 60:715-724, 1988.

112. Tanaka TT: *Head, neck and TMD management*, San Diego, 1989, Clinical Research Foundation.

113. Tanaka TT: *TMJ microanatomy: an approach to current controversies*, Chula Vista, Calif, 1998, Terry T. Tanaka (DVD).

114. Luder HU, Bobst P, Schroeder HE: Histometric study of synovial cavity dimension of human temporomandibular joints with normal and anterior disc position, *J Orofac Pain* 7:263-274, 1993.

115. Roberts CA, Tallents RH, Espeland MA, Handelman SL, Katzberg RW: Mandibular range of motion versus arthrographic diagnosis of the temporomandibular joint, *Oral Surg Oral Med Oral Pathol* 60:244-251, 1985.

116. Tallents RH, Hatala M, Katzberg RW, Westesson PL: Temporomandibular joint sounds in asymptomatic volunteers, *J Prosthet Dent* 69:298-304, 1993.

117. Dibbets JMH, van der Weele LT: The prevalence of joint noises as related to age and gender, *J Craniomandib Disord* 6:157-160, 1992.

118. Katzberg RW, Westesson PL, Tallents RH, Drake CM: Anatomic disorders of the temporomandibular joint disc in asymptomatic subjects, *J Oral Maxillofac Surg* 54:147-153, 1996.

119. Isberg A, Isacsson G, Johansson AS, Larson O: Hyperplastic soft-tissue formation in the temporomandibular joint associated with internal derangement. A radiographic and histologic study, *Oral Surg Oral Med Oral Pathol* 61:32-38, 1986.

120. Holumlund AB, Gynther GW, Reinholt FP: Disk derangement and inflammatory changes in the posterior disk attachment of the temporomandibular joint, *Oral Surg Oral Med Oral Pathol* 73:9-18, 1992.

121. Harkins SJ, Marteney JL: Extrinsic trauma: a significant precipitating factor in temporomandibular dysfunction, *J Prosthet Dent* 54:271-272, 1985.

122. Moloney F, Howard JA: Internal derangements of the temporomandibular joint. III. Anterior repositioning splint therapy, *Aust Dent J* 31:30-39, 1986.

123. Weinberg S, Lapointe H: Cervical extension-flexion injury (whiplash) and internal derangement of the temporomandibular joint, *J Oral Maxillofac Surg* 45:653-656, 1987.

124. Pullinger AG, Seligman DA: Trauma history in diagnostic groups of temporomandibular disorders, *Oral Surg Oral Med Oral Pathol* 71:529-534, 1991.

125. Westling L, Carlsson GE, Helkimo M: Background factors in craniomandibular disorders with special reference to general joint hypermobility, parafunction, and trauma, *J Craniomandib Disord* 4:89-98, 1990.

126. Pullinger AG, Seligman DA: Association of TMJ subgroups with general trauma and MVA, *J Dent Res* 67:403-414, 1988.

127. Pullinger AG, Monteriro AA: History factors associated with symptoms of temporomandibular disorders, *J Oral Rehabil* 15:117-124, 1988.

128. Skolnick J, Iranpour B, Westesson PL, Adair S: Prepubertal trauma and mandibular asymmetry in orthognathic surgery and orthodontic patients, *Am J Orthod Dentofacial Orthop* 105:73-77, 1994.

129. Braun BL, DiGiovanna A, Schiffman E et al: A cross-sectional study of temporomandibular joint dysfunction in post-cervical trauma patients, *J Craniomandib Disord* 6:24-31, 1992.

130. Burgess J: Symptom characteristics in TMD patients reporting blunt trauma and/or whiplash injury, *J Craniomandib Disord* 5:251-257, 1991.

131. De Boever JA, Keersmaekers K: Trauma in patients with temporomandibular disorders: frequency and treatment outcome, *J Oral Rehabil* 23:91-96, 1996.

132. Yun PY, Kim YK: The role of facial trauma as a possible etiologic factor in temporomandibular joint disorder, *J Oral Maxillofac Surg* 63:1576-1583, 2005.

133. Seals RR Jr, Morrow RM, Kuebker WA, Farney WD: An evaluation of mouthguard programs in Texas high school football, *J Am Dent Assoc* 110:904-909, 1985.

134. Garon MW, Merkle A, Wright JT: Mouth protectors and oral trauma: a study of adolescent football players, *J Am Dent Assoc* 112:663-665, 1986.

135. Luz JGC, Jaeger RG, de Araujo VC, de Rezende JRV: The effect of indirect trauma on the rat temporomandibular joint, *Int J Oral Maxillofac Surg* 20:48-52, 1991.

136. Knibbe MA, Carter JB, Frokjer GM: Postanesthetic temporomandibular joint dysfunction, *Anesth Prog* 36:21-25, 1989.

137. Gould DB, Banes CH: Iatrogenic disruptions of right temporomandibular joints during orotracheal intubation causing permanent closed lock of the jaw, *Anesth Analg* 81:191-194, 1995.

138. Oofuvong M: Bilateral temporomandibular joint dislocations during induction of anesthesia and orotracheal intubation, *J Med Assoc Thai* 88:695-697, 2005.

139. Mangi Q, Ridgway PF, Ibrahim Z, Evoy D: Dislocation of the mandible, *Surg Endosc* 18:554-556, 2004.

140. Barnsley L, Lord S, Bogduk N: Whiplash injury; a clinical review, *Pain* 58:283-307, 1994.

141. Kronn E: The incidence of TMJ dysfunction in patients who have suffered a cervical whiplash injury following a traffic accident, *J Orofac Pain* 7:209-213, 1993.

142. Goldberg HL: Trauma and the improbable anterior displacement, *J Craniomandib Disord* 4:131-134, 1990.

143. McKay DC, Christensen LV: Whiplash injuries of the temporomandibular joint in motor vehicle accidents: speculations and facts, *J Oral Rehabil* 25:731-746, 1998.

144. Kasch H, Hjorth T, Svensson P, Nyhuus L, Jensen TS: Temporomandibular disorders after whiplash injury: a controlled, prospective study, *J Orofac Pain* 16:118-128, 2002.

145. Klobas L, Tegelberg A, Axelsson S: Symptoms and signs of temporomandibular disorders in individuals with chronic whiplash-associated disorders, *Swed Dent J* 28:2 9-36, 2004.

146. Howard RP, Hatsell CP, Guzman HM: Temporomandibular joint injury potential imposed by the low-velocity extension-flexion maneuver, *J Oral Maxillofac Surg* 53:256-262, 1995.

147. Howard RP, Benedict JV, Raddin JH Jr, Smith HL: Assessing neck extension-flexion as a basis for temporomandibular joint dysfunction, *J Oral Maxillofac Surg* 49:1210-1213, 1991.

148. Szabo TJ, Welcher JB, Anderson RD et al: Human occupant kinematic response to low speed rear-end impacts. In Society of Automotive Engineers: *Occupant containment and methods of assessing occupant protection in the crash environment*, Warrendale, Pa, 1994, SAE, p SP-1045.

149. Heise AP, Laskin DM, Gervin AS: Incidence of temporomandibular joint symptoms following whiplash injury, *J Oral Maxillofac Surg* 50:825-828, 1992.

150. Probert TCS, Wiesenfeld PC, Reade PC: Temporomandibular pain dysfunction disorder resulting from road traffic accidents—an Australian study, *Int J Oral Maxillofac Surg* 23:338-341, 1994.

151. Stegenga B: *Temporomandibular joint osteoarthrosis and internal derangement: diagnostic and therapeutic outcome assessment*, Groningen, The Netherlands, 1991, Drukkerij Van Denderen BV, p 500.

152. Dijkgraaf LC, de Bont LG, Boering G, Liem RS: The structure, biochemistry, and metabolism of osteoarthritic cartilage: a review of the literature, *J Oral Maxillofac Surg* 53:1182-1192, 1995.

153. Nitzan DW, Nitzan U, Dan P, Yedgar S: The role of hyaluronic acid in protecting surface-active phospholipids from lysis by exogenous phospholipase A(2), *Rheumatology (Oxford)* 40:336-340, 2001.

154. Nitzan DW: The process of lubrication impairment and its involvement in temporomandibular joint disc displacement: a theoretical concept, *J Oral Maxillofac Surg* 59:36-45, 2001.

155. Nitzan DW, Marmary Y: The "anchored disc phenomenon": a proposed etiology for sudden-onset, severe, and persistent closed lock of the temporomandibular joint, *J Oral Maxillofac Surg* 55:797-802, 1997; discussion 802-803.

156. Zardeneta G, Milam SB, Schmitz JP: Iron-dependent generation of free radicals: plausible mechanisms in the progressive deterioration of the temporomandibular joint, *J Oral Maxillofac Surg* 58:302-308, 2000; discussion 309.

157. Nitzan DW, Etsion I: Adhesive force: the underlying cause of the disc anchorage to the fossa and/or eminence in the temporomandibular joint—a new concept, *Int J Oral Maxillofac Surg* 31:94-99, 2002.

158. Nitzan DW: 'Friction and adhesive forces'—possible underlying causes for temporomandibular joint internal derangement, *Cells Tissues Organs* 174:6-16, 2003.

159. Tomida M, Ishimaru JI, Murayama K, Kajimoto T, Kurachi M et al: Intra-articular oxidative state correlated with the pathogenesis of disorders of the temporomandibular joint, *Br J Oral Maxillofac Surg* 42:405-409, 2004.

160. Dan P, Nitzan DW, Dagan A, Ginsburg I, Yedgar S: H2O2 renders cells accessible to lysis by exogenous phospholipase A2: a novel mechanism for cell damage in inflammatory processes, *FEBS Lett* 383:75-78, 1996.

161. Milam SB, Schmitz JP: Molecular biology of temporomandibular joint disorders: proposed mechanisms of disease, *J Oral Maxillofac Surg* 53:1448-1454, 1995.

162. Milam SB, Zardeneta G, Schmitz JP: Oxidative stress and degenerative temporomandibular joint disease: a proposed hypothesis, *J Oral Maxillofac Surg* 56:214-223, 1998.

163. Aghabeigi B, Haque M, Wasil M, Hodges SJ, Henderson B et al: The role of oxygen free radicals in idiopathic facial pain, *Br J Oral Maxillofac Surg* 35:161-165, 1997.

164. Yamaguchi A, Tojyo I, Yoshida H, Fujita S: Role of hypoxia and interleukin-1beta in gene expressions of matrix metalloproteinases in temporomandibular joint disc cells, *Arch Oral Biol* 50:81-87, 2005.

165. Israel HA, Diamond B, Saed-Nejad F, Ratcliffe A: The relationship between parafunctional masticatory activity and arthroscopically diagnosed temporomandibular joint pathology, *J Oral Maxillofac Surg* 57:1034-1039, 1999.

166. Nitzan DW: Intraarticular pressure in the functioning human temporomandibular joint and its alteration by uniform elevation of the occlusal plane, *J Oral Maxillofac Surg* 52:671-679, 1994.

167. Milam SB, Schmitz JP: Molecular biology of temporomandibular joint disorders: proposed mechanisms of disease, *J Oral Maxillofac Surg* 12:1448-1454, 1995.

168. Monje F, Delgado E, Navarro MJ, Miralles C, Alonso del Hoyo JR: Changes in temporomandibular joint after mandibular subcondylar osteotomy: an experimental study in rats, *J Oral Maxillofac Surg* 51:1221-1234, 1993.

169. Shaw RM, Molyneux GS: The effects of induced dental malocclusion on the fibrocartilage disc of the adult rabbit temporomandibular joint, *Arch Oral Biol* 38:415-422, 1993.

170. Isberg A, Isacsson G: Tissue reactions associated with internal derangement of the temporomandibular joint. A radiographic, cryomorphologic, and histologic study, *Acta Odontol Scand* 44:160-164, 1986.

171. Wright WJ Jr: Temporomandibular disorders: occurrence of specific diagnoses and response to conservative management. Clinical observations, *Cranio* 4:150-155, 1986.

172. Seligman DA, Pullinger AG: Association of occlusal variables among refined TM patient diagnostic groups, *J Craniomandib Disord* 3:227-236, 1989.

173. Solberg WK, Bibb CA, Nordstrom BB, Hansson TL: Malocclusion associated with temporomandibular joint changes in young adults at autopsy, *Am J Orthod* 89:326-330, 1986.

174. Tsolka P, Walter JD, Wilson RF, Preiskel HW: Occlusal variables, bruxism and temporomandibular disorder: a clinical and kinesiographic assessment, *J Oral Rehabil* 22:849-956, 1995.

175. Celic R, Jerolimov V: Association of horizontal and vertical overlap with prevalence of temporomandibular disorders, *J Oral Rehabil* 29:588-593, 2002.

176. Williamson EH, Simmons MD: Mandibular asymmetry and its relation to pain dysfunction, *Am J Orthod* 76:612-617, 1979.

177. De Boever JA, Adriaens PA: Occlusal relationship in patients with pain-dysfunction symptoms in the temporomandibular joint, *J Oral Rehabil* 10:1-7, 1983.

178. Brandt D: Temporomandibular disorders and their association with morphologic malocclusion in children. In Carlson DS, McNamara JA, Ribbens KA, editors: *Developmental aspects of temporomandibular joint disorders*, Ann Arbor, 1985, University of Michigan Press, pp 279-291.

179. Bernal M, Tsamtsouris A: Signs and symptoms of temporomandibular joint dysfunction in 3 to 5 year old children, *J Pedod* 10:127-140, 1986.

180. Nilner M: Functional disturbances and diseases of the stomatognathic system. A cross-sectional study, *J Pedod* 10:211-238, 1986.

181. Stringert HG, Worms FW: Variations in skeletal and dental patterns in patients with structural and functional alterations of the temporomandibular joint: a preliminary report, *Am J Orthod* 89:285-297, 1986.

182. Gunn SM, Woolfolk MW, Faja BW: Malocclusion and TMJ symptoms in migrant children, *J Craniomandib Disord* 2:196-200, 1988.

183. Dworkin SF, Huggins KH, LeResche L, Von Korff M, Howard J et al: Epidemiology of signs and symptoms in temporomandibular disorders: clinical signs in cases and controls, *J Am Dent Assoc* 120:273-281, 1990.

184. Glaros AG, Brockman DL, Acherman RJ: Impact of overbite on indicators of temporomandibular joint dysfunction, *J Craniomandib Pract* 10:277-289, 1992.

185. McNamara JA Jr, Seligman DA, Okeson JP: Occlusion, orthodontic treatment, and temporomandibular disorders: a review, *J Orofac Pain* 9:73-90, 1995.

186. Ronquillo HI, Guay J, Tallents RH, Katzberg R, Murphy W et al: Comparison of internal derangements with condyle-fossa relationships, horizontal and vertical overlap, and angle class, *J Craniomandib Disord* 2:137-140, 1988.

187. Pullinger AG, Seligman DA, Solberg WK: Temporomandibular disorders. Part II: occlusal factors associated with temporomandibular joint tenderness and dysfunction, *J Prosthet Dent* 59:363-367, 1988.

188. Pullinger AG, Seligman DA: Overbite and overjet characteristics of refined diagnostic groups of temporomandibular disorders patients, *Am J Orthod Dentofac Orthop* 100:401-409, 1991.

189. Hirsch C, John MT, Drangsholt MT, Mancl LA: Relationship between overbite/overjet and clicking or crepitus of the temporomandibular joint, *J Orofac Pain* 19:218-225, 2005.

190. John MT, Hirsch C, Drangsholt MT, Mancl LA, Setz JM: Overbite and overjet are not related to self-report of temporomandibular disorder symptoms, *J Dent Res* 81:164-169, 2002.

191. Ohta M, Minagi S, Sato T, Okamoto M, Shimamura M: Magnetic resonance imaging analysis on the relationship between anterior disc displacement and balancing-side occlusal contact, *J Oral Rehabil* 30:30-33, 2003.

192. Farrar WB, McCarty WL: *A clinical outline of temporomandibular joint diagnosis and treatment*, Montgomery, Ala, 1983, Normandie Publications.

193. Wilson HE: Extraction of second permanent molars in orthodontic treatment, *Orthodontist* 3:18-24, 1971.

194. Witzig JW, Spahl TH: *The clinical management of basic maxillofacial orthopedic appliances*, Littleton, Mass, 1987, PSG Publishing.

195. Witzig JW, Yerkes IM: Functional jaw orthopedics: mastering more technique. In Gelb H, editor: *Clinical management of head, neck and TMJ pain and dysfunction*, Philadelphia, 1985, Saunders, pp 207-235.

196. Sadowsky C, BeGole EA: Long-term status of temporomandibular joint function and functional occlusion after orthodontic treatment, *Am J Orthod* 78:201-212, 1980.

197. Larsson E, Ronnerman A: Mandibular dysfunction symptoms in orthodontically treated patients ten years after the completion of treatment, *Eur J Orthod* 3:89-94, 1981.

198. Sadowsky C, Polson AM: Temporomandibular disorders and functional occlusion after orthodontic treatment: results of two long-term studies, *Am J Orthod* 86:386-390, 1984.

199. Dibbets JM, van der Weele LT: Orthodontic treatment in relation to symptoms attributed to dysfunction of the temporomandibular joint. A 10-year report of the

University of Groningen study, *Am J Orthod Dentofacial Orthop* 91:193-199, 1987.

200. Dahl BL, Krogstad BS, Ogaard B, Eckersberg T: Signs and symptoms of craniomandibular disorders in two groups of 19-year-old individuals, one treated orthodontically and the other not, *Acta Odontol Scand* 46:89-93, 1988.

201. Wadhwa L, Utreja A, Tewari A: A study of clinical signs and symptoms of temporomandibular dysfunction in subjects with normal occlusion, untreated, and treated malocclusions, *Am J Orthod Dentofac Orthop* 103:54-61, 1993.

202. Henrikson T, Nilner M: Temporomandibular disorders and the need for stomatognathic treatment in orthodontically treated and untreated girls, *Eur J Orthod* 22: 283-292, 2000.

203. Henrikson T, Nilner M, Kurol J: Signs of temporomandibular disorders in girls receiving orthodontic treatment. A prospective and longitudinal comparison with untreated Class II malocclusions and normal occlusion subjects, *Eur J Orthod* 22:271-281, 2000.

204. Conti A, Freitas M, Conti P, Henriques J, Janson G: Relationship between signs and symptoms of temporomandibular disorders and orthodontic treatment: a cross-sectional study, *Angle Orthod* 73:411-417, 2003.

205. Kim MR, Graber TM, Viana MA: Orthodontics and temporomandibular disorder: a meta-analysis, *Am J Orthod Dentofacial Orthop* 121:438-446, 2002.

206. How CK: Orthodontic treatment has little to do with temporomandibular disorders, *Evid Based Dent* 5:75, 2004.

207. Henrikson T, Nilner M: Temporomandibular disorders, occlusion and orthodontic treatment, *J Orthod* 30:129-137, 2003; discussion 127.

208. Dibbets JM, van der Weele LT: Extraction, orthodontic treatment, and craniomandibular dysfunction, *Am J Orthod Dentofacial Orthop* 99:210-219, 1991.

209. Dibbets JM, van der Weele LT: Long-term effects of orthodontic treatment, including extraction, on signs and symptoms attributed to CMD, *Eur J Orthod* 14:16-20, 1992.

210. Dibbets JM, van der Weele LT, Meng HP: The relationships between orthodontics and temporomandibular joint dysfunction. A review of the literature and longitudinal study, *Schweiz Monatsschr Zahnmed* 103:162-168, 1993.

211. Katzberg RW, Westesson PL, Tallents RH, Drake CM: Orthodontics and temporomandibular joint internal derangement, *Am J Orthod Dentofacial Orthop* 109: 515-520, 1996.

212. Sadowsky C, Theisen TA, Sakols EI: Orthodontic treatment and temporomandibular joint sounds—a longitudinal study, *Am J Orthod Dentofacial Orthop* 99:441-447, 1991.

213. Beattie JR, Paquette DE, Johnston LE Jr: The functional impact of extraction and nonextraction treatments: a long-term comparison in patients with borderline, equally susceptible Class II malocclusions, *Am J Orthod Dentofacial Orthop* 105:444-449, 1994.

214. Luppanapornlarp S, Johnston LE Jr: The effects of premolar-extraction: a long-term comparison of outcomes in clear-cut extraction and nonextraction Class II patients, *Angle Orthod* 63:257-272, 1993.

215. Kremenak CR, Kinser DD, Harman HA, Menard CC, Jakobsen JR: Orthodontic risk factors for temporomandibular disorders (TMD). I: premolar extractions, *Am J Orthod Dentofacial Orthop* 101:13-20, 1992.

216. Kundinger KK, Austin BP, Christensen LV, Donegan SJ, Ferguson DJ: An evaluation of temporomandibular joints and jaw muscles after orthodontic treatment involving premolar extractions, *Am J Orthod Dentofacial Orthop* 100:110-115, 1991.

217. Nitzan DW, Dolwick MF: An alternative explanation for the genesis of closed-lock symptoms in the internal derangement process, *J Oral Maxillofac Surg* 49:810-815, 1991.

218. Nitzan DW, Mahler Y, Simkin A: Intra-articular pressure measurements in patients with suddenly developing, severely limited mouth opening, *J Oral Maxillofac Surg* 50:1038-1042, 1992.

219. Murakami K, Segami N, Moriya Y, Iizuka T: Correlation between pain and dysfunction and intra-articular adhesions in patients with internal derangement of the temporomandibular joint, *J Oral Maxillofac Surg* 50: 705-708, 1992.

220. Bell WE: *Temporomandibular disorders: classification, diagnosis, management,* ed 3, Chicago, 1990, Year Book Medical, p 395.

221. Kavuncu V, Sahin S, Kamanli A, Karan A, Aksoy C: The role of systemic hypermobility and condylar hypermobility in temporomandibular joint dysfunction syndrome, *Rheumatol Int* 26:257-260, 2006.

222. Bell WE: *Temporomandibular disorders: classification, diagnosis, management,* ed 3, Chicago, 1990, Year Book Medical, p 158.

223. Kai S, Kai H, Nakayama E, Tabata O, Tashiro H et al: Clinical symptoms of open lock position of the condyle. Relation to anterior dislocation of the temporomandibular joint, *Oral Surg Oral Med Oral Pathol* 74: 143-148, 1992.

224. Nitzan DW: Temporomandibular joint "open lock" versus condylar dislocation: signs and symptoms, imaging, treatment, and pathogenesis, *J Oral Maxillofac Surg* 60:506-511, 2002; discussion 512-513.

225. Bell WE: *Temporomandibular disorders: classification, diagnosis, management,* ed 3, Chicago, 1990, Year Book Medical, p 77.

226. Hall MB, Gibbs CC, Sclar AG: Association between the prominence of the articular eminence and displaced TMJ disks, *Cranio* 3:237-239, 1985.

227. Kerstens HC, Tuinzing DB, Golding RP, Van der Kwast WA: Inclination of the temporomandibular joint eminence and anterior disc displacement, *Int J Oral Maxillofac Surg* 18:228-232, 1989.

228. Ren YF, Isberg A, Wesetessen PL: Steepness of the articular eminence in the temporomandibular joint, *Oral Surg Oral Med Oral Pathol* 80:258-266, 1995.

229. Galante G, Paesani D, Tallents RH, Hatala MA, Katzberg RW et al: Angle of the articular eminence in patients with temporomandibular joint dysfunction and asymptomatic volunteers, *Oral Surg Oral Med Oral Pathol Oral Radiol Endod* 80:242-249, 1995.

230. Alsawaf M, Garlapo DA, Gale EN, Carter MJ: The relationship between condylar guidance and temporomandibular joint clicking, *J Prosthet Dent* 61:349-356, 1989.

231. Solberg WK, Hansson TL, Nordstrom B: The temporomandibular joint in young adults at autopsy: a morphologic classification and evaluation, *J Oral Rehabil* 12:303-310, 1985.

232. Maeda Y, Korioth T, Wood W: Stress distribution on simulated mandibular condyles of various shapes, *J Dent Res* 69:337, 1990 (abstract).

233. Gage JP: Collagen biosynthesis related to temporomandibular joint clicking in childhood, *J Prosthet Dent* 53:714-717, 1985.

234. Aufdemorte TB, Van Sickels JE, Dolwick MF, Sheridan PJ, Holt GR et al: Estrogen receptors in the temporomandibular joint of the baboon (Papio cynocephalus): an autoradiographic study, *Oral Surg Oral Med Oral Pathol* 61:307-314, 1986.

235. Milam SB, Aufdemorte TB, Sheridan PJ, Triplett RG, Van Sickels JE et al: Sexual dimorphism in the distribution of estrogen receptors in the temporomandibular joint complex of the baboon, *Oral Surg Oral Med Oral Pathol* 64:527-532, 1987.

236. McCarroll RS, Hesse JR, Naeije M, Yoon CK, Hansson TL: Mandibular border positions and their relationships with peripheral joint mobility, *J Oral Rehabil* 14:125-131, 1987.

237. Bates RE Jr, Stewart CM, Atkinson WB: The relationship between internal derangements of the temporomandibular joint and systemic joint laxity, *J Am Dent Assoc* 109:446-447, 1984.

238. Waite PD: Evaluation of 49 mitral valve prolapse patients for maxillofacial skeletal deformities and temporomandibular joint dysfunction, *Oral Surg Oral Med Oral Pathol* 62:496-499, 1986.

239. Westling L: Craniomandibular disorders and general joint mobility, *Acta Odontol Scand* 47:293-299, 1989.

240. Plunkett GA, West VC: Systemic joint laxity and mandibular range of movement, *Cranio* 6:320-326, 1988.

241. Johansson AS, Isberg A: The anterosuperior insertion of the temporomandibular joint capsule and condylar mobility in joints with and without internal derangement: a double-contrast arthrotomographic investigation, *J Oral Maxillofac Surg* 49:1142-1148, 1991.

242. Buckingham RB, Braun T, Harinstein DA, Oral K, Bauman D et al: Temporomandibular joint dysfunction syndrome: a close association with systemic joint laxity (the hypermobile joint syndrome), *Oral Surg Oral Med Oral Pathol* 72:514-519, 1991.

243. Westling L, Mattiasson A: General joint hypermobility and temporomandibular joint derangement in adolescents, *Ann Rheum Dis* 51:87-90, 1992.

244. Adair SM, Hecht C: Association of generalized joint hypermobility with history, signs, and symptoms of temporomandibular joint dysfunction in children, *Pediatr Dent* 15:323-326, 1993.

245. Perrini F, Tallents RH, Katzberg RW, Ribeiro RF, Kyrkanides S et al: Generalized joint laxity and temporomandibular disorders, *J Orofac Pain* 11:215-221, 1997.

246. De Coster PJ, Van den Berghe LI, Martens LC: Generalized joint hypermobility and temporomandibular disorders: inherited connective tissue disease as a model with maximum expression, *J Orofac Pain* 19:47-57, 2005.

247. Chun DS, Koskinen-Moffett L: Distress, jaw habits, and connective tissue laxity as predisposing factors to TMJ sounds in adolescents, *J Craniomandib Disord* 4:165-176, 1990.

248. Blasberg B, Hunter T, Philip S: Peripheral joint hypermobility in individuals with and without temporomandibular disorders, *J Dent Res* 70:278, 1991 (abstract).

249. Dijkstra PU, de Bont LGM, Stegenga B, Boering G: Temporomandibular joint osteoarthrosis and generalized joint hypermobility, *J Craniomandib Pract* 10:221-232, 1992.

250. Dijkstra PU, de Bont LGM, de Leeuw R, Stegenga B, Boering G: Temporomandibular joint osteoarthrosis and temporomandibular joint hypermobility, *J Craniomandib Pract* 11:268-275, 1993.

251. Khan FA, Pedlar J: Generalized joint hypermobility as a factor in clicking of the temporomandibular joint, *Int J Oral Maxillofac Surg* 25:101-104, 1996.

252. Winocur E, Gavish A, Halachmi M, Bloom A, Gazit E: Generalized joint laxity and its relation with oral habits and temporomandibular disorders in adolescent girls, *J Oral Rehabil* 27:614-622, 2000.

253. Elfving L, Helkimo M, Magnusson T: Prevalence of different temporomandibular joint sounds, with emphasis on disc-displacement, in patients with temporomandibular disorders and controls, *Swed Dent J* 26:9-19, 2002.

254. Conti PC, Miranda JE, Araujo CR: Relationship between systemic joint laxity, TMJ hypertranslation, and intra-articular disorders, *Cranio* 18:192-197, 2000.

255. Dickson-Parnell B, Zeichner A: The premenstrual syndrome: psychophysiologic concomitants of perceived stress and low back pain, *Pain* 34:161-173, 1988.

256. Olson GB, Peters CJ, Franger AL: The incidence and severity of premenstrual syndrome among female craniomandibular pain patients, *Cranio* 6:330-338, 1988.

257. Wardrop RW, Hailes J, Burger H, Reade PC: Oral discomfort at menopause, *Oral Surg Oral Med Oral Pathol* 67:535-544, 1989.

258. LeResche L, Mancl L, Sherman JJ, Gandara B, Dworkin SF: Changes in temporomandibular pain and other symptoms across the menstrual cycle, *Pain* 106:253-261, 2003.

259. LeResche L, Saunders K, Von Korff MR, Barlow W, Dworkin SF: Use of exogenous hormones and risk of temporomandibular disorder pain, *Pain* 69:153-160, 1997.

260. Mogil JS, Sternberg WF, Kest B, Marek P, Liebeskind JC: Sex differences in the antagonism of swim stress-induced analgesia: effects of gonadectomy and estrogen replacement, *Pain* 53:17-25, 1993.

261. Flake NM, Bonebreak DB, Gold MS: Estrogen and inflammation increase the excitability of rat temporomandibular joint afferent neurons, *J Neurophysiol* 93:1585-1597, 2005.

262. Kiliaridis S et al: Endurance test and fatigue recovery of the masticatory system, *J Dent Res* 70:342, 1991 (abstract).

263. Wongwatana S, Kronman JH, Clark RE, Kabani S, Mehta N: Anatomic basis for disk displacement in temporomandibular joint (TMJ) dysfunction, *Am J Orthod Dentofacial Orthop* 105:257-264, 1994.

264. Stegenga B, de Bont LG, Boering G, van Willigen JD: Tissue responses to degenerative changes in the temporomandibular joint: a review, *J Oral Maxillofac Surg* 49:1079-1088, 1991.

265. Gynther GW, Holmlund AB, Reinholt FP: Synovitis in internal derangement of the temporomandibular joint: correlation between arthroscopic and histologic findings, *J Oral Maxillofac Surg* 52:913-917, 1994.

266. Holmlund A, Hellsing G, Axelsson S: The temporomandibular joint: a comparison of clinical and arthroscopic findings, *J Prosthet Dent* 62:61-65, 1989.

267. Holmlund AB, Gynther GW, Reinholt FP: Disk derangement and inflammatory changes in the posterior disk attachment of the temporomandibular joint. A histologic study, *Oral Surg Oral Med Oral Pathol* 73:9-12, 1992.

268. Luder HU, Bobst P, Schroeder HE: Histometric study of synovial cavity dimensions of human temporomandibular joints with normal and anterior disc position, *J Orofac Pain* 7:263-74, 1993.

269. Stegenga B, de Bont LG, Boering G: Osteoarthrosis as the cause of craniomandibular pain and dysfunction: a unifying concept, *J Oral Maxillofac Surg* 47:249-256, 1989.

270. De Bont LGM, Boering G, Liem RSB, Eulderink F, Westesson PL: Osteoarthritis and internal derangement of the temporomandibular joint: a light microscopic study, *J Oral Maxillofac Surg* 44:634-643, 1986.

271. Mills DK, Daniel JC, Herzog S, Scapino RP: An animal model for studying mechanisms in human temporomandibular joint disc derangement, *J Oral Maxillofac Surg* 52:1279-1292, 1994.

272. Helmy E, Bays R, Sharawy M: Osteoarthrosis of the temporomandibular joint following experimental disc perforation in Macaca fascicularis, *J Oral Maxillofac Surg* 46:979-990, 1988.

273. Boering G: *Temporomandibular joint arthrosis: a clinical and radiographic investigation: thesis*, Groningen, The Netherlands, 1966, University of Groningen.

274. Farrar WB, McCarty WL: *A clinical outline of temporomandibular joint diagnosis and treatment*, Montgomery, Ala, 1983, Normandie Publications, pp 191-201.

275. McCarty WL, Farrar WB: Surgery for internal derangements of the temporomandibular joint, *J Prosthet Dent* 42:191-196, 1979.

276. Wilkes CH: Arthrography of the temporomandibular joint in patients with the TMJ pain-dysfunction syndrome, *Minn Med* 61:645-652, 1978.

277. Bell WE: *Temporomandibular disorders: classification, diagnosis, management*, ed 3, Chicago, 1990, Year Book Medical, pp 182-195.

278. Akerman S, Kopp S, Rohlin M: Histological changes in temporomandibular joints from elderly individuals. An autopsy study, *Acta Odontol Scand* 44:231-239, 1986.

279. Kircos LT, Ortendahl DA, Mark AS, Arakawa M: Magnetic resonance imaging of the TMJ disc in asymptomatic volunteers, *J Oral Maxillofac Surg* 45:852-854, 1987.

280. Zander HA, Muhlemann HR: The effects of stress on the periodontal structures, *Oral Surg Oral Med Oral Pathol* 9:380-387, 1956.

281. Glickman I: Inflammation and trauma from occlusion, *J Periodontol* 34:5-15, 1963.

282. Ramfjord SP, Ash MM: *Occlusion*, ed 3, Philadelphia, 1983, Saunders.

283. Svanberg G, Lindhe J: Experimental tooth hypermobility in the dog: a methodologic study, *Odontol Rev* 24:269-277, 1973.

284. Ericsson I, Lindhe J: Effect of longstanding jiggling on experimental marginal periodontitis in the beagle dog, *J Clin Periodontol* 9:497-503, 1982.

285. Polson AM, Meitner SW, Zander HA: Trauma and progression of marginal periodontitis in squirrel monkeys. III. Adaption of interproximal alveolar bone to repetitive injury, *J Periodontal Res* 11:279-289, 1976.

286. Ettala-Ylitalo UM, Markkanen H, Yli-Urpo A: Influence of occlusal interferences on the periodontium in patients treated with fixed prosthesis, *J Prosthet Dent* 55:252-255, 1986.

287. Kenney EB: A histologic study of incisal dysfunction and gingival inflammation in the rhesus monkey, *J Periodontol* 11:290, 1972.

288. Sirirungrojying S, Kerdpon D: Relationship between oral tori and temporomandibular disorders, *Int Dent J* 49:101-104, 1999.

289. Clifford T, Lamey PJ, Fartash L: Mandibular tori, migraine and temporomandibular disorders, *Br Dent J* 180:382-384, 1996.

290. Jainkittivong A, Langlais RP: Buccal and palatal exostoses: prevalence and concurrence with tori, *Oral Surg Oral Med Oral Pathol Oral Radiol Endod* 90:48-53, 2000.

291. Ikeda T, Nakano M, Bando E: The effect of traumatic occlusal contact on tooth pain threshold, *J Dent Res* 70:330, 1991 (abstract).

292. Ramfjord SP, Ash MM: *Occlusion*, ed 3, Philadelphia, 1983, Saunders, pp 313-314.

293. Okeson JP, Kemper JT: Clinical examination of 168 general dental patients in 1982 (unpublished).

294. Pullinger AG, Seligman DA: The degree to which attrition characterizes differentiated patient groups of temporomandibular disorders, *J Orofac Pain* 7:196-208, 1993.

295. Kois JC, Phillips KM: Occlusal vertical dimension: alteration concerns, *Compend Contin Educ Dent* 18:1169-1174, 1176-1177, 1997; quiz 1180.

296. Cook NR, Evans DA, Funkenstein HH, Scherr PA, Ostfeld AM et al: Correlates of headache in a population-based cohort of elderly, *Arch Neurol* 46:1338-1344, 1989.

297. Sternbach RA: Survey of pain in the United States: the Nuprin Pain Report, *Clin J Pain* 2:49-53, 1986.

298. Cacchiotti DA, Plesh O, Bianchi P, McNeill C: Signs and symptoms in samples with and without temporomandibular disorders, *J Craniomandib Disord* 5:167-172, 1991.

299. Gelb H, Tarte J: A two-year clinical dental evaluation of 200 cases of chronic headache: the craniocervical mandibular syndrome, *J Am Dent Assoc* 91:1230-1239, 1975.

300. Kreisberg MK: Headache as a symptom of craniomandibular disorders. II: management, *Cranio* 4:219-228, 1986.

301. Schokker RP, Hansson TL, Ansink BJ: Craniomandibular disorders in patients with different types of headache, *J Craniomandib Disord* 4:47-51, 1990.

302. Jensen R, Rasmussen BK, Pedersen B, Lous I, Olesen J: Prevalence of oromandibular dysfunction in a general population, *J Orofac Pain* 7:175-182, 1993.

303. Wanman A, Agerberg G: Recurrent headaches and craniomandibular disorders in adolescents: a longitudinal study, *J Craniomandib Disord* 1:229-236, 1987.

304. Reik L Jr, Hale M: The temporomandibular joint pain-dysfunction syndrome: a frequent cause of headache, *Headache* 21:151-156, 1981.

305. Graff-Radford SB: Oromandibular disorders and headache. A critical appraisal, *Neurol Clin* 8:929-945, 1990.

306. Forssell H, Kangasniemi P: Correlation of the frequency and intensity of headache to mandibular dysfunction in headache patients, *Proc Finn Dent Soc* 80:223-226, 1984.

307. Forssell H, Kirveskari P, Kangasniemi P: Response to occlusal treatment in headache patients previously treated by mock occlusal adjustment, *Acta Odontol Scand* 45:77-80, 1987.

308. Nassif NJ, Talic YF: Classic symptoms in temporomandibular disorder patients: a comparative study, *Cranio* 19:33-41, 2001.

309. Ciancaglini R, Radaelli G: The relationship between headache and symptoms of temporomandibular disorder in the general population, *J Dent* 29:93-98, 2001.

310. Liljestrom MR, Le Bell Y, Anttila P, Aromaa M, Jamsa T et al: Headache children with temporomandibular disorders have several types of pain and other symptoms, *Cephalalgia* 25:1054-1060, 2005.

311. Bernhardt O, Gesch D, Schwahn C, Mack F, Meyer G et al: Risk factors for headache, including TMD signs and symptoms, and their impact on quality of life. Results of the Study of Health in Pomerania (SHIP), *Quintessent Int* 36:55-64, 2005.

312. Kemper JT Jr, Okeson JP: Craniomandibular disorders and headaches, *J Prosthet Dent* 49:702-705, 1983.

313. Schokker RP, Hansson TL, Ansink BJ: The result of treatment of the masticatory system of chronic headache patients, *J Craniomandib Disord* 4:126-130, 1990.

314. Vallerand WP, Hall MB: Improvement in myofascial pain and headaches following TMJ surgery, *J Craniomandib Disord* 5:197-204, 1991.

315. Vallon D, Ekberg EC, Nilner M, Kopp S: Short-term effect of occlusal adjustment on craniomandibular disorders including headaches, *Acta Odontol Scand* 49:89-96, 1991.

316. Vallon D, Ekberg E, Nilner M, Kopp S: Occlusal adjustment in patients with craniomandibular disorders including headaches. A 3- and 6-month follow-up, *Acta Odontol Scand* 53:55-59, 1995.

317. Quayle AA, Gray RJ, Metcalfe RJ, Guthrie E, Wastell D: Soft occlusal splint therapy in the treatment of migraine and other headaches, *J Dent* 18:123-129, 1990.

318. Magnusson T, Carlsson GE: A 2½-year follow-up of changes in headache and mandibular dysfunction after stomatognathic treatment, *J Prosthet Dent* 49:398-402, 1983.

319. Haley D, Schiffman E, Baker C, Belgrade M: The comparison of patients suffering from temporomandibular disorders and a general headache population, *Headache* 33:210-213, 1993.

320. Ekberg E, Vallon D, Nilner M: Treatment outcome of headache after occlusal appliance therapy in a randomized controlled trial among patients with temporomandibular disorders of mainly arthrogenous origin, *Swed Dent J* 26:115-124, 2002.

321. Jokstad A, Mo A, Krogstad BS: Clinical comparison between two different splint designs for temporomandibular disorder therapy, *Acta Odontol Scand* 63:218-226, 2005.

322. Olesen J: The International Classification for Headache Disorders, *Cephalalgia* 24(suppl 1):1-160, 2004.

323. Okeson J: *Orofacial pain: guidelines for classification, assessment, and management*, Chicago, 1996, Quintessence, pp 53-60.

324. Okeson JP: *Bell's orofacial pains*, ed 6, Chicago, 2005, Quintessence, pp 141-196.

325. Hudzinski LG, Lawrence GS: Significance of EMG surface electrode placement models and headache findings, *Headache* 28:30-35, 1988.

326. Pritchard DW: EMG cranial muscle levels in headache sufferers before and during headache, *Headache* 29:103-108, 1989.

327. Van Boxtel A, Goudswaard P, Janssen K: Absolute and proportional resting EMG levels in muscle contraction and migraine headache patients, *Headache* 23:215-222, 1983.

328. Rugh JD, Hatch JP: The effects of psychological stress on electromyographic activity and negative affect in ambulatory tension-type headache patients, *Headache* 30:216-219, 1990.

329. Diamond S: Muscle contraction headaches. In Dalessio D, editor: *Wolff's headache and other head pain*, New York, 1987, Oxford University Press, pp 172-189.

330. Olesen J: Clinical and pathophysiological observations in migraine and tension-type headache explained by

integration of vascular, supraspinal and myofascial inputs, *Pain* 46:125-132, 1991.

331. Okeson JP: *Bell's orofacial pains*, ed 6, Chicago, 2005, Quintessence, pp 401-448.

332. Wolff HG: *Headache and other head pain*, New York, 1963, Oxford University Press, pp 35-47.

333. Hanington E, Jones RJ, Amess JA, Wachowicz B: Migraine: a platelet disorder, *Lancet* 2:720-723, 1981.

334. Sicuteri F: Migraine, a central biochemical dysnociception, *Headache* 16:145-159, 1976.

335. Olesen J, Edvinsson L: *Basic mechanisms of headache*, Amsterdam, 1988, Elsevier, pp 223-227.

336. Moskowitz MA: Neurogenic inflammation in the pathophysiology and treatment of migraine, *Neurology* 43: S16-20, 1993.

337. Rasmussen BK, Jensen R, Schroll M, Olesen J: Epidemiology of headache in a general population—a prevalence study, *J Clin Epidemiol* 44:1147-1157, 1991.

338. Lance JW, Anthony M: Some clinical aspects of migraine, *Arch Neurol* 15:356-361, 1966.

339. Selby G, Lance JW: Observations on 500 cases of migraine and allied vascular headache, *J Neurol Neurosurg Psychiatry* 23:23-32, 1960.

340. Steele JG, Lamey PJ, Sharkey SW, Smith GM: Occlusal abnormalities, pericranial muscle and joint tenderness and tooth wear in a group of migraine patients, *J Oral Rehabil* 18:453-458, 1991.

341. Jensen R, Rasmussen BK, Pedersen B, Olesen J: Prevalence of oromandibular dysfunction in a general population, *J Orofac Pain* 7:175-182, 1993.

342. Kuttila S, Kuttila M, Le Bell Y, Alanen P, Jouko S: Aural symptoms and signs of temporomandibular disorder in association with treatment need and visits to a physician, *Laryngoscope* 109:1669-1673, 1999.

343. Ciancaglini R, Loreti P, Radaelli G: Ear, nose, and throat symptoms in patients with TMD: the association of symptoms according to severity of arthropathy, *J Orofac Pain* 8:293-297, 1994.

344. Brookes GB, Maw AR, Coleman MJ: 'Costen's syndrome'—correlation or coincidence: a review of 45 patients with temporomandibular joint dysfunction, otalgia and other aural symptoms, *Clin Otolaryngol* 5: 23-36, 1980.

345. Gelb H, Calderone JP, Gross SM, Kantor ME: The role of the dentist and the otolaryngologist in evaluating temporomandibular joint syndromes, *J Prosthet Dent* 18: 497-503, 1967.

346. DuBrul EL: *Sicher's oral anatomy*, St Louis, 1980, Mosby, pp 531-532.

347. Malkin DP: The role of TMJ dysfunction in the etiology of middle ear disease, *Int J Orthod* 25:20-21, 1987.

348. Williamson EH: Interrelationship of internal derangements of the temporomandibular joint, headache, vertigo, and tinnitus: a survey of 25 patients, *Cranio* 8:301-306, 1990.

349. Parker WS, Chole RA: Tinnitus, vertigo, and temporomandibular disorders, *Am J Orthod Dentofacial Orthop* 107:153-158, 1995.

350. Vernon J, Griest S, Press L: Attributes of tinnitus that may predict temporomandibular joint dysfunction, *Cranio* 10:282-287, 1992.

351. Kelly HT, Goodfriend DJ: Medical significance of equilibration of the masticating mechanism, *J Prosthet Dent* 10:496-515, 1960.

352. Kelly HT, Goodfriend DJ: Vertigo attributable to dental and temporomandibular joint causes, *J Prosthet Dent* 14:159-173, 1964.

353. Myrhaug H: *The theory of otosclerosis and morbus meniere (labyrinthine vertigo) being caused by the same mechanism: physical irritants, an oto-gnathic syndrome: thesis*, Bergen, Norway, 1969, Staudia.

354. Myrhaug H: Para functions in gingival mucosa as cause of an otodental syndrome, *Quintessence Int* 1:81-94, 1970.

355. Rubinstein B, Axelsson A, Carlsson GE: Prevalence of signs and symptoms of craniomandibular disorders in tinnitus patients, *J Craniomandib Disord* 4:186-192, 1990.

356. Ren YF, Isberg A: Tinnitus in patients with temporomandibular joint internal derangement, *Cranio* 13:75-80, 1995.

357. Bernhardt O, Gesch D, Schwahn C, Bitter K, Mundt T et al: Signs of temporomandibular disorders in tinnitus patients and in a population-based group of volunteers: results of the Study of Health in Pomerania, *J Oral Rehabil* 31:311-319, 2004.

358. Upton LG, Wijeyesakere SJ: The incidence of tinnitus in people with disorders of the temporomandibular joint, *Int Tinnitus J* 10:174-176, 2004.

359. Camparis CM, Formigoni G, Teixeira MJ, de Siqueira JT. Clinical evaluation of tinnitus in patients with sleep bruxism: prevalence and characteristics, *J Oral Rehabil* 32: 808-814, 2005.

360. Penkner K, Kole W, Kainz J, Schied G, Lorenzoni M: The function of tensor veli palatini muscles in patients with aural symptoms and temporomandibular disorder. An EMG study, *J Oral Rehabil* 27:344-348, 2000.

361. Rubenstein B, Carlsson GF: Effects of stomatognathic treatment of tinnitus: a retrospective study, *J Craniomandib Pract* 5:254-259, 1987.

362. Bush FM: Tinnitus and otalgia in temporomandibular disorders, *J Prosthet Dent* 58:495-498, 1987.

363. Marasa FK, Ham BD: Case reports involving the treatment of children with chronic otitis media with effusion via craniomandibular methods, *Cranio* 6:256-270, 1988.

364. Kempf HG, Roller R, Muhlbradt L: Correlation between inner ear disorders and temporomandibular joint diseases (see comments), *HNO* 41:7-10, 1993.

365. Wright EF, Bifano SL: Tinnitus improvement through TMD therapy, *J Am Dent Assoc* 128:1424-1432, 1997

366. Gelb H, Gelb ML, Wagner ML: The relationship of tinnitus to craniocervical mandibular disorders, *Cranio* 15:136-143, 1997.

367. Steigerwald DP, Verne SV, Young D: A retrospective evaluation of the impact of temporomandibular joint arthroscopy on the symptoms of headache, neck pain, shoulder pain, dizziness, and tinnitus, *Cranio* 14:46-54, 1996.

368. Wright EF, Syms CA, Bifano SL: Tinnitus, dizziness, and nonotologic otalgia improvement through temporomandibular disorder therapy, *Mil Med* 165:733-736, 2000.

369. Loughner BA, Larkin LH, Mahan PE: Discomalleolar and anterior malleolar ligaments: possible causes of middle ear damage during temporomandibular joint surgery, *Oral Surg Oral Med Oral Pathol* 68:14-22, 1989.

370. Turp JC: Correlation between myoarthropathies of the masticatory system and ear symptoms (otalgia, tinnitus), *HNO* 46:303-310, 1998.

371. Toller MO, Juniper RP: Audiological evaluation of the aural symptoms in temporomandibular joint dysfunction, *J Craniomaxillofac Surg* 21:2-8, 1993.

372. Lam DK, Lawrence HP, Tenenbaum HC: Aural symptoms in temporomandibular disorder patients attending a craniofacial pain unit, *J Orofac Pain* 15:146-157, 2001.

History of and Examination for Temporomandibular Disorders

9

CHAPTER

"Nothing is more critical to success than beginning with all the necessary data."

—JPO

The signs and symptoms of temporomandibular disorders (TMDs) are extremely common. The epidemiologic studies described in Chapter 7 suggest that 50% to 60% of the general population has a sign of some functional disturbance of the masticatory system. Some of these appear as significant symptoms that motivate the patient to seek treatment. Many, however, are subtle and not even at a level of clinical awareness by the patient. As described earlier, signs of which the patient is unaware are said to be subclinical. Some subclinical signs can later become apparent and represent more significant functional disturbances if left unattended. Therefore it is important to identify any and all signs and symptoms of functional disturbances in each patient.

This is not to suggest that all signs indicate a need for treatment. The significance of the sign and the etiology, as well as the prognosis of the disorder, are factors that determine the need for treatment. The significance of a sign, however, cannot be evaluated until that sign has been identified. Because many of the signs are subclinical, many disturbances can progress and remain undiagnosed and therefore untreated by the clinician. The effectiveness and success of treatment lie in the ability of the clinician to establish the proper diagnosis. This can be established only after a thorough examination of the patient for the signs and symptoms of functional disturbances. Each sign represents a portion of information needed to establish a proper diagnosis. Therefore it is extremely important that each sign and symptom be identified by means of a thorough history and examination procedure. This is the essential foundation for successful treatment.

The purpose of a history and examination is to identify any area or structure of the masticatory system that shows breakdown or pathologic change. To be effective, the examiner must have a sound understanding of the clinical appearance and function of the healthy masticatory system (see Part I). Breakdown in the masticatory system is generally signified by pain and/or dysfunction. History and examination procedures should therefore be directed toward the identification of masticatory pain and dysfunction.

When the patient's chief complaint is pain, it is important to identify the source of the problem. The dentist's primary role in therapy is the treatment of masticatory pains. As already described, masticatory pains have their sources in and emanate from masticatory structures. Masticatory structures are the teeth, periodontium, supporting structures of the teeth, temporomandibular joints (TMJs), and muscles that move the mandible. By virtue of training, the dentist is best suited for treating these structures. Unfortunately, however, disorders of the head and neck can frequently lead to heterotopic pains that are felt in the masticatory structures but do not have their sources within masticatory structures (see Chapter 2). These types of pains must be properly identified during an examination so that an accurate diagnosis can be established. To be effective, treatment must be directed toward the source of pain and not toward the site. For dental treatment to be effective, the pain must be of masticatory origin.

A general rule in identifying masticatory pain is that jaw function usually aggravates or accentuates the problem. In other words, the functional activities of chewing and talking increase the pain. This rule is not always true, however, because some nonmasticatory pains can produce secondary hyperalgesia in masticatory structures, and thus function will increase the pain. At the same time one must be suspicious of the patient who reports the location of the pain to be TMJ or masticatory muscles yet whose history and examination reveal no alteration in range of jaw movement or increase in pain during function. When this circumstance exists, therapy directed toward the masticatory structures is likely to be useless. The examiner must find the true source of pain before effective treatment can be provided.

SCREENING HISTORY AND EXAMINATION

Because the prevalence of TMDs is high, it is recommended that each patient who comes to the dental office be screened for these problems, regardless of the apparent need or lack of need for treatment. The purpose of the screening history and examination is to identify patients with subclinical signs, as well as symptoms that the patient may not relate but are commonly associated with functional disturbances of the masticatory system (e.g., headaches, ear symptoms). The screening history consists of several questions that will help orient the clinician to any TMDs. These can be asked personally by the clinician or may be included in a general health and dental questionnaire that the patient completes before being seen by the dentist.

The following can be used to identify functional disturbances[1]:

1. Do you have difficulty and/or pain when opening your mouth, for instance, when yawning?
2. Does your jaw get "stuck" or "locked" or "go out"?
3. Do you have difficulty and/or pain when chewing, talking, or using your jaws?
4. Are you aware of noises in the jaw joints?
5. Do your jaws regularly feel stiff, tight, or tired?
6. Do you have pain in or about the ears, temples, or cheeks?
7. Do you have frequent headaches, neckaches, or toothaches?
8. Have you had a recent injury to your head, neck, or jaw?
9. Have you been aware of any recent changes in your bite?
10. Have you previously been treated for any unexplained facial pain or a jaw joint problem?

Accompanying the screening history is a short screening examination. This should be brief and is an attempt to identify any variation from normal anatomy and function. It begins with an inspection of the facial symmetry. Any variation from the general bilateral symmetry should raise suspicion and indicate the need for further examination. The screening examination also includes observations of jaw movement. Restriction or irregular mandibular movements are indications for a more thorough examination.

Several important structures of the masticatory system are palpated for pain or tenderness during the screening examination. The temporal and masseter muscles are palpated bilaterally along with the lateral aspects of the TMJs. Any pain or tenderness should be viewed as a potential indicator of a TMD.

If the screening history and examination reveal positive findings, a more thorough history and examination for TMDs is completed. Three basic structures should be examined for pain and/or dysfunction: the muscles, TMJs, and dentition. Before the examination, a complete history of the problem, both past and present, is obtained from the patient.

HISTORY TAKING FOR TEMPOROMANDIBULAR DISORDERS

The importance of taking a thorough history can hardly be overemphasized. When the clinician is examining a patient for dental disease (e.g., caries), a relatively small percentage of the information needed for diagnosis will be gained through the history; most of it will come from the examination. Diagnosing pain, however, is quite different. With pain disorders, as much as 70% to 80% of the information needed to make the diagnosis will come from the history, with the examination contributing a smaller part.

Most often the patient will provide essential information that cannot be acquired from the examination procedures. The history is key in making an accurate diagnosis, and often patients will tell the examiner the diagnosis in their own words.

The history can be obtained by one of two manners. Some clinicians prefer to *converse directly* with the patient concerning the history of the problem. This allows them to direct questions that appropriately follow the patient's previous response. Although this method of seeking vital facts is effective, it relies heavily on the clinician's ability to pursue *all* areas of concern. A more thorough and consistent history can be taken by a *written questionnaire* that includes all areas of concern. This method assures that each bit of necessary information is obtained. Although it is usually more complete, some patients have difficulty expressing their problem using a standard form. Therefore in most cases the best history taking consists of having the patient complete a predeveloped questionnaire so that the clinician can review it with the patient and discuss the findings.

It is helpful to have the patient complete the questionnaire in a quiet area with no particular time constraints. As the clinician reviews the questionnaire with the patient, any discrepancies or major concerns can be discussed with the patient to gain additional information. At this time the patient is freely allowed to expound on concerns that were not expressed in the questionnaire.

The history begins with a complete medical questionnaire identifying any major medical problems of the patient. Major medical problems can play an important role in functional disturbances. For example, a patient's generalized arthritic condition can also affect the TMJ. Even when symptoms are not closely related to a major medical problem, the existence of such a problem may play an important role in selecting a treatment method.

An effective history centers on the patient's chief complaint. This is a good starting point in obtaining needed information. The patient is allowed to describe, in his or her own words, the chief complaint. If the patient has more than one complaint, each complaint is initially recorded and detailed information on each is collected separately. A complete history obtains information in the following specific areas.

PAIN

When pain is present, it is evaluated according to the patient's description of the chief complaint; location; onset; characteristics; any aggravating and alleviating factors; past treatments; and any relationship to other complaints as to location, behavior, quality, duration, and degree. Each of these factors is discussed in this section and highlighted in Box 9-1.

Chief Complaint

A good starting point in history taking is to obtain an accurate description of the patient's chief complaint. This should first be taken in the patient's own words and then restated in technical language as indicated. If the patient has more than one pain complaint, each complaint should be noted and, when possible, placed in a list according to its significance to the patient. Each complaint needs to be evaluated according to each factor listed in the history outline. Once this has been accomplished, each pain complaint should be assessed regarding its relationship to any of the other complaints. Some complaints may be secondary to another complaint, whereas others may be independent. Determining these relationships is basic to management.

Location of Pain. The patient's ability to locate the pain with accuracy has diagnostic value. The examiner, however, should always guard against assuming that the site of pain necessarily identifies the true source of pain—the structure from which the pain actually emanates. The patient's description of the location of his or her complaint identifies only the site of pain. It is the examiner's responsibility to determine whether it is also the true source of the pain. Sometimes, what

Features to Be Included in a Thorough Orofacial Pain History

I. Chief complaint (may be more than one)
   A. Location of pain
   B. Onset of pain
      1. Associated with other factors
      2. Progression
   C. Characteristics of pain
      1. Quality of pain
      2. Behavior of pain
         a. Temporal
         b. Duration
         c. Localization
      3. Intensity of pain
      4. Concomitant symptoms
      5. Flow of pain
   D. Aggravating and alleviating factors
      1. Function and parafunction
      2. Physical modalities
      3. Medications
      4. Emotional stress
      5. Sleep disturbances
      6. Litigation
   E. Past consultations and/or treatments
   F. Relationship to other pain complaints
II. Past medical history
III. Review of systems
IV. Psychologic assessment

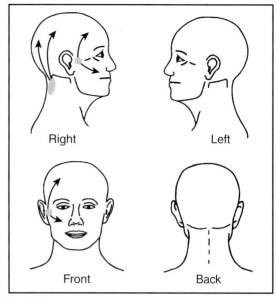

Fig. 9-1 The patient should be asked to draw the location and radiating pattern of the pain.

appears to be adequate cause at the site of pain may mislead both patient and doctor, such as visible superficial herpetic lesions in an area that also happens to be the site of pain referral from the cervical area. The clinician needs to perform the needed diagnostic tests to determine the true source of the pain (see Chapter 10).

It can be helpful to provide the patient with a drawing of the head and neck and ask him or her to outline the location of the pain (Fig. 9-1). This allows the patient to reflect in his or her own way any and all of the pain sites. The patient can also draw arrows revealing any patterns of pain referral. These drawing can give the clinician significant insight regarding the location and even the type of pain the patient is experiencing.

Onset of Pain. Assessing any circumstances that were associated with the initial onset of the pain complaint is important. These circumstances can give great insight as to cause. For example, in some instances the pain complaint began immediately following a motor vehicle accident. Trauma is a frequent cause of a pain condition and provides not only insight about cause but also considerations such as other injuries, related emotional trauma, and possible litigation. The onset of some pain conditions is associated with systemic illnesses or jaw function, or it may even be wholly spontaneous. Having the patient present the circumstances associated with the initial onset in chronologic order is important for the proper relationships to be evaluated.

Asking the patient what he or she believes caused the pain condition is equally important. This may provide great insight into the patient's view of his or her pain. In many instances the patient knows precisely what caused the condition. Even if the patient is confused as to cause, the examiner may gain valuable information that is useful in management. For example, this question may reveal anger associated with blame for the pain condition.

Importantly, the examiner should know whether the patient believes mistreatment or another practitioner has caused the pain. This type of anger may greatly affect future treatment outcome.

Characteristics of Pain. The characteristics of the pain need to be precisely described by the patient as to its quality, behavior, intensity, concomitant symptoms, and manner of flow.

Quality of pain. The quality of pain should be classified according to how it makes the patient feel. This classification is usually termed *bright* or *dull*. When pain has a stimulating or exciting effect on the patient, it is classified as bright. When the pain has a depressing effect that causes the patient to withdraw to some extent, it is classified as dull. Such judgment should be wholly independent of pain intensity, variability, temporal characteristics, or any accompanying lancinating exacerbations that may punctuate the basic underlying painful sensation.

Further evaluation of the quality of pain should be made to classify it as pricking, itching, stinging, burning, aching, or pulsating. Many pains, of course, require more than a single designation. Bright, tingling pain is classified as a *pricking* sensation, especially when mild and stimulating. Superficial discomfort that does not reach pain threshold intensity may be described as *itching*. As intensity increases, it may take on a pricking, stinging, aching, or burning quality. Deep discomfort that does not reach pain threshold intensity may be described as a vague, diffuse sensation of pressure, warmth, or tenderness. As intensity increases, the pain may take on a sore, aching, throbbing, or burning quality. When the discomfort has an irritating, hot, raw, caustic quality, it is usually described as *burning*. Most pains have an aching quality. Some noticeably increase with each heartbeat and are described as *pulsating* or *throbbing*.

Behavior of pain. The behavior of the pain should be evaluated according to frequency or temporal behavior, as well as its duration and localizability.

Temporal behavior. Temporal behavior reflects the frequency of the pain, as well as the periods between episodes of the pain. If the suffering distinctly comes and goes, leaving pain-free intervals of noticeable duration, it is classified as *intermittent*. If such pain-free intervals do not occur, the suffering is classified as *continuous*. Intermittency should not be confused with *variability*, in which there may be alternate periods of high- and low-level discomfort. *Intermittent* pain implies the occurrence of true intermissions or pain-free periods during which comfort is complete. This temporal behavior should not be confused with the effect of medications that induce periods of comfort by analgesic action. When episodes of pain, whether continuous or intermittent, are separated by an extended period of freedom from discomfort, only to be followed by another similar episode of pain, the syndrome is said to be *recurrent*.

Pain duration. The duration of individual pains in an episode is an important descriptive feature that aids in pain identification. A pain is said to be *momentary* if its duration can be expressed in seconds. Longer-lasting pains are classified in minutes, hours, or a day. A pain that continues from one day to the next is said to be *protracted*.

Localization. The localization behavior of the pain should be included in its description. If the patient can define the pain to an exact anatomic location, it is classified as *localized pain*. If such description is less well defined and somewhat vague and variable anatomically, it is termed *diffuse pain*. Rapidly changing pain is classified as *radiating*. A momentary cutting exacerbation is usually described as *lancinating*. More gradually changing pain is described as *spreading*, and if it progressively involves adjacent anatomic areas, the pain is called *enlarging*. If it changes from one location to another, the complaint is described as *migrating*. Referred pain and secondary hyperalgesia are clinical expressions of secondary or heterotopic pain.

Intensity of pain. The intensity of pain should be established by distinguishing between mild and severe pain. This can be based on how the patient appears to react to his or her suffering. Mild pain is associated with pain that is described by the patient, but there is no display of visible physical reactions. Severe pains are associated with significant reactions of the patient to provocation of the painful area. One of the best methods of assessing the intensity of the pain is with a visual analog scale. The patient is present with a line that has "no pain" written on one end and "the most severe pain possible" written on the other end. The patient is then asked to place a mark on the location of the line that best describes his or her pain today. A scale of 0 to 5 or 0 to 10 can be used to assess the intensity of the pain, 0 being no pain and 10 being the most pain possible. This scale is not only helpful for the initial assessment of pain but is also useful at follow-up appointments to evaluate the success or failure of therapies.

Concomitant symptoms. All concomitant symptoms such as sensory, motor, or autonomic effects that accompany the pain should be included. Sensations such as hyperesthesia, hypoesthesia, anesthesia, paresthesia, or dysesthesia should be mentioned. Any concomitant change in the special senses affecting vision, hearing, smell, or taste should be noted. Motor changes expressed as muscular weakness, muscular contractions, or actual spasm should be recognized. Various localized autonomic symptoms should be observed and described. Ocular symptoms may include lacrimation, injection of the conjunctiva, pupillary changes, and edema of the lids. Nasal symptoms include nasal secretion and congestion. Cutaneous symptoms involve skin temperature, color, sweating, and piloerection. Gastric symptoms include nausea and indigestion.

Manner of flow of pain. The manner of flow yields important information by determining whether the individual pains are steady or paroxysmal. A flowing type of pain, even though variable in intensity or distinctly intermittent, is described as *steady.* Such pain is to be distinguished from *paroxysmal* pain, which characteristically consists of sudden volleys or jabs. The volleys may vary considerably in both intensity and duration. When they occur frequently, the pain may become nearly continuous.

Aggravating and Alleviating Factors

Effect of functional activities. The effect of functional activities should be observed and described. Common biomechanical functions include such activities as movement of the face, jaw, or tongue and the effects of swallowing, head position, and body position. The effect of activities such as talking, chewing, yawning, brushing the teeth, shaving, washing the face, turning the head, stooping over, or lying down should be noted. The effect of emotional stress, fatigue, and time of day also should be recorded.

The pain may be triggered by minor superficial stimulation such as touch or movement of the skin, lips, face, tongue, or throat. When triggered by such activities, it is wise to distinguish between stimulation of overlying tissues that are only incidentally stimulated and the result of functioning of the joints and muscles themselves. The former is true triggering, whereas the latter is pain induction. This distinction can usually be made by stabilizing the joints and muscles with a bite block to prevent their movement while the other structures are stimulated or moved. If uncertainty exists, the distinction can be made more positively by using local anesthesia. Topical anesthesia of the throat effectively arrests triggering in the glossopharyngeal nerve distribution. Mandibular block anesthesia stops triggering from the lower lip and tongue. Infraorbital anesthesia arrests triggering from the upper lip and maxillary skin. None of these procedures prevents the induction of true masticatory pain.

Parafunctional activities should also be assessed. The patient should be questioned regarding bruxism, clenching, or any other oral habit. One should remember that often these activities occur at subconscious levels and the patient may not be accurate with the reporting (i.e., clenching and bruxing). Other habits are more readily reported (e.g., holding objects between the teeth, such as a pipe, pencils, or occupational implements). Habits that introduce extraoral forces are also identified, such as holding a telephone between the chin and shoulder, resting the mandible in the hands while sitting at a table, or playing certain musical instruments.[2,3] Any force applied to the jaw (either intraorally or extraorally) must be identified as a potential contributing factor to the functional disturbance.[4]

Effect of physical modalities. The patient should be questioned regarding the effectiveness of hot or cold on the pain condition. The patient should be asked if other modalities such as massage or TENS (transcutaneous electrical neural stimulation) therapy have been tried and, if so, what the results were. The results of such therapies may shed light of the type and therapeutic responsiveness of the pain condition.

Medications. The patient should review all past and present medications taken for the pain condition.

Dosages should be reported along with the frequency taken and effectiveness in altering the chief complaint. It is also helpful to know who prescribed these medications because his or her input may also shed light on the pain condition. Some commonly used medications such as oral contraceptives and estrogen replacements may play a role in some pain conditions,[5,6] although this is still debated.[7]

Emotional stress. As previously mentioned, emotional stress can play a significant role in functional disturbances of the masticatory system. While taking the history, the clinician should attempt to assess the level of emotional stress being experienced by the patient. This is often difficult to do. No conclusive questionnaires can be used to identify whether high levels of emotional stress relate to the patient's problem, nor can any emotional stress test be used to help diagnose or determine an effective treatment. Sometimes the course of the symptoms can be helpful. When symptoms are periodic, the patient should be questioned for any correlation between symptoms and high levels of emotional stress. A positive correlation is an important finding and will affect diagnosis and treatment. This represents another factor that can only be identified by taking a thorough history. The effect of emotional stress on the patient is also ascertained by questioning for the presence of other psychophysiologic disorders (e.g., gastritis, hypertension, colitis). The presence of these types of disorders helps document the effect of stress on the patient.

Sleep quality. Relationships exist between some pain conditions and the quality of the patient's sleep.[8-11] Therefore it is important that the quality of the patient's sleep be reviewed. Patients who report poor-quality sleep should be questioned regarding the relationship of this finding with the pain condition. Particular notice should be taken when the patient reports awaking during the night in pain or when the pain actually awakes the patient.

Litigation and disability. During the interview it is important to inquire whether the patient is involved in any form of litigation related to the pain complaint. This information may help the clinician better appreciate all the conditions that surround the pain complaint. The presence of litigation does not directly imply secondary gains, but this condition may be present.

A similar condition may exist with disability. If the patient is either receiving or applying for disability that will allow him or her not to work yet receive compensation, it may have a powerful effect on the individual's desire to get well and return to work. Secondary gains may have a direct effect on the success or failure of the clinician's treatment.

Past Consultations and Treatments. During the interview all previous consultations and treatments should be thoroughly discussed and reviewed. This information is extremely important so that repetition of tests and therapies are avoided. If information is incomplete or unclear, the previous treating clinician should be contacted and appropriate information requested. Clinical notes from previous treating clinicians can be extremely helping in deciding future treatments.

When a patient reports previous treatments such as an occlusal appliance, the patient should be asked to bring the appliance to the evaluation appointment. The previous success of this treatment should be reported and the appliance evaluated. This evaluation may shed light on future treatment considerations.

Relationship to Other Pain Complaints. As previously discussed, some patients may report more than one pain complaint. When more than one complaint is reported, the clinician needs to evaluate each aspect of each complaint separately. Once each complaint is evaluated according to the previously mentioned criteria, the relationship of one complaint to the others should be ascertained. Sometimes a pain complaint may actually be secondary to another complaint. In these instances, effective management of the primary pain complaint will likely also resolve the secondary pain complaint. In other instances, one complaint may be totally independent of another complaint. When this exists, individual therapy may need to be directed to each complaint. Identifying the relationship between these complaints is essential and best determined by the history.

Medical History

Because pain can be a symptom related to many physical illnesses and disorders, it is essential that the past and present medical condition be carefully evaluated. Any past serious illnesses, hospitalizations, operations, medications, or other significant treatments should be discussed in light of the present pain complaint. When indicated, treating physicians should be contacted for additional information. It may also be appropriate to discuss the suggested treatment with the patient's physician when significant health problems are present.

Review of Systems

A complete history should also include appropriate questions concerning the present status of the patient's general body systems. Questions should investigate the present health status of the following systems: cardiovascular (including lungs), digestive, renal, liver, and peripheral and central nervous systems. Any abnormalities should be noted, and any relationship with the pain complaint should be determined.

Psychologic Assessment

As pain becomes more chronic, psychologic factors relating to the pain complaint become more common. Routine psychologic evaluation may not be necessary with acute pain; however, with chronic pain it becomes essential. It may be difficult for the general practitioner to confidently evaluate psychologic factors. For this reason, chronic pain patients are best evaluated and managed by a multidisciplinary approach.

A variety of measuring tools can be used to assess the psychologic status of the patient. Turk and Rudy[12] have developed the Multidimensional Pain Inventory (MPI). This scale evaluates how the pain experience is affecting the patient. It classifies the patient into three pain profiles: adaptive coping, interpersonal distress, and dysfunctional chronic pain. Dysfunctional chronic pain is a profile of severe pain, functional disability, psychologic impairment, and low perceived life control.

Another useful tool is the Symptom Check List 90 (SCL-90).[13] This evaluation provides an assessment of the following eight psychologic states: somatization, obsessive-compulsive behavior, interpersonal sensitivity, depression, anxiety, hostility, phobic anxiety, paranoid ideation, and psychoticism.

Assessing these factors is essential when evaluating the chronic pain patient.

Often the general practitioner may not have immediate access to psychologic evaluation support. In this instance the practitioner may elect to use IMPATH[14] or the TMJ Scale.[15,16] These two scales have been developed for use in the private dental practice to assist in evaluating clinical and certain psychologic factors associated with orofacial pains. These scales can assist the dentist in identifying whether psychologic issues are an important aspect of the patient's pain condition. Although these scales are helpful, they are not as complete as the previously mentioned psychologic tests and certainly do not replace the personal evaluation of a clinical psychologist.

CLINICAL EXAMINATION

Once the history has been obtained and thoroughly discussed with the patient, a clinical examination is performed. It should identify any variations from the normal health and function of the masticatory system.

Because of the complexity of head and neck pain disorders, it is important that certain nonmasticatory structures be at least grossly examined for the purpose of ruling out other possible disorders.[17] Even before one examines the masticatory structures, it is important to evaluate gross function of the cranial nerves and the eyes, ears, and neck. If abnormal findings are identified, an immediate referral to the appropriate specialist is indicated.

CRANIAL NERVE EXAMINATION

The 12 cranial nerves supply sensory information to and receive motor impulses from the brain. Any gross problem relating to their function must be identified so that abnormal conditions can be immediately and appropriately addressed. Treating a neurologic problem with dental techniques will not only fail to solve the problem but also is likely to be hazardous because appropriate treatment may then be delayed. The dentist need not be trained as a neurologist. In fact, the cranial nerve examination does not need to be complex. Any therapist who regularly evaluates pain problems can test the gross function of the cranial nerves to rule out neurologic disorders. The following simple evaluation procedures can be used to assess each nerve.

Olfactory Nerve (I)

The first cranial nerve has sensory fibers originating in the mucous membrane of the nasal cavity and provides the sensation of smell. It is tested by asking the patient to detect differences among the odors of peppermint, vanilla, and chocolate. (Having these available in the office for testing is helpful.) The clinician must also determine whether the patient's nose is obstructed. This can be done by asking the patient to exhale nasally onto a mirror. Fogging of the mirror from both nostrils denotes adequate air flow.

Optic Nerve (II)

The second cranial nerve, also sensory, with fibers originating in the retina, provides for sight. It is tested by having the patient cover one eye and read a few sentences. The other eye is checked in the same manner. The visual field is assessed by standing behind the patient and slowly bringing your fingers from behind around into view (Fig. 9-2). The patient should report when the fingers first appear.

Normally no variation exists between when they are seen on the right and on the left.

Oculomotor, Trochlear, and Abducent Nerves (III, IV, VI)

The third, fourth, and sixth cranial nerves, supplying motor fibers to the extraocular muscles, are tested by having the patient follow a finger while the clinician makes an X (Fig. 9-3). Both eyes should move smoothly and similarly as they follow the finger. The pupils should be of equal size and rounded and should react to light by constricting. The accommodation reflex is tested by having the patient change focus from a distant to a near object. The pupils should constrict as the object (the finger) approaches the patient's face. Not only should they both constrict to direct light, but each should also constrict to light directed in the other eye (consensual light reflex) (Fig. 9-4).

Trigeminal Nerve (V)

The fifth cranial nerve is both sensory (from the face, scalp, nose, and mouth) and motor (to the muscles of mastication). Sensory input is tested by lightly stroking the face with a cotton tip bilaterally in three regions: forehead, cheek, and lower jaw (Fig. 9-5). This will give a rough idea of the function

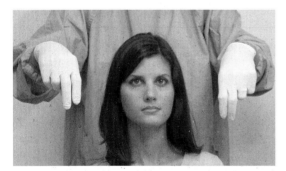

Fig. 9-2 CHECKING THE PATIENT'S VISUAL FIELD (i.e., optic nerve). With the patient looking forward, the examiner's fingers are brought around to the front from behind. The initial position at which the fingers are seen marks the extent of the visual field. Right and left fields should be similar.

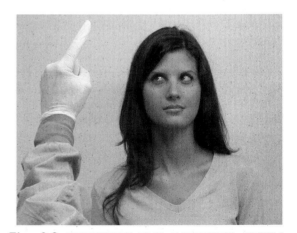

Fig. 9-3 CHECKING THE PATIENT'S EXTRA-OCULAR MUSCLES. Without moving the patient's head, the examiner asks her to follow the finger as it makes an X in front of the patient. Any variation in right or left eye movement is noted.

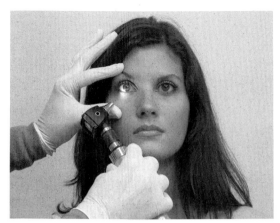

Fig. 9-4 Constriction of the pupil can be seen when light is directed toward the eye. The opposite pupil should also constrict, demonstrating the consensual light reflex.

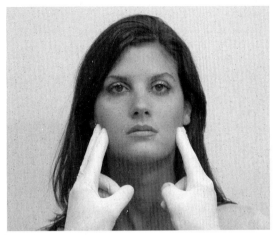

Fig. 9-6 Motor function of the trigeminal nerve is tested by evaluating the strength of masseter muscle contraction. The patient is asked to clench the teeth together while the clinician feels for equal contraction of the right and left masseter muscles. This is also done for the temporalis muscles.

of the ophthalmic, maxillary, and mandibular branches of the trigeminal nerve. The patient should describe similar sensations on each side. The trigeminal nerve also contains sensory fibers from the cornea. The corneal reflexes can be tested by observing the patient's blink in response to a light touch on the cornea with a sterile cotton pledget or tissue. Gross motor input is tested by having the patient clench while you feel both masseter and

temporal muscles (Fig. 9-6). The muscles should contract equally bilaterally.

Facial Nerve (VII)

The seventh cranial nerve is also sensory and motor. The sensory component, supplying taste sensations from the anterior portion of the tongue, is tested by asking the patient to distinguish between sugar and salt using just the tip of the tongue. The motor component, which innervates the muscles of facial expression, is tested by asking the patient to raise both eyebrows, smile, and show the lower teeth. During these movements, any bilateral differences are recorded.

Acoustic Nerve (VIII)

Also called *vestibulocochlear*, the eighth cranial nerve supplies the senses of balance and hearing. The patient should be questioned regarding any recent changes in upright posture or in hearing, especially if they were associated with the problem that initiated the office visit. If there is a question regarding balance, ask the patient to walk heel to toe along a straight line. Gross hearing can be evaluated by rubbing a strand of hair between your first finger and thumb near the patient's ear

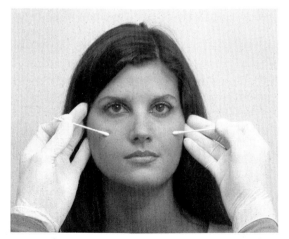

Fig. 9-5 Cotton tip applicators are used to compare light touch discrimination between the right and left maxillary branches of the trigeminal nerve. The ophthalmic and mandibular branches are also tested.

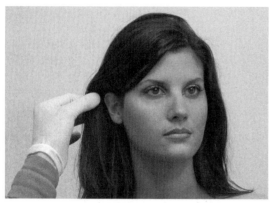

Fig. 9-7 Gross hearing can be evaluated by rubbing a strand of hair between the finger and thumb near the patient's ear and noting any difference between right and left hearing sensitivities.

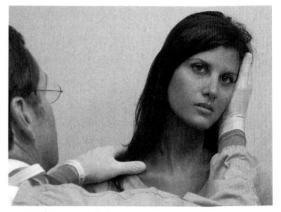

Fig. 9-8 The spinal accessory nerve function (motor) to the sternocleidomastoid is tested by having the patient move the head first to the right and then to the left against resistance. The right and left sides should be relatively equal in strength.

and noting any difference between right and left sensitivities (Fig. 9-7).

Glossopharyngeal and Vagus Nerves (IX, X)

The ninth and tenth cranial nerves are tested together because they both supply fibers to the back of the throat. The patient is asked to say "ah," and the soft palate is observed for symmetric elevations. The gag reflex is tested by touching each side of the pharynx.

Accessory Nerve (XI)

The spinal accessory nerve supplies fibers to the trapezius and sternocleidomastoid (SCM) muscles. The motor input to the trapezius is tested by asking the patient to shrug the shoulders against resistance. The SCM is tested by having the patient move the head first to the right and then to the left against resistance (Fig. 9-8). The clinician should note any differences in muscle strength.

Hypoglossal Nerve (XII)

The twelfth cranial nerve supplies motor fibers to the tongue. To test it, ask the patient to protrude the tongue and note any uncontrolled or consistent lateral deviation. The strength of the tongue can also be evaluated by having the patient push laterally against a tongue blade.

As previously stated, any abnormalities found during the cranial nerve examination should be

viewed as important and appropriate medical referral should be made.

EYE EXAMINATION

The patient is questioned regarding his or her vision and any recent changes, especially any associated with the reason for seeking treatment. As in the cranial nerve examination, simple techniques will be sufficient in testing gross vision. The patient's left eye is covered, and he or she is asked to read a few sentences from a paper. The other eye is then similarly examined. Any diplopia or blurriness of vision is noted, as well as whether this relates to the pain problem. Pain felt in or around the eyes and whether reading affects the pain are noted. Reddening of the conjunctivae should be recorded along with any tearing or swelling of the eyelids.

EAR EXAMINATION

Approximately 70% of patients reporting with TMJ pain also complain of ear discomfort. The proximity of the ear to the TMJ and muscles of mastication, as well as their common trigeminal innervation, creates a frequent condition for referral of pain. Although few of these patients have actual ear disease, when present it is important to identify it and refer the patient for proper treatment. Any dentist

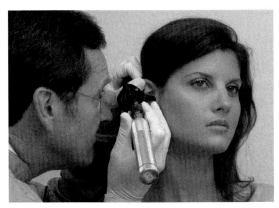

Fig. 9-9 An otoscope is used to visualize the external ear canal and the tympanic membrane for any unusual findings. If abnormal findings are suspected, the patient should be referred to an otolaryngologist for a thorough evaluation.

who treats TMDs should become proficient at examining the ear for gross pathology. Hearing should be checked as in the eighth cranial nerve examination. Infection of the external auditory meatus (otitis externa) can be identified by simply pushing inward on the tragus. If this causes pain, there could be an external ear infection and the patient should be referred to an otolaryngologist. An otoscope will be necessary to visualize the tympanic membrane for inflammation, perforations, or fluid (Fig. 9-9).

Remember that the dentist's role should be merely to attempt to rule out gross ear disease with an otologic examination. Any questionable findings should be referred to an otolaryngologist for a more thorough evaluation. On the other hand, normal findings from an otologic examination may be taken as encouragement to continue to search for the true source of pain or dysfunction.

CERVICAL EXAMINATION

As described in Chapter 2, cervicospinal pain and dysfunction can be referred to the masticatory apparatus. Because this is a frequent occurrence, it is important to evaluate the neck for pain or movement difficulties. A simple screening examination for craniocervical disorders is easily accomplished. The mobility of the neck is examined for range and symptoms. The patient is asked to look first to the

right and then to the left (Fig. 9-10, *A*). At least 70 degrees of rotation should exist in each direction.[18] Next the patient is asked to look upward as far as possible (extension) (Fig. 9-10, *B*) and then downward as far as possible (flexion) (Fig. 9-10, *C*). The head should normally extend backward some 60 degrees and flex downward 45 degrees.[18] Finally, the patient is asked to bend the neck to the right and left (Fig. 9-10, *D*). This should be possible to approximately 40 degrees each way.[18] Any pain is recorded, and any limitation of movement carefully investigated to determine whether its source is a muscular or vertebral problem. When patients with limited range of movement can be passively stretched to a greater range, the source is usually muscular. Patients with vertebral problems cannot normally be stretched to a greater range. If the clinician suspects that the patient has a craniocervical disorder, proper referral for a more complete (cervicospinal) evaluation is indicated. This is important because craniocervical disorders can be closely associated with TMD symptoms.[19]

Once the cranial nerves, eyes, ears, and cervicospinal area have been evaluated, the masticatory apparatus is examined. The masticatory examination consists of evaluating three major structures: muscles, joints, and teeth. A muscle examination is used to evaluate the health and function of the muscles. A TMJ examination is used to evaluate the health and function of the joints. An occlusal examination is used to evaluate the health and function of the teeth and their supportive structures.

MUSCLE EXAMINATION

Pain is not associated with the normal function or palpation of a healthy muscle. In contrast, a frequent clinical sign of compromised muscle tissue is pain. The condition that brings about compromise or unhealthy muscle tissue may be muscle overuse or physical trauma such as overstretching or receiving a blow to the muscle tissue itself. Most often the muscles of mastication become compromised through increased activity. As the number and duration of contractions increase, so also do the physiologic needs of the muscle tissues. Increased muscle tonicity or hyperactivity,

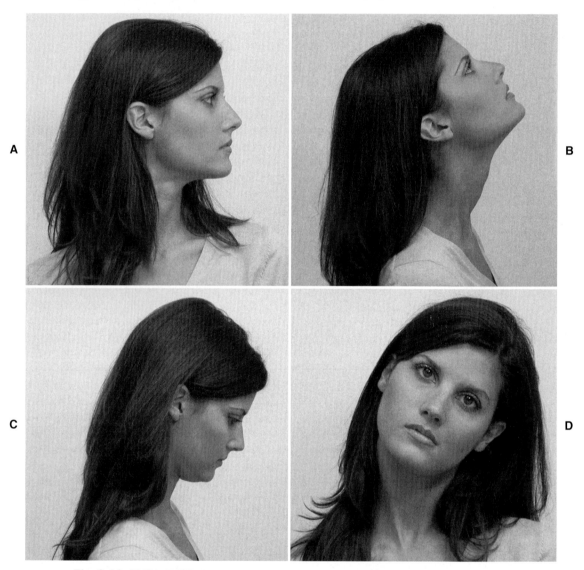

Fig. 9-10 EXAMINATION FOR CRANIOCERVICAL DISORDERS. The patient is asked to look to the extreme right and the extreme left **(A)**, look upward fully **(B)**, look downward fully **(C)**, and bend the neck to the right and left **(D)**.

however, can lead to a decrease in blood flow to the muscle tissues, lowering the inflow of nutrient substances needed for normal cell function while accumulating metabolic waste products. This accumulation of metabolic waste products and of other algogenic substances is thought to cause the muscle pain.[20,21] With time it is now appreciated that the central nervous system

can contribute to the myalgia with neurogenic inflammation.[20,22]

In its early stages myalgia is noticed only during function of the muscle. If sustained hyperactivity continues, it can be long lasting and result in dull aching pain that often radiates over the entire muscle. The pain can eventually become severe enough to limit mandibular function. The degree and location of muscle pain and tenderness are identified during a muscle examination. The muscle can be examined by direct palpation or by functional manipulation.

Muscle Palpation

A widely accepted method of determining muscle tenderness and pain is by digital palpation.[23-25] A healthy muscle does not elicit sensations of tenderness or pain when palpated. Deformation of compromised muscle tissue by palpation can elicit pain.[26] Therefore if a patient reports discomfort during palpation of a specific muscle, it can be deduced that the muscle tissue has been compromised by either trauma or fatigue.

Palpation of the muscle is accomplished mainly by the palmar surface of the middle finger, with the index finger and forefinger testing the adjacent areas. Soft but firm pressure is applied to the designated muscles, with the fingers compressing the adjacent tissues in a small circular motion. A single firm thrust of 1 or 2 seconds' duration is usually better than several light thrusts. During palpation the patient is asked whether it hurts or is just uncomfortable.

For the muscle examination to be most helpful, the degree of discomfort is ascertained and recorded. This is often a difficult task. Pain is subjective and is perceived and expressed quite differently from patient to patient. Yet the degree of discomfort in the structure can be important to recognizing the patient's pain problem, as well as an excellent method of evaluating treatment effects. Therefore an attempt is made to not only identify the affected muscles but also to classify the degree of pain in each. When a muscle is palpated, the patient's response is placed in one of four categories.[27,28] A zero (0) is recorded when the muscle is palpated and there is no pain or tenderness reported by the patient. A number 1 is recorded if the patient responds that the palpation is uncomfortable (tenderness or soreness). A number 2 is recorded if the patient experiences definite discomfort or pain. A number 3 is recorded if the patient shows evasive action or eye tearing or verbalizes a desire not to have the area palpated again. The pain or tenderness of each muscle is recorded on an examination form, which will assist

diagnosis and later be used in the evaluation and assessment of progress.

A thorough muscle examination should identify not only generalized muscle tenderness and pain but also the small hypersensitive trigger points associated with myofascial pain. As stated in Chapters 2 and 8, trigger points act as sources of deep pain input that can produce central excitatory effects. These areas must be identified and recorded. To locate trigger points, the examiner palpates the entire body of each muscle. Generalized muscle pain may not exist in a muscle with trigger points. When recording examination findings, it is important to differentiate between generalized muscle pain and trigger point pain because the diagnosis and treatment are often different.

When trigger points are located, an attempt should be made to determine whether there is any pattern of pain referral. Pressure should be applied to the trigger point for 4 to 5 seconds, and the patient is asked whether the pain is felt to radiate in any direction. If a pattern of referred pain is reported, it should be noted on a drawing of the face for future reference. Patterns of referred pain are often helpful in identifying and diagnosing certain pain conditions.

A routine muscle examination includes *palpation* of the following muscles or muscle groups: temporalis, masseter, sternocleidomastoideus, and posterior cervical (e.g., the splenius capitis and trapezius). For increased efficiency of the examination, both right and left muscles are palpated simultaneously. The technique of palpating each muscle is described. An understanding of the anatomy and function of the muscles is essential for proper palpation (see Chapter 1).

The muscle examination also includes evaluation of the medial and lateral pterygoids by *functional manipulation*. This technique is used for muscles that are impossible or nearly impossible to palpate manually.

Temporalis. The temporalis is divided into three functional areas, and therefore each area is independently palpated. The *anterior* region is palpated above the zygomatic arch and anterior to the TMJ (Fig. 9-11, *A*). Fibers of this region run essentially in a vertical direction. The *middle* region is palpated directly above the TMJ and superior to

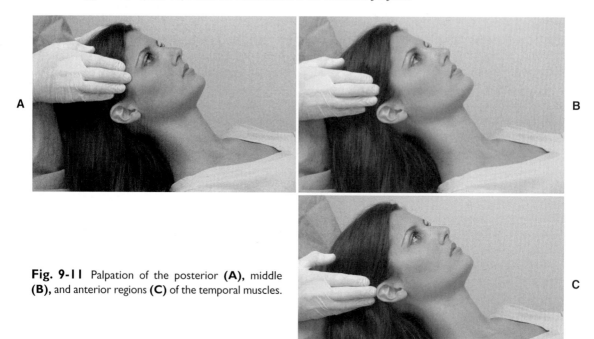

Fig. 9-11 Palpation of the posterior **(A)**, middle **(B)**, and anterior regions **(C)** of the temporal muscles.

the zygomatic arch (Fig. 9-11, *B*). Fibers in this region run in an oblique direction across the lateral aspect of the skull. The *posterior* region is palpated above and behind the ear (Fig. 9-11, *C*). These fibers run in an essentially horizontal direction.

If uncertainty arises regarding the proper finger placement, the patient is asked to clench the teeth together. The temporalis will contract, and the fibers should be felt beneath the fingertips. It is helpful to be positioned behind the patient and to use the right and left hands to palpate respective muscle areas simultaneously. During palpation of each area the patient is asked whether it hurts or is just uncomfortable, and the response is classified as 0, 1, 2, or 3, according to the previously described criteria. If a trigger point is located, it should be identified on the examination form along with any pattern of referral.

When evaluating the temporalis muscle, it is also important to palpate its tendon. The fibers of the temporalis muscle extend inferiorly to converge into a distinct tendon that attaches to the coronoid

process of the mandible. Some TMDs commonly produce a temporalis tendonitis, which can create pain in the body of the muscle, as well as referred pain behind the adjacent eye (retroorbital pain). The tendon of the temporalis is palpated by placing the finger of one hand intraorally on the anterior border of the ramus and the finger of the other hand extraorally on the same area. The intraoral finger is moved up the anterior border of the ramus until the coronoid process and the tendon are palpated (Fig. 9-12). The patient is asked to report any discomfort or pain.

Masseter. The masseter is palpated bilaterally at its superior and inferior attachments. First, the fingers are placed on each zygomatic arch (just anterior to the TMJ). They are then dropped down slightly to the portion of the masseter attached to the zygomatic arch, just anterior to the joint (Fig. 9-13, *A*). Once this portion (the deep masseter) has been palpated, the fingers drop to the inferior attachment on the inferior border of the ramus. The area of palpation is directly above

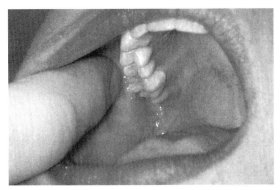

Fig. 9-12 PALPATION OF THE TENDON OF THE TEMPORALIS. The finger is moved up the anterior border of the ramus until the coronoid process and the attachment of the tendon of the temporalis are felt.

the attachment of the body of the masseter (i.e., the superficial masseter) (Fig. 9-13, *B*). The patient's response is recorded.

Sternocleidomastoideus. Although the SCM does not function directly in moving the mandible, it is specifically mentioned because it often becomes symptomatic with TMDs and it is easily palpated. The palpation is done bilaterally near its insertion on the outer surface of the mastoid fossa, behind the ear (Fig. 9-14, *A*). The entire length of the muscle is palpated, down to its origin near the clavicle (Fig. 9-14, *B*). The patient is asked to report any discomfort during the procedure. Also, any

trigger points found in this muscle are noted because they are frequent sources of referred pain to the temporal, joint, and ear area.

Posterior Cervical Muscles. The posterior cervical muscles (trapezius, longissimus [capitis and cervicis], splenius [capitis and cervicis], and levator scapulae) do not directly affect mandibular movement; however, they do become symptomatic during certain TMDs and therefore are routinely palpated. They originate at the posterior occipital area and extend inferiorly along the cervicospinal region. Because they are layered over each other, they are sometimes difficult to identify individually.

In palpating these muscles, the examiner's fingers slip behind the patient's head. Those of the right hand palpate the right occipital area, and those of the left hand palpate the left (Fig. 9-15, *A*) at the origins of the muscles. The patient is questioned regarding any discomfort. The fingers move down the length of the neck muscles through the cervical area (Fig. 9-15, *B*), and any patient discomfort is recorded. It is important to be aware of trigger points in these muscles because they are a common source of frontal headache.

The *splenius capitis* is palpated for general pain or tenderness, as well as for trigger points. Its attachment to the skull is a small depression just posterior to the attachment of the SCM (Fig. 9-16). Palpation is begun at this point and moves inferiorly until the muscle blends into the other

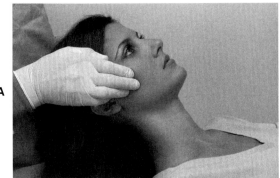
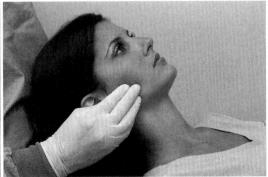

A

B

Fig. 9-13 A, Palpation of the masseter muscles at their superior attachment to the zygomatic arches. **B,** Palpation of the superficial masseter muscles near the lower border of the mandible.

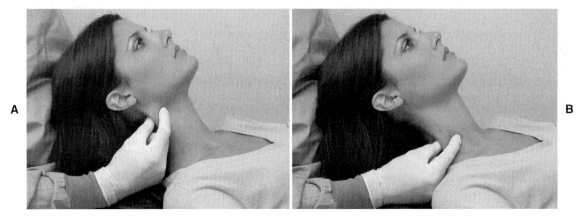

Fig. 9-14 Palpation of the sternocleidomastoideus high near the mastoid process **(A)** and low near the clavicle **(B).**

neck muscles. Any pain, tenderness, or trigger points are recorded.

The *trapezius* is an extremely large muscle of the back, shoulder, and neck that (like the SCM and the splenius) does not directly affect jaw function but is a common source of headache pain and is easily palpated. The major purpose of its palpation is not to evaluate shoulder function but to search for active trigger points that may be producing referred pain. The trapezius commonly has trigger points that refer pain to the face. In fact, when facial pain is the patient's chief complaint, this muscle should be one of the first sources investigated. The upper part is palpated from behind the

SCM, inferolaterally to the shoulder (Fig. 9-17), and any trigger points are recorded.

Clinical Significance of Trigger Points. As discussed in Chapter 2, trigger points can be either *active* or *latent*. When active, they are clinically identified as specific hypersensitive areas within the muscle tissue. Often a small, firm, tight band of muscle tissue can be felt. When latent, trigger points are not detectable. Active trigger points are frequently a source of constant deep pain and produce central excitatory effects.[29,30] When referred (heterotopic) pain is detected, therefore, it is wholly dependent on the conditions of the trigger points (the source of the pain). This means that if

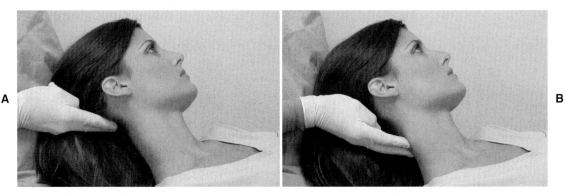

Fig. 9-15 A, Palpation of muscular attachments in the occipital region of the neck. **B,** The fingers are brought inferiorly down the cervical area, and the muscles are palpated for pain and tenderness.

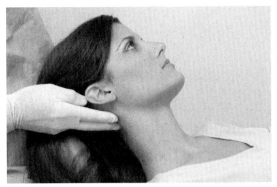

Fig. 9-16 The splenius capitis is palpated at its attachment to the skull just posterior to the attachment of the sternocleidomastoideus.

active referring trigger points are provoked, the referred pain will usually be increased, which becomes a significant diagnostic observation in relating pain complaints to their source. For example, when a patient's chief complaint is headache, careful palpation of the aforementioned neck muscles for trigger points will demonstrate its source. When a trigger point is located, applying pressure to it will usually increase the headache (referred) pain.

The specific pattern of referred pain from various trigger point locations has been outlined by Travell and Simons (see Chapter 8).[30] An understanding

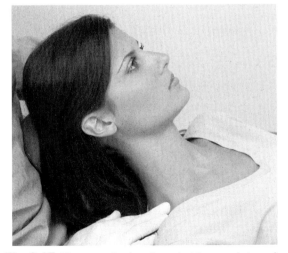

Fig. 9-17 The trapezius is palpated as it ascends into the neck structures.

of these common referral sites may help the clinician who is attempting to diagnose a facial pain problem. As discussed in Chapter 10, anesthetic blocking of the trigger point often eliminates the referred headache pain and thus becomes a helpful diagnostic tool.

Functional Manipulation

Three muscles that are basic to jaw movement but impossible or nearly impossible to palpate are the inferior lateral pterygoid, superior lateral pterygoid, and medial pterygoid. The inferior and superior lateral pterygoids reside deep within the skull, originating on the lateral wing of the sphenoid bone and the maxillary tuberosity and inserting on the neck of the mandibular condyle and the TMJ capsule. The medial pterygoid has a similar origin, but it extends downward and laterally to insert on the medial surface of the angle of the mandible. Although the medial pterygoid can be palpated by placing the finger in the lateral aspect of the pharyngeal wall of the throat, this palpation is difficult and sometimes uncomfortable for the patient. All three muscles receive their innervation from the mandibular branch of the trigeminal (V) nerve.

For years, an intraoral technique was suggested for palpating the lateral pterygoid, but this has not been proved effective.[31,32] Because the location of this muscle made palpation impossible, a second method for evaluating muscle symptoms, called *functional manipulation*, was developed on the basis of the principle that as a muscle becomes fatigued and symptomatic, further function only elicits pain.[20,26,33,34] Thus a muscle that is compromised by excessive activity is painful both during contraction and when being stretched, and in these cases functional manipulation is the only technique for evaluating whether it is indeed a source of deep pain.

In some instances palpation in the region of the lateral and medial pterygoids may elicit pain, but functional manipulation does not. A study[35] comparing the results of palpation and functional manipulation of the inferior lateral pterygoid showed that 27% of a control group had tenderness to intraoral palpation, but none had symptoms following functional manipulation. This implied that 27% of the time a false-positive result was being reported with palpation. In the same study a group of orofacial pain patients was similarly examined; 69% were found to have lateral pterygoid pain with a palpation technique, yet only 27% had pain with functional manipulation. In this case the implication was that when palpation was used, the lateral pterygoid might be blamed for pain 42% of the time when it was not actually the source. There is no question that when the area posterior to the maxillary tuberosity is palpated, a high incidence of pain occurs; functional manipulation merely suggests that this pain is not from the lateral pterygoids but that other structures are likely responsible.

During functional manipulation each muscle is contracted and then stretched. If the muscle is a true source of pain, both activities will increase the pain. The following section reviews the functional manipulation techniques for evaluation of three muscles that are difficult to reliably palpate: inferior lateral pterygoid, superior lateral pterygoid, and medial pterygoid.

Functional Manipulation of the Inferior Lateral Pterygoid Muscle

Contraction. When the inferior lateral pterygoid contracts, the mandible is protruded and/or the mouth is opened. Functional manipulation is best accomplished by having the patient make a protrusive movement because this muscle is the primary protruding muscle. It is also active during opening, but so are other muscles, which adds confusion to the findings. The most effective manipulation therefore is to have the patient protrude against resistance provided by the examiner (Fig. 9-18). If the inferior lateral pterygoid is the source of pain, this activity will increase the pain.

Stretching. The inferior lateral pterygoid stretches when the teeth are in maximum intercuspation. Therefore if it is the source of pain when the teeth are clenched, the pain will increase. When a tongue blade is placed between the posterior teeth, the intercuspal position (ICP) cannot be reached and therefore the inferior lateral pterygoid does not fully stretch. Consequently, biting on a separator does not increase the pain but may even decrease or eliminate it.

Functional Manipulation of the Superior Lateral Pterygoid Muscle

Contraction. The superior lateral pterygoid contracts with the elevator muscles (temporalis,

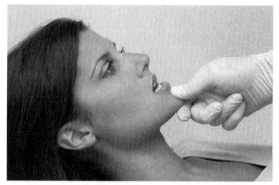

Fig. 9-18 FUNCTIONAL MANIPULATION OF THE INFERIOR LATERAL PTERYGOID. The patient is asked to protrude against resistance provided by the examiner.

masseter, and medial pterygoid), especially during a power stroke (clenching). Therefore if it is the source of pain, clenching will increase the pain. If a tongue blade is placed between the posterior teeth bilaterally (Fig. 9-19) and the patient clenches on the separator, pain again increases with contraction of the superior lateral pterygoid. These observations are exactly the same as for the elevator muscles. Stretching is necessary to enable superior lateral pterygoid pain to be distinguished from elevator pain.

Stretching. As with the inferior lateral pterygoid, stretching of the superior lateral pterygoid occurs at maximum intercuspation. Therefore stretching

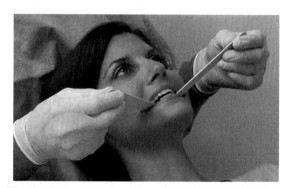

Fig. 9-19 Functional manipulation of the superior lateral pterygoid is achieved by asking the patient to bite on a tongue blade bilaterally.

and contracting of this muscle occur during the same activity, clenching. If the superior lateral pterygoid is the source of pain, clenching will increase it. Superior lateral pterygoid pain can be differentiated from elevator pain by having the patient open wide. This will stretch the elevator muscles but not the superior lateral pterygoid. If opening elicits no pain, then the pain of clenching is from the superior lateral pterygoid. If the pain increases during opening, then both the superior lateral pterygoid and the elevators may be involved. Differentiating pain in the former from pain in the latter is often difficult unless the patient can isolate the location of the sore muscle.

Functional Manipulation of the Medial Pterygoid Muscle

Contraction. The medial pterygoid is an elevator muscle and therefore contracts as the teeth are coming together. If it is the source of pain, clenching the teeth together will increase the pain. When a tongue blade is placed between the posterior teeth and the patient clenches against it, the pain is still increased because the elevators are still contracting.

Stretching. The medial pterygoid also stretches when the mouth is opened wide. Therefore if it is the source of pain, opening the mouth wide will increase pain.

Functional manipulation of muscles that are impossible to palpate can provide accurate information regarding the source of masticatory pain. All the information necessary is obtained by having the patient open wide, protrude against resistance, clench the teeth together, and then bite on a separator. The response of each muscle to functional manipulation is summarized in Table 9-1.

If a muscle is a true source of pain, functional manipulation will be helpful in identifying this source. However, the fact that pain is produced during functional manipulation does not necessarily mean a source of pain has been identified. Referred symptoms such as secondary hyperalgesia can create painful symptoms during muscle function. In this instance functional manipulation identifies only the site of pain and not the source.[36] Anesthetic blocking may be necessary to differentiate the source of pain from the site (see Chapter 10).

Intracapsular Disorders. Another source of pain can confuse these functional manipulation findings. Intracapsular disorders of the TMJ (e.g., a functional dislocation of the disc, an inflammatory disorder) can elicit pain with increased interarticular pressure and movement. Functional manipulation both increases interarticular pressure and moves the condyle. Therefore this pain is easily confused with muscle pain. For example, if an inflammatory disorder exists and the patient opens wide, pain is increased as a result of movement and function of the inflamed structures. If the mandible is protruded against resistance, pain is also increased because movement and interarticular pressure are causing force to be applied to the inflamed structures. If the teeth are clenched together, pain is again increased with the increased interarticular pressure and force to the inflamed structures. If, however, the patient

---

TABLE 9-1

Functional Manipulation by Muscle

	Contracting	Stretching
Inferior lateral pterygoid muscle	Protruding against resistance, ↑ pain	Clenching on teeth, ↑ pain Clenching on separator, no pain
Superior lateral pterygoid muscle	Clenching on teeth, ↑ pain Clenching on separator, ↑ pain	Clenching on teeth, ↑ pain Clenching on separator, ↑ pain Opening mouth, no pain
Medial pterygoid muscle	Clenching on teeth, ↑ pain Clenching on separator, ↑ pain	Opening mouth, ↑ pain

clenches unilaterally on a separator, the interarticular pressure is decreased on the ipsilateral side and pain in that joint will be decreased.

These results are logical but confusing because they are the same results found when the inferior lateral pterygoid is the site of pain. Therefore a fifth test must be administered to differentiate inferior lateral pterygoid from intracapsular pain. This can be done by placing a separator between the posterior teeth on the painful side. The patient is asked to close on the separator and then protrude against resistance. If an intracapsular disorder is the site of pain, the pain will not increase (or possibly will even decrease) because closing on a separator decreases the interarticular pressure and thus reduces the forces to the inflamed structures. Contraction of the inferior lateral pterygoid, however, is increased during resistant protrusive movement and therefore pain will increase if this is its source of origin.

The four basic functional manipulation activities, along with the activity necessary to differentiate intracapsular pain, are listed in Table 9-2 (see also Table 9-1). The potential sites or sources of pain are also listed, as well as how each will react to functional manipulation.

Maximum Interincisal Distance

A muscle examination is not complete until the effect of muscle function on mandibular movement has been evaluated. The normal range[37] of mouth opening when measured interincisally is between 53 and 58 mm. Even a 6-year-old child can normally open a maximum of 40 mm or more.[38,39] Because muscle symptoms are often accentuated during function, it is common for people to assume a restricted pattern of movement. The patient is asked to open slowly until pain is first felt (Fig. 9-20, *A*). At that point the distance between the incisal edges of the maxillary and mandibular anterior teeth is measured. This is the maximum comfortable opening. The patient is next asked to open the mouth maximally (Fig. 9-20, *B*). This is recorded as the maximum opening. In the absence of pain the maximum comfortable opening and maximum opening are the same.

A restricted mouth opening is considered to be any distance less than 40 mm. Only 1.2% of young adults[40] open less than 40 mm. One must remember, however, that 15% of the healthy elderly population[40] opens less than 40 mm. Less than 40 mm of mouth opening therefore seems to represent a reasonable point to designate restriction, but one should always consider the patient's age and body size. This distance is measured by observing the incisal edge of the mandibular central incisor traveling away from its position at maximum intercuspation. If a person has a 5-mm vertical overlap of the anterior teeth and the maximum interincisal distance is 57 mm, the mandible has actually moved 62 mm in opening. In people who have extremely deep bites, these measurements must be considered when determining normal range of movement.

TABLE **9-2**

Functional Manipulation by Activity

	Medial Pterygoid Muscle	Inferior Lateral Pterygoid Muscle	Superior Lateral Pterygoid Muscle	Intracapsular Disorder
Opening widely	Pain ↑	Pain ↑ slightly	No pain	Pain ↑
Protruding against resistance	Pain ↑ slightly	Pain ↑	No pain	Pain ↑
Clenching on teeth	Pain ↑	Pain ↑	Pain ↑	Pain ↑
Clenching on separator (unilaterally)	Pain ↑	No pain	Pain ↑	No pain
Protruding against resistance with unilateral separator	Pain ↑ slightly	Pain ↑	Pain ↑ slightly (if clenching on unilateral separator)	No pain

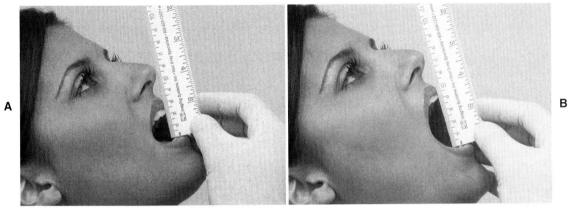

Fig. 9-20 MEASURING MOUTH OPENING. A, The patient is asked to open the mouth until pain is first felt. At this point the distance between the incisal edges of the anterior teeth is measured. This measurement is called the *maximum comfortable mouth opening.* **B,** The patient is then asked to open as wide as possible even in the presence of pain. This measurement is called the *maximum mouth opening.*

If mouth opening is restricted, it is helpful to test the "end feel." The end feel describes the characteristics of the restriction that limits the full range of joint movement.[41] The end feel can be evaluated by placing the fingers between the patient's upper and lower teeth and applying gentle but steady force in an attempt to passively increase the interincisal distance (Fig. 9-21). If the end feel is "soft,"

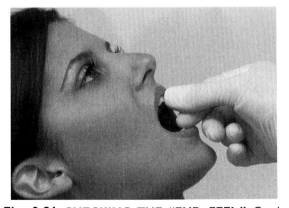

Fig. 9-21 CHECKING THE "END FEEL." Gentle but steady pressure is placed on the lower incisors for approximately 10 to 15 seconds. Increased mandibular opening indicates a soft end feel (usually associated with a masticatory muscle disorder).

increased opening can be achieved but must be done slowly. A soft end feel suggests muscle-induced restriction.[42] If no increase in opening can be achieved, the end feel is said to be "hard." Hard end feels are more likely associated with intracapsular sources (e.g., a disc dislocation).

The patient is next instructed to move his or her mandible laterally. Any lateral movement less than 8 mm is recorded as a restricted movement (Fig. 9-22). Protrusive movement is also evaluated in a similar manner.

The path taken by the midline of the mandible during maximum opening is observed next. In the healthy masticatory system there is no alteration in the straight opening pathway. Any alterations in opening are recorded. Two types of alteration can occur: deviations and deflections. A *deviation* is any shift of the jaw midline during opening that disappears with continued opening (a return to midline) (Fig. 9-23, *A*). It is usually caused by a disc derangement in one or both joints and is a result of the condylar movement necessary to get past the disc during translation. Once the condyle has overcome this interference, the straight midline path is resumed. A *deflection* is any shift of the midline to one side that becomes greater with opening and does not disappear at

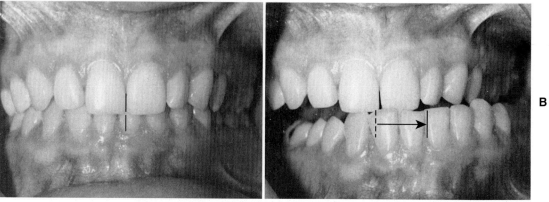

Fig. 9-22 EXAMINING FOR LATERAL MOVEMENT OF THE MANDIBLE.
A, The patient is observed in the maximum intercuspal position, and the area of the mandibular incisor directly below the midline between the maxillary central incisors is noted. This can be marked with a pencil. **B,** The patient makes a maximum left movement and then a maximum right laterotrusive movement, and the distance that the mark has moved from the midline is measured. This will reveal the distance the mandible has moved in each direction.

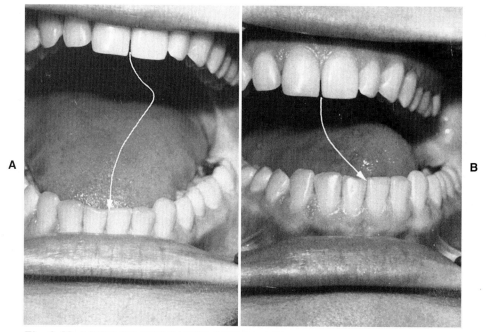

Fig. 9-23 ALTERATIONS IN THE OPENING PATHWAY. **A,** Deviation. The opening pathway is altered but returns to a normal midline relationship at maximum opening. **B,** Deflection. The opening pathway is shifted to one side and becomes greater with opening. At maximum opening the midline is deflected to its greatest distance.

maximum opening (does not return to midline) (Fig. 9-23, *B*). It is caused by restricted movement in one joint. The source of the restriction varies and must be investigated.

Restricted movements of the mandible are caused by either extracapsular or intracapsular sources. The former are generally the muscles and therefore relate to a muscle disorder. The latter are generally associated with disc-condyle function and the surrounding ligaments and thus are usually related to a disc derangement disorder. Extracapsular and intracapsular restrictions present different characteristics.

Extracapsular Restrictions. Extracapsular restrictions typically occur with elevator muscle spasms and pain. These muscles tend to restrict translation and thus limit opening. Pain in the elevator muscles, however, does not restrict lateral and protrusive movements. Therefore with this type of restriction, normal eccentric movements are present but opening movement is restricted, primarily because of pain. The point of restriction can range anywhere from 0 to 40 mm interincisally. With this type of restriction, the patient is usually able to increase opening slowly, but the pain is intensified (soft end feel).

Extracapsular restrictions often create a deflection of the incisal path during opening. The direction of the deflection depends on the location of the muscle that causes the restriction. If the restricting muscle is lateral to the joint (as with the masseter), the deflection during opening will be to the ipsilateral side. If the muscle is medial (as with the medial pterygoid), the deflection will be to the contralateral side.

Intracapsular Restrictions. Intracapsular restrictions typically present a different pattern. A disc derangement disorder (e.g., functional dislocation) decisively restricts translation of that joint. Typically the restriction is in only one joint and limits mandibular opening in that joint primarily to rotation (25 to 30 mm interincisally). At this point, further movement is restricted not because of pain but because of structural resistances in the joint. When intracapsular restrictions are present, deflection of the incisal path during opening is always to the ipsilateral (affected) side.

TEMPOROMANDIBULAR JOINT EXAMINATION

The TMJs are examined for any signs or symptoms associated with pain and dysfunction. Radiographs and other imaging techniques can also be useful (see Additional Diagnostic Tests).

Temporomandibular Joint Pain

Pain or tenderness of the TMJs is determined by digital palpation of the joints when the mandible is both stationary and during dynamic movement. The fingertips are placed over the lateral aspects of both joint areas simultaneously. If uncertainty exists regarding the proper position of the fingers, the patient is asked to open and close a few times. The fingertips should feel the lateral poles of the condyles passing downward and forward across the articular eminences. Once the position of the fingers over the joints has been verified, the patient relaxes and medial force is applied to the joint areas (Fig. 9-24, *A*). The patient is asked to report any symptoms, and they are recorded with the same numeric code that is used for the muscles. Once the symptoms are recorded in a static position, the patient opens and closes, and any symptoms associated with this movement are recorded (Fig. 9-24, *B*). As the patient opens maximally, the fingers should be rotated slightly posteriorly to apply force to the posterior aspect of the condyle (Fig. 9-24, *C*). Posterior capsulitis and retrodiscitis are clinically evaluated in this manner.

To evaluate the TMJ effectively, one must have a sound understanding of the anatomy in the region. When the fingers are placed properly over the lateral poles of the condyles and the patient is asked to clench, little to no movement is felt. However, if the fingers are misplaced only 1 cm anterior to the lateral pole and the patient is asked to clench, the deep portion of the masseter can be felt contracting. This slight difference in positioning of the fingers may influence the examiner's interpretation regarding the origin of the pain. The clinician must also be aware that a portion of the parotid gland extends to the region of the joint and parotid symptoms can arise from this area. The examiner must be astute in identifying whether the symptoms are originating from joint, muscle, or gland.

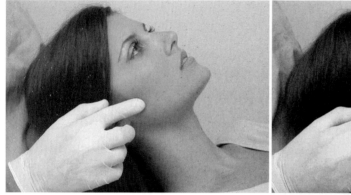

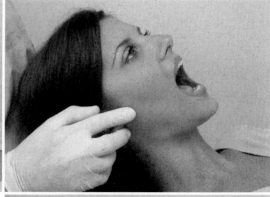

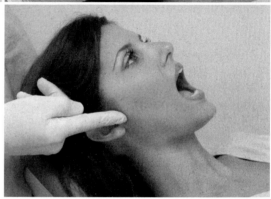

Fig. 9-24 PALPATION OF THE TEMPORO-MANDIBULAR JOINT. A, Lateral aspect of the joint with the mouth closed. **B,** Lateral aspect of the joint during opening and closing. **C,** With the mouth fully open, the finger is moved behind the condyle to palpate the posterior aspect of the joint.

The basis of treatment will be determined by this evaluation.

Temporomandibular Joint Dysfunction

Dysfunction of the TMJs can be separated into two types: joint sounds and joint restrictions.

Joint Sounds. As mentioned in Chapter 8, joint sounds are either clicks or crepitation. A click is a single sound of short duration. If it is relatively loud, it is sometimes referred to as a *pop*. Crepitation is a multiple gravel-like sound described as *grating and complicated*. Crepitation is most commonly associated with osteoarthritic changes of the articular surfaces of the joint.[43]

Joint sounds can be perceived by placing the fingertips over the lateral surfaces of the joint and having the patient open and close. Often they may be felt by the fingertips. A more careful examination can be performed by placing a stethoscope over the joint area. If a stethoscope is used, the clinician must appreciate that this instrument will detect many more sounds than mere palpation

and the significance of these sounds needs to be assessed. Not all joint sounds should be considered a problem worthy of treatment (see Chapter 13). In most instances, palpation techniques are adequate to record joint sounds.

Not only should the character of any joint sounds be recorded (e.g., clicking, crepitation), but also the degree of mandibular opening (i.e., interincisal distance) associated with the sound. Of equal importance is whether the sound occurs during opening or closing or can be heard (or felt) during both these movements (i.e., a reciprocal click; see Chapter 8).

Examining the joint for sounds by placing the fingers in the patient's ears is not wise. It has been demonstrated that this technique can actually produce joint sounds that are not present during normal function of the joint.[44] It is thought that this technique forces the ear canal cartilage against the posterior aspect of the joint and either this tissue produces sounds or this force displaces the disc, which produces the additional sounds.

The presence or absence of joint sounds gives insight regarding disc position. One should be aware, however, that the absence of sounds does not always mean normal disc position. In one study[45] 15% of silent, asymptomatic joints were found to have disc displacements on arthrograms. Information received during examination of the joints needs to be evaluated with respect to all other examination findings.

Joint Restrictions. The dynamic movements of the mandible are observed for any irregularities or restrictions. The characteristics of intracapsular restrictions have already been described in connection with the muscle examination. Any mandibular movements that either are restricted or have unusual pathway characteristics are recorded.

The key findings of both muscle and TMJ examinations are recorded on a treatment outcome form (Fig. 9-25). This form has room available for recording information received at subsequent appointments once therapy is initiated, thus allowing the therapist to make a quick evaluation of the effect of treatment on the symptoms.

DENTAL EXAMINATION

In evaluating a patient for TMDs, the dental structures must be carefully examined. The most important feature to evaluate is the orthopedic stability between the ICP of the teeth and the TMJ positions. Evaluating the dental structures for any breakdown that might suggest the presence of a functional disturbance is also important.

To examine a patient's occlusal condition, it is necessary to have an appreciation of what is normal (see Chapters 1, 3, 4, and 6) and what is functionally optimal (see Chapter 5). As stated in Chapter 7, these two conditions are not identical. For example, a patient may have a single posterior tooth contacting when the mandible is closed in centric relation (CR). This is common if the clinician retrudes the mandible during the examination. There may also be a 2-mm shift or slide from this CR position to the ICP (maximum intercuspation). Although this condition may be common, it is not considered functionally ideal. The question that cannot be answered during an occlusal examination is whether the difference between

optimal and normal is a contributing factor of the functional disturbance. Remember, the occlusal condition is *not always* a factor in the disturbance. Although some studies[46-48] have suggested a relationship between the types and severities of malocclusions and the symptoms of TMDs, others[49-51] do not seem to corroborate this idea (see Chapter 7). Thus merely examining an occlusal condition cannot determine its influence on function of the masticatory system.

When a patient presents an occlusal condition that is neither optimal nor normal, the tendency is to assume that it is the major contributing factor. Although this may seem logical, this assumption cannot be substantiated by research studies. Therefore during the occlusal examination one can merely observe the interrelationships of the teeth and record the findings relative to normal and optimal. These findings must accompany other examination findings to determine their relationship, if any, to a TMD.

The dental examination begins with inspection of the teeth and their supportive structures for any indications of breakdown. Common signs and symptoms are tooth mobility, pulpitis, and tooth wear.

Mobility

Tooth mobility can result from two factors: loss of bony support (periodontal disease) and unusually heavy occlusal forces (traumatic occlusion). Whenever it is observed, both factors must be considered. Mobility is identified by applying intermittent buccal and lingual force to each tooth. This is best accomplished by using two mirror handles or a mirror handle and a finger (Fig. 9-26). Usually two fingers will not permit proper evaluation. One mirror handle is placed to the buccal or labial of the tooth to be tested, and the other to the lingual. Force is applied first toward the lingual and then toward the buccal. The tooth is observed for any movement.

Remember, all teeth exhibit a small degree of mobility. This is often observed with the mandibular incisors. Any movement greater than 0.5 mm is noted. A commonly used classification[52] for mobility uses a scoring form of 1 to 3. A rating of 1 is given to a tooth that is slightly more mobile than normal. A rating of 2 is given when 1 mm of movement

Date								
Type of treatment								
Temporalis R								
Temporalis L								
Tendon of temporalis R								
Tendon of temporalis L								
Masseter R								
Masseter L								
Posterior cervical (neck) R								
Posterior cervical (neck) L								
Sternocleido-mastoideus R								
Sternocleido-mastoideus L								
Splenius capitis R								
Splenius capitis L								
Trapezius R								
Trapezius L								
Maximum comfortable opening (mm) R								
Maximum comfortable opening (mm) L								
Maximum opening (mm) R								
Maximum opening (mm) L								
TMJ pain R								
TMJ pain L								
TMJ sounds R								
TMJ sounds L								
Headaches per week								
Other (specify)								

Fig. 9-25 MUSCLE AND TEMPOROMANDIBULAR JOINT EXAMINATION AND TREATMENT OUTCOME FORM. Objective measurements are recorded for the initial as well as subsequent appointments. This form assists in evaluating treatment effects over time. The pain scores (0, 1, 2, and 3) are appropriately recorded along with interincisal distances (in millimeters). Trigger points identified in a muscle are recorded as *TP*. *TMJ*, Temporomandibular joint.

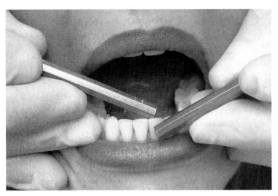

Fig. 9-26 Testing for tooth mobility.

occurs in any direction from the normal position. A rating of 3 indicates mobility that is greater than 1 mm in any direction. When mobility is present, it is extremely important to evaluate the periodontal health and gingival attachment of the tooth. This information leads to the determination of either primary or secondary traumatic occlusion. The former results when unusually heavy occlusal forces exceed the resistance of the healthy periodontium, thereby creating mobility. The latter results when light to normal forces exceed the resistance of a weakened periodontium, creating mobility. The weakened condition is the result of bone loss.

Often heavy occlusal forces can cause radiographic changes in the teeth and their supportive structures. Standard periapical radiographs are evaluated for three signs that frequently correlate with heavy occlusal forces and/or mobility: a widened periodontal space, condensing osteitis (osteosclerosis), and hypercementosis. It should be noted that these changes alone are not evidence of traumatic occlusal forces. They must be correlated with clinical findings to aid in the establishment of a proper diagnosis.

Widening of the Periodontal Space. Increased mobility is directly related to resorption of the bone supporting the lateral aspects of the tooth. This resorption creates a wider area for the periodontal ligament, apparent on the radiograph as increased space. The increase is normally greater at the crestal bone area and narrows apically, and its effect has been termed *funneling* of the bone (Fig. 9-27).

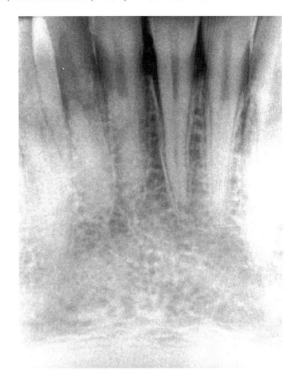

Fig. 9-27 WIDENING OF THE PERIODONTAL SPACE. The mesial aspect of the mandibular central incisor reveals "funneling."

Osteosclerosis. Generally when tissue is subjected to heavy force, one of two processes is likely to occur. Either it is destroyed, becoming atrophic, or it responds to the irritation by becoming hypertrophic. The same processes occur in the bony supportive structures of the teeth. Bone can be lost, creating a widened periodontal space. In other instances, it can respond with hypertrophic activity and osteosclerosis results. Osteosclerosis is an increase in the density of the bone and is seen as a more radiopaque area of the bone (Fig. 9-28).

Hypercementosis. Hypertrophic activity can also occur at the cementum level, with an apparent proliferation of cementum. This is often seen radiographically as a widening of the apical areas of the root (Fig. 9-29).

Pulpitis

An extremely common complaint of persons who come to the dental office is tooth sensitivity or pulpitis. Several major causative factors can lead

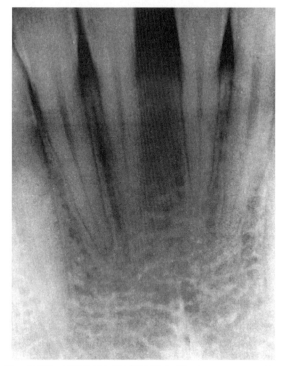

Fig. 9-28 OSTEOSCLEROSIS. The bone surrounding the apical half of the left mandibular lateral incisor root is of increased density. This is called *osteosclerosis*.

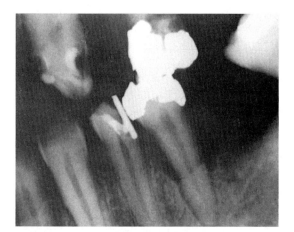

Fig. 9-29 HYPERCEMENTOSIS. The increased amount of cementum is associated with the root of the mandibular second premolar.

to these symptoms. By far the most common is the advancement of dental caries toward the pulpal tissue. Therefore it is important to rule out this factor with a dental examination and appropriate radiographs. On occasion, however, persons come in with pulpitis that has no apparent dental or periodontal etiology. They complain of sensitivity to temperature changes, especially cold. When all other obvious causative factors have been ruled out, one must consider heavy occlusal forces. The mechanism by which heavy occlusal forces create pulpitis is not clear. It has been suggested[53] that heavy forces applied to a tooth can increase blood pressure and passive congestion within the pulp, causing pulpitis. Chronic pulpitis can lead to pulpal necrosis. Although some studies[54] do not support this concept, clinical observations do appear to pinpoint a relationship between pulpitis and heavy occlusal forces.

Another confusing diagnosis that can present as pulpal symptoms is a small, minute fracture or crack in the tooth. This type of fracture is rarely seen radiographically and therefore is easily overlooked. Although sensitivity is a common complaint, other signs can help locate the problem. Having the patient bite on a small wooden separator over each cusp tip will cause a shearing effect at the fracture site and elicit a sharp pain. This diagnostic test is helpful in ruling out root fracture.

The examiner must be aware that tooth pain can exist that does not originate within the tooth itself. When a patient reports toothache and the examiner cannot find any local cause of the problem, distant sites should be considered. Toothache of nondental origin can come from muscular, vascular, neural, or sinus sources.[55,56] The most common of these is muscular. Trigger points that develop in certain muscles can create central excitatory effects that refer pain to the teeth. Three muscles can do this: the temporalis, masseter, and anterior belly of the digastric.[30] As shown in Fig. 9-30, *A*, *B*, and *C*, each muscle has specific referral patterns. The temporalis usually refers pain only to the maxillary teeth but may also refer to the anterior or posterior teeth, depending on the location of the trigger point. The masseter refers only to posterior teeth but may also refer to either maxillary or mandibular teeth, depending on the location of the

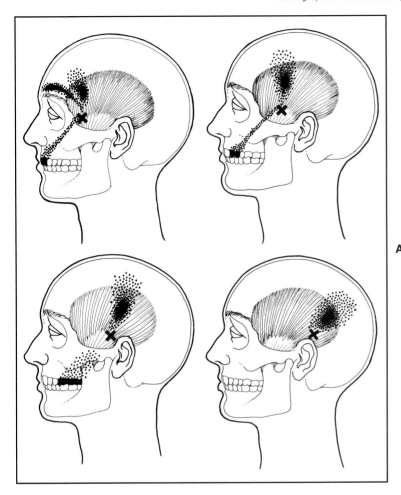

A

Fig. 9-30 REFERRAL OF MYO-FASCIAL TRIGGER POINT PAIN TO THE TEETH. A, The temporalis refers only to the maxillary teeth.

Continued

trigger point. The anterior digastric refers pain to the mandibular anterior teeth only.

The key to identifying referred tooth pain is that *local provocation of the painful tooth does not increase the symptoms.* In other words, hot, cold, and/or biting on the tooth do not increase or change the pain. However, local provocation of the active trigger point will increase the toothache symptoms. When the examiner is suspicious of referred pain to a tooth, local anesthetic blocking of the tooth and/or muscle is helpful in confirming the diagnosis (discussed in Chapter 10). Infiltration of local anesthetic around the painful tooth will not decrease the pain, but blocking the trigger point with the anesthetic will both obtund the trigger point and eliminate the toothache.

Tooth Wear

Tooth wear is by far the most common sign of breakdown in the dentition. It is probably seen more often than any other functional disturbance in the masticatory system. The vast majority of such wear is a direct result of parafunctional activity. When it is observed, either functional or parafunctional activity must be identified. This is done by examining the position of the wear facets on the teeth (Fig. 9-31).

Functional wear should occur near fossa areas and centric cusp tips. These facets occur on the inclines that guide the mandible in the final stages of mastication. Wear found during eccentric movements is almost always caused by parafunctional activity. To identify this type of wear, it is necessary

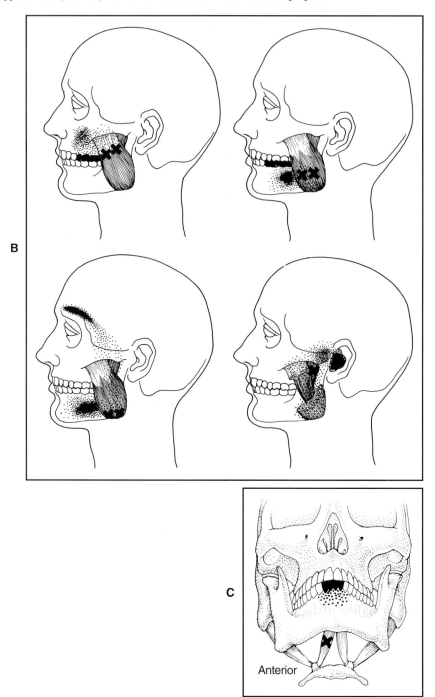

Fig. 9-30, cont'd B, The masseter refers only to the posterior teeth. **C,** The digastricus anterior refers only to the mandibular incisors. *(From Travell JG, Simons DG: Myofascial pain and dysfunction. The trigger point manual, Baltimore, 1983, Williams & Wilkins, pp 220, 237, and 274.)*

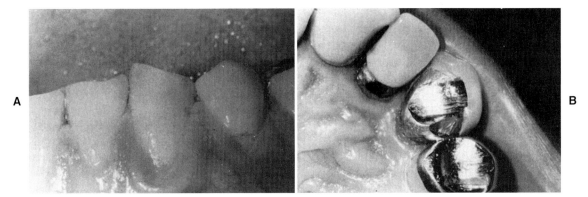

Fig. 9-31 TYPICAL WEAR PATTERN. A, The canine has been flattened compared with its original shape. **B,** Wear facets on several crowns.

merely to have the patient close on the opposing wear facets and visualize the mandibular position (Fig. 9-32). If the mandibular position is close to the ICP, it is likely to be functional wear. However, if an eccentric position is assumed, the cause is more often parafunctional activity.

If tooth wear is present but opposing wear cannot be made to contact, other etiologic factors must be considered. The patient should be questioned regarding any oral habits such as biting on a pipe or bobby pins (Fig. 9-33, *A*). One must also be aware that some teeth that appear worn may, in fact, be chemically abraded. Holding strong citric acid fruits (e.g., lemons) in the mouth or chronic acid regurgitation (heartburn) can create chemical abrasion (Fig. 9-33, *B* and *C*).

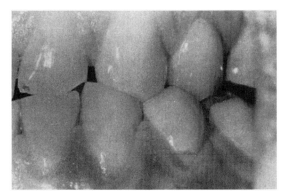

Fig. 9-32 When the patient closes on the wear facets, a laterotrusive position of the mandible is assumed. This is indicative of parafunctional activity.

The patient should be questioned regarding the presence of parafunctional (bruxing) activity. Patients who have a diurnal bruxing habit may acknowledge this, but unfortunately nocturnal bruxism often goes unnoticed.[57] Studies[58,59] show a poor correlation between awareness of bruxism and severity of the tooth wear. The examination therefore becomes an important part of the diagnosis. However, the presence of tooth wear does not mean that the patient is currently bruxing his or her teeth. The tooth wear may have occurred years ago. Therefore the history of symptoms and the examination findings need to be combined to evaluate the present level of bruxism. As one can see, bruxism is not always an easy diagnosis to establish.

Abfractions

Abfractions are noncarious cervical lesions or wedge-shaped defects in a tooth (Fig. 9-34). Most abfractions appear in the facial or buccal cervical areas of the first premolars followed by the second premolars. Maxillary and mandibular teeth seem to be equally affected by abfractions, with the exception of mandibular canines, which have a much lower estimated risk of incurring abfractions than do maxillary canines.[60] The prevalence of developing abfractions generally increases with age.[60] The etiology of abfractions is quite debated. Some have suggested that abfractions are the results of flexing of the root at the cervical region when the tooth is placed under heavy occlusal loading.[60,61] If this is accurate, then bruxing activity

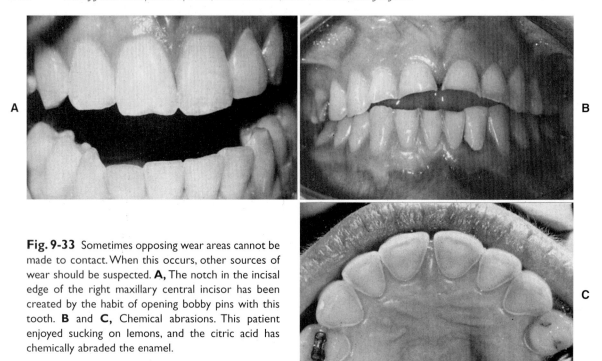

Fig. 9-33 Sometimes opposing wear areas cannot be made to contact. When this occurs, other sources of wear should be suspected. **A,** The notch in the incisal edge of the right maxillary central incisor has been created by the habit of opening bobby pins with this tooth. **B** and **C,** Chemical abrasions. This patient enjoyed sucking on lemons, and the citric acid has chemically abraded the enamel.

is a likely cause. Others, however, have not found a strong correlation between occlusal loading and abrasions.[62] Some believe abrasions are caused by aggressive tooth brushing.[63] Because the cause of abrasions is still uncertain, management is unpredictable. However, when a patient demonstrates

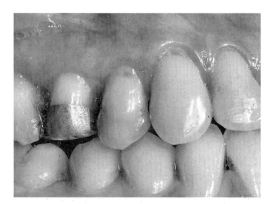

Fig. 9-34 Defects or abrasions in the cervical regions of the maxillary canine and first premolar are thought by some investigators to be related to heavy occlusal loading.

significant occlusal wear facets on a tooth that also has an abrasion, one might be suspicious of the relationship. In this situation one might consider protecting the tooth by reducing the loading (occlusal appliance therapy).

Occlusal Examination

The occlusal contact pattern of the teeth is examined in all possible positions and movements of the mandible: the CR position, the ICP, protrusive movement, and right and left laterotrusive movements. In evaluating the occlusal condition, one should keep in mind the criteria for optimum functional occlusion (see Chapter 5). Any variation from that could (but does not necessarily) play a contributing factor in the cause of a functional disturbance.

A variety of techniques can be used to locate the occlusal contacts on the teeth. Sometimes it is helpful to question the patient regarding the presence and location of tooth contacts. It is best to verify the patient's response by marking the contacts with articulating paper on ribbon. When articulating paper is used, it is best to dry the teeth well before marking so that they will accept the marking. Shim stock (0.0005-inch-thick Mylar strip) is also helpful in identifying the presence of occlusal contacts. This technique is described in the section Mediotrusive Contacts.

During an occlusal examination, remember that the masticatory system is composed of tissues that are able to flex, compress, and change position when force is applied. Examining diagnostic casts on a rigid articulator has led dentists to believe that the masticatory system is rigid. However, this is not a true assumption. Occlusal contacts cause teeth to move slightly as the periodontal ligaments and bone are compressed. Therefore to assess the occlusal condition accurately, one must be careful to have the patient close the mouth almost to the point of tooth contact and then evaluate. As heavier force is applied, the initial tooth contact may shift. This will allow multiple tooth contacts, which will mask the initial contact and make it impossible to locate the initial point of occlusion, especially in CR.

Centric Relation Contacts. The occlusal examination begins with an observation of the occlusal contacts when the condyles are in their optimum functional relationship. This is when they are in the musculoskeletally stable (MS) position, located most superoanteriorly in the mandibular fossae and braced against the posterior slopes of the articular eminences, with the discs properly interposed (CR). The mandible can then be purely rotated, opened, and closed approximately 20 mm interincisally while the condyles remain in their MS position. The MS position is located, and the mandible is closed to identify the occlusal relationship of the teeth in this joint position (CR).

Locating the centric relation position. Locating the CR position can sometimes be difficult. To guide the mandible into this position, one must first understand that the neuromuscular control system governs all movement. The functional concept to consider is that the neuromuscular system acts in a protective manner when the teeth are threatened by damaging contacts. Because in some instances closure of the mandible in CR leads to a single tooth contact on cuspal inclines, the neuromuscular control system perceives this as potentially damaging to that tooth. Therefore care must be

taken in positioning the mandible to assure the patient's neuromuscular system that damage will not occur.

In attempting to locate CR, it is important that the patient be relaxed. This can be aided by having the patient recline comfortably in the dental chair. One's choice of words can also help. Demanding "relaxation" in a harsh voice does not encourage it. The patient is approached in a soft, gentle, reassuring, and understanding manner. Encouragement is given when success is achieved.

Dawson[64] has described an effective technique for guiding the mandible into CR. It begins with the patient lying back with the chin pointed upward (Fig. 9-35, *A*). Lifting the chin upward places the head in an easier position to locate the condyles near the CR position. The dentist sits behind the patient, and the four fingers of each hand are placed on the lower border of the mandible with the smallest finger behind the angle of the mandible. It is important that the fingers be located on the bone and not in the soft tissues of the neck (Fig. 9-35, *B* and *C*). Next, both thumbs are placed over the symphysis of the chin so that they touch each other between the chin and the lower lip (Fig. 9-35, *D* and *E*). When the hands are in this position, the mandible is guided by upward force placed on its lower border and angle with the fingers, while at the same time the thumbs press downward and backward on the chin. The overall force on the mandible is directed so that the condyles will be seated in their most superoanterior position braced against the posterior slopes of the eminences (Fig. 9-36). Firm but gentle force is necessary to guide the mandible so as not to elicit any protective reflexes.

Locating CR begins with the anterior teeth no more than 10 mm apart to ensure that the temporomandibular ligaments have not forced translation of the condyles (see Chapter 1). The mandible is positioned with a gentle arcing until it freely rotates around the MS (CR) position. This arcing consists of short movements of 2 to 4 mm. Once it is rotating around the CR position, force is firmly applied by the fingers to seat the condyles in their most superoanterior position.

In this superoanterior position the condyle-disc complexes are in proper relation to accept forces.

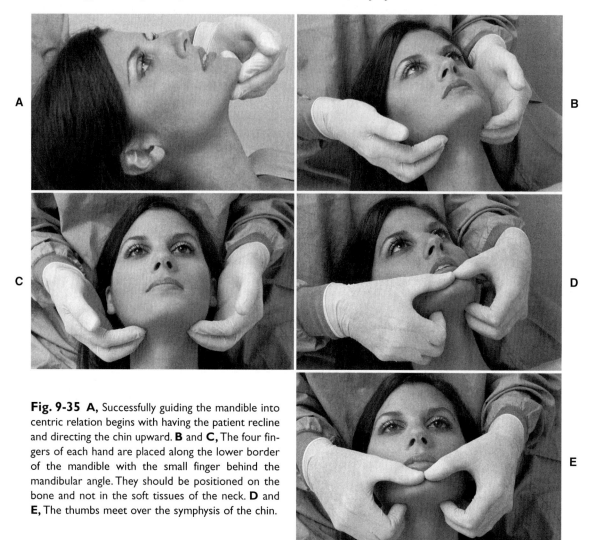

Fig. 9-35 A, Successfully guiding the mandible into centric relation begins with having the patient recline and directing the chin upward. **B** and **C,** The four fingers of each hand are placed along the lower border of the mandible with the small finger behind the mandibular angle. They should be positioned on the bone and not in the soft tissues of the neck. **D** and **E,** The thumbs meet over the symphysis of the chin.

When such a relationship exists, guiding the mandible to CR creates no pain. If pain is produced, it is likely that an intracapsular disorder exists. TMJ symptoms during bilateral manual manipulation are likely the results of loading the retrodiscal tissues secondary to a functionally displaced or dislocated disc. Inflammatory disorders of the TMJ can also elicit discomfort when, in guiding the mandible, force is applied to inflamed structures. If either of these conditions exists, an accurate reproducible CR position will not likely be achieved. Because these symptoms aid in establishing a

proper diagnosis, they are important and are therefore recorded.

Another method of finding the MS (CR) position is by using the muscles themselves to seat the condyles. This can be accomplished with a leaf gauge (Fig. 9-37, *A* and *B*).[65] The concept behind a leaf gauge is that when only the anterior teeth occlude (disengaging the posterior teeth), the directional force provided by the elevator muscles (temporalis, masseter, medial pterygoid) seats the condyles in a superoanterior position within the fossae. The anterior stop provided by the leaf

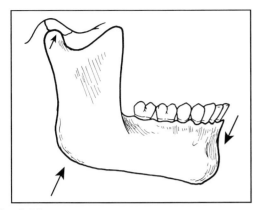

Fig. 9-36 When downward force is applied to the chin (thumbs) *(arrow)* and upward force is applied to the angle of the mandible (fingers), the condyles are seated in a superoanterior position in the fossae.

gauge acts as a fulcrum, allowing the condyles to be pivoted to an MS position in the fossae. A leaf gauge must be used carefully so that the condyle will not be deflected away from CR. If the leaf gauge is too rigid, it may provide a posterior slope, deflecting the mandible posteriorly as the elevator muscles contract. Another error may result if the patient attempts to bite on the leaf gauge in a slightly forward position as though biting into a sandwich. This will lead to protruding of the mandible from the CR position.

For effective use of the leaf gauge, the patient must close down on the posterior teeth with mild force. Enough leaves are placed between the anterior teeth to separate the posterior teeth slightly.

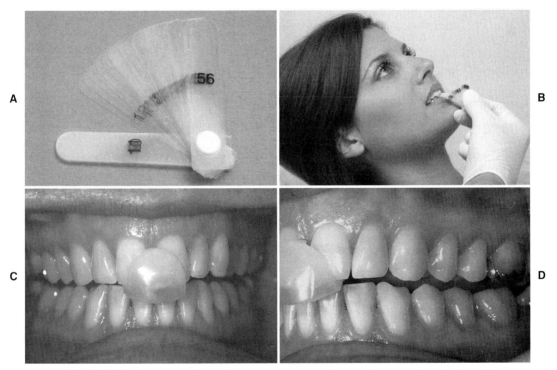

Fig. 9-37 A, Leaf gauge. **B,** Leaf gauge used to assist locating the musculoskeletally stable (MS) position. The patient is asked to close, and enough leaves are placed between the anterior teeth to separate the posterior teeth slightly. As the patient tries to seat the posterior teeth, the condyles will move to the centric relation (CR) position. Care should be taken to ensure that the patient does not protrude while closing or that the leaf gauge does not exert a retruding force on the condyles. Once the position has been located, the leaves are removed one at a time so that the initial contact in CR can be identified. **C,** An anterior jig can be used to help locate the MS position. **D,** A lateral view of the jig and the disoccluded posterior teeth. *(Anterior jig by Great Lakes Orthodontics Products, 199 Fire Tower Drive, Tonawanda, NY, 14151-5111.)*

The patient is instructed to close by trying to use only the temporal muscles, avoiding any heavy masseter contraction. At first this is a difficult request but by having the patient place two fingers over these muscles, the examiner can demonstrate how they feel when contracting. The patient will quickly learn to contract the temporal muscles predominantly, which will minimize protrusive forces. Once this has been mastered, the leaves are removed one by one until tooth contact is achieved. The first tooth contact is the initial one in CR.

Another method of finding the MS position is by using an anterior jig (see Fig. 9-37, *C* and *D*). An anterior jig is a small piece of acrylic that is adapted to the maxillary anterior teeth, providing an occlusal stop for a lower incisor. The stop needs to be developed so that it is flat and perpendicular to the long axis of the mandibular incisor in order to not deflect the mandibular position when force is applied. When the patient is asked to close on the posterior teeth, the anterior tooth contact on the jig will stop the mandible from complete closure and the condyles will then be seated to the MS position by the elevator muscles. This technique can be coupled with the bilateral mandibular manipulation technique that has already been discussed. The combination of the bilateral manual manipulation technique and the anterior jig is especially helpful when acquiring an occlusal record for mounting the patient's cast on an articular area (see Chapter 18).

Identifying the initial centric relation contact. Once the MS position is located, the mandible is closed so that the occlusion can be evaluated. Remember that the initial contact in CR may be perceived by the neuromuscular control system as damaging to that tooth and this threat of damage, along with the instability of the mandibular position, may activate the protective reflexes to seek a more stable position (i.e., maximum intercuspation). Therefore the mandible is raised slowly until the first tooth contacts lightly. The patient is asked to identify the location of this contact. The teeth on this side are then dried. Articulating paper is positioned between the teeth, and the mandible is again guided and closed until contact is reestablished.

Once the contact is located, light force can be applied by the patient to help mark the contact

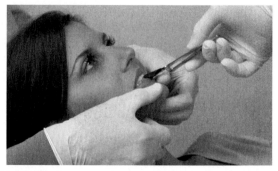

Fig. 9-38 To assist in locating the initial contact in centric relation, the dental assistant positions articulating paper (held in forceps) between the teeth during closure.

with the articulating paper. Forceps are used to hold the marking paper or ribbon (Fig. 9-38). If the patient is asked to help with closure, the condyles must be maintained in their most superoanterior position and the patient merely aids by raising the teeth into contact.

When the initial contact is identified, the procedure is repeated to verify or confirm this contact. It should be very reproducible. If it recurs on another tooth, CR has not been accurately located and efforts must continue until a reproducible contact is located. Once the initial contact in CR has been accurately located, a record of the teeth involved is made, as well as the exact location of the contact. This is referred to as the *initial CR contact*.

Once the initial CR contact has been recorded, the condyles are again repositioned in CR and the mandible is closed onto this contact. The patient holds the mandible securely on the contact, and the relationship of the maxillary and mandibular teeth is noted. Then the patient is requested to apply force to the teeth, and any shifting of the mandible is observed. If the occlusion is not stable in the CR position, shifting will occur that carries the condyles away from their MS positions to the more stable maximum ICP. This shifting is called the *centric slide* and represents a lack of orthopedic stability. Past literature suggests that when a retruded position of the mandible is used, the slide is present in approximately 8 of 10 patients[66] with an average distance of 1 to 1.5 mm.[38,67] As discussed in Chapter 5, the most retruded position of the mandible is no longer commonly used.

Instead the profession has embraced the concept of using the MS position as CR. Presently we do not have general population studies that examine the amount of slide from the MS position to the ICP. My opinion is that this slide would be less than that from the retruded position because this is how nature has established orthopedic stability in the masticatory system. However, when a centric slide is observed, orthopedic instability is present.

Observing the horizontal and vertical components of the slide is important. Some slides occur in a straight anterosuperior direction into the ICP. Others have a lateral component. Some reports[38,66] indicate that slides that deflect the mandible to the left or right are more commonly associated with dysfunction than are slides that create a straight anterovertical movement. The vertical steepness of the slide can be a significant feature in determining treatment when therapy is indicated. If the patient is asked to apply force to the teeth and no shift occurs, the ICP is said to be coincident with CR.

Intercuspal Position. Several characteristics of the ICP are closely evaluated: acute malocclusion, occlusal stability, arch integrity, and vertical dimension.

Acute malocclusion. An acute malocclusion is a sudden change in the ICP directly related to a functional disturbance. The patient is fully aware of this change and reports it on request. Acute malocclusions can be induced by muscle disorders and intracapsular disorders.

Muscle spasms can alter the postural position of the mandible. When this occurs and the teeth are brought into contact, an altered occlusal condition is felt by the patient. Spasms of the inferior lateral pterygoid cause the condyle on the affected side to be pulled anteriorly and medially, resulting in disocclusion of the posterior teeth on the ipsilateral side and heavy anterior tooth contacts on the contralateral side (Fig. 9-39). Complete spasm of an elevator muscle disallows opening of the mouth; however, partial spasm of an elevator muscle has a less dramatic effect. Partial spasm of an elevator muscle causes only slight changes that may not be observed clinically. Even though not clinically noticeable, the patient often complains that the "teeth don't fit together correctly."

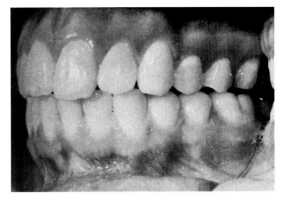

Fig. 9-39 ACUTE POSTERIOR MALOCCLUSION. This change was caused by unilateral spasms of the inferior lateral pterygoid. The patient described a loss of tooth contact on the ipsilateral posterior teeth and heavy contact on the contralateral canines.

Intracapsular disorders that cause a rapid change in the relationship of the articular surfaces of the joint can create an acute malocclusion. Change may include functional displacements and functional dislocations of the disc, retrodiscitis, and any acute bony alterations. When the changes create a condition that permits the bony structures to come closer together, as with a functionally dislocated disc or bone loss associated with osteoarthritis, the ipsilateral posterior teeth are felt to contact heavily (Fig. 9-40). When the changes create a condition that separates the bony structures, such as retrodiscitis or an injection of fluid to the joint (i.e., arthrography), the contralateral posterior teeth are felt to contact heavily.

The clinician should note that functional manipulation techniques are also helpful in identifying the origin of the acute malocclusion.

Maximum intercuspal stability versus joint stability. No gross discrepancy should exist between the MS position of the joints and the stable ICP of the teeth. It has already been mentioned that small discrepancies (1 to 2 mm) commonly exist between CR and the ICP. Although these do not necessarily disrupt mandibular stability, larger discrepancies can do so.[59,68,69]

Occlusal stability is examined by placing the patient in an upright and relaxed position. The patient closes slowly until the first tooth contacts. This is maintained while the examiner observes the

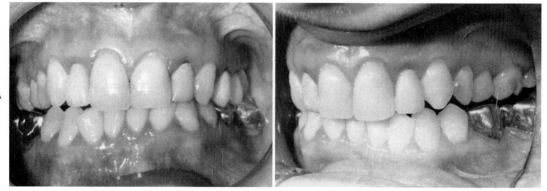

Fig. 9-40 ACUTE MALOCCLUSION. A, Severe loss of bony articular support in the left condyle as a result of osteoarthritis. With this loss an acute malocclusion has resulted. The patient complains that she can contact only on the left posterior teeth. With the loss of condylar support, the mandible has shifted and there are heavy contacts on that side. These act as a fulcrum, pivoting the mandible and separating the posterior teeth on the opposite side. **B,** Mirror view of the right side. No posterior tooth contacts appear on this side.

occlusal relationship. Then the patient clenches. If a significant shift occurs in the mandibular position from light tooth contact to the clenched position, one should suspect a lack of stability between joint and tooth positions. Because this shift depends on various features that are under the patient's control, such as head position and posture, it is repeated several times for verification of results. The lack of stability between intercuspation and the joint positions can be a major contributing factor to disc derangement disorders. When this test reveals an orthopedic instability, it should be verified by the other examination techniques previously discussed. Although this technique may be helpful, it should not be relied on as the sole determiner of orthopedic instability.

Arch integrity. The quality of the ICP is evaluated next. Any loss of arch integrity (through missing teeth or carious loss of tooth structure) is noted (Fig. 9-41). Any drifting, tipping, or supereruption of teeth is also recorded.

Vertical dimension of occlusion. The vertical dimension of occlusion represents the distance between the maxillary and mandibular arches when the teeth are in occlusion. It can be affected by loss of teeth, caries, drifting, and occlusal wear. A common condition that results in a loss of vertical dimension is created when a significant number of posterior

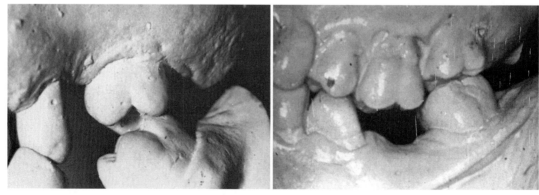

Fig. 9-41 POOR ARCH INTEGRITY AND STABILITY. Missing teeth and the subsequent drifting of adjacent teeth are demonstrated.

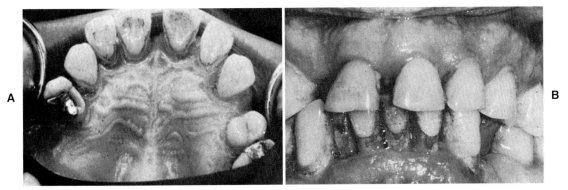

Fig. 9-42 CHRONIC LOSS IN VERTICAL DIMENSION (i.e., posterior bite collapse). **A,** The anterior teeth flair labially. This creates an increase in the interdental spaces. **B,** Labial flair of the maxillary anterior teeth and the resulting increased interdental spaces are demonstrated.

teeth are lost and the anterior teeth become the functional stops for mandibular closure. The maxillary anterior teeth are not in position to accept heavy occlusal forces, and often they flair labially. Space is created between the anterior teeth as the vertical dimension decreases (Fig. 9-42). This is referred to as a *posterior bite collapse* and can be associated with functional disturbances.[70,71] On occasion, the vertical dimension is iatrogenically increased by the placement of restorations that are too high.[72] Any alterations in the vertical dimension of occlusion, whether an increase or a decrease, are noted during examination.

Eccentric Occlusal Contacts. The superior eccentric border movements of the mandible are dictated by the occlusal surfaces of the teeth. For most patients the anterior teeth influence or guide the mandible during eccentric movements. The characteristics of the guidance are closely evaluated.

When anterior teeth occlude during an eccentric mandibular movement, they often provide immediate guidance for the rest of the dentition. In some instances they do not contact in maximum intercuspation (anterior open bite). Therefore eccentric guidance is provided by the posterior teeth. When they do contact in the ICP, the horizontal and vertical overlaps of the teeth determine the effectiveness of the guidance.

The guidance must be evaluated for its efficacy in disoccluding the posterior teeth during eccentric movements (Fig. 9-43). In some instances vertical overlap is adequate, but a significant horizontal

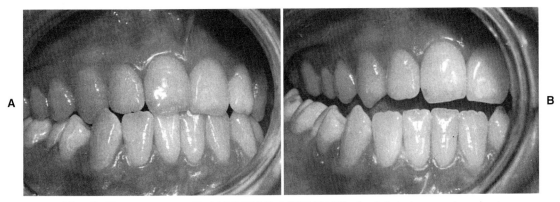

Fig. 9-43 INEFFECTIVE ANTERIOR GUIDANCE. A, Relatively normal occlusal condition. However, the position and occlusal relationship of the right maxillary canine should be noted. **B,** During a right laterotrusive movement the canine cannot provide anterior guidance, resulting in an undesirable mediotrusive contact on the contralateral side.

overlap exists that keeps the anterior teeth from contacting in maximum intercuspation. Then the mandible must move a distance before the anterior teeth occlude and guidance is achieved. The guidance in such a patient is not immediate and therefore not considered effective (see Chapter 5). The effectiveness of the eccentric guidance is recorded.

Protrusive contacts. The patient is asked to move the mandible from the ICP into the protrusive position. The occlusal contacts are observed until the mandibular anterior teeth have passed completely over the incisal edges of the maxillary anterior teeth or a distance of 8 to 10 mm, whichever comes first (Fig. 9-44). Two colors of articulating paper are helpful in identifying these contacts. Blue paper can be placed between the teeth, and the patient is asked to close and protrude several times. Next, red paper is placed and the patient again closes and taps the teeth together in the ICP. The red marks will denote centric occlusal contacts, and any blue marks left uncovered by the red will denote protrusive contacts. The exact position of all the protrusive contacts is recorded.

Laterotrusive contacts. The patient is asked to move the mandible laterally until the canines pass beyond end-to-end relation or 8 to 10 mm, whichever comes first. The buccal-to-buccal laterotrusive contacts are easily visualized, and the type of laterotrusive guidance is noted (e.g., canine guidance, group function,

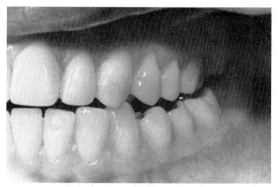

Fig. 9-45 LATEROTRUSIVE CONTACTS. The patient is asked to move the mandible laterally until the end-to-end relationship of the canines is passed. The type of guidance is observed. This patient reveals a canine guidance that disoccludes the posterior teeth.

posterior teeth only) (Fig. 9-45). The laterotrusive contacts on the lingual cusps are also identified. These cannot be clinically visualized and therefore must be located by red and blue articulating paper or by observing mounted diagnostic casts. All laterotrusive contacts are recorded.

Mediotrusive contacts. Some experts have suggested that mediotrusive contacts contribute significantly to functional disturbances.[73-75] These contacts should therefore be examined carefully. They can easily elude the casual examiner as a result of the neuromuscular control system. When the mandible moves in a lateral direction, mediotrusive contacts are perceived by the neuromuscular system as damaging and there is a reflex movement that attempts to disengage these teeth. The orbiting condyle is lowered in its orbiting pathway to avoid any mediotrusive contacts.

When contact areas between the teeth are only slight, the neuromuscular system successfully avoids them. If they are heavy, however, this activity is less effective and the contacts prevail (Fig. 9-46).[76] Because these contacts may play a significant role in functional disturbances, it is important that they be identified and not masked by the neuromuscular system.

Mediotrusive contacts should be evaluated first by asking the patient to move the mandible in the appropriate mediotrusive direction. Contacts identified during this movement are considered

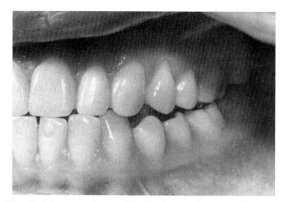

Fig. 9-44 PROTRUSIVE CONTACTS. The patient is asked to protrude until the anterior teeth reach an end-to-end relationship. The location of protrusive contacts is observed. Posterior protrusive contacts are especially noted.

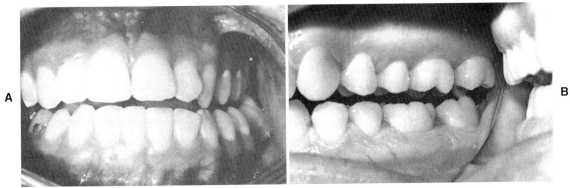

Fig. 9-46 MEDIOTRUSIVE CONTACTS. A, Between the maxillary and mandibular second molars. **B,** Sometimes prominent, actually providing the eccentric mandibular guidance. In this patient a casual look would suggest the presence of a canine guidance. However, a careful examination reveals that the left maxillary and mandibular canines are not actually contacting during this laterotrusive movement. The guidance is being provided by a mediotrusive contact on the right mandibular third molar.

unassisted mediotrusive contacts. Next, firm force is placed on the mandibular angle in a superomedial direction and the patient is again asked to move in the mediotrusive direction (Fig. 9-47). This force is often adequate to overcome the neuromuscular protection, revealing mediotrusive contacts not found during the unassisted movement. These contacts are called *assisted mediotrusive contacts.*

In a study[77] in which 103 patients (206 sides) were observed, only 29.9% revealed unassisted mediotrusive contacts. When the movement was assisted, the number increased to 87.8%. Both assisted and unassisted mediotrusive contacts need to be identified because their influence on masticatory function may be quite different.

Gross unassisted mediotrusive contacts appear to affect masticatory function adversely and therefore represent a potential etiologic factor in a functional disturbance. On the other hand, mediotrusive contacts that are only present with significant assisted force may actually protect the ipsilateral joint during heavy loading, such as during bruxism or when sleeping on the stomach. One study[75] demonstrated that subjects with assisted mediotrusive contacts actually had fewer TMJ sounds compared with a group that had no mediotrusive contacts. In another study[78] mediotrusive contacts were found to be more common in a control group than a group with TMD symptoms. The idea that assisted and unassisted mediotrusive contacts affect masticatory function differently has not received much attention in dentistry. This concept needs further investigation because treatment ramifications are great.

Mediotrusive contacts can be identified by questioning the patient, but they should be verified with articulating paper (the red and blue technique). Shim stock or a Mylar strip is also helpful. It is placed between the posterior teeth and the

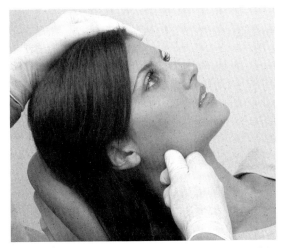

Fig. 9-47 Assisted mandibular movement is helpful in identifying mediotrusive contacts.

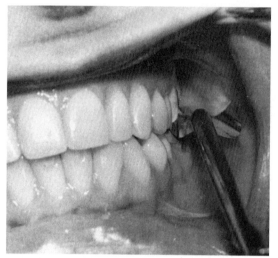

Fig. 9-48 Shim stock or a Mylar strip can assist in locating mediotrusive contacts.

patient is instructed to clench. While a constant pulling force is maintained on the shim stock, the patient moves in a mediotrusive direction (Fig. 9-48). If the mandible moves less than 1 mm and the shim stock is disengaged, no mediotrusive contact exists. If the shim stock continues to bind when the mandible moves beyond 1 mm, a mediotrusive contact does exist. This technique can be used for all posterior teeth. Any mediotrusive contacts are recorded on an occlusal examination form.

ADDITIONAL DIAGNOSTIC TESTS

The most important information for establishing a proper TMD diagnosis comes from the history and examination. Once this information is accumulated, a clinical diagnosis should be established. Sometimes other diagnostic tests can provide additional information that might help verify or challenge the established clinical diagnosis. It should always be remembered that these additional tests are only used to gain additional information and never to establish the diagnosis.

Imaging of the Temporomandibular Joint

Various types of imaging techniques can be used to gain additional insight regarding the health and function of the TMJs. When painful symptoms arise

from the joints and there is reason to believe that a pathologic condition exists, TMJ radiographs should be obtained. These will provide information regarding (1) the morphologic characteristics of the bony components of the joint and (2) certain functional relationships between the condyle and the fossa.

Radiographic Techniques. Radiographs of the TMJs are complicated by several anatomic and technical circumstances that hinder clear and unobstructed visualization of the joints. A pure lateral view of the condyle is impossible with conventional x-ray equipment because of superimposition of the bony structures of the midface (Fig. 9-49). Therefore to achieve a successful projection of the TMJs, the x-rays must be directed across the head either from below the midface in a superior direction (infracranial or transpharyngeal view) or through the skull directed inferiorly above the midface to the condyle (transcranial). Only through a specialized tomographic projection can the pure lateral view of the condyle be obtained.

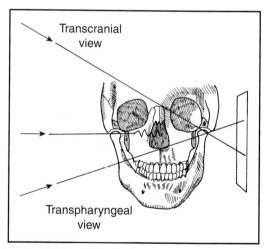

Fig. 9-49 CONVENTIONAL RADIOGRAPHIC TECHNIQUES USED TO VIEW THE CONDYLE. A pure lateral view is obstructed by the bony structures of the midface. However, a projection can be obtained by passing the x-rays from a superior position across the cranium to the condyle (i.e., *transcranial view*). Another projection can be obtained by passing the rays from inferiorly below the opposite side or between the coronoid process and neck of the condyle to the opposite side (i.e., *transpharyngeal* or *infracranial view*).

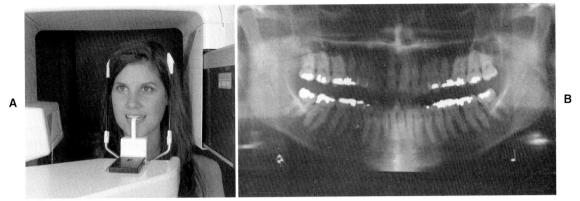

Fig. 9-50 PANORAMIC RADIOGRAPHY. A, Patient positioning. **B,** Typical projection, which is an excellent screening view of all the teeth and surrounding structures. The condyles are also clearly visible.

Four basic radiographic techniques can be used in most dental offices for evaluating the TMJs: (1) panoramic, (2) lateral transcranial, (3) transpharyngeal, and (4) transmaxillary (anteroposterior [AP]) views. Other, more sophisticated techniques can be used when additional information is necessary.

Panoramic view. The panoramic radiograph has become widely used in dental offices. With slight variations in the standard technique, it can provide screening of the condyles (Fig. 9-50). It is a good screening tool because its use results in minimum superimposition of structures over the condyles.

Although the bony structures of the condyle can be evaluated well, the panoramic view has some limitations. To view the condyle best, it is often necessary for the patient to open maximally so that the structures of the articular fossae will not be superimposed on the condyle. If the patient has only limited mandibular opening, superimposition is likely. With this technique the condyles are the only structures that are visualized well. The articular fossae are often partially, if not totally, obscured.

Because the panoramic radiograph is an infracranial view, the lateral pole of the condyle becomes superimposed over the condylar head. Therefore the area that appears to represent the superior subarticular surface of the condyle is actually only the subarticular surface of the medial pole (Fig. 9-51). This must be understood before interpretation can begin.

Lateral transcranial view. The lateral transcranial view can provide good visualization of both the condyle and the fossa. In past years this technique was popular because with minimal expense it can be adapted to most general dental radiographic techniques.

The patient is placed in a head positioner, and the x-rays are directed inferiorly across the skull (above the midface) to the contralateral TMJ and recorded (Fig. 9-52). Usually several projections of each joint are taken so that the function can

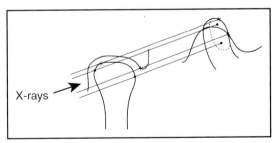

Fig. 9-51 TRANSPHARYNGEAL (INFRACRA-NIAL) PROJECTION. The area that appears to be the superior subarticular surface of the condyle is actually the medial pole. The lateral pole is superimposed inferiorly over the body of the condyle. The fossa is also superimposed over the condyle, which complicates interpretation of the radiograph.

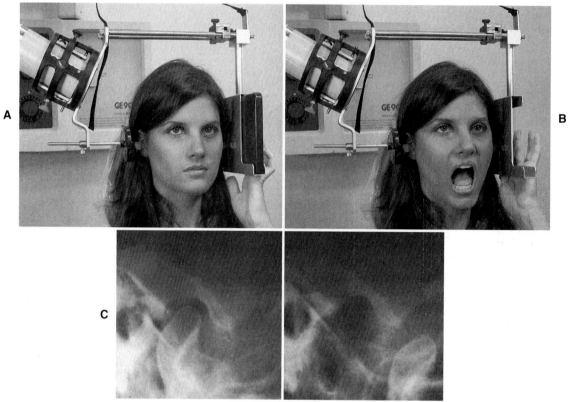

Fig. 9-52 TRANSCRANIAL PROJECTION. A, Teeth together. **B,** Maximum open position. **C,** The condyle can be visualized in the fossa with the articular eminence directly anterior. Posterior to the condyle a relatively round *(dark)* area is the external auditory meatus. The condyle has translated out of the fossa during an opening movement.

be evaluated. For example, one projection is obtained with the teeth together in maximum intercuspation and another with the mouth maximally opened. Interpretation of the transcranial view begins with an understanding of the angle by which the projection is made.

Because the x-rays are passing downward across the skull, this angulation superimposes the medial pole of the condyle below the central subarticular surface and lateral pole (Fig. 9-53). Therefore when the film is viewed, the apparent superior subarticular surface of the condyle is actually only the lateral aspect of the lateral pole. However, this projection is more acceptable than the infracranial view for visualizing the articular fossae.

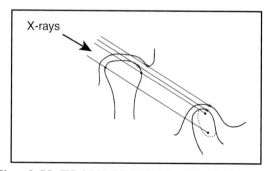

Fig. 9-53 TRANSCRANIAL PROJECTION. The area that appears to be the superior subarticular surface of the condyle is actually the lateral pole. The medial pole is superimposed inferiorly over the body of the condyle. In this projection the fossa is not superimposed over the condyle; thus a clearer view of the condyle is usually obtained.

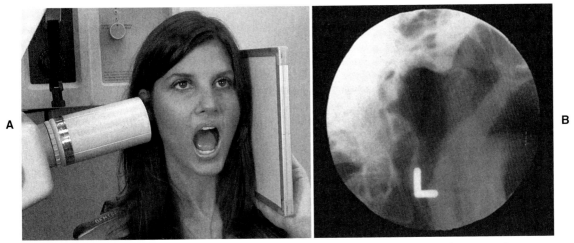

Fig. 9-54 TRANSPHARYNGEAL PROJECTION. A, Patient positioned for a view of the left temporomandibular joint. **B,** Typical view of the condyle.

Transpharyngeal projection. This view is similar to the panoramic view. However, because the x-rays are directed either from below the angle of the mandible or through the sigmoid notch, the angle at which they project the condyle is not as great as in the panoramic view. This means that the projection is closer to a true lateral view (Fig. 9-54). Although the technique demonstrates the condyle satisfactorily, the mandibular fossa is not usually visualized as well as the transcranial view.

Anteroposterior transmaxillary projection. This view can also be helpful. It is obtained from anterior to posterior with the mouth wide open and the condyles translated out of the fossae[79] (Fig. 9-55). If the condyle cannot be translated to the crest of the eminence, superimposition of the subarticular

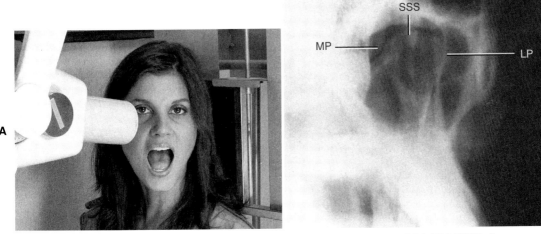

Fig. 9-55 ANTEROPOSTERIOR TRANSMAXILLARY RADIOGRAPHY. A, Positioning for the left temporomandibular joint. **B,** Typical view of a condyle. In this projection the medial *(MP)* and lateral *(LP)* poles can be easily visualized along with the superior subarticular surfaces *(SSS)* of the condyle.

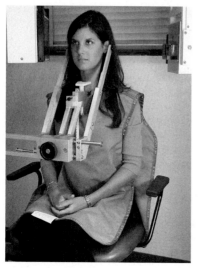

Fig. 9-56 Patient seating in a tomography unit in the proper position to take a lateral temporomandibular joint tomogram.

bone results and much of the usefulness of this radiograph is lost. When this projection can be correctly taken, it offers a good view of the superior subarticular bone of the condyle, as well as the medial and lateral poles. The AP projection also affords an excellent view for evaluating a fracture in the neck of the condyle.

Tomography. The previously mentioned imaging techniques can be routine dental office procedures and are most helpful in evaluating joint structures. On occasion, however, these screening films will not provide enough information and more sophisticated techniques are necessary. The lateral tomographic view provides a more accurate view of the TMJs.[80] It uses controlled movement of the head of the x-ray tube and the film to obtain a radiograph of the desired structures that deliberately blurs out other structures (Fig. 9-56). These radiographs are not infracranial or transcranial projections but true lateral projections (Fig. 9-57, *A* and *B*). AP views

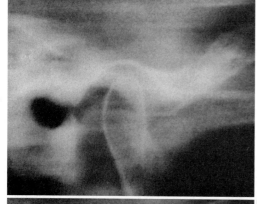

A

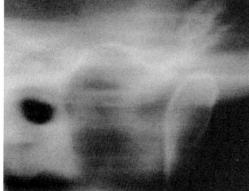

B

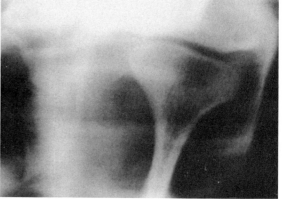

C

Fig. 9-57 LATERAL TOMOGRAPHY VIEW OF THE TEMPOROMANDIBULAR JOINT. A, Closed position. **B,** Open position. **C,** Anteroposterior tomogram. The tomography provides fine clarity. *(Courtesy Dr. Jay Mackman, Radiology and Dental Imaging Center of Wisconsin, Milwaukee.)*

can also be taken with tomography, revealing the lateral and medial poles without any superimposition (Fig. 9-57, C). This view may also be helpful in evaluating the articular surface of the condyle.

The tomogram can be obtained at precise sagittal intervals, so true sections of the joint are seen (lateral, middle, and medial poles). Bony changes and functional relationships of the joint can also be easily visualized.

The advantage of tomography is that it is generally more accurate than panoramic or transcranial radiographs for identifying bony abnormalities or changes.[80,81] Because it is a true sagittal view, one can evaluate condylar position in the fossae more accurately than with the transcranial view.[82,83] The disadvantages of tomography are cost and inconvenience. Although some dentists have tomographic units in their offices, the cost is great and may be difficult to justify in a general practice. The patient must therefore be sent to an outpatient clinic or hospital for the procedure. Another disadvantage is that the patient is exposed to higher levels of radiation than with other techniques. These disadvantages, however, are minimal when additional information is necessary to assist in diagnosis. If necessary, the tomogram is usually the first specialized film requested.

Arthrography. Arthrography was a radiographic technique in which contrast medium was injected into the joint spaces to outline important soft tissue structures. This technique became popular in the mid-1980s when the importance of the soft tissues was appreciated (especially disc position). Routine radiographic techniques and tomography only depict bony structures and their interrelationships, with no regard for the soft tissues. Through careful analysis of the joint spaces outlined by the contrast medium, the position and sometimes the condition of the articular disc could be ascertained (Fig. 9-58).[81,84-86] Because arthrography used a fluoroscope, one could visualize the dynamic movements of the disc and condyle, which was helpful in identifying condyle-disc dysfunction and perforations of the disc.[81,86,87] Unfortunately, this procedure was technique sensitive and, with the onset of better soft tissue imaging techniques (magnetic resonance imaging [MRI]), arthrograms became obsolete.

Computed tomography. Another technique that has been developed in the past decade is computed tomographic (CT) scanning. CT scanners produce digital data measuring the extent of x-ray transmission through various tissues. These data may be transformed into a density scale and used to generate or reconstruct a visual image[88] (Fig. 9-59, A). This technology can reconstruct the TMJ in a three-dimensional image that can offer even more diagnostic information to the clinician (Fig. 9-59, B).

The latest advancement in this technology is called *cone beam tomography.*[89] Cone beam tomography allows for viewing the condyle in multiple planes so that all surfaces can be visualized (Fig. 9-60). This technology is also capable of reconstructing three-dimensional images of the patient that can be rotated on the computer screen for more complete viewing (Fig. 9-61). Cone beam tomography can image both hard and soft tissues; therefore the disc-condyle relationship can be observed and evaluated without disturbing the existing anatomic relationships.[90-97]

However, CT scans have some disadvantages. The equipment is relatively expensive and therefore not always accessible. Often CT scans expose the patient to more radiation than simpler films, but the new cone beam technology has offered better images with far less radiation. This technology is certainly offering many features to assist the clinician in better understanding the patient's condition.

Magnetic Resonance Imaging. MRI has become the gold standard for evaluating the soft tissue of the TMJ, especially disc position. It uses a strong magnetic field to create changes in the energy level of the soft tissue molecules (principally hydrogen ions). These changes in energy levels create an image in a computer similar to a CT scan. MRI of the TMJs (Fig. 9-62) has demonstrated better visualization of the soft tissues than CT scans[98-101] and has the major advantage of not introducing radiation that might produce tissue damage to the patient. Thus far it has shown no harmful effects.

The disadvantages of MRI are similar to those of CT scanning. MRI units are usually quite expensive and not available in a traditional dental setting. The technology may also vary from site to site, and thus

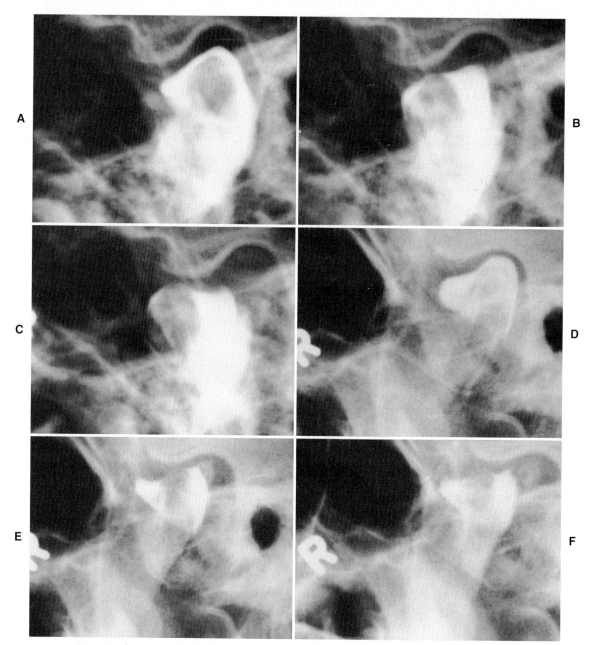

Fig. 9-58 ARTHROGRAPHIC PROJECTION. A radiopaque contrast medium has been injected into the inferior joint space outlining the inferior surface of the articular disc in this normal joint. In the closed mouth position of a normal joint **(A)**, the contrast medium can be visualized throughout the inferior joint space. As the mouth opens **(B)**, the disc rotates posteriorly, forcing the contrast medium into the posterior region of the inferior joint space. When the mouth is fully opened **(C)**, the disc is rotated to its maximum posterior position on the condyle, forcing the contrast medium completely out of the anterior region of the joint space. In this position the contrast medium is only seen in the posterior region of the inferior joint space. **D** to **F**, An anterior dislocated disc without reduction. During mouth opening the contrast medium remains in the anterior portion of the inferior joint space. The medium remains here because the disc is dislocated and cannot rotate posteriorly on the condyle. *(Courtesy Dr. Jay Mackman, Radiology and Dental Imaging Center of Wisconsin, Milwaukee.)*

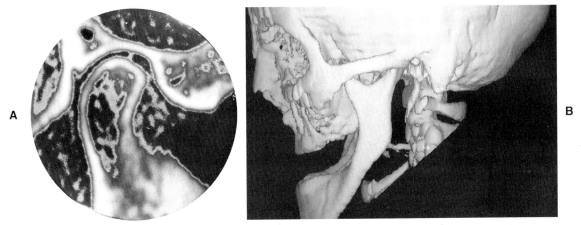

Fig. 9-59 COMPUTED TOMOGRAPHIC (CT) SCAN. A, Typical CT projection of the temporomandibular joint. Hard tissue (bone) is visualized better than the soft tissues with this technique. **B,** A three-dimensional CT reconstruction of an edentulous patient. *(A from Wilkinson T, Maryniuk G: The correlation between sagittal anatomic sections and computerized tomography of the TMJ,* J Craniomandib Pract *1:37, 1983.)*

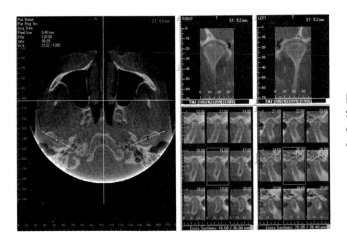

Fig. 9-60 CONE BEAM TOMOGRAPHIC SCAN. This technology allows for viewing of the condyle in multiple planes. *(Courtesy Drs. Allan Farmer and William Scarf, Louisville, Ky.)*

the quality of images may differ greatly. Another disadvantage of the MRI is that it is normally a static image, although more recently cine MRI has begun providing information on disc and joint movement.[102-104] This technology is becoming more refined and is replacing many of the existing imaging modalities.

The clinician should note that the presence of a displaced disc in an MRI does not suggest a pathologic finding. It has been demonstrated that between 26% and 38% of normal, asymptomatic subjects reveal disc position abnormality on MRIs.[105-112]

These studies reveal that false positives and false negatives are common with these imaging techniques, and therefore care must be taken regarding their interruption.

Bone Scanning. In certain clinical conditions it is helpful to know whether there is an active inflammatory process in the TMJs. Standard radiographs may reveal that the morphology of a condyle has changed, but they are not helpful in determining whether the process is active (osteoarthritis) or dormant (osteoarthrosis). When this information is important for treatment, a bone scan can be helpful.

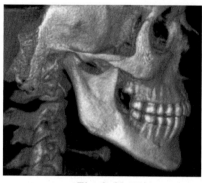
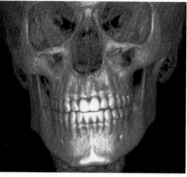
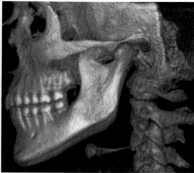

Fig. 9-61 These images have been reconstructed using cone beam technology. These three-dimensional images can be rotated on the computer screen so that the clinician can visualize the precise area of interest. *(Courtesy Drs. Allan Farmer and William Scarf, Louisville, Ky.)*

A bone scan is obtained by injecting a radiolabeled material into the blood stream that concentrates in areas of rapid bone turnover (Fig. 9-63). Once the material has had an opportunity to move to the areas of increased bone activity, an emission image is taken.[113,114] A similar technique uses single-photon emission computed tomography (SPECT) to identify increased areas of activity in bone.[115-119] Importantly, these techniques cannot discriminate between bone remodeling and degeneration. Therefore the information must be combined with clinical findings to have meaning.

Radiographic Interpretation. For radiographs to be useful in the diagnosis and treatment of TMDs, accurate interpretation is essential.

Because of the varying conditions of the joint and limitations of the techniques, however, TMJ radiographs often invite misinterpretation or even overinterpretation.

Limiting conditions. Three limiting conditions need to be considered before interpretation of standard radiographs can begin: (1) absence of articular surfaces, (2) superimposition of subarticular surfaces, and (3) variations in normal.

The primary structures visualized with most radiographs are the bony components in the joint. The characteristic form of bony structures may provide insight into the pathology of the joint; however, the clinician should remember that change in bony form may not always imply pathology.

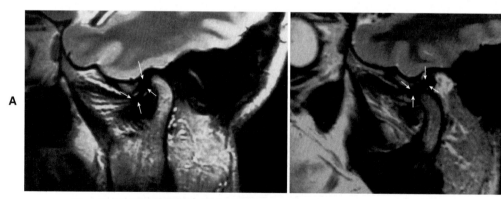

Fig. 9-62 MAGNETIC RESONANCE IMAGE. A, When the mouth is closed, the articular disc *(dark areas surrounded by arrows)* is dislocated anterior to the condyle. **B,** During opening, the disc *(arrows)* is recaptured into its normal position on the condyle.

midface (tomograms, CT scans, and MRIs are the exception), these so-called flat plates can have the subarticular surface superimposed on the condylar head (see Figs. 9-51 and 9-53).

When interpreting such radiographs, one must be aware that the entire subarticular surface of the condyle does not lie adjacent to the joint space as it would if the exposure were taken from a straight lateral view. In the transcranial view the subarticular surface adjacent to joint space is the lateral aspect of the lateral pole. In the panoramic or infracranial view, it is the medial aspect of the medial pole (Fig. 9-64). When a tomogram is taken, the view is a true lateral projection. These are important features to understand when

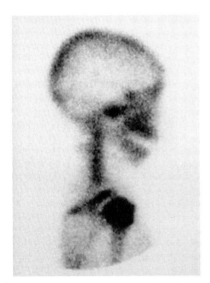

Fig. 9-63 A bone scan of the head and neck reveals a high concentration of radiolabeled material present in the temporomandibular joint and maxillary regions. This finding suggests an increased cellular activity in these regions.

Absence of articular surfaces. The articular surfaces of all joints are normally smooth and consistent. When irregularities are found, it must be suspected that pathologic changes have occurred. The articular surfaces of the condyle, disc, and fossa, however, cannot be visualized on standard radiographs. The surfaces of the condyle and fossa are made up of dense fibrous connective tissues supported by a small area of undifferentiated mesenchyme and growth cartilage,[33,120,121] which is not visible radiographically. The surface seen is actually subarticular bone. The articular disc, likewise, is composed of dense fibrous connective tissue, which also is not visible on standard radiographs. Therefore the surfaces actually seen are the subarticular bones of the condyle and fossa, with space between them. This space, known as the *radiographic joint space*, contains the vital soft tissues that are so important to joint function and dysfunction. Thus routine radiographs of the joint do not give insight into the health and function of these tissues.

Superimposition of subarticular surfaces. The superimposition of subarticular surfaces can limit the helpfulness of radiographs. Because most routine projections of the TMJs are single images taken at an angle to avoid the structures of the

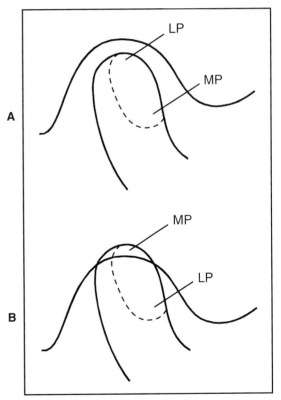

Fig. 9-64 When interpreting temporomandibular joint radiographs, one must always remember the projection being used to achieve the image. The subarticular bone that appears to be the superior articular surface of the condyle in the transcranial view **(A)** is actually the lateral pole of the condyle *(LP)*, whereas in the transpharyngeal view **(B)**, it is the medial pole *(MP)*.

interpreting these radiographs. Fig. 9-65 compares these different views in the same patient, showing that the findings are different depending on the location of the pathology.

Variations in normal. When viewing a radiograph, one has a tendency to consider all features that do not exhibit normal morphology as abnormal and therefore pathologic. Although this may sometimes be true, one must appreciate that a great degree of variation exists from patient to patient in the appearance of a normal and healthy joint. Variation from normal does not necessarily indicate a pathologic condition. The angulation at which the radiograph is obtained, the head position, and the

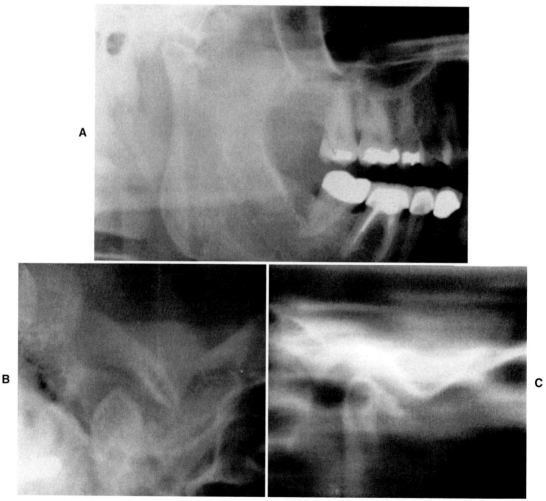

Fig. 9-65 These radiographs compare the same right temporomandibular joint using three techniques. **A,** Panoramic (i.e., transpharyngeal) view. The bony mass is observed in the anterior region of the condyle. **B,** The same joint in a transcranial view. In this view no abnormality is found. **C,** Tomogram of the same joint. This true lateral view reveals that there is a bony abnormality anterior to the condyle. This abnormality is on the medial aspect of the condyle and therefore is not seen in the transcranial view. This series demonstrates the need for several views when pathology is suspected. *(Courtesy Dr. Jay Mackman, Radiology and Dental Imaging Center of Wisconsin, Milwaukee.)*

normal anatomic rotation of the condyle can all influence the image that is projected. With such anatomic variations, one must be cautious in radiographic interpretation.

The limitations of the TMJ radiograph pose a significant handicap in the accurate interpretation of the joint. Radiographs should not be used to diagnose a TMD. Rather, they should be used as a source of additional information to either support or negate an already established clinical diagnosis.

Interpretation of the bony structures. Once it is understood that the soft tissues are missing in a radiograph, the morphology of the bony components of the joint can be evaluated. The radiographic appearance of the bony surface of the joint is normally smooth and continuous. Any disruption should be viewed with suspicion that bony changes have occurred. Both the articular fossa and the condyle should be examined because changes can occur in either structure.

Several changes commonly occur in the subarticular surfaces of the condyle and fossa. Erosions appear as pitted and irregular contours of the bony surfaces (Fig. 9-66). As they progress, larger concavities can be seen. In some instances the bony

surfaces become flattened (Fig. 9-67). If the condyle is flattened, a condition called *lipping* is created and small bone projections (osteophytes) may form (Figs. 9-68 and 9-69).[122] Occasionally, subarticular bone becomes thickened and osteosclerosis is seen adjacent to the articular surfaces of the joint. Subchondral cysts can also appear as radiolucent areas in the subarticular bone.

All of these radiographic findings are commonly associated with osteoarthritic changes of the joint.[122,123]

Although such changes are often indicative of pathosis, evidence[80,124-126] suggests that osteoarthritic changes are common in adult patients. The TMJ is capable of changing according to the chronic forces that are applied to it. These changes are known as *remodeling*, and remodeling can be in the form of bone addition (called *progressive remodeling*) or in the resolution of bone *(regressive remodeling)*.[127] Therefore when osteoarthritic changes are noted on a radiograph, it is difficult to determine whether the condition is destructive (as with osteoarthritis) or a normal remodeling process (Fig. 9-70).

Assuming that remodeling occurs as a result of mild forces applied over a long period is logical.

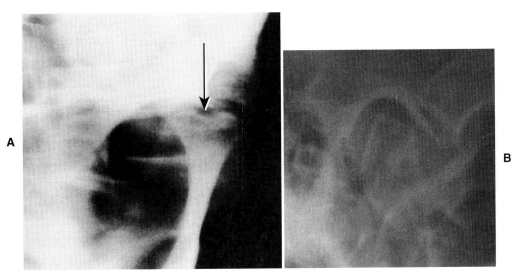

Fig. 9-66 EROSION OF THE ARTICULAR SURFACE OF THE CONDYLE *(arrow).* **A,** Anteroposterior tomography view. **B,** Lateral pole of the condyle (i.e., transcranial view). *(Courtesy Dr. Jay Mackman, Radiology and Dental Imaging Center of Wisconsin, Milwaukee.)*

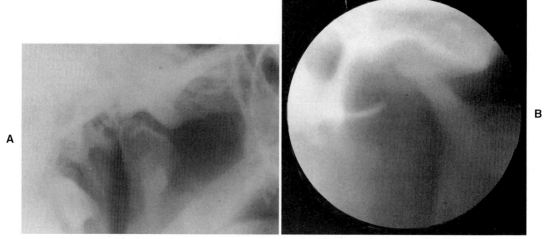

Fig. 9-67 FLATTENING OF THE ARTICULAR SURFACE OF THE CONDYLE.
A, Transpharyngeal view. **B,** Lateral tomographic projection.

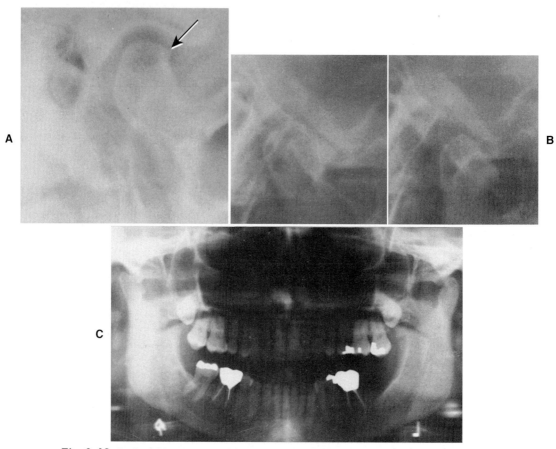

Fig. 9-68 A, Condylar osteophyte (lipping) of the lateral pole. **B,** Transcranial views showing the generalized flattening of the articular surfaces. This is best visualized in the open joint position. **C,** Panoramic view of the right condyle with osteoarthritic changes. *(Courtesy Dr. L.R. Bean, University of Kentucky College of Dentistry, Lexington.)*

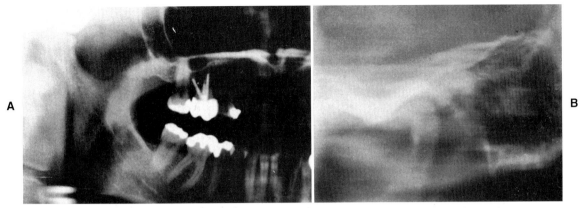

Fig. 9-69 Condylar osteophyte as depicted in panoramic view **(A)** and in the tomographic view **(B)**. *(Courtesy Dr. Jay Mackman, Radiology and Dental Imaging Center of Wisconsin, Milwaukee.)*

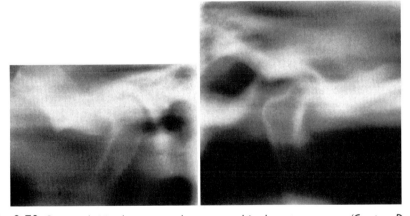

Fig. 9-70 Osteoarthritic changes are demonstrated in these tomograms. *(Courtesy Dr. Jay Mackman, Radiology and Dental Imaging Center of Wisconsin, Milwaukee.)*

If these forces become too great, remodeling breaks down and the destructive changes associated with osteoarthritis are seen. Often with these changes come symptoms of joint pain. It is difficult to determine whether the process is active or caused by a previous condition that has now resolved and left an abnormal form (osteoarthrosis).[128] A series of radiographs taken over time can help determine the activity of the changes. Of note is that radiographic changes in the shape of the condyle or fossa may have little relationship to symptoms.[129-131]

Several other observations of bony structures can be made while examining radiographs. The steepness of the articular eminence can be easily evaluated on the transcranial radiograph. This is done by drawing a line through the supraarticular crest of the zygoma, which is nearly parallel to the Frankfort horizontal plane. The steepness of the eminence is determined by the angle that this reference line makes with a line drawn through the posterior slope of the eminence (Fig. 9-71). As previously discussed, the steeper the angle of the eminence, the greater the rotational movement of the disc on the condyle during mouth opening. Some authors[132,133] have found this feature to be related to certain disc derangement disorders, whereas others have not.[134-136] Therefore this feature

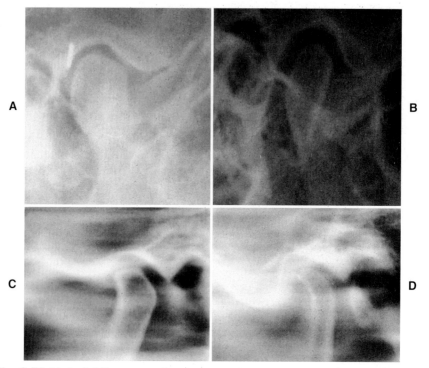

Fig. 9-71 Marked differences in the steepness of the articular eminences in these four patients are demonstrated. **A** and **B,** Transcranial projections. **C** and **D,** Tomographic projections. The steepness may contribute to certain disc derangement disorders. *(Tomography views courtesy Dr. Jay Mackman, Radiology and Dental Imaging Center of Wisconsin, Milwaukee.)*

may not relate well with clinical symptoms, and caution should be used regarding diagnosis and planning treatment.

Another bony abnormality that can be easily identified is the relative size of the condyle to the fossa (Fig. 9-72). Smaller condyles may be less able to tolerate heavy loading forces and therefore more likely to reveal osteoarthritic changes. The presence of a small condyle, however, does not represent a pathologic condition. These findings must be correlated with clinical findings.

Radiographs are also helpful in screening bony tissues for structural abnormalities that may create symptoms, which mimic TMDs. The panoramic view is especially useful for this purpose. Cysts and tumors of dental and bony origins can be identified. The maxillary sinuses can also be visualized. The styloid process should be observed, especially for unusual length. On occasion, the styloid

ligament will become calcified and appear radiographically to be quite long (Fig. 9-73). An elongated styloid process can elicit painful symptoms when it is forced into adjacent soft tissues of the neck during normal head movements. This condition is called *Eagle syndrome*[137-139] and can be confused with TMD symptoms.

Interpretation of the condylar position. Because the soft tissues of the joint are not seen on a radiograph, the so-called joint space is visualized between the subarticular surfaces of the condyle and fossa. In the transcranial projection the joint space is easily visualized. Some experts[140] have suggested that the condyle should be centered within the articular fossa. This implies that the radiographic joint space must be of equal dimensions in the anterior, middle, and posterior regions. It has even been suggested that treatment should be rendered to patients when joint spaces are not

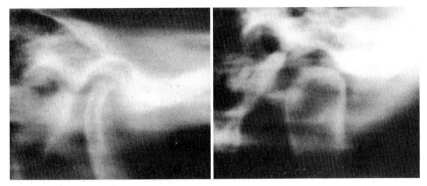

Fig. 9-72 These tomograms demonstrate the marked difference in condylar size and fossa. Condylar size should be noted but by itself does not represent pathology. This finding must be correlated with clinical findings. *(Courtesy Dr. Jay Mackman, Radiology and Dental Imaging Center of Wisconsin, Milwaukee.)*

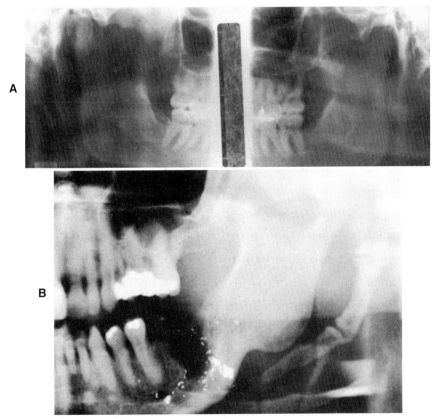

Fig. 9-73 EAGLE SYNDROME. A, An extremely long and calcified styloid process is observed in this panoramic projection. This patient was suffering from submandibular neck pain, especially with head movement. **B,** In this panoramic projection a large styloid process has been fractured. The large radiolucency in the mandibular molar region is secondary to a gunshot wound. *(Courtesy Dr. Jay Mackman, Radiology and Dental Imaging Center of Wisconsin, Milwaukee.)*

equal so that concentricity of the joint can be achieved.[141] Little evidence exists, however, to support the claim that equal joint space is either normal or desirable. In fact, evidence[142-145] shows that the thickness of the dense fibrous tissues covering the articular surface of the condyle can vary significantly. Because this tissue is not visualized radiographically, the subarticular bone may appear closer to or farther from the fossa depending on the tissue thickness. It also seems that large anatomic variations can exist among patients, which suggests[83,145-154] that one should not place too much emphasis on the position of the condyle in the fossa. Furthermore, the transcranial projection of the condyle can be used in evaluating only the lateral joint space and therefore may be misleading for the entire joint.[83,148,154]

Another factor that needs to be considered is head position. Slight positional changes of the head may alter the radiographic joint space (Fig. 9-74).[155] Variations in the anatomy of the lateral pole may also influence the joint space because this is the structure responsible for the space. Evidently, therefore, assessment of the joint space on transcranial radiographs has limited diagnostic value.

In tomographic projections a true lateral position can be obtained of any desired area of the joint. With this technique the joint space can be more accurately evaluated (Fig. 9-75).[83] Yet even with tomography there may be great variation among normal subjects.[142,147,148,150]

In one study a significant correlation existed between narrowing of the posterior joint space (posterior condylar displacement) and the existence of a disc derangement disorder.[156] This correlation did not exist with muscle disorders, which would suggest that tomograms and perhaps CT scans may be of some help in identifying posterior displacements of the condyle.[90] Although such a conclusion makes clinical sense, the clinician should not overinterpret these films. Radiographs are best used to help confirm an already established clinical diagnosis and not to establish the diagnosis. Clinicians who are guided predominantly by

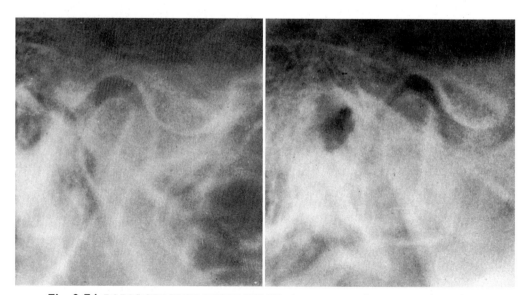

Fig. 9-74 RADIOGRAPHIC JOINT SPACE. In a transcranial projection, the angle at which the condyle is projected by the x-ray beam has a significant effect on the width of the radiographic joint space. This angulation is altered by the positioning of some transcranial units and even more commonly by the position of the head in the unit. Two transcranial projections of the same joint with the teeth occluded ensure no condylar movement. The variation in radiographic joint space is entirely caused by an approximately 7-degree turn of the head toward the film. This subtle change was not perceived by the technician.

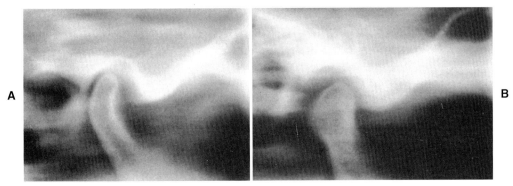

Fig. 9-75 One condyle appears to be positioned more posteriorly in the fossa **(A)**, whereas the other appears more anteriorly positioned **(B).** Although these tomograms represent a true lateral view, the difference in joint spaces does not necessarily represent a pathologic condylar position. The thickness of the disc (not seen) may explain the unequal joint spaces. These findings must be correlated with clinical symptoms to have meaning. *(Courtesy Dr. Jay Mackman, Radiology and Dental Imaging Center of Wisconsin, Milwaukee.)*

radiographs will inevitably have high percentages of misdiagnosis. Information gained from radiographs must be carefully scrutinized.[157]

Interpretation of joint function. Some radiographs (e.g., the transcranial view) can be used to assess joint function. This is accomplished by comparing the position of the condyle in the closed joint position with that in the open joint position.

In a normally functioning TMJ the condyle is seen to travel down the articular eminence to the height of the crest and, in many instances, even beyond it.[158,159] If the condyle cannot move to this extent, some type of restriction must be suspected. This may result from extracapsular sources (i.e., muscles) or intracapsular sources (i.e., ligaments, discs).

Radiographic evidence of extracapsular restrictions usually originates within the muscles. Such restrictions may be created by co-contraction or spasms of the elevator muscles, which prevent full mouth opening. However, elevator muscle restrictions do not inhibit lateral movement. Therefore the condyle will appear to be restricted on the radiograph of an opening movement but will seem to move within normal limits if a lateral movement is made and another is film taken.[160]

Radiographic evidence of intracapsular restrictions is usually caused by a loss of normal condyle-disc function. Frequently, disc derangement disorders restrict translatory movement of the involved joint. Therefore in the involved joint, little forward movement of the condyle is seen between the closed and opened joint positions. The unaffected side is usually normal. Unlike extracapsular restrictions, intracapsular restrictions will reveal the same limited pattern of movement on lateral movement radiographs as on opening radiographs.

Sometimes functional transcranial radiographs are helpful in confirming an anteriorly dislocated disc. In the normal joint the disc is maintained between the condyle and fossa, and the result is a consistent joint space in the closed and opened positions. However, when the disc is anteriorly and medially dislocated, the condyle is forced to translate, jamming the disc against the posterior slope of the eminence. As the condyle continues to jam the disc, it is displaced away from the eminence. This may create an increase in the radiographic anterior joint space.[161] The diagnosis of an anteriorly dislocated disc may sometimes be assisted radiographically by comparing the anterior joint space in the closed and opened positions. If the joint space increases in the opened position, an anteriorly dislocated disc should be suspected.

Importantly, the patient's head position should remain constant for both the open and closed exposures to ensure that variation in joint spaces is not created.

Intracapsular restrictions can also be created by ankylosis or capsular fibrosis. These types of restrictions tightly bind the condyle to the mandibular fossa and normally cause the condyle to become restricted in all movements. Thus the condyle shows no positional changes radiographically in any forward or lateral movements. Likewise, no change occurs in the joint spaces.[160]

These radiographic findings of joint restrictions should only assist in, and not be solely responsible for, diagnosis. History and clinical findings should be used in collaboration with radiographic findings to establish the diagnosis. Lack of condylar movement on a radiograph is meaningless without corroboration of these clinical findings. For example, a patient has severe muscle pain that is intensified on opening. A TMJ radiograph reveals little condylar movement. Radiographic evidence alone implies a restricted joint when actually there is a normal healthy joint being restricted by a muscle disorder.

A second patient may have a fibrotic ankylosis of the condyle that restricts movement of the TMJ. Because this fibrous unit consists of soft tissue and cannot be visualized radiographically, the radiographs appear similar to those of the first patient. Only clinical findings can differentiate the true restricted joint (intracapsular) in the second patient from the normal joint with extracapsular restriction in the first.

When evaluating joint function it is helpful to compare the patient's right and left sides. The movements should be similar. In ankylosis or an anteriorly dislocated disc, the affected side will reveal considerably less movement than the unaffected side. However, one common error during the radiographic technique will result in a false-positive reading of the functional movement. During the radiographic technique the patient is instructed to open wide for the exposure of the right TMJ. This wide opening may intensify the pain. Next, the head position is changed so that a left-side exposure can be made. Again, the patient opens wide. Realizing the pain that was elicited earlier, however, the patient is likely to open less wide during the left exposure. If the examiner is unaware of the reason for this variation, the left condyle will appear radiographically to be more restricted than the right when actually there is no difference. To avoid such discrepancy, a standard wedge is placed between teeth during both opening exposures so that an equal movement of both condyles will be ensured and thus allow radiographic comparisons of the two sides.

Any true restriction of the joint is verified by clinical evidence. When one joint is restricted, mandibular opening deflects the mandible toward the affected side. When restriction is noted radiographically, the patient is clinically observed for this type of movement.

Summary of the Uses of Temporomandibular Joint Imaging. Radiographs have limited use in the identification and treatment of TMDs.[43,162-164] Only through collaboration with clinical findings and history do they gain significance. When there is reason to believe that an organic joint pathosis exists, radiographs of the TMJs are obtained. Transcranial and panoramic views are used as screening devices for general assessment of bony abnormalities and osteoarthritic changes. Functional movements are also evaluated and correlated with clinical findings. Tomography is reserved for patients in whom the screening radiographs reveal a possible abnormality that needs closer visualization and investigation. CT, MRI, and bone scans are reserved for times when additional information will significantly improve the establishment of a proper diagnosis and treatment plan.

Importantly, the clinician should remember that abnormal radiographic findings must be viewed with caution. A well-designed clinical study failed to reveal a statistically significant relationship between radiographic findings and clinical symptoms.[165] Also, the information gained from radiographic interruption has not been demonstrated to be useful in determining the outcome of treatment.[166]

Mounted Cast

If during the examination the clinician identifies significant orthopedic instability, accurately mounted study casts may be helpful to further assess the occlusal condition. Mounted casts are not indicated for all patients being examined for TMDs. Mounted casts may be necessary when future dental treatment will be provided (e.g., prosthodontics, orthodontics).

Dental study casts can be of value, not only as a baseline record for tooth and jaw relations but also for evaluating the effects of bruxism over time.[144] The clinician should keep in mind that acute muscle and joint pain and joint edema can decrease the accuracy of the mountings.[167] Therefore occlusal analysis is most reliable after acute disease processes are resolved.

Because the relationship between occlusion and TMD symptoms cannot be reliably determined at the time of the initial examination (see Chapter 7), mounted casts are not extremely useful in initially diagnosing a TMD or other forms of orofacial pain. The significance of the occlusal condition as a contributing factor to a TMD may become verified by therapeutic trials (discussed in later chapters). For this reason mounted casts may be most useful when taken after the clinician has significant clinical evidence that the occlusal condition is related to the TMD symptoms.

When mounted casts are indicated, the casts should be mounted on either a semiadjustable or a fully adjustable articulator. Mounted casts provide better visualization of the occlusal contacts (especially in the lingual view) and remove the influence of neuromuscular control from eccentric movements. The casts should be mounted with the aid of an accurate facebow transfer and CR record. Diagnostic casts are always mounted in the MS (CR) position so that the full range of mandibular movement can be examined on the articulator (see Chapter 18.)

Electromyography

In recent years much attention has been drawn to the use of electromyograhic (EMG) recordings in the diagnosis and treatment of TMDs.[168,169] Experts originally believed that if a painful muscle was in spasm, increased EMG activity would be recorded from the involved muscle. Although this is likely true for myospasms, studies[170-173] now demonstrate that muscle pain is often not associated with any significant increase in EMG activity. Most muscle pain seems to be a result of local muscle soreness, myofascial pain, or centrally mediated myalgia. As described in Chapter 8, these conditions are not directly associated with muscle contraction (and muscle contraction is necessary to produce an increase in EMG activity). Although some studies do demonstrate that patients with muscle pain have higher EMG activity than controls, most of these differences are small.[174,175] In fact, the differences are often less than the variations that occur between patients (e.g., male versus female, thin face versus overweight face).[176]

It has also been demonstrated that relatively small variations in electrode placement can significantly change EMG recordings.[177] This means that recordings taken during multiple visits cannot be compared unless extreme care is taken to place the electrode in the exact same location for each recording.[178] With such slight differences and such great variations, EMG recordings should not be used to diagnose or monitor treatment of TMDs.[179-184] This is not to suggest that EMG records are invalid or have no use. Electromyography has been proved to provide excellent information on muscle function under research conditions. It is also useful with various biofeedback techniques to enable the patient to monitor muscle tension during relaxation training.[185] These techniques are discussed in Chapter 11.

Mandibular Tracking Devices

Certain TMDs can produce alterations in the normal movements of the mandible. One such disorder is a disc displacement with reduction. During opening, the condyle and disc move together until the disc is reduced. During this reduction a click is often felt (see Chapter 8), and the mandibular opening pathway will deviate (see Chapter 9). If a jaw-tracking device is used, the exact movement of the mandible can be recorded. Some experts have suggested that these tracking devices can be used to diagnose and monitor treatment of TMDs. Unfortunately, many intracapsular and extracapsular disorders create deviations and deflections in mandibular movement pathways. Because a particular deviation may not be specific for a particular disorder, this information should only be used in conjunction with history and examination findings. No evidence suggests that the sensitivity and specificity of jaw-tracking devices are reliable enough to be used for diagnosis and management.[184,186-189]

Sonography

Sonography is the technique of recording and graphically demonstrating joint sounds. Some techniques use audio amplifying devices, whereas others rely on ultrasound echo recordings (Doppler ultrasonography). Although these devices may accurately record joint sounds, the significance of these sounds has not been well established. As described in Chapter 8, joint sounds are often related to specific disc derangements and therefore their presence may have meaning. On the other hand, the presence of joint sounds does not, in itself, denote a problem. Many healthy joints can produce sounds during certain movements. If sonography is to have meaning, it must be able to separate sounds that have significance to treatment from those that do not. Presently sonography does not provide the clinician with any additional diagnostic information over manual palpation or stethoscopic evaluation.[180,184,190,191]

Vibration Analysis

Vibration analysis has been suggested to help in diagnosing intracapsular TMD, and internal derangements in particular.[192,193] This technique measures the minute vibrations made by the condyle as it translates and has been shown to be reliable.[194] Some specific parameters of vibration analysis appear to be sensitive and specific for identifying disc displacement patients compared with other TMD patients.[195]

A negative analysis finding is highly accurate for identifying a normal joint, and a positive finding is more accurate for identifying a reducing disc displacement than a clinical examination for joint sounds or a patient's perception of joint sounds.[196] Nevertheless, the technique diagnoses up to 25% of normal joints as derangements and misclassifies many deranged joints as normal, especially if the joint sounds are not audible or if the derangement has advanced to a nonreducing stage.[192,196,197] Although some studies do report encouraging accuracy in detection joint vibrations, data demonstrating that vibration analysis is a useful adjunct in the selection of appropriate patient therapy are lacking. Therefore one must question the cost benefit of such instrumentation. Thus at this time, vibration analysis is not the test of choice for suspected internal derangement.

Thermography

Thermography is a technique that records and graphically illustrates surface skin temperatures. Various temperatures are recorded by different colors, producing a map that depicts the surface being studied. It has been suggested that normal subjects have bilaterally symmetric thermograms.[198] From this concept some have suggested that thermograms that are not symmetric reveal a problem such as a TMD.[199,200] Although some studies do demonstrate that asymmetric thermograms are associated with TMD, another study does not.[201-203] One also finds that there is great variability of normal facial surface temperature between sides.[204,205] The sensitivity and specificity of identifying myofascial trigger points with thermography has not been demonstrated to be reliable.[206] The great variation among sides, patients, and reports suggests that, at this time, thermography is not a useful technique for the diagnosis and management of TMDs.[185]

References

1. Okeson J: Assessment of orofacial pain disorders. In Okeson J, editor: *Orofacial pain: guidelines for assessment, diagnosis, and management*, Chicago, 1996, Quintessence, pp 19-44.
2. Howard JA: Temporomandibular joint disorders, facial pain and dental problems of performing artists. In Sataloff R, Brandfonbrener A, Lederman R, editors: *Textbook of performing arts medicine*, New York, 1991, Raven, pp 111-169.
3. Bryant GW: Myofascial pain dysfunction and viola playing, *Br Dent J* 166:335-336, 1989.
4. Chun DS, Koskinen-Moffett L: Distress, jaw habits, and connective tissue laxity as predisposing factors to TMJ sounds in adolescents, *J Craniomandib Disord* 4:165-176, 1990.
5. LeResche L, Saunders K, Von Korff MR, Barlow W, Dworkin SF: Use of exogenous hormones and risk of temporomandibular disorder pain, *Pain* 69:153-60, 1997.
6. Nekora-Azak A: Temporomandibular disorders in relation to female reproductive hormones: a literature review, *J Prosthet Dent* 91:491-493, 2004.
7. Hatch JP, Rugh JD, Sakai S, Saunders MJ: Is use of exogenous estrogen associated with temporomandibular signs and symptoms? *J Am Dent Assoc* 132:319-326, 2001.

8. Moldofsky H, Scarisbrick P, England R, Smythe H: Musculoskeletal symptoms and non-REM sleep disturbance in patients with fibrositis syndrome and healthy subjects, *Psychosom Med* 37:341-351, 1975.

9. Moldofsky H, Scarisbrick P: Induction of neurasthenic musculoskeletal pain syndrome by selective sleep stage deprivation, *Psychosom Med* 38:35-44, 1976.

10. Molony RR, MacPeek DM, Schiffman PL, Frank M, Neubauer JA et al: Sleep, sleep apnea and the fibromyalgia syndrome, *J Rheumatol* 13:797-800, 1986.

11. Saletu A, Parapatics S, Saletu B, Anderer P, Prause W et al: On the pharmacotherapy of sleep bruxism: placebo-controlled polysomnographic and psychometric studies with clonazepam, *Neuropsychobiology* 51:214-225, 2005.

12. Turk DC, Rudy TE: Toward a comprehensive assessment of chronic pain patients: a multiaxial approach, *Behav Res Ther* 25:237-249, 1987.

13. Derogatis LR: *The SCL 90R: administration, scoring and procedure manual*, Baltimore, 1977, Clinical Psychology Research.

14. Fricton JR, Nelson A, Monsein M: IMPATH: microcomputer assessment of behavioral and psychosocial factors in craniomandibular disorders, *Cranio* 5:372-381, 1987.

15. Levitt SR, McKinney MW, Lundeen TF: The TMJ scale: cross-validation and reliability studies, *Cranio* 6:17-25, 1988.

16. Levitt SR, McKinney MW: Validating the TMJ scale in a national sample of 10,000 patients: demographic and epidemiologic characteristics, *J Orofac Pain* 8:25-35, 1994.

17. Drum RK, Fornadley JA, Schnapf DJ: Malignant lesions presenting as symptoms of craniomandibular dysfunction, *J Orofac Pain* 7:294-299, 1993.

18. Clark GT: Examining temporomandibular disorder patients for cranio-cervical dysfunction, *J Craniomandib Pract* 2:55-63, 1983.

19. Clark GT, Green EM, Dornan MR, Flack VF: Craniocervical dysfunction levels in a patient sample from a temporomandibular joint clinic, *J Am Dent Assoc* 115:251-256, 1987.

20. Mense S: Nociception from skeletal muscle in relation to clinical muscle pain, *Pain* 54:241-289, 1993.

21. Keele KD: A physician looks at pain. In Weisenberg M, editor: *Pain; clinical and experimental perspectives*, St Louis, 1975, Mosby, pp 45-52.

22. Mense S: Considerations concerning the neurobiological basis of muscle pain, *Can J Physiol Pharmacol* 69:610-616, 1991.

23. Burch JG: Occlusion related to craniofacial pain. In Alling CC, Mahan PE, editors: *Facial pain*, Philadelphia, 1977, Lea & Febiger, pp 165-180.

24. Krogh-Poulsen WG, Olsson A: Management of the occlusion of the teeth. In Schwartz L, Chayes CM, editors: *Facial pain and mandibular dysfunction*, Philadelphia, 1969, Saunders, pp 236-280.

25. Schwartz L, Chayes CM: The history and clinical examination. In Schwartz L, Chayes CM, editors: *Facial pain and mandibular dysfunction*, Philadelphia, 1969, Saunders, pp 159-178.

26. Frost HM: Musculoskeletal pains. In Alling CC, Mahan PE, editors: *Facial pain*, Philadelphia, 1977, Lea & Febiger, pp 140-152.

27. Moody PM, Calhoun TC, Okeson JP, Kemper JT: Stress-pain relationship in MPD syndrome patients and non-MPD syndrome patients, *J Prosthet Dent* 45:84-88, 1981.

28. Okeson JP, Kemper JT, Moody PM: A study of the use of occlusion splints in the treatment of acute and chronic patients with craniomandibular disorders, *J Prosthet Dent* 48:708-712, 1982.

29. Travell JG, Rinzler SH: The myofascial genesis of pain, *Postgrad Med* 11:425-434, 1952.

30. Simons DG, Travell JG, Simons LS: *Travell & Simons' myofascial pain and dysfunction: the trigger point manual*, ed 2, Baltimore, 1999, Lippincott Williams & Wilkins.

31. Johnstone DR, Templeton M: The feasibility of palpating the lateral pterygoid muscle, *J Prosthet Dent* 44:318-323, 1980.

32. Stratmann U, Mokrys K, Meyer U, Kleinheinz J, Joos U et al: Clinical anatomy and palpability of the inferior lateral pterygoid muscle, *J Prosthet Dent* 83:548-554, 2000.

33. Bell WE: *Temporomandibular disorders*, Chicago, 1986, Year Book Medical.

34. Svensson P, Arendt-Nielsen L, Nielsen H, Larsen JK: Effect of chronic and experimental jaw muscle pain on pain-pressure thresholds and stimulus-response curves, *J Orofac Pain* 9:347-356, 1995.

35. Thomas CA, Okeson JP: Evaluation of lateral pterygoid muscle symptoms using a common palpation technique and a method of functional manipulation, *Cranio* 5:125-129, 1987.

36. Okeson JP: *Bell's orofacial pains*, ed 6, Chicago, 2005, Quintessence, pp 63-94.

37. Agerberg G: Maximal mandibular movement in young men and women, *Swed Dent J* 67:81-100, 1974.

38. Solberg W: Occlusion-related pathosis and its clinical evaluation. In Clark JW, editor: *Clinical dentistry*, New York, 1976, Harper & Row, pp 1-29.

39. Vanderas AP: Mandibular movements and their relationship to age and body height in children with or without clinical signs of craniomandibular dysfunction: part IV. A comparative study, *ASDC J Dent Child* 59:338-341, 1992.

40. Bitlar G et al: Range of jaw opening in an elderly non-patient population, *J Dent Res* 70:419, 1991 (abstract).

41. McCarroll RS, Hesse JR, Naeije M, Yoon CK, Hansson TL: Mandibular border positions and their relationships with peripheral joint mobility, *J Oral Rehabil* 14:125-131, 1987.

42. Hesse JR, Naeije M, Hansson TL: Craniomandibular stiffness toward maximum mouth opening in healthy subjects: a clinical and experimental investigation, *J Craniomandib Disord* 4:257-266, 1990.

43. Bezuur JN, Habets LL, Hansson TL: The recognition of craniomandibular disorders—a comparison between clinical, tomographical, and dental panoramic radiographical findings in thirty-one subjects, *J Oral Rehabil* 15:549-554, 1988.

44. Hardison JD, Okeson JP: Comparison of three clinical techniques for evaluating joint sounds, *Cranio* 8:307-311, 1990.

45. Westesson PL, Eriksson L, Kurita K: Reliability of a negative clinical temporomandibular joint examination: prevalence of disk displacement in asymptomatic temporomandibular joints, *Oral Surg Oral Med Oral Pathol* 68:551-554, 1989.

46. Ricketts RM: Clinical interferences and functional disturbances of the masticatory system, *Am J Orthodont Dentofac Orthop* 52:416-439, 1966.

47. Geering AH: Occlusal interferences and functional disturbances of the masticatory system, *J Clin Periodontol* 1:112-119, 1974.

48. Lieberman MA, Gazit E, Fuchs C, Lilos P: Mandibular dysfunction in 10-18 year old school children as related to morphological malocclusion, *J Oral Rehabil* 12:209-214, 1985.

49. Egermark-Eriksson I, Carlsson GE, Magnusson T: A long-term epidemiologic study of the relationship between occlusal factors and mandibular dysfunction in children and adolescents, *J Dent Res* 66:67-71, 1987.

50. De Boever JA, Adriaens PA: Occlusal relationship in patients with pain-dysfunction symptoms in the temporomandibular joint, *J Oral Rehabil* 10:1-7, 1983.

51. Lous I, Sheik-Ol-Eslam A, Moller E: Postural activity in subjects with functional disorders of the chewing apparatus, *Scand J Dent Res* 78:404-410, 1970.

52. Miller SC: *Textbook of periodontia*, Philadelphia, 1938, Blakiston.

53. Ramfjord SP, Ash MM: *Occlusion*, ed 3, Philadelphia, 1983, Saunders.

54. Landay MA, Nazimov H, Seltzer S: The effects of excessive occlusal force on the pulp, *J Periodontol* 41:3-11, 1970.

55. Okeson JP: *Bell's orofacial pains*, ed 6, Chicago, 2005, Quintessence, pp 287-328.

56. Okeson JP, Falace DA: Nonodontogenic toothache, *Dent Clin North Am* 41:367-383, 1997.

57. Marbach JJ, Raphael KG, Dohrenwend BP, Lennon MC: The validity of tooth grinding measures: etiology of pain dysfunction syndrome revisited, *J Am Dent Assoc* 120:327-333, 1990.

58. Seligman DA, Pullinger AG, Solberg WK: The prevalence of dental attrition and its association with factors of age, gender, occlusion, and TMJ symptomatology, *J Dent Res* 67:1323-1333, 1988.

59. Pullinger AG, Seligman DA: The degree to which attrition characterizes differentiated patient groups of temporomandibular disorders, *J Orofac Pain* 7:196-208, 1993.

60. Bernhardt O, Gesch D, Schwahn C, Mack F, Meyer G et al: Epidemiological evaluation of the multifactorial aetiology of abfractions, *J Oral Rehabil* 33:17-25, 2006.

61. Miller N, Penaud J, Ambrosini P, Bisson-Boutelliez C, Briancon S: Analysis of etiologic factors and periodontal conditions involved with 309 abfractions, *J Clin Periodontol* 30:828-832, 2003.

62. Litonjua LA, Andreana S, Bush PJ, Tobias TS, Cohen RE: Noncarious cervical lesions and abfractions: a re-evaluation, *J Am Dent Assoc* 134:845-850, 2003.

63. Piotrowski BT, Gillette WB, Hancock EB: Examining the prevalence and characteristics of abfractionlike cervical lesions in a population of U.S. veterans, *J Am Dent Assoc* 132:1694-1701; quiz 1726-1727, 2001.

64. Dawson PE: *Evaluation, diagnosis and treatment of occlusal problems*, St Louis, 1989, Mosby.

65. Carroll WJ, Woelfel JB, Huffman RW: Simple application of anterior jig or leaf gauge in routine clinical practice, *J Prosthet Dent* 59:611-617, 1988.

66. Rieder C: The prevalence and magnitude of mandibular displacement in a survey population, *J Prosthet Dent* 39:324-329, 1978.

67. Posselt U: Studies in the mobility of the human mandible, *Acta Odontol Scand* 10(suppl):19, 1952.

68. McNamara JA Jr, Seligman DA, Okeson JP: Occlusion, orthodontic treatment, and temporomandibular disorders: a review, *J Orofac Pain* 9:73-90, 1995.

69. Okeson JP: Occlusion and functional disorders of the masticatory system, *Dent Clin North Am* 39:285-300, 1995.

70. McNamara D: Variance of occlusal support in temporomandibular pain-dysfunction patients, *J Dent Res* 61:350, 1982.

71. Fonder AC: *The dental physician*, Blacksburg, Va, 1977, University Publications.

72. Mahn P: *Pathologic manifestations in occlusal disharmony II*, New York, 1981, Science & Medicine.

73. Ramfjord S: Bruxism: a clinical and electromyographic study, *J Am Dent Assoc* 62:21-28, 1961.

74. Williamson EH, Lundquist DO: Anterior guidance: its effect on electromyographic activity of the temporal and masseter muscles, *J Prosthet Dent* 49:816-823, 1983.

75. Minagi S, Watanabe H, Sato T, Tsuru H: Relationship between balancing-side occlusal contact patterns and temporomandibular joint sounds in humans: proposition of the concept of balancing-side protection, *J Craniomandib Disord* 4:251-256, 1990.

76. Rugh JD, Katz JO: The effect of verbal instruction on identification of balancing contacts, *J Dent Res* 65:189, 1986 (abstract).

77. Okeson JP, Dickson JL, Kemper JT: The influence of assisted mandibular movement on the incidence of nonworking tooth contact, *J Prosthet Dent* 48:174-177, 1982.

78. Kahn J, Tallents RH, Katzberg RW, Ross ME, Murphy WC: Prevalence of dental occlusal variables and intraarticular temporomandibular disorders: molar relationship, lateral guidance, and nonworking side contacts, *J Prosthet Dent* 82:410-415, 1999.

79. Bean LR: The transmaxillary projection in temporomandibular joint radiography, *Dentomaxillofac Radiol* 6:90, 1975.

80. Bean LR, Omnell KA, Oberg T: Comparison between radiologic observations and macroscopic tissue changes in temporomandibular joints, *Dentomaxillofac Radiol* 6:90-106, 1977.

81. Watt-Smith S, Sadler A, Baddeley H, Renton P: Comparison of arthrotomographic and magnetic resonance images of 50 temporomandibular joints with operative findings, *Br J Maxillofac Surg* 31:139-143, 1993.

82. Ludlow JB, Nolan PJ, McNamara JA: Accuracy of measures of temporomandibular joint space and condylar position with three tomographic imaging techniques, *Oral Surg Oral Med Oral Pathol* 72:364-370, 1991.

83. Knoernschild KL, Aquilino SA, Ruprecht A: Transcranial radiography and linear tomography: a comparative study, *J Prosthet Dent* 66:239-250, 1991.

84. Dolwick MF, Sanders B: *TMJ internal derangement and arthrosis*, St Louis, 1985, Mosby.

85. Lydiatt D, Kaplan P, Tu H, Sleder P: Morbidity associated with temporomandibular joint arthrography in clinically normal joints, *J Oral Maxillofac Surg* 44:8-10, 1986.

86. Rohrer FA, Palla S, Engelke W: Condylar movements in clicking joints before and after arthrography, *J Oral Rehabil* 18:111-123, 1991.

87. Delfino JJ, Eppley BL: Radiographic and surgical evaluation of internal derangements of the temporomandibular joint, *J Oral Maxillofac Surg* 44:260-267, 1986.

88. Manzione JV, Katzberg RW, Manzione TJ: Internal derangements of the temporomandibular joint. II. Diagnosis by arthrography and computed tomography, *Int J Periodont Restor Dent* 4:16-27, 1984.

89. Marmulla R, Wortche R, Muhling J, Hassfeld S: Geometric accuracy of the NewTom 9000 Cone Beam CT, *Dentomaxillofac Radiol* 34:28-31, 2005.

90. Christiansen EL, Thompson JR, Zimmerman G, Roberts D, Hasso AN et al: Computed tomography of condylar and articular disk positions within the temporomandibular joint, *Oral Surg Oral Med Oral Pathol* 64:757-767, 1987.

91. Hoffman DC, Berliner L, Manzione J, Saccaro R, McGivern BE Jr: Use of direct sagittal computed tomography in diagnosis and treatment of internal derangements of the temporomandibular joint, *J Am Dent Assoc* 113:407-411, 1986.

92. Manco LG, Messing SG: Splint therapy evaluation with direct sagittal computed tomography, *Oral Surg Oral Med Oral Pathol* 61:5-11, 1986.

93. Van Ingen JM, de Man K, Bakri I: CT diagnosis of synovial chondromatosis of the temporomandibular joint, *Br J Maxillofac Surg* 28:164-167, 1990.

94. Paz ME, Carter LC, Westesson PL, Katzberg RW, Tallents R et al: CT density of the TMJ disk: correlation with histologic observations of hyalinization, metaplastic cartilage, and calcification in autopsy specimens, *Am J Orthod Dentofacial Orthop* 98:354-357, 1990.

95. Honda K, Larheim TA, Maruhashi K, Matsumoto K, Iwai K: Osseous abnormalities of the mandibular condyle: diagnostic reliability of cone beam computed tomography compared with helical computed tomography based on an autopsy material, *Dentomaxillofac Radiol* 35:152-157, 2006.

96. Scarfe WC, Farman AG, Sukovic P: Clinical applications of cone-beam computed tomography in dental practice, *J Can Dent Assoc* 72:75-80, 2006.

97. Honda K, Matumoto K, Kashima M, Takano Y, Kawashima S et al: Single air contrast arthrography for temporomandibular joint disorder using limited cone beam computed tomography for dental use, *Dentomaxillofac Radiol* 33:271-273, 2004.

98. Katzberg RW, Schenck J, Roberts D, Tallents RH, Manzione JV et al: Magnetic resonance imaging of the temporomandibular joint meniscus, *Oral Surg Oral Med Oral Pathol* 59:332-335, 1985.

99. Wilk RM, Harms SE, Wolford LM: Magnetic resonance imaging of the temporomandibular joint using a surface coil, *J Oral Maxillofac Surg* 44:935-943, 1986.

100. Manzione JV, Katzberg RW, Tallents RH, Bessette RW, Sanchez-Woodworth RE et al: Magnetic resonance imaging of the temporomandibular joint, *J Am Dent Assoc* 113:398-402, 1986.

101. Donlon WC, Moon KL: Comparison of magnetic resonance imaging, arthrotomography and clinical and surgical findings in temporomandibular joint internal derangements, *Oral Surg Oral Med Oral Pathol* 64:2-5, 1987.

102. Bell KA, Jones JP: Cine magnetic resonance imaging of the temporomandibular joint, *J Craniomandib Pract* 10:313-317, 1992.

103. Quemar JC, Akoka S, Romdane H, de Certaines JD: Evaluation of a fast pseudo-cinematic method for magnetic resonance imaging of the temporomandibular joint, *Dentomaxillofac Radiol* 22:61-68, 1993.

104. Yustin DC, Rieger MR, McGuckin RS, Connelly ME: Determination of the existence of hinge movements of the temporomandibular joint during normal opening by Cine-MRI and computer digital addition, *J Prosthodont* 2:190-195, 1993.

105. Moore JB, Choe KA, Burke RH, DiStefano GR: Coronal and sagittal TMJ meniscus position in asymptomatic subjects by MRI, *J Oral Maxillofac Surg* 47(suppl 1):75-76, 1989.

106. Hatala M, Westesson PL, Tallents RH, Katzberg RW: TMJ disc displacement in asymptomatic volunteers detected by MR imaging (abstract), *J Dent Res* 70:278, 1991 (abstract).

107. Tallents RH, Hatala MP, Hutta J et al: Temporomandibular joint sounds in normal volunteers, *J Dent Res* 70:371, 1991.

108. Kircos LT, Ortendahl DA, Mark AS, Arakawa M: Magnetic resonance imaging of the TMJ disc in asymptomatic volunteers, *J Oral Maxillofac Surg* 45:852-854, 1987.

109. Katzberg RW, Westesson PL, Tallents RH, Drake CM: Anatomic disorders of the temporomandibular joint disc in asymptomatic subjects, *J Oral Maxillofac Surg* 54:147-153, 1996.

110. Katzberg RW, Westesson PL, Tallents RH, Drake CM: Orthodontics and temporomandibular joint internal derangement, *Am J Orthod Dentofacial Orthop* 109:515-520, 1996.

111. Tasaki MM, Westesson PL, Isberg AM, Ren YF, Tallents RH: Classification and prevalence of temporomandibular joint disk displacement in patients and symptom-free volunteers, *Am J Orthod Dentofacial Orthop* 109:249-262, 1996.

112. Ribeiro RF, Tallents RH, Katzberg RW, Murphy WC, Moss ME et al: The prevalence of disc displacement in symptomatic and asymptomatic volunteers aged 6 to 25 years, *J Orofac Pain* 11:37-47, 1997.

113. Goldstein HA, Bloom CY: Detection of degenerative disease of the temporomandibular joint by bone scintigraphy: concise communication, *J Nucl Med* 21:928-930, 1980.

114. Kircos LT, Ortendahl DA, Hattner RS, Faulkner D, Chafetz NI et al: Emission imaging of patients with craniomandibular dysfunction, *Oral Surg Oral Med Oral Pathol* 65:249-254, 1988.

115. Collier BD Jr, Hellman RS, Krasnow AZ: Bone SPECT, *Semin Nucl Med* 17:247-266, 1987.

116. Engelke W, Tsuchimochi M, Ruttimann UE, Hosain F: Assessment of bone remodeling in the temporomandibular joint by serial uptake measurement of technetium 99m-labeled methylene diphosphonate with a cadmium telluride probe, *Oral Surg Oral Med Oral Pathol* 71:357-363, 1991.

117. Harris SA, Rood JP, Testa HJ: Post-traumatic changes of the temporomandibular joint by bone scintigraphy, *Int J Oral Maxillofac Surg* 17:173-176, 1988.

118. Katzberg RW, O'Mara RE, Tallents RH, Weber DA: Radionuclide skeletal imaging and single photon emission computed tomography in suspected internal derangements of the temporomandibular joint, *J Oral Maxillofac Surg* 42:782-787, 1984.

119. Krasnow AZ, Collier BD, Kneeland JB, Carrera GF, Ryan DE et al: Comparison of high-resolution MRI and SPECT bone scintigraphy for noninvasive imaging of the temporomandibular joint, *J Nucl Med* 28:1268-1274, 1987.

120. Oberg T, Carlsson GE: Macroscopic and microscopic anatomy of the temporomandibular joint. In Zarb GA, Carlsson GE, editors: *Temporomandibular joint; function and dysfunction*, St Louis, 1979, Mosby, pp 101-118.

121. Stegenga B, de Bont LG, Boering G, van Willigen JD: Tissue responses to degenerative changes in the temporomandibular joint: a review, *J Oral Maxillofac Surg* 49:1079-1088, 1991.

122. Worth HM: Radiology of the temporomandibular joint. In Zarb GA, Carlsson GE, editors: *Temporomandibular joint function and dysfunction*, St Louis, 1979, Mosby, pp 321-372.

123. Hatcher DC: Craniofacial imaging, *J Calif Dent Assoc* 19:27-34, 1991.

124. Oberg T, Carlsson GE, Fajers CM: The temporomandibular joint. A morphologic study on a human autopsy material, *Acta Odontol Scand* 29:349-384, 1971.

125. Hansson T, Oberg T: Clinical survey on occlusal physiology in 67-year-old persons in Dalby (Sweden), *Tandlakartidningen* 63:650-655, 1971.

126. Toller PA: Osteoarthrosis of the mandibular condyle, *Br Dent J* 134:223-231, 1973.

127. Durkin JF: Cartilage of the mandibular condyle. In Zarb GA, Carlsson GE, editors: *Temporomandibular joint; function and dysfunction*, St Louis, 1979, Mosby.

128. Boering G: *Temporomandibular joint arthrosis: a clinical and radiographic investigation*, Groningen, The Netherlands, 1966, University of Groningen, p 500.

129. De Leeuw R, Boering G, Stegenga B, de Bont LG: TMJ articular disc position and configuration 30 years after initial diagnosis of internal derangement, *J Oral Maxillofac Surg* 53:234-241; discussion 241-242, 1995.

130. De Leeuw R, Boering G, Stegenga B, de Bont LG: Temporomandibular joint osteoarthrosis: clinical and radiographic characteristics 30 years after nonsurgical treatment: a preliminary report, *Cranio* 11:15-24, 1993.

131. De Leeuw R, Boering G, Stegenga B, de Bont LG: Clinical signs of TMJ osteoarthrosis and internal derangement 30 years after nonsurgical treatment, *J Orofac Pain* 8: 18-24, 1994.

132. Hall MB, Gibbs CC, Sclar AG: Association between the prominence of the articular eminence and displaced TMJ disks, *Cranio* 3:237-239, 1985.

133. Kerstens HC, Tuinzing DB, Golding RP, Van der Kwast WA: Inclination of the temporomandibular joint eminence and anterior disc displacement, *Int J Oral Maxillofac Surg* 18:228-232, 1989.

134. Ren YF, Isberg A, Westesson PL: Steepness of the articular eminence in the temporomandibular joint. Tomographic comparison between asymptomatic volunteers with normal disk position and patients with disk displacement, *Oral Surg Oral Med Oral Pathol Oral Radiol Endod* 80:258-266, 1995.

135. Galante G, Paesani D, Tallents RH, Hatala MA, Katzberg RW et al: Angle of the articular eminence in patients with temporomandibular joint dysfunction and asymptomatic volunteers, *Oral Surg Oral Med Oral Pathol* 80:242-249, 1995.

136. Alsawaf M, Garlapo DA, Gale EN, Carter MJ: The relationship between condylar guidance and temporomandibular joint clicking, *J Prosthet Dent* 61:349-354, 1989.

137. Eagle WW: Elongated styloid process: symptoms and treatment, *Arch Otolaryngol* 67:172-176, 1958.

138. Keur JJ, Campbell JP, McCarthy JF, Ralph WJ: The clinical significance of the elongated styloid process, *Oral Surg Oral Med Oral Pathol* 61:399-404, 1986.

139. Zaki HS, Greco CM, Rudy TE, Kubinski JA: Elongated styloid process in a temporomandibular disorder sample: prevalence and treatment outcome, *J Prosthet Dent* 75:399-405, 1996.

140. Weinberg LA: Role of condylar position in TMJ dysfunction-pain syndrome, *J Prosthet Dent* 41:636-643, 1979.

141. Weinberg LA: The etiology, diagnosis, and treatment of TMJ dysfunction-pain syndrome. Part III: treatment, *J Prosthet Dent* 43:186-196, 1980.

142. Hatcher DC, Blom RJ, Baker CG: Temporomandibular joint spatial relationships: osseous and soft tissues, *J Prosthet Dent* 56:344-353, 1986.

143. Baldioceda F, Pullinger AG, Bibb CA: Relationship of condylar bone profiles and dental factors to articular soft-tissue thickness, *J Craniomandib Disord* 4:71-79, 1990.

144. Pullinger AG, Bibb CA, Ding X, Baldioceda F: Contour mapping of the TMJ temporal component and the relationship to articular soft tissue thickness and disk displacement, *Oral Surg Oral Med Oral Pathol* 76:636-646, 1993.

145. Ren YF, Isberg A, Westesson PL: Condyle position in the temporomandibular joint. Comparison between asymptomatic volunteers with normal disk position and patients with disk displacement, *Oral Surg Oral Med Oral Pathol Oral Radiol Endod* 80:101-107, 1995.

146. Lindblom G: Anatomy and function of the temporomandibular joint, *Acta Odontol Scand* 17(suppl 28): 1-287, 1960.

147. Berry DC: The relationship between some anatomical features of the human mandibular condyle and its appearance on radiographs, *Arch Oral Biol* 2:203-208, 1960.

148. Blaschke DD, White SC: Radiology. In Sarnat GB, Laskin DM, editors: *The temporomandibular joint*, Springfield, Ill, 1979, Charles C Thomas, pp 240-276.

149. Bean LR, Thomas CA: Significance of condylar positions in patients with temporomandibular disorders, *J Am Dent Assoc* 114:76-77, 1987.

150. Pullinger A, Hollender L: Assessment of mandibular condyle position: a comparison of transcranial radiographs and linear tomograms, *Oral Surg Oral Med Oral Pathol* 60:329-334, 1985.

151. Jumean F, Hatjigiorgis CG, Neff PA: Comparative study of two radiographic techniques to actual dissections of the temporomandibular joint, *Cranio* 6:141-147, 1988.

152. Aquilino SA, Matteson SR, Holland GA, Phillips C: Evaluation of condylar position from temporomandibular joint radiographs, *J Prosthet Dent* 53:88-97, 1985.

153. Alexander SR, Moore RN, DuBois LM: Mandibular condyle position: comparison of articulator mountings and magnetic resonance imaging [see comments], *Am J Orthod Dentofacial Orthop* 104:230-239, 1993.

154. Petersson A: *Radiography of the temporomandibular joint. A comparison of information obtained from different radiographic techniques*, Malmo, Sweden, 1976, University of Malmo, p 500.

155. Smith SR, Matteson SR, Phillips C, Tyndall DA: Quantitative and subjective analysis of temporomandibular joint radiographs, *J Prosthet Dent* 62:456-463, 1989.

156. Pullinger AG, Solberg WK, Hollender L, Guichet D: Tomographic analysis of mandibular condyle position in diagnostic subgroups of temporomandibular disorders, *J Prosthet Dent* 55:723-729, 1986.

157. Okeson J: Assessment of orofacial pain disorders. In Okeson J, editor: *Orofacial pain: guidelines for assessment, diagnosis, and management*, Chicago, 1996, Quintessence, pp 32-34.

158. Obwegeser HL, Farmand M, Al-Majali F, Engelke W: Findings of mandibular movement and the position of the mandibular condyles during maximal mouth opening, *Oral Surg Oral Med Oral Pathol* 63:517-525, 1987.

159. Muto T, Kohara M, Kanazawa M, Kawakami J: The position of the mandibular condyle at maximal mouth opening in normal subjects, *J Oral Maxillofac Surg* 52:1269-1272, 1994.

160. Bell WE: *Temporomandibular disorders: classification, diagnosis, management*, ed 3, Chicago, 1990, Year Book Medical.

161. Farrar WB: Characteristics of the condylar path in internal derangements of the TMJ, *J Prosthet Dent* 39:319-323, 1978.

162. Bezuur JN, Habets LL, Jimenez Lopez V, Naeije M, Hansson TL: The recognition of craniomandibular disorders—a comparison between clinical and radiographic findings in eighty-nine subjects, *J Oral Rehabil* 15:215-221, 1988.

163. Muir CB, Goss AN: The radiologic morphology of asymptomatic temporomandibular joints, *Oral Surg Oral Med Oral Pathol* 70:349-354, 1990.

164. Muir CB, Goss AN: The radiologic morphology of painful temporomandibular joints, *Oral Surg Oral Med Oral Pathol* 70:355-359, 1990.

165. Schiffman EL, Anderson GC, Fricton JR, Lindgren BR: The relationship between level of mandibular pain and dysfunction and stage of temporomandibular joint internal derangement, *J Dent Res* 71:1812-1815, 1992.

166. Eliasson S, Isacsson G: Radiographic signs of temporomandibular disorders to predict outcome of treatment, *J Craniomandib Disord* 6:281-287, 1992.

167. Dyer EH: Importance of a stable maxillomandibular relation, *J Prosthet Dent* 30:241-251, 1973.

168. Glaros AG, McGlynn FD, Kapel L: Sensitivity, specificity, and the predictive value of facial electromyographic data in diagnosing myofascial pain-dysfunction, *Cranio* 7:189-193, 1989.

169. Gervais RO, Fitzsimmons GW, Thomas NR: Masseter and temporalis electromyographic activity in asymptomatic, subclinical, and temporomandibular joint dysfunction patients, *Cranio* 7:52-57, 1989.

170. Carlson CR, Okeson JP, Falace DA, Nitz AJ, Curran SL: Comparison of psychological and physiological functioning between patients with masticatory muscle pain and matched controls, *J Orofac Pain* 7:15-22, 1993.

171. Yemm R: A neurophysiological approach to the pathology and aetiology of temporomandibular dysfunction, *J Oral Rehabil* 12:343-353, 1985.

172. Majewski RF, Gale EN: Electromyographic activity of anterior temporal area pain patients and non-pain subjects, *J Dent Res* 63:1228-1231, 1984.

173. Lund JP, Donga R, Widmer CG, Stohler CS: The pain-adaptation model: a discussion of the relationship between chronic musculoskeletal pain and motor activity, *Can J Physiol Pharmacol* 69:683-694, 1991.

174. Lous I, Sheikoleslam A, Moller E: Muscle hyperactivity in subjects with functional disorders of the chewing apparatus, *Scand J Dent Res* 78:404-410, 1970.

175. Dahlstrom L, Carlsson SG, Gale EN, Jansson TG: Stress-induced muscular activity in mandibular dysfunction: effects of biofeedback training, *J Behav Med* 8:191-200, 1985.

176. Oltjen JM, Goldreich HN, Rugh JD: Masseter surface EMG levels in overweight and normal subjects, *J Dent Res* 69:149, 1990 (abstract).

177. Rugh JD, Santos JA, Harlan JA, Hatch JP: Distribution of surface EMG activity over the masseter muscle, *J Dent Res* 67:513, 1988.

178. Oltjen JM, Palla S, Rugh JD: Evaluation of an invisible UV ink for EMG surface electrode placement repeatability, *J Dent Res* 70:513, 1991.

179. Lund JP, Widmer CG: An evaluation of the use of surface electromyography in the diagnosis, documentation, and treatment of dental patients, *J Craniomandib Disord Facial Oral Pain* 3:125-137, 1988.

180. Mohl ND, Lund JP, Widmer CG, McCall WD Jr: Devices for the diagnosis and treatment of temporomandibular disorders. Part II: electromyography and sonography [published erratum appears in *J Prosthet Dent* 63:13A, 1990], *J Prosthet Dent* 63:332-336, 1990.

181. Rugh JD, Davis SE: Accuracy of diagnosing MPD using electromyography, *J Dent Res* 69:273, 1990.

182. Lund JP, Widmer CG, Feine JS: Validity of diagnostic and monitoring tests used for temporomandibular disorders [see comments], *J Dent Res* 74:1133-43, 1995.

183. Mohl ND: Reliability and validity of diagnostic modalities for temporomandibular disorders, *Adv Dent Res* 7: 113-119, 1993.

184. Widmer CG, Lund JP, Feine JS: Evaluation of diagnostic tests for TMD, *J Calif Dent Assoc* 18:53-60, 1990.

185. Mohl ND, Ohrbach RK, Crow HC, Gross AJ: Devices for the diagnosis and treatment of temporomandibular disorders. Part III: thermography, ultrasound, electrical stimulation, and electromyographic biofeedback [published erratum appears in *J Prosthet Dent* 63:13A, 1990], *J Prosthet Dent* 63:472-477, 1990.

186. Mohl ND, McCall WS, Lund JP, Plesh O: Devises for the diagnosis and treatment of temporomandibular disorders: part I. Introduction, scientific evidence, and jaw tracking, *J Prosthet Dent* 63:198-201, 1990.

187. Feine JS, Hutchins MO, Lund JP: An evaluation of the criteria used to diagnose mandibular dysfunction with the mandibular kinesiograph, *J Prosthet Dent* 60:374-380, 1988.

188. Theusner J, Plesh O, Curtis DA, Hutton JE: Axiographic tracings of temporomandibular joint movements, *J Prosthet Dent* 69:209-215, 1993.

189. Tsolka D, Preiskel HW: Kinesiographic and electromyographic assessment of the effects of occlusal adjustment therapy on craniomandibular disorders by a double-blind method, *J Prosthet Dent* 69:85-92, 1993.

190. Toolson GA, Sadowsky C: An evaluation of the relationship between temporomandibular joint sounds and mandibular movements, *J Craniomandib Disord* 5:187-196, 1991.

191. Widmer CG: Temporomandibular joint sounds: a critique of techniques for recording and analysis, *J Craniomandib Disord* 3:213-217, 1989.

192. Christensen LV, Donegan SJ, McKay DC: Temporomandibular joint vibration analysis in a sample of non-patients, *Cranio* 10:35-41, 1992.

193. Paiva G, Paiva PF, de Oliveira ON: Vibrations in the temporomandibular joints in patients examined and treated in a private clinic, *Cranio* 11:202-205, 1993.

194. Ishigaki S, Bessette RW, Maruyama T: Diagnostic accuracy of TMJ vibration analysis for internal derangement and/or degenerative joint disease, *Cranio* 12:241-245, 1994.

195. Wabeke KB, Spruijt RJ, van der Zaag J: The reliability of clinical methods for recording temporomandibular joint sounds, *J Dent Res* 73:1157-1162, 1994.

196. Ishigaki S, Bessette RW, Maruyama T: Vibration analysis of the temporomandibular joints with meniscal displacement with and without reduction, *J Craniomandib Pract* 11:192-201, 1993.

197. Tallents RH, Hatala M, Katzberg RW, Westesson PL: Temporomandibular joint sounds in asymptomatic volunteers, *J Prosthet Dent* 69:298-304, 1993.

198. Feldman F, Nickoloff EL: Normal thermographic standards for the cervical spine and upper extremities, *Skeletal Radiol* 12:235-249, 1984.

199. Gratt BM, Sickles EA, Ross JB: Electronic thermography in the assessment of internal derangement of the temporomandibular joint. A pilot study, *Oral Surg Oral Med Oral Pathol* 71:364-370, 1991.

200. Steed PA: The utilization of contact liquid crystal thermography in the evaluation of temporomandibular dysfunction [published erratum appears in *Cranio* 9: preceding 183, 1991], *Cranio* 9:120-128, 1991.

201. Berry DC, Yemm R: Variations in skin temperature of the face in normal subjects and in patients with mandibular dysfunction, *Br J Oral Surg* 8:242-247, 1971.

202. Berry DC, Yemm R: A further study of facial skin temperature in patients with mandibular dysfunction, *J Oral Rehabil* 1:255-264, 1974.

203. Finney JW, Holt CR, Pearce KB: Thermographic diagnosis of temporomandibular joint disease and associated neuromuscular disorders, *Postgrad Med J* Special Report: 93-95, 1986.

204. Johansson A, Kopp S, Haraldson T: Reproducibility and variation of skin surface temperature over the temporomandibular joint and masseter muscle in normal individuals, *Acta Odontol Scand* 43:309-313, 1985.

205. Gratt BM, Sickles EA: Thermographic characterization of the asymptomatic temporomandibular joint, *J Orofac Pain* 7:7-14, 1993.

206. Swerdlow B, Dieter JN: An evaluation of the sensitivity and specificity of medical thermography for the documentation of myofascial trigger points [see comments], *Pain* 48:205-213, 1992.

Diagnosis of Temporomandibular Disorders

10
CHAPTER

"The most important thing you can do for your patient is to make the correct diagnosis. It is the foundation for success."

—JPO

To manage masticatory disorders effectively, one must understand the numerous types of problems that can exist and the variety of etiologies that cause them. Separating these disorders into common groups of symptoms and etiologies is a process called *diagnosis*. The clinician must keep in mind that for each diagnosis there is an appropriate treatment. No single treatment is appropriate for all temporomandibular disorders (TMDs). Therefore making a proper diagnosis becomes an extremely important part of managing the patient disorder. In many instances the success of the therapy depends not on how well the treatment is performed but instead on how appropriate the therapy is for the disorder. In other words, proper diagnosis is the key to successful treatment.

A diagnosis is achieved by careful evaluation of information derived through the history and examination procedures. This information should lead to the identification of a specific disorder. If a person has a single disorder, diagnosis becomes a relatively routine procedure. The clinician should remember, however, that there are no rules limiting an individual to just one disorder at a time. In fact, many persons who have suffered for more than several months are likely to present with more than one disorder. It is the clinician's responsibility to identify each disorder and then (when

possible) prioritize them in order of their significance. This can be a complex task, considering, for example, the possible relationships between just two general problems: a disc derangement disorder and a masticatory muscle disorder. If the person reports with only joint pain or only muscle pain, diagnosis becomes routine. However, many persons will have both joint and muscle pain and it then becomes important to identify the relationships of these because treatment is quite different.

Suppose a person falls and sustains a blow to the chin and jaw. A disc derangement disorder can develop. After several days of joint pain, the muscles become secondarily involved as a mechanism of restricting jaw movement (protective co-contraction). When the person reports to the office, both joint pain (i.e., pain in the intracapsular tissues) and muscle pain are present. The information received during the history and examination should assist in determining that the patient has a primary problem with the joint and a secondary problem with the muscles. Once proper treatment is extended to the joint, the joint symptoms will resolve and so will the secondary muscle pain. If in this instance the muscle pain is treated but not the joint pain, the treatment will likely fail because the primary disorder has not been managed.

The same problem can occur, in reverse, with a masticatory muscle disorder that increases the clinical symptom of clicking in the joint. The person reports with muscle pain and joint clicking. If the clicking alone is treated, the painful muscle will remain. Treatment should be directed toward the primary, not secondary, diagnosis. The history and examination must assist the clinician in determining this order. The clinician should also realize that the person may be suffering from both a muscle disorder and a joint disorder that are unrelated to each other. Generally, in this instance, the chief complaint should be addressed first.

DIAGNOSING PAIN DISORDERS

In disorders that have pain as a primary symptom, it is imperative that the source of the pain be identified. If it is primary pain, this will not be difficult because the source and the site are in the same location (see Chapter 2). With primary pain the patient is pointing directly to the source of pain. However, if the pain is heterotopic, the patient will be directing attention to the site of pain, which may be quite remote from the actual source of the pain. Remember, treatment is effective only if it is directed at the source, not at the site of pain.

One key in locating the source of pain is that local provocation should accentuate it. Although this rule does not always apply, one should be suspicious that when local provocation does not increase the pain it may be heterotopic. In other words, if a patient is complaining of temporomandibular joint (TMJ) area pain, he or she should also complain that it hurts to open and chew (local provocation). If the patient does not report any functional problem with jaw movement, the TMJ may be merely a site of pain and not pathologically involved. It is the clinician's job in this instance to continue to examine the patient for the source of the pain.

When pain symptoms become complex, it is sometimes necessary to use selective local anesthetic blockade of tissues to help differentiate the site from the source. Anesthetic blocking should be a routine diagnostic procedure for the clinician.

Local anesthetic blockade of the source of pain will at least temporarily eliminate the symptoms because it blocks the nociceptive input originating from the true source of the pain (Fig. 10-1, *A*). Local anesthetic blockade of the site will have no effect because there is no nociceptive input coming from that site (Fig. 10-1, *B*). Heterotopic

pains are the result of the central excitatory effect in the brainstem produced by a distance source of nociception (see Chapter 2). An example is a patient whose chief complaint is a tension-type headache in the temporal region. The clinician may discover that it is produced by central excitatory effects from a trigger point in the trapezius. The patient points to the temple as the chief complaint, but palpation of this area (local provocation) does not accentuate the headache. Local anesthetic blockade of the temporal muscle fails to reduce the pain because this is a site and not the source. As the clinician continues the examination, an active trigger point is found in the trapezius. Local provocation of the trigger point not only increases the pain felt in the trapezius but also increases the temporal headache (site of referred pain) (Fig. 10-1, *C*). Local anesthetic blockade of the trapezius trigger point eliminates not only the trigger point pain but also the temporal headache (the referred pain is wholly dependent on the source of pain) (Fig. 10-1, *D*). The clinician has now identified the source of the headache and thus made a diagnosis. Diagnostic blocking of a muscle trigger point may be extremely helpful when myofascial trigger point pain is suspected.

Compared with referred pain, secondary hyperalgesia responds differently to local anesthetic blockade. When the original source of pain is blocked, referred pain resolves immediately but secondary hyperalgesia may remain for hours. Therefore the effect of a local anesthetic injection on secondary hyperalgesia should not be evaluated until the following day.

The following four rules (depicted in Fig. 10-1, *A* to *D*) summarize the examination techniques used to differentiate primary pain from referred pain:

1. Local provocation of the site of pain does not increase the pain.
2. Local provocation at the source of pain increases the pain not only at the source but also increases the pain at the site.
3. Local anesthetic blocking of the site of pain does not decrease the pain.
4. Local anesthetic blocking of the source of the pain decreases the pain at the source, as well as the site.

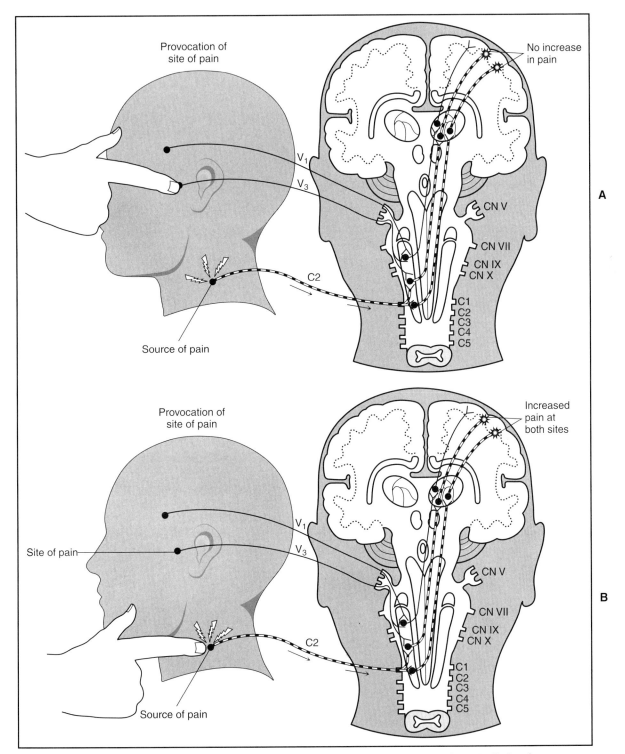

Fig. 10-1 A, Local provocation of the site of pain does not increase the pain. **B,** Local provocation of the source of pain increases the pain not only at the source but may also increase it at the site.

Continued

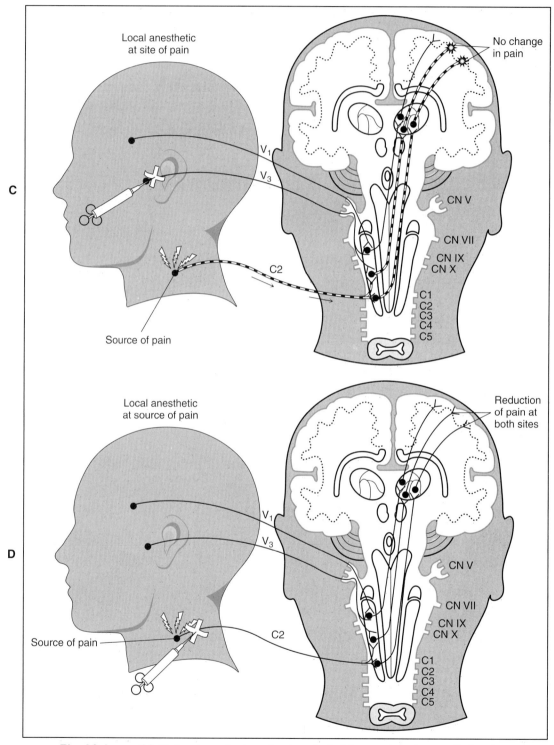

Fig. 10-1, cont'd C, Local anesthesia at the site of pain fails to reduce the pain. **D,** Local anesthesia at the source of pain reduces the pain at the source and site. *(Redrawn from Okeson JP:* Bell's orofacial pains, *ed 6, Chicago, 2005, Quintessence, pp 154-155.)*

DIAGNOSTIC ANALGESIC BLOCKING

INDICATIONS FOR ANALGESIC BLOCKING

The value of local anesthetic injections and application of topical anesthetics to identify and localize pain cannot be overemphasized. It is essential when differentiating primary from secondary pains. It is equally useful to identify the pathways that mediate peripheral pain and to localize pain sources. Often when the source of pain is difficult to identify, local anesthetic blocking of related tissues is the key to making the proper diagnosis. The examiner should therefore become skilled in the use of this valuable diagnostic tool. Muscle injections can also be useful for diagnostic purposes, as well as for therapy. Local anesthetic blocking not only provides valuable diagnostic information but in some pain disorders can also provide therapeutic value. This is especially true for myofascial pain and myospasm.

Another indication for analgesic blocking is to help educate the patient to the source of his or her pain problem. Often patients do not appreciate the concept of pain referral, and it can be quite convincing to the patient when blocking a remote site reduces or even eliminates the chief complaint. This can be a valuable educational tool.

ARMAMENTARIUM

The armamentarium needed to provided anesthetic blocks is already present in most dental offices. It begins with an aspirating syringe and both short and long 27-gauge needles. The length needed depends on the structure that is targeted. Alcohol and/or Betadine swipes are also required to clean the site to be injected. Sterile 2 × 2 gauzes should also be available to apply to the injection site to control bleeding. Clean disposable gloves are also necessary.

The type of local anesthetic used may vary according to the type and purpose of the particular injection. When only diagnostic information is necessary, the use of short-acting drugs is most desirable. Usually a solution without a vasoconstricting agent is best. Good anesthesia for skeletal muscle requires a nonvasoconstricting solution because of the vasodilating effect of epinephrine-like substances on such tissue. This reverse effect on muscle tissue is sometimes forgotten and may account for the transient anesthesia of poor quality sometimes obtained when muscles are injected for diagnostic purposes.

Local anesthetics have been demonstrated to have a measure of myotoxicity. Procaine appears to be the least myotoxic of the local anesthetics in common use.[1] Mild inflammatory reactions follow the injection of 1% and 2% procaine hydrochloride, as well as isotonic sodium chloride.[2] Single injections of either procaine or isotonic saline cause no muscle necrosis.[3] The longer-acting and stronger anesthetics induce more severe inflammation and occasional coagulation necrosis of muscle tissue.[4] Regeneration takes place in approximately 7 days. Solutions containing epinephrine cause greater muscle damage.[5] To minimize the danger of muscle damage in analgesic blocking for both diagnostic and therapeutic purposes, low concentrations of procaine are advisable and such injections should be spaced at least 7 days apart. Because procaine is not available in dental carpules, the dentist may select 2% lidocaine (Xylocaine) or 3% mepivacaine (Carbocaine)[6] without a vasoconstrictor. When a longer-acting anesthetic is indicated, 0.5% bupivacaine (Marcaine) may be used.[7] Although bupivacaine is sometimes indicated for joint pain (auriculotemporal nerve block), it should not be routinely used with muscle injections because of its myotoxicity.[8]

The diagnostic use of local anesthetics in muscles should be curtailed to actual need. It should be noted that, despite some myotoxicity, the diagnostic and therapeutic use of local anesthesia in the management of myogenous pain disorders is clinically justified. Many diagnostic procedures and therapeutic modalities are attended by some risk. Radiation in radiography has destructive effects. All anesthetics and most medications are toxic to some degree. The inherent risks therefore must be weighed against the benefits derived. Reasonable judgment should be exercised in the application of all procedures that entail a measure of risk to the patient

GENERAL RULES TO FOLLOW

When any injection is to be performed, the clinician should observe the following fundamental rules:

1. The clinician should have a sound knowledge of the anatomy of all structures in the region that is to be injected. The purpose of an injection is to isolate the particular structure that is to be blocked. Therefore the clinician must know the precise location and appropriate technique used to get the needle tip to the desired structure. Equally important is that the clinician should have a sound understanding of all the important structures in the area that should be avoided during the injection.
2. The clinician should have a sound knowledge of the pharmacology of all solutions that will be used.
3. The clinician should avoid injecting into inflamed or diseased tissues.
4. The clinician should maintain strict asepsis at all times.
5. The clinician should always aspirate before injecting solution so as to be sure the needle is not in a blood vessel.

TYPES OF INJECTIONS

Diagnostic and therapeutic anesthetic blocks are divided into three types according to the structures that are targeted: muscle injections, nerve block injections, and intracapsular injections. Each of these is discussed separately because the indications and techniques vary.

Muscle Injections

Injecting a muscle can be valuable in determining the source of a pain disorder. In some instances muscle injections can provide therapeutic value. For example, the injection of local anesthetic into a myofascial trigger point can result in significant pain reduction long after the anesthetic has been metabolized.[9-11] In myofascial pain the patient presents with a firm, taut band of muscle tissue that is quite painful to palpate. This is known as a *trigger point* and is often responsible for producing a pattern of pain referral[9] (see Chapter 8). When this is suspected, the trigger point can be injected with

local anesthetic and the resulting pattern of pain referral is shut down. The precise mechanisms of trigger point pain and the indications for treatment are reviewed in Chapter 12. When it has been determined that injection of the trigger point is indicated, the following sequence should be followed:

- The trigger point is located by placing the finger over the muscle, and firm pressure is applied to locate the tight band. The finger is moved across the band so that it can be felt to "snap" under the pressure of the finger. Once the band is identified, the finger is moved up and down the band until the most painful area is located (Fig. 10-2, *A*).
- Once the trigger point is located, the tissue over the trigger point is cleaned with alcohol. The trigger point is then trapped between two fingers so that when the needle is placed into the area, the tight ban will not move away (Fig. 10-2, *B*).
- The needle tip is then inserted into the tissue superficial to the trigger point and is penetrated to the depth of the tight band (Fig. 10-2, *C*). Receiving feedback from the patient regarding the accuracy of needle placement is often helpful. Usually the patient can tell immediately when the clinician has entered the trigger point. Once the needle tip is at the proper depth, the syringe is aspirated to ensure it is not in located in a vessel. Then a small amount of anesthetic is deposited in the area (¼ of a carpule).
- Once the initial anesthetic is deposited, it is useful to "fan" the needle tip slightly. This is done by withdrawing the needle halfway, changing the needle direction slightly, and reentering into the firm band to the same depth (Fig. 10-2, *D*). The needle tip should not be completely removed from the tissue. This manipulation of the needle tip should be repeated several times, especially if the patient has not confirmed that the needle tip has been in the area of exquisite tenderness. At each site a syringe is aspirated and a small amount of anesthetic can be deposited. In some instances the muscle will be felt to quickly contract. This is known as the "twitch response" and usually helps confirm that the needle is properly placed. Although the presence of a twitch response is favorable, not all

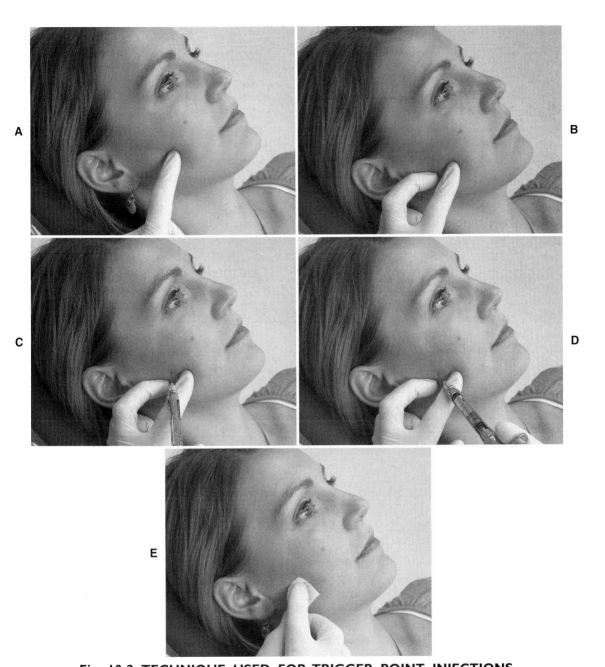

Fig. 10-2 TECHNIQUE USED FOR TRIGGER POINT INJECTIONS.
A, The trigger point is located by placing the finger over the muscle and applying firm pressure to locate the tight band. **B,** The trigger point is then trapped between two fingers so that when the needle is placed into the area, the tight ban will not slip away. **C,** The needle tip is then inserted into the tissue superficial to the trigger point, and it is penetrated to the depth of the tight band. **D,** Once the initial anesthetic is deposited, it is useful to "fan" the needle tip slightly. This is done by withdrawing the needle slightly, changing the needle direction 10 to 15 degrees, and reentering the firm band to the same depth. **E,** Once the injection is completed, the needle is withdrawn and a sterile gauze is held over the injection site with slight pressure for 10 to 20 seconds to ensure good hemostasis. *(Modified from the original model developed by JP Okeson, DA Falace, CR Carlson, A Nitz, and DT Anderson, Orofacial Pain Center, University of Kentucky in 1991.)*

muscles demonstrate this and successful pain reduction can often be achieved without it.

- Once the injection is completed, the needle is fully withdrawn and a sterile gauze is held over the injection site with slight pressure for 20 to 30 seconds to ensure good hemostasis (Fig. 10-2, *E*).

This general technique is used for most muscle injections; however, the unique anatomy of each muscle may demand slight variations. Extremely important is that the clinician is familiar with the anatomy of the muscle to be injected so as to avoid disturbing any neighboring structures. This text cannot review the anatomy of all the muscles that may need to be injected, and therefore it is recommended that appropriate gross anatomy texts be reviewed before the clinician proceeds with an injection. Some of the muscles that can be easily injected are the masseter (Fig. 10-3), temporalis (Fig. 10-4), sternocleidomastoid (Fig. 10-5), splenius capitis (Fig. 10-6), posterior occipital (Fig. 10-7), and trapezius (Fig. 10-8). The orofacial pain specialist should become familiar with the anatomic features of these muscles and surrounding structures so that safe and predictable injections can be routinely performed.

Nerve Block Injections

Diagnostic nerve blocks can be useful in identifying whether a painful structure is actually a site or source of pain. When diagnosis is the primary purpose for the injection, a short-acting local anesthetic should be used without a vasoconstrictor.

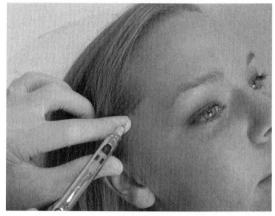

Fig. 10-4 Injection of the temporalis muscle.

In some instances long-term pain relief may be therapeutically indicated. This may be appropriate for certain chronic pain conditions when prolonged relief of pain can be used to interrupt pain cycling and hopefully reduce central sensitization. When long-term anesthesia is indicated, a long-term local anesthetic such as bupivacaine with a vasoconstrictor may be a better choice.

Important nerve blocks that should be considered are dental blocks, the auriculotemporal nerve block, and the infraorbital nerve block.

Dental Blocks. The practicing dentist uses nerve blocks routinely in dental treatments. The clinician should remember that these same injections can provide valuable diagnostic information. The common nerve blocks used are the inferior

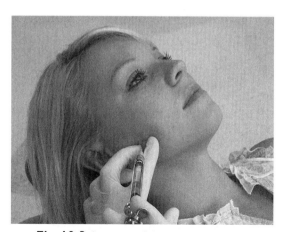

Fig. 10-3 Injection of the masseter muscle.

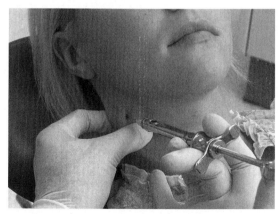

Fig. 10-5 Injection of the sternocleidomastoid muscle from an anterior approach so as to avoid vital deep structures.

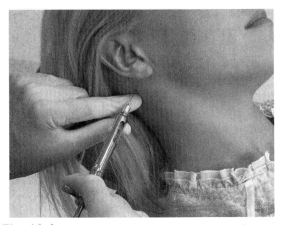

Fig. 10-6 Injection of the splenius capitis muscle at its attachment to the skull slightly distal to the mastoid process.

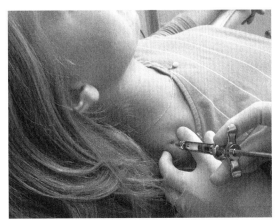

Fig. 10-8 Injection of a common site for a trigger point in the trapezius muscle.

alveolar nerve block, the posterior superior nerve block, the mental nerve block, and infiltration blocks often administered in various areas of the maxillary arch. The techniques used for these blocks will not be reviewed here because they are routinely used in the dental office. Although these blocks are mostly used for anesthesia during dental procedures, their diagnostic value should not be overlooked. For example, an inferior alveolar nerve block will completely eliminate any source of pain coming from the mandibular teeth on the side of the injection. This block is useful in separating

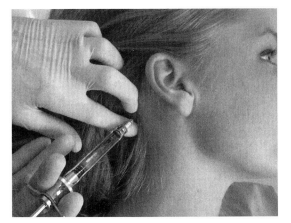

Fig. 10-7 Injection of the posterior occipital muscles at their attachments to the skull.

dental pain from muscle or joint pain because it only blocks the dental structures. This is important diagnostic information, especially when a patient's chief complaint is toothache. If a mandibular toothache is truly of dental origin, an inferior alveolar nerve block will eliminate the pain. If, however, the toothache is actually a referred pain to the tooth, the block will not change the pain.

When attempting to localize a particular tooth as a source of pain, it is important to consider local infiltration of the anesthetic first before a total nerve block (i.e., mandibular block). Isolating a single tooth with local anesthetic is far more specific than blocking an entire quadrant of teeth. Once the entire nerve has been blocked, it may be difficult to identify the specific tooth until the anesthesia has been metabolized. As a general rule for diagnosing tooth pain, begin by using localized areas of anesthesia and moving to broader areas as needed. Starting with a total nerve block can be confusing, especially if one tooth is referring to another and both are blocked at the same time.

Importantly, when identifying pain sources, the clinician must ask the patient the proper question. If the patient has a nonodontogenic toothache and an inferior alveolar nerve block is administered, the pain will not be resolved even though the tissues become anesthetized. If the doctor asks whether the area is numb, the patient will respond positively.

This may lead the clinician to assume the pain has resolved, which is not the case. The clinician needs to carefully phrase the question after giving the patient local anesthesia. The clinician should ask the question in this manner: "Now, I realize that your jaw is numb, but does it still hurt?" The patient will certainly feel numb, but the important question is, "Does it still hurt?" This is a critical concept to appreciate when differentiating the odontogenic toothache from the nonodontogenic toothache.

Auriculotemporal Nerve Block. An important nerve block that all orofacial pain clinicians should become familiar with is the auriculotemporal nerve block. This nerve block has significant diagnostic value. The primary innervation of the TMJ is from the auriculotemporal nerve, with secondary innervation coming from the masseteric and posterior deep temporal nerves.[12] Therefore if the TMJ is a source of pain, this nerve block will quickly eliminate the pain. Because the TMJ area is a frequent site of pain referral, this block is valuable and indicated to help identify when the joint is actually a source of pain. In fact, any time there is irreversible treatment planned for the TMJ, such as surgery, this block can help confirm the need for such treatment. If an auriculotemporal nerve block does not resolve the pain, aggressive therapies should not be considered until the true source of the pain is identified.

Some clinicians anesthetize the TMJ by injecting directly into the joint or into the retrodiscal structures. Although this may be effective, it also can traumatize delicate joint structures. A less traumatic method is to anesthetize the joint structures by blocking the auriculotemporal nerve before its fibers reach the joint. The auriculotemporal nerve can be blocked by first cleaning the tissue (Fig. 10-9, *A*) and then passing a 27-gauge needle through the skin just anterior to and slightly above the junction of the tragus and the earlobe (Fig. 10-9, *C*). The needle is then advanced until it touches the posterior neck of the condyle. The needle is then repositioned in a more posterior direction until the tip of the needle is able to pass behind the posterior neck of the condyle (Fig. 10-9, *D*). Once the neck of the condyle is felt, the tip of the needle is carefully moved slightly behind the

posterior aspect of the condyle in an anteromedial direction to a depth of 1 cm (Fig. 10-9, *E*). The syringe is then aspirated and if no blood is seen, the solution is deposited.[13] If the true source of pain is the joint, the pain should be eliminated or certainly significantly decreased in 4 to 5 minutes.

Intracapsular Injections

On occasion it is indicated to inject directly into the TMJ. This type of injection would be indicated for therapeutic, not diagnostic, reasons. Diagnostic information is derived from performing the auriculotemporal nerve block. A therapeutic injection would be indicated when it is appropriate to introduce some medication to the joint structures. The types of medications that may be considered are discussed in Chapter 11.

Normally the superior joint space is the target for an intracapsular (intraarticular) injection because it is the largest joint space and is the simplest to consistently locate. The joint can be entered by first locating the lateral pole of the condyle. This can be assisted by asking the patient to open and close the mouth (Fig. 10-10, *A*). Once the pole is located, the clinician should ask the patient to open slightly and palpate directly above to locate the zygomatic arch. The tissue is cleaned, and the tip of the needle is placed just below the zygomatic arch and slightly behind the posterior and superior aspect of the condyle. The needle is angulated slightly anterior superiorly to avoid the retrodiscal tissues (Fig. 10-10, *B*). Once the capsule is penetrated, the tip of the needle will be in the superior joint space. The solution is then deposited and the needle removed. A sterile gauze is held over the injection site for a few seconds to ensure hemostasis. The patient is then asked to open and close the mouth a few times to distributed the solution throughout the joint space.

Often a successful intraarticular injection will leave the patient with an immediate acute malocclusion on the ipsilateral side. Because there is little area in the superior joint space, the introduction of additional fluid will temporally cause an increase in the joint space that leads to the separation of the posterior teeth on the same side of the injection. This will resolve in a few hours. The patient should be made aware of this condition so

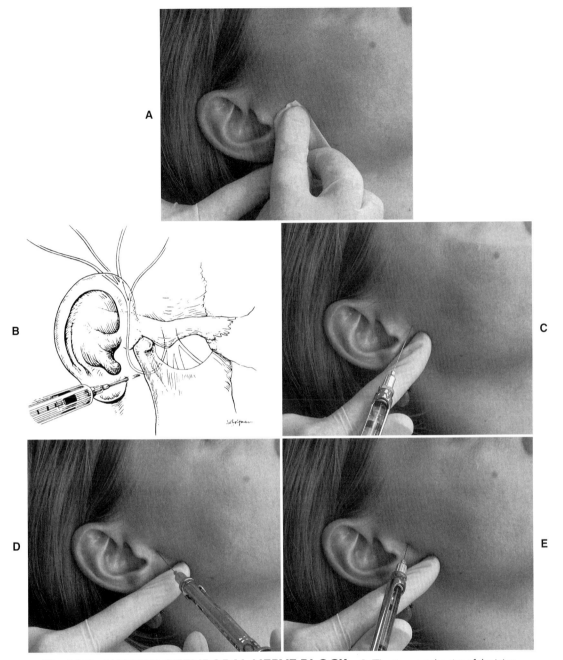

Fig. 10-9 AURICULOTEMPORAL NERVE BLOCK. A, The tissue at the site of the injection is thoroughly cleaned. **B,** This drawing shows the position of the auriculotemporal nerve as it transverses around the posterior aspect of the condyle. It also demonstrates the proper needle placement for an auriculotemporal nerve block. **C,** The needle is placed slightly anterior to the junction of the tragus and ear lobule and is penetrated until the posterior neck of the condyle is felt. **D,** The needle is then repositioned in a more posterior direction until the tip of the needle is able to pass behind the posterior neck of the condyle. **E,** Once the needle tip passes beyond the neck of the condyle, the syringe is again positioned in a more anterior direction and the tip is inserted behind the neck of the condyle. The total depth of the needle is approximately 1 cm. The syringe is then aspirated, and if there is no blood drawn back into the syringe, the anesthetic solution is deposited. Placement of the needle in this manner will minimize anesthetizing the facial nerve. (*B from Donlon WC, Truta MP, Eversole LR: A modified auriculotemporal nerve block for regional anesthesia of the temporomandibular joint,* J Oral Maxillofac Surg *42:544-545, 1984.*)

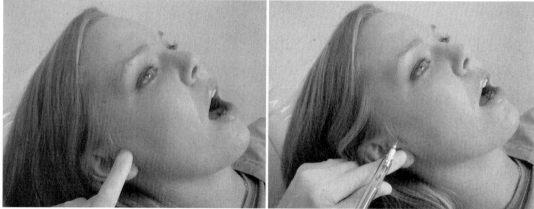

Fig. 10-10 AN INTRACAPSULAR TEMPOROMANDIBULAR JOINT INJECTION. The joint can be entered by first locating the lateral pole of the condyle. This can be assisted by asking the patient to open and close the mouth **(A).** Once the pole is located, the clinician should ask the patient to open slightly and palpate directly above to locate the zygomatic arch. The tissue is cleaned, and the tip of the needle is placed just below the zygomatic arch and slightly behind the posterior and superior aspect of the condyle. The needle is angulated slightly anterior superiorly to avoid the retrodiscal tissues **(B).** Once the capsule is penetrated, the tip of the needle will be in the superior joint space.

that it does not lead to any unnecessary concern or emotional stress.

Infraorbital Nerve Block. The infraorbital nerve transverses below the eye to exit from the infraorbital foramen located in the inferior border of the orbit. This nerve goes on to innervate the facial structures below the eye and some of the lateral aspects of the nose. In cases of trauma to the face this nerve can be injured, resulting in a continuous neuropathic pain. Blocking this nerve may have some therapeutic value. The nerve can be blocked by either an extraoral or intraoral approach. When the extraoral approached is used the foramen is identified by palpation of the inferior border of the orbit, feeling for a slight notch. The notch represents the exit of the infraorbital nerve. Once the notch is located, the tissue is cleaned and the needle is place to the depth of the notch and into the foreman when possible (Fig. 10-11, *A*). When the intraoral approach is used, the notch is found in the same manner as previously described. The middle finger is used to maintain the position of the notch, while the index finger and thumb are used to retract the lip.

The needle is placed into the mouth, and the tip is inserted into the vestibule and directed upward to the notch (Fig. 10-11, *B*). In some instances a long 27-gauge needle may be necessary to reach the foramen with this technique.

KEYS IN MAKING A DIFFERENTIAL DIAGNOSIS

As stated in previous chapters, the two most common masticatory problems (other than odontalgia) that present in a dental office are masticatory muscle disorders and intracapsular joint disorders. It is extremely important that they be differentiated because their treatments are quite different. The clinician who cannot routinely separate them is likely to have relatively poor success in managing TMDs.

Although muscle and joint disorders have some common clinical findings, seven areas of information acquired during the history and examination will assist in separating them. These keys in diagnosis are the following: (1) history,

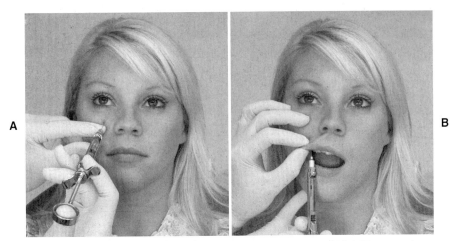

Fig. 10-11 INJECTION OF THE INFRAORBITAL NERVE. A, When performing an extraoral approach, the infraorbital foramen is palpated (notch) and the needle tip is placed directly into the opening of the foramen. **B,** During the intraoral approach, the foramen is first located extraorally and the position is maintained by a finger. The needle is placed into the vestibule and moved superiorly until the tip is located at the foramen. For this injection a long-gauge needle is used.

(2) mandibular restriction, (3) mandibular interference, (4) acute malocclusion, (5) loading of the joint, (6) functional manipulation, and (7) diagnostic anesthetic blockade.

1. *History.* The history is always helpful in distinguishing joint from muscle disorders.[14,15] Listen for an event that seemed to initiate the disorder. When a joint is traumatized, the symptoms are likely to begin in association with the trauma and be relatively constant or worsen from that time forward. Muscle disorders, on the other hand, appear to fluctuate and cycle from severe to mild with no apparent initiating event. Muscle problems are more closely related to changes in levels of emotional stress, and therefore periods of total remission are not uncommon when stress is low.

2. *Mandibular restriction.* Restriction of mouth opening and eccentric movements are common findings with both joint disorders and muscle disorders. The character of the restrictions, however, can be quite different. Restriction in mouth opening because of intracapsular problems (e.g., a dislocated disc without reduction) usually occurs at 25 to 30 mm. At that point the mouth cannot be opened wider, even with mild passive force. This hard "end feel" is commonly associated with a dislocated disc blocking translation of the condyle. Restricted mouth opening as a result of muscle disorders can occur anywhere during the opening movement. For example, a restricted opening of 8 to 10 mm is most certainly of muscle origin. When the mouth opening is restricted by muscles, mild passive force will usually lengthen the muscles slightly and result in a small increase in opening. This represents a soft "end feel" and is typical of muscle restrictions. Combining these clinical findings with the onset of the limited mouth opening obtained in the history is helpful in understanding the reason for the restriction.

   Mandibular restriction should also be evaluated by observing the patient move in left and right eccentric positions. In patients with an intracapsular restriction (i.e., disc dislocation without reduction), a contralateral eccentric movement will be limited but an ipsilateral movement will be normal. However, with muscle disorders the elevators (temporalis, masseter, medial pterygoid) are responsible for the limited mouth opening and, because eccentric movements do not generally lengthen these muscles, a normal range of eccentric movement exists.

3. *Mandibular interference.* When the mouth is opened, the pathway of the mandible is observed for any deviations or deflections. If the deviation occurs during opening and the jaw then returns to midline before 30 to 35 mm of total opening, it is likely to be associated with a disc derangement disorder (Fig. 10-12). If the speed of opening alters the location of the deviation, it is likely to be discal movement such as disc displacement with reduction. If the speed of opening does not alter the interincisal distance of the deviation and if the location of the deviation is the same for opening and closing, then a structural incompatibility is a likely diagnosis. Muscle disorders that cause deviation of

mandibular opening pathways are commonly large, inconsistent, sweeping movements not associated with joint sounds. These deviations are a result of muscle engrams. Deviation can also occur because of subluxation at the wide-open position. This is an intracapsular disorder, but not necessarily a pathologic condition.

Deflection of the mandibular opening pathway results when one condyle does not translate (Fig. 10-13). This may be caused by an intracapsular problem such as a disc dislocation without reduction or an adhesion problem. With these problems the mandible will deflect to the ipsilateral side during the late stages of opening. Deflection during opening can also result if a unilateral elevator muscle, such as the masseter, becomes shortened (myospasm). This condition can be separated from intracapsular disorders by observing the protrusive and lateral

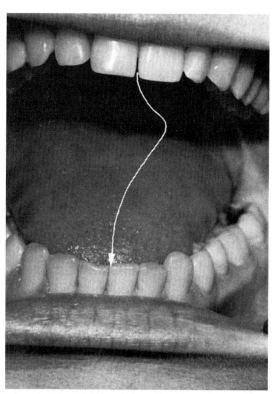

Fig. 10-12 DEVIATION. The opening pathway is altered but returns to a normal midline relationship at maximum opening.

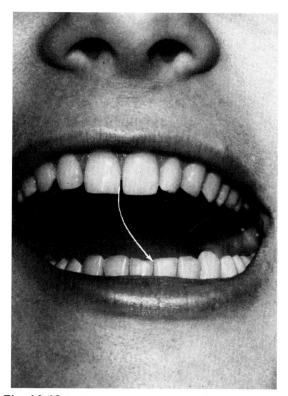

Fig. 10-13 Deflection of the opening path is commonly associated with a disc dislocation without reduction or a unilateral muscle restriction.

eccentric movements. If the problem is intracapsular, the mandible will deflect to the side of the involved joint during protrusion and be restricted during a contralateral movement (normal movement to the ipsilateral side). If the problem is extracapsular (i.e., muscle), there will be no deflection during the protrusive movement and no restrictions in lateral movements.

When deflection of the mandible is caused by an intracapsular source, the mandible will always move toward the involved joint. If the deflection is the result of a shortened muscle, the direction in which the mandible moves will depend on the position of the involved muscle with respect to the joint. If the muscle is lateral to the joint (i.e., masseter or temporalis), the deflection will be toward the involved muscle. If it is medial to the joint (i.e., medial pterygoid), deflection will be away from the involved muscle (in a contralateral direction).

4. *Acute malocclusion.* As stated earlier, an acute malocclusion is a sudden alteration of the occlusion condition secondary to a disorder. An acute malocclusion caused by a muscle disorder will vary according to the muscles involved. If the inferior lateral pterygoid is in spasm and shortens, the condyle will be brought slightly forward in the fossa on the involved side. This will result in a disocclusion of the ipsilateral posterior teeth and heavy contact on the contralateral canines. If the spasms are in the elevator muscles, the patient is likely to report a feeling that the teeth "suddenly don't fit right," yet clinically it may be difficult to visualize any change. An acute malocclusion resulting from an intracapsular disorder is usually closely related to the event that changed the joint function. If the disc is suddenly displaced, the thicker posterior border may be superimposed between the condyle and fossa and cause a sudden increase in the discal space. This appears clinically as a loss of ipsilateral posterior tooth contact. If the disc becomes suddenly dislocated, collapse of the discal space can occur as the condyle compresses the retrodiscal tissues. The patient notes this as a sudden change in the occlusion characterized as heavy posterior contact on the ipsilateral side. If this condition continues, retrodiscitis may result and cause tissue inflammation with swelling of the retrodiscal tissues. The resulting acute malocclusion may now change to one characterized by loss of posterior tooth contacts on the ipsilateral side.

5. *Loading the joint.* As mentioned in Chapter 9, positioning the condyles to their musculoskeletally stable position and loading the structures with manipulative force does not produce pain in a healthy joint. When pain is produced, one should be suspicious of an intracapsular source of pain (Fig. 10-14).

6. *Functional manipulation.* As stated in Chapter 9, functional manipulation can be helpful in identifying the location of pain. Functional manipulation procedures that do not produce pain tend to rule out muscle disorders as the source of the problem.

7. *Diagnostic anesthetic blockade.* For patients in whom the preceding six procedures have not convincingly assisted in making a differential diagnosis between joint and muscle disorders, anesthetic blockade is indicated. Anesthetic blocking of the auriculotemporal nerve can quickly rule in or out an intracapsular disorder. The dentist working with pain disorders should be familiar with this injection technique and use it without hesitation to assist in diagnosis.

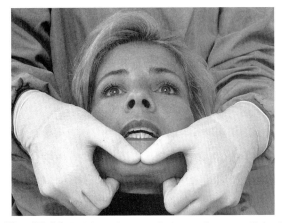

Fig. 10-14 A bilateral manipulation technique will load the joints and help determine whether pain is from an intracapsular or an extracapsular source.

CLASSIFICATION OF TEMPOROMANDIBULAR DISORDERS

For years, classifying TMDs has been a confusing issue. There have been almost as many classifications as there have been texts on the subject. Then Welden Bell[16] presented a classification that logically categorizes these disorders, and the American Dental Association[17] adopted it with few changes. It has, in fact, become a "road map" helping clinicians toward a precise and well-defined diagnosis.

This chapter presents the basic classification of TMDs developed by Bell but incorporates some additional modifications of my own. It begins by separating all TMDs into four broad categories having similar clinical characteristics: (1) masticatory muscle disorders, (2) TMJ disorders, (3) chronic mandibular hypomobility disorders, and (4) growth disorders. Each of these categories is further divided according to dissimilarities that are clinically identifiable. The result is a relatively intricate classification system that initially might appear to be almost too complex. However, this classification is important because treatment indicated for each subcategory varies greatly. In fact, treatment that is indicated for one may be contraindicated for another. Therefore it is important that these subcategories be identified and clearly defined so that proper treatment will be initiated.

Treatment failures are commonly attributed to the utilization of one mode for all patients in a major category. This, however, demonstrates improper diagnostic technique and almost always leads to treatment failure. It is virtually impossible to overemphasize the importance of proper diagnosis as the key to successful treatment. Dentistry is indebted to Dr. Bell for his major contribution to the diagnostic classification of TMDs.

Each broad category can be described according to the symptoms that are common to it, whereas each subdivision is characterized by the clinical characteristics that differentiate it from the others. In this chapter each disorder is discussed according to causes, history, and examination findings that lead to establishing a diagnosis. Once a diagnosis is established, appropriate treatment must be provided. Treatment for each disorder is discussed in Chapters 11 to 16. The classification used for diagnosing TMDs is summarized in Box 10-1.

MASTICATORY MUSCLE DISORDERS

Certainly the most frequent complaint given by patients with functional disturbances of the masticatory system is muscle pain (myalgia). Patients commonly report that the pain is associated with functional activities such as chewing, swallowing, and speaking. The pain is also aggravated by manual palpation or functional manipulation of the muscles. Restricted mandibular movement is common. Muscle pain is of extracapsular origin and may be primarily induced by the inhibitory effects of deep pain input. The restriction is most often not related to any structural change in the muscle itself. Sometimes accompanying these muscle symptoms is an acute malocclusion. Typically, the patient will report that his or her bite has changed. As previously stated, muscle pain disorders can so alter the resting mandibular position that when the teeth are brought into contact the patient perceives a change in the occlusion.

All masticatory muscle disorders are not clinically the same. At least five different types are known, and being able to distinguish among them is important because the treatment of each is quite different. The five types are (1) protective co-contraction (muscle splinting), (2) local muscle soreness, (3) myofascial (trigger point) pain, (4) myospasm, and (5) centrally mediated myalgia. A sixth condition known as *fibromyalgia* also needs to be discussed. The first three conditions (protective co-contraction, local muscle soreness, and myofascial pain) are commonly seen in the dental office. Myospasm and centrally mediated myalgia are less frequently seen. Because most of these masticatory muscle disorders occur and recover in a relatively short period of time, they are generally considered acute myalgic disorders. When these conditions are not resolved, more chronic pain disorders that are often more complicated to manage may result. Centrally mediated myalgia and fibromyalgia are examples of chronic myalgic disorders. In some patients myofascial pain can also become chronic. Chronic myofascial pain and

BOX 10-1

Classification System Used for Diagnosing Temporomandibular Disorders

I. Masticatory muscle disorders
   A. Protective co-contraction (11.8.4)*
   B. Local muscle soreness (11.8.4)
   C. Myofascial pain (11.8.1)
   D. Myospasm (11.8.3)
   E. Centrally mediated myalgia (11.8.2)
II. Temporomandibular joint (TMJ) disorders
   A. Derangement of the condyle-disc complex
      1. Disc displacements (11.7.2.1)
      2. Disc dislocation with reduction (11.7.2.1)
      3. Disc dislocation without reduction (11.7.2.2)
   B. Structural incompatibility of the articular surfaces
      1. Deviation in form (11.7.1)
         a. Disc
         b. Condyle
         c. Fossa
      2. Adhesions (11.7.7.1)
         a. Disc to condyle
         b. Disc to fossa
      3. Subluxation (hypermobility) (11.7.3)
      4. Spontaneous dislocation (11.7.3)
   C. Inflammatory disorders of the TMJ
      1. Synovitis/capsulitis (11.7.4.1)
      2. Retrodiscitis (11.7.4.1)
      3. Arthritides (11.7.6)

   a. Osteoarthritis (11.7.5)
   b. Osteoarthrosis (11.7.5)
   c. Polyarthritides (11.7.4.2)
      4. Inflammatory disorders of associated structures
         a. Temporal tendonitis
         b. Stylomandibular ligament inflammation
III. Chronic mandibular hypomobility
   A. Ankylosis (11.7.6)
      1. Fibrous (11.7.6.1)
      2. Bony (11.7.6.2)
   B. Muscle contracture (11.8.5)
      1. Myostatic
      2. Myofibrotic
   C. Coronoid impedance
IV. Growth disorders
   A. Congenital and developmental bone disorders
      1. Agenesis (11.7.1.1)
      2. Hypoplasia (11.7.1.2)
      3. Hyperplasia (11.7.1.3)
      4. Neoplasia (11.7.1.4)
   B. Congenital and developmental muscle disorders
      1. Hypotrophy
      2. Hypertrophy (11.8.6)
      3. Neoplasia (11.8.7)

Adapted from Okeson JP: *Orofacial pain: guidelines for assessment, diagnosis, and, management,* ed 3, Chicago, 1996, Quintessence, pp 45-52.
*The code number after each disorder has been established by the American Academy of Orofacial Pain in cooperation with the International Headache Society.

centrally mediated myalgia are *regional* pain disorders, whereas fibromyalgia is a chronic *systemic* myalgic disorder. Fibromyalgia is not primarily a masticatory problem, and therefore the dentist needs to be able to recognize it for referral to the appropriate medical personnel.

In Chapter 8, a masticatory muscle model was described showing the relationship between the acute myalgic disorders and certain events that are experienced by the masticatory system. This model also depicts how a nonresolving acute myalgic disorder can become chronic when certain perpetuating conditions are present (Fig. 10-15). This section does not review the model but instead

concentrates on a detailed description of each disorder so that a proper diagnosis can be established. If the model needs to be reviewed, please refer to Chapter 8.

Protective Co-Contraction (Muscle Splinting)

The first response of the masticatory muscles to one of the previously described events is protective co-contraction. Protective co-contraction is a central nervous system (CNS) response to injury or threat of injury. In the past this response was referred to as *muscle splinting.*[16] In the presence of an event, the activity of appropriate muscles seems to be altered so as to protect the injured part from

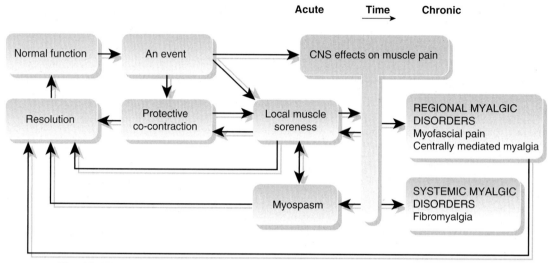

Fig. 10-15 The masticatory muscle model is explained in detail in Chapter 8. *(Modified from the original model developed by J.P. Okeson, D.A. Falace, C.R. Carlson, A. Nitz, and D.T. Anderson, Orofacial Pain Center, University of Kentucky, 1991.)*

further injury.[18-22] As described in Chapter 2, all muscles are maintained in a mildly contracted state known as *tonus*. Tonus persists without fatigue by virtue of the alternating contractions and relaxations of the muscle fibers, which keep the overall muscle length unchanged and resist any sudden elongation.

When protective co-contraction occurs, the CNS increases the activity of the antagonist muscle during contraction of the agonist muscle. It is important to recognize that co-contraction[23] is observed during many normal functional activities, such as bracing the arm when attempting a task with the fingers. In the presence of altered sensory input or pain, however, antagonistic muscle groups seem to fire during movement in an attempt to protect the injured part. In the masticatory system, for example, a patient who is experiencing protective co-contraction will demonstrate a small increased amount of muscle activity in the elevator muscles during mouth opening.[20,24] During closing of the mouth, increased activity is noted in the depressing muscles. This reflex-like activity is not a pathologic condition but a normal protective or guarding mechanism that needs to be identified and appreciated by the clinician. Importantly, the clinician must recognize that this increase in muscle activity is slight and therefore not clinically identifiable with electromyographic (EMG) output,

except under stringent experimental conditions. This increased EMG output is much smaller than the clinical error encountered from patient variability, as well as electrode placement variability (see Chapter 9).

Causes. Three conditions can lead to protective co-contraction:

1. *Altered sensory or proprioceptive input.* Protective co-contraction may be initiated by any change in the occlusal condition that significantly alters sensory input, such as the introduction of a poorly fitting crown. If a crown is placed with a high occlusal contact, it tends to alter the sensory and proprioceptive input to the CNS. Consequently, the elevator muscles (temporalis, masseter, medial pterygoid) may become protectively co-contracted in an attempt to prevent the crown from contacting the opposing tooth. Protective co-contraction can also result from any event that alters the oral structures, such as opening too wide or a long dental appointment. It may follow a dental injection that traumatized tissues.

2. *Constant deep pain input.* As already discussed, the presence of deep pain input felt in local structures can produce protective co-contraction of associated muscles (Fig. 10-16). This phenomenon occurs by way of the central excitatory effects described in Chapter 2. It is important to

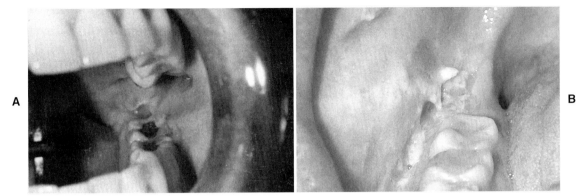

Fig. 10-16 A, This patient reported symptoms of protective co-contraction. The soft tissue surrounding the second molar and the erupting third molar was inflamed and tender to palpation (pericoronitis). **B,** This patient reports chronically biting the soft tissues of the cheek. This tissue injury is painful, which results in protective co-contraction.

note that the source of the deep pain need not be muscle tissue itself but can be any associated structure such as tendons, ligaments, joints, or even the teeth.

3. *Increased emotional stress.* Clinical observations strongly demonstrate that emotional stress can greatly influence masticatory muscle activity[25-29] (see Chapter 7). When an individual experiences increased levels of emotional stress, a common response is for the gamma efferent system to alter the sensitivity of the muscle spindle. This increases the sensitivity of the muscle to lengthening, resulting in an increased tonicity of the muscle. The clinical response of the muscle is seen as protective co-contraction. Increased emotional stress also has the ability to initiate parafunctional activities such as nocturnal bruxism and clenching. As previously discussed, these activities can lead to muscle symptoms.

History. The history reported by the patient reveals a recent event associated with one of the causes that has just been discussed. The patient may report an increase in emotional stress or the presence of a source of deep pain. The key to the history is that the event has been recent, usually within a day or two.

Clinical Characteristics. Myalgia, although often present, is not usually the major complaint associated with protective muscle co-contraction.

The following four clinical characteristics identify this clinical condition:

1. *Structural dysfunction.* In the presence of protective co-contraction, the velocity and range of mandibular movement is decreased. This results from the co-contraction that has already been described. Any restriction of mandibular movement is secondary to the pain; therefore slow and careful opening of the mouth often reveals a near-normal range of movement.

2. *No pain at rest.* Individuals who experience protective co-contraction have little to no pain when the muscle is allowed to rest. Co-contraction may represent a slight increase in tonicity of the muscle, but an increase in tonicity, especially for a short period of time, does not produce myalgia. As already mentioned, it is unlikely that this slight increase in activity can be measured by EMG output, especially when considering the great variability of resting activity among patients.[30-33]

3. *Increased pain with function.* Individuals who experience protective co-contraction often report an increase in myogenous pain during function of the involved muscles. When the individual attempts to function normally, the co-contraction or splinting is increased, resisting jaw movement. This antagonistic activity can lead to myalgic complaints. It is often only through

function that the individual becomes aware of the altered muscle condition.

4. *Feeling of muscle weakness.* Individuals experiencing protective co-contraction commonly report a feeling of muscle weakness. They often complain that their muscles seem to tire quickly. No clinical evidence has been found, however, that the muscles are actually weakened.

Local Muscle Soreness (Noninflammatory Myalgia)

Local muscle soreness is a primary, noninflammatory, myogenous pain disorder and is often the first response of the muscle tissue to continued protective co-contraction. Whereas co-contraction represents a CNS-induced muscle response, local muscle soreness represents a change in the local environment of the muscle tissues. This change may be the result of prolonged co-contraction or excessive use of the muscle producing fatigue.[34,35] When unaccustomed use is the cause, the symptoms may be delayed (delayed-onset muscle soreness). Local muscle soreness may also result from direct tissue damage (trauma).

Causes. Four principal conditions lead to local muscle soreness:

1. *Protracted co-contraction.* As already described, continued co-contraction will lead to local muscle soreness. Because this muscle soreness itself is a source of deep pain, an important clinical event can occur. Deep pain produced by local muscle soreness can in fact produce protective co-contraction. This additional co-contraction can, of course, produce more local muscle soreness. Therefore a cycle can be created whereby local muscle soreness produces more co-contraction and so on. This cyclic muscle pain has already been discussed in Chapter 2.

   The clinician needs to be aware of the complications this might pose on a clinical basis. For example, trauma to a muscle will produce local muscle soreness. The pain experienced from the muscle soreness in turn produces protective co-contraction. Because protective co-contraction can lead to local muscle soreness, a cycle begins. During this cycling, the original tissue damage produced by the trauma can resolve. When tissue repair is complete, the original source of pain is eliminated; however, the patient may continue to suffer with a cyclic muscle pain disorder. Because the original cause of the pain is no longer part of the clinical picture, the clinician can be easily confused during the examination. The clinician needs to recognize that even though the original cause has resolved, a cyclic muscle pain condition exists and needs to be treated. This condition is an extremely common clinical finding and often leads to mismanagement of the patient.

2. *Trauma.* A muscle can sustain at least two types of trauma:

   a. *Local tissue injury:* As has already been discussed, local injury of tissue can occur through events such as local anesthetic injections or tissue strains.

   b. *Unaccustomed use:* Trauma to muscle tissue can be created by abusive or unaccustomed use of muscle tissues.[36-39] This may result from bruxing or clenching the teeth or even from unaccustomed chewing of gum. Importantly, unaccustomed use of muscles often results in delayed-onset muscle soreness. The delay of symptoms is normally 24 to 48 hours after the event. Most individuals are familiar with this phenomenon by experiencing delayed-onset muscle soreness in other muscles. For example, if one attempts to overuse back muscles by unaccustomed work during a weekend, stiffness and pain will follow 1 to 2 days after the event. Therefore it is logical to assume that unaccustomed activity such as bruxing can also produce pain 1 to 2 days after the event.

3. *Increased emotional stress.* As already discussed, continued increased levels of emotional stress can lead to prolonged co-contraction and muscle pain. This cause is common and may be difficult for the dentist to control.

4. *Idiopathic myogenous pain.* An idiopathic origin of myogenous pain must be included in this discussion because a complete understanding of muscle pain is not presently available.[40] It is hoped that as our knowledge expands, this origin of pain will be better explained.

   History. The history reported by the patient reveals that the pain complaint began several hours or 1 day following an event associated with one of the causes that has just been discussed. The patient may report that the pain began following an increase in emotional stress or the presence of another source of deep pain.

Clinical Characteristics. A patient experiencing local muscle soreness will present with the following clinical characteristics:

1. *Structural dysfunction.* When masticatory muscles experience local muscle soreness, there is a decrease in the velocity and range of mandibular movement. This alteration is secondary to the inhibitory effect of pain (protective co-contraction). Unlike co-contraction, however, slow and careful mouth opening still reveals limited range of movement. Passive stretching by the examiner can often achieve a more normal range (soft end feel).
2. *Minimum pain at rest.* Local muscle soreness does not generally produce pain when the muscle is at rest.
3. *Increased pain to function.* Individuals experiencing local muscle soreness report an increase in pain when the involved muscle functions.
4. *Actual muscle weakness.* Local muscle soreness results in an overall reduction in the strength of the affected muscles.[41,42] This reduction in strength appears to be related to the presence of pain and is returned to normal when the pain is eliminated.[42,43] This phenomenon is another effect of protective co-contraction.
5. *Local muscle tenderness.* Muscles experiencing local muscle soreness reveal increased tenderness and pain to palpation. Generally the entire body of the involved muscle is tender to palpation.

Central Nervous System Effects on Muscle Pain

The muscle pain conditions described to this point are relatively simple, having their origins predominately in the local muscle tissues. Unfortunately muscle pain can become much more complex. In many instances, activity within the CNS can either influence or actually *be* the origin of the muscle pain. This may occur either secondary to ongoing deep pain input or altered sensory input, or it may arise from central influences such as upregulation of the autonomic nervous system (i.e., emotional stress). This occurs when conditions within the CNS excite peripheral sensory neurons (primary afferents), creating the antidromic release of algogenic substances into the peripheral tissues, resulting in muscle pain (i.e., neurogenic inflammation).[40,44-46] These central excitatory effects can also lead to motor effects (i.e., primary efferents), resulting in an increase in muscle tonicity (i.e., co-contraction).[47]

Therapeutically, it is important that the clinician appreciates that the muscle pain now has a central origin. The CNS responds in this manner secondary to either (1) the presence of ongoing deep pain input; (2) increased levels of emotional stress (i.e., an upregulation of the autonomic nervous system); or (3) changes in the descending inhibitory system that lead to a decrease in the ability to counter the afferent input, whether nociceptive or not.

Centrally influenced muscle pain disorders are therapeutically divided into *acute myalgic disorders* such as myospasm or *chronic myalgic disorders*, which are further divided into *regional myalgic disorders* or *systemic myalgic disorders*. Regional myalgic disorders are subdivided into *myofascial pain* and *chronic centrally mediated myalgia*. An example of a systemic myalgic disorder is fibromyalgia.

Myospasm (Tonic Contraction Myalgia)

Myospasm is an involuntary, CNS-induced tonic muscle contraction. For many years dentists believed that myospasms were a significant source of myogenous pain. Recent studies, however, shed new light on muscle pain and myospasms. It is reasonable to expect that a muscle in spasm or tonic contraction would reveal a relatively high level of EMG activity. Studies, however, do not support that painful muscles have a significant increase in their EMG output.[47-49] These studies have forced us to rethink the classification of muscle pain and differentiate myospasms from other muscle pain disorders. Although muscle spasms do occur in the muscles of mastication, this condition is not common and, when present, is usually easily identified by clinical characteristics.

Causes. The cause of myospasm has not been well documented. Several factors are likely to combine to promote myospasms:

1. *Local muscle conditions.* Local muscle conditions certainly seem to foster myospasm. These conditions

may involve muscle fatigue and changes in local electrolyte balance.

2. *Systemic conditions.* Some individuals are apparently more prone to myospasm than others. This may represent some systemic factor or the presence of another musculoskeletal disorder.[50]

3. *Deep pain input.* The presence of deep pain input can encourage myospasm. This deep pain may arise from local muscle soreness, abusive trigger point pain, or any associated structure (e.g., TMJ, ear, tooth).

History. Because myospasms result in a sudden shortening of a muscle, a significant history is evident. The patient will report a sudden onset of pain, tightness, and often a change in jaw position. Mandibular movement will be difficult.

Clinical Characteristics. Individuals experiencing myospasms present with the following clinical characteristics:

1. *Structural dysfunction.* Two clinical findings noted regarding structural dysfunction are as follows:
   a. There is marked restriction in the range of movement determined by the muscle or muscles in spasm. For example, if an elevator muscle such as the masseter were in spasm, there would be marked restriction in mouth opening.
   b. Structural dysfunction may also present as an acute malocclusion. An acute malocclusion is a sudden change in the occlusal contact pattern of the teeth secondary to a disorder. This may occur as a result of a myospasm in the inferior lateral pterygoid muscle. A spasm and subsequent shortening of the left lateral pterygoid muscle will produce a shifting of the mandible into a right lateral eccentric position. This will result in heavy occlusal contact of the right anterior teeth and loss of occlusal contact between the left posterior teeth.

2. *Pain at rest.* Myospasms usually produce significant pain when the mandible is at rest.

3. *Increased pain with function.* When a patient attempts to function with a muscle in spasm, the pain will be increased.

4. *Local muscle tenderness.* Palpation of the muscle or muscles experiencing myospasm reveals significant tenderness.

5. *Muscle tightness.* The patient reports a sudden tightening or knotting up of the entire muscle. Palpation of the muscle or muscles experiencing myospasm reveals them to be firm and hard.

Acute versus Chronic Muscle Disorders

The myalgic disorders that have been described are commonly seen in the general practice of dentistry and usually represent problems of short duration. With proper therapy, these disorders can be completely resolved. However, when myogenous pain persists, more chronic and often complex muscle pain disorders can develop. With chronicity, myogenous pain disorder symptoms become less local and more regional or even occasionally global. Often cyclic muscle pain becomes an important factor that perpetuates the condition. Other conditions have been presented in Chapter 8.

As a general rule, chronic pain is considered pain that has been present for 6 months or longer. The duration of pain, however, is not the only factor that determines chronicity. Some pains are experienced for years but never become chronic pain conditions. Likewise, some pain conditions become clinically chronic in a matter of months. An additional factor that must be considered is the continuity of the pain. When a pain experience is constant, with no periods of relief, the clinical manifestations of chronicity develop quickly. On the other hand, if the pain is interrupted with periods of remission (no pain), the condition may never become a chronic pain disorder. For example, migraine is an extremely painful neurovascular condition that may last for years and never develop into a chronic pain disorder. The reason for this is the significant periods of relief between episodes of pain. Conversely, the constant pain associated with centrally mediated myalgia, when left untreated, can develop the clinical manifestations of chronicity within several months.

The dentist should recognize that when myalgic complaints progress from an acute condition to a more chronic condition, the effectiveness of local treatment is greatly reduced. The reason for this failure of treatment is because the origin of the condition becomes more central. Chronic pain disorders often need to be managed by a multidisciplinary approach. In many instances the dentist alone is not equipped to manage these disorders. Therefore it is important for the dentist to recognize chronic pain disorders and consider referring the patient to a team of appropriate therapists who are better able to manage the pain condition.

Regional Myalgic Disorders

The two types of regional myalgic disorders are *myofascial pain* and *centrally mediated myalgia*. Both conditions reveal peripheral symptoms but are greatly influenced by the CNS. Understanding this concept is paramount to treatment.

Myofascial Pain (Trigger Point Myalgia). Myofascial pain is a regional myogenous pain condition characterized by local areas of firm, hypersensitive bands of muscle tissue known as *trigger points*. This condition is sometimes referred to as *myofascial trigger point pain*. This type of muscle disorder is not widely appreciated or completely understood, yet it commonly occurs in patients with myalgic complaints. In one study[51] more than 50% of the patients reporting to a university pain center were diagnosed as having this type of pain.

Myofascial pain may occur periodically for some patients and therefore represent an acute myalgic disorder. However, myofascial pain may also be associated with other ongoing pain disorders, thereby becoming a chronic pain condition demanding more therapeutic efforts for resolution. The clinician needs to learn by the history whether the condition is acute or chronic so that proper management will be instituted.

Travell and Rinzler[52] first described myofascial trigger point pain in 1952, yet the dental and medical communities were slow to appreciate its significance. In 1969 Laskin[53] published an important paper expressing to the dental community that there are many patients with muscle pain complaints in which the cause is not the occlusal condition. He emphasized the importance of emotional stress and other factors. Although Laskin referenced the term *myofascial pain* in his article, he was not actually describing the same clinical characteristics reported by Travell. From this article the dental profession began using the term *myofascial pain dysfunction* (MPD) syndrome. Today MPD syndrome is often used in dentistry as a general term to denote any muscle disorder (not an intracapsular disorder). Because the term is so broad and general, it is not useful in the specific diagnosis and management of masticatory muscle disorders. MPD syndrome should not be confused with Travell and Rinzler's description, which is used in this textbook.

Myofascial pain arises from hypersensitive areas in muscles called *trigger points*. These localized areas in muscle tissues or their tendinous attachments are often felt as taut bands when palpated, which elicits pain.[54-56] The exact nature of a trigger point is not known. Some experts[41,56-58] have suggested that certain nerve endings in the muscle tissues may become sensitized by algogenic substances that create a localized zone of hypersensitivity. There may be a local temperature rise at the site of the trigger point, suggesting an increase in metabolic demand and/or reduction of blood flow to these tissues.[59,60]

A trigger point is a circumscribed region in which just a relatively few motor units are contracting. If all the motor units of a muscle contract, the muscle will of course shorten in length (see Chapter 2). This condition, called *myospasm*, is discussed later in this section. Because a trigger point has only a select group of motor units contracting, no overall shortening of the muscle will occur as with myospasm.

The unique characteristic of trigger points is that they are a source of constant deep pain and therefore can produce central excitatory effects (see Chapter 2). If a trigger point centrally excites a group of converging afferent interneurons, referred pain will often result, generally in a predictable pattern according to the location of the involved trigger point.[61]

Causes. Although myofascial pain is seen clinically as trigger points in the skeletal muscles, this condition is certainly not derived solely from the muscle tissue. Evidence indicates that the CNS plays a significant role in the cause of this pain condition.[40,56] The combination of both central and peripheral factors makes this condition more difficult to manage. Simons and Travell[62] have described certain etiologic factors that seem to be associated with myofascial pain. Unfortunately we lack a complete understanding of this myogenous pain condition. Therefore it is difficult to be specific concerning all etiologic factors. The following conditions are clinically related to myofascial pain:

1. *Protracted local muscle soreness.* Muscles that experience continued muscle soreness are likely to develop myofascial trigger points and subsequently develop the clinical characteristics of myofascial pain.

2. *Constant deep pain.* As discussed in Chapter 2, constant deep pain input can create central excitatory effects in remote sites. If the central excitatory effect involves an efferent (motor) neuron, two types of muscle effects can be observed: (1) protective co-contraction and (2) the development of trigger points. When a trigger point develops, it becomes a source of deep pain and can produce additional central excitatory effects. These secondary trigger points are called *satellite trigger points.*[63] This expansion of the myofascial pain condition complicates diagnosis and management and can create a cyclic condition similar to the cyclic muscle pain that has already been discussed.

3. *Increased emotional stress.* Increased emotional stress can greatly exacerbate myofascial pain. This may occur by way of increased activity of the gamma efferent neurons to the muscle spindles or by a generalized increase in sympathetic nervous system activity (see Chapter 2).

4. *Sleep disturbances.* Studies[64,65] suggest that disruptions of the normal sleep cycle can create musculoskeletal symptoms. Whether sleep disturbances cause musculoskeletal pain or musculoskeletal pain causes sleep disturbances (or both) is not clear. What is clear is that a relationship does exist and needs to be appreciated by the clinician. The clinician must therefore be able to recognize common complaints associated with related sleep disorders.

5. *Local factors.* Certain local conditions that influence muscle activity such as habits, posture, strains, and even chilling seem to affect myofascial pain.

6. *Systemic factors.* It appears that certain systemic factors can influence or even produce myofascial pain. Systemic factors such as hypovitaminosis, poor physical conditioning, fatigue, and viral infections have been reported.[62]

7. *Idiopathic trigger point mechanism.* The precise cause of trigger points has not been determined. Therefore a category of unknown factors must be included in the overall cause of this myogenous pain disorder. Continued investigation will lead to a better understanding of not only cause but also the mechanisms involved in myofascial pain.

History. Patients suffering with myofascial pain will often present with a misleading history. The patient's chief complaint will often be the heterotopic pain and not the actual source of pain (the trigger points). Therefore the patient will direct the clinician to the location of the tension-type headache or protective co-contraction. If the clinician is not careful, he or she may direct treatment to the secondary pains, which, of course, will fail. The clinician must have the knowledge and diagnostic skills necessary to identify the primary source of pain so that proper treatment can be selected.

Clinical characteristics. An individual suffering with myofascial pain will commonly reveal the following clinical characteristics:

1. *Structural dysfunction.* Muscles experiencing myofascial pain reveal a decrease in the velocity and range of movement secondary to the inhibitory effect of pain (protective co-contraction). This decreased range of movement is often less than that observed with local muscle soreness.

2. *Pain at rest.* Patients experiencing myofascial pain report pain even when the muscles are at rest. The pain, however, is not commonly related to the location of the trigger points, but instead represents referred pain. The chief complaint therefore is reported as tension-type headache.[54]

3. *Increased pain with function.* Although pain is increased with function of the involved muscles, the amount of pain reported is usually less than with local muscle soreness. The pain is only increased when the trigger point area is provoked by function.

4. *Presence of trigger points.* Palpation of the muscle reveals local areas of firm, hypersensitive bands of muscle tissue called *trigger points.* Although palpation of trigger points produces pain, local

muscle sensitivity is not the most common complaint of patients suffering from myofascial trigger point pain. As previously mentioned, the most common complaints center around the central excitatory effects created by the trigger points. In many instances patients may be aware only of the referred pain and not even acknowledge the trigger points. A perfect example is the patient suffering from trigger point pain in the semispinalis capitis in the posterior occipital region of the neck. Trigger points in this region commonly refer pain to the anterior temple region just above the eye (Fig. 10-17).[66] The patient's chief complaint is temporal headache, with little acknowledgment of the trigger point in the posterior cervical region. This clinical presentation can easily distract the clinician from the source of the problem. The patient will draw the clinician's attention to the site of pain (the temporal headache) and not the source. The clinician must always remember that for treatment to be effective, it must be directed toward the source of the pain, not the site, and therefore clinicians must constantly be searching for the true source of the pain.

Because trigger points can create central excitatory effects, it is also important to be acutely aware of the possible clinical manifestations. As stated in Chapter 2, central excitatory effects can appear as referred pain, secondary hyperalgesia, protective co-contraction, or even autonomic responses. These conditions must be considered when evaluating the patient.

An interesting clinical feature of a trigger point is that it may present in an active or latent state. In the active state it produces central excitatory effects. Therefore when a trigger point is active, a tension-type headache is commonly felt.[54] When a trigger point is latent, the patient does not report the headache complaint.

Because referred pain is wholly dependent on its original source, palpation of an active trigger point (local provocation) often increases such pain.[61] Although not always present, when this characteristic appears it is an extremely helpful diagnostic aid. In the latent state a trigger point is no longer sensitive to palpation and therefore does not produce referred pain. When trigger points are latent, they are difficult to find by palpation and the patient does not complain of heterotopic pain.

Experts believe that trigger points do not resolve without treatment. They may in fact become latent or dormant, creating a temporary relief of the referred pain. Trigger points may be activated by various factors[67] such as increased use of a muscle, strain on the muscle, emotional stress, or even an upper respiratory infection. When trigger points are activated, the tension-type headache returns. This is a common finding with patients who complain of regular late-afternoon tension-type headaches following a trying and stressful day.

Along with referred pain, other central excitatory effects may be felt. When secondary hyperalgesia is present, it is commonly felt as sensitivity to touch of the scalp. Some patients will even report that their "hair hurts" or that it is painful to brush their hair. Protective co-contraction is another common condition associated with myofascial trigger point pain. Trigger points in the shoulder or cervical muscles can produce co-contraction in the muscles of mastication. If this continues, local

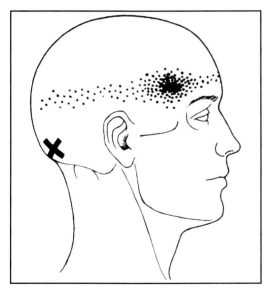

Fig. 10-17 A trigger point *(X)* in the semispinalis capitis muscle will refer pain to the anterior temporal region slightly above the eye. (*From Travell JG, Simons DG:* Myofascial pain and dysfunction. The trigger point manual, *Baltimore, 1983, Williams & Wilkins, p 306.*)

muscle soreness in masticatory muscles can develop. Treatment of the masticatory muscles will not resolve the condition because its source is the trigger points of the cervicospinal and shoulder muscles. However, treatment of the trigger points in the shoulder muscle will resolve the masticatory muscle disorder. Management may become difficult when local muscle soreness has been present for a period of time because it can initiate cyclic muscle pain (see Chapter 2). In these cases, treatment extended to both the muscles of mastication and the trigger points in the cervicospinal and shoulder muscles will usually resolve the problem.

On occasion, autonomic effects are created by deep pain input from trigger points. These may result in such clinical findings as tearing or drying of the eye. Vascular changes such as blanching and/or reddening of tissues may occur. Sometimes the conjunctiva will become red. Mucosal changes may produce nasal discharge similar to an allergic response. The key to determining whether the autonomic effects are related to central excitatory effects or to a local reaction such as allergies is the unilateral appearance. Central excitatory effects in the trigeminal area rarely cross the midline. Therefore if the deep pain is unilateral, the autonomic effects will be on the same side as the pain. In other words, one eye will be red and the other normal, one nostril draining mucus and the other not. With allergic responses both eyes or both nostrils will be involved.

By way of summary, the chief clinical symptoms reported with myofascial trigger point pain are not the trigger points themselves but more commonly the symptoms associated with the central excitatory effects created by the trigger points. The clinician must be aware of this and find the involved trigger points. When these are palpated, they appear as hypersensitive areas often felt as taut bands within the muscle. Usually no local pain exists when the muscle is at rest, but some pain exists when the muscle is used. Often slight structural dysfunction will be seen in the muscle harboring the trigger points. This is commonly reported as a "stiff neck."

Centrally Mediated Myalgia (Chronic Myositis). Centrally mediated myalgia is a chronic, continuous muscle pain disorder originating predominantly from CNS effects that are felt peripherally in the muscle tissues. This disorder clinically presents with symptoms similar to an inflammatory condition of the muscle tissue and therefore is sometimes referred to as *myositis*. This condition, however, is not characterized by the classic clinical signs associated of inflammation (e.g., reddening, swelling). Chronic centrally mediated myalgia results from a source of nociception found in the muscle tissue that has its origin in the CNS (neurogenic inflammation).

The clinician should note that centrally mediated myalgia is more closely associated with a continuity of muscle pain than the actual duration. Many muscle pain disorders are episodic, leaving intermediate times of no muscle pain. Periodic episodes of muscle pain do not produce centrally mediated myalgia. A prolonged and constant period of muscle pain, however, is likely to lead to centrally mediated myalgia.

Causes. The pain associated with centrally mediated myalgia has its cause more in the CNS than in the muscle tissue itself. As the CNS becomes more involved, antidromic neural impulses are sent out to the muscular and vascular tissues, producing local neurogenic inflammation. This neurogenic inflammation produces pain in these tissues even though the main cause is the CNS, hence the term *centrally mediated myalgia*. It is important that the clinician understand this concept because the only manner to effectively manage this condition is to address the central mechanism. Therefore the clinician can not only treat the peripheral structures, such as teeth, muscles, and joints, but must direct therapy to the CNS. This is neither an instinctive nor traditional approach for most dentists. The most common cause of chronic centrally mediated myalgia is protracted local muscle soreness or myofascial pain. In other words, the longer the patient complains of myogenous pain, the greater the likelihood of chronic centrally mediated myalgia.

A clinical characteristic of chronic centrally mediated myalgia is the presence of constant, aching myogenous pain. The pain is present during rest and increases with function. The muscles are tender to palpate, and structural dysfunction is common. The most common clinical feature is the extended duration of the symptoms.

History. Two significant features present in the history of a patient with centrally mediated myalgia.

The first is the duration of the pain problem. As already discussed, centrally mediated myalgia takes time to develop. Therefore the patient will report a long history of myogenous pain. Typically, the pain will have been present for at least 4 weeks and often several months. The second feature of centrally mediated myalgia is the constancy of the pain. Pains that last for months or even years but come and go with periods of total remission are not characteristic of centrally mediated myalgia. Patients will commonly report that even if the jaw is at rest, the pain is present. This reflects an inflammatory condition of the tissue.

Clinical characteristics. The following six clinical characteristics are common with centrally mediated myalgia:

1. *Structural dysfunction.* Patients experiencing centrally mediated myalgia present with a significant decrease in the velocity and range of mandibular movement. This decreased range is secondary to the inhibitory effect of pain (normal range cannot be achieved). The neurogenic inflammation associated with centrally mediated myalgia may lead to a "sterile" inflammatory response of the muscle tissue, which will further reduce range of mandibular movement.

2. *Pain at rest.* As just mentioned, patients with centrally mediated myalgia report myogenous pain even when the muscles are at rest. Pain during rest is a key clinical characteristic of centrally mediated myalgia and is likely caused by the sensitization of muscle nociceptors by the algogenic substances released in the neurogenic inflammation process.[41,68,69]

3. *Increased pain with function.* Function of the affected muscles greatly increases the patient's pain.

4. *Local muscle tenderness.* Muscle tissues are painful when palpated.

5. *Feeling of muscle tightness.* Patients suffering with centrally mediated myalgia will commonly complain of a feeling of muscle tightness.

6. *Muscle contracture.* Prolonged centrally mediated myalgia can lead to a muscle condition known as contracture. *Contracture* refers to a painless shortening of the functional length of a muscle. As discussed in Chapter 2, stretching a muscle to full length stimulates the Golgi tendon organ, which in turn produces relaxation

in the same muscle (inverse stretch reflex). Periodic stretching or lengthening of a muscle is necessary to maintain its working length. When the inverse stretch reflex is not stimulated, the muscle will functionally shorten. This state of contracture will resist any sudden attempt to lengthen the muscle. Contracture is common with centrally mediated myalgia because in order for patients to reduce their pain, they will limit their mouth opening. The treatment of contracture is discussed in Chapter 12.

Systemic Myalgic Disorders

Certain muscle pain complaints have their origin almost entirely within the CNS. Because of this feature, the symptoms are widespread. One such condition is fibromyalgia.

Fibromyalgia (Fibrositis). Fibromyalgia is a chronic, global, musculoskeletal pain disorder. In the past fibromyalgia was referred to in the medical literature as *fibrositis*. According to a 1990 consensus report,[70] fibromyalgia is a widespread musculoskeletal pain disorder in which there is tenderness at 11 or more of 18 specific tender sites throughout the body. Pain must be felt in three of the four quadrants of the body and be present for at least 3 months. Fibromyalgia is not a masticatory pain disorder and therefore needs to be recognized and referred to appropriate medical personnel.

Causes. The cause of fibromyalgia has not been well documented. The continued presence of etiologic factors related to acute myalgic disorders such as constant deep pain and increased emotional stress may be significant. Certainly the hypothalamic-pituitary-adrenal (HPA) axis has been implicated.[71] An ongoing musculoskeletal pain source such as a whiplash injury may have some influence on the development of fibromyalgia, although this is not clear. When this occurs, the condition is referred to as *secondary fibromyalgia.* Certainly other unidentified conditions also lead to fibromyalgia. Presently a reasonable explanation of the cause of fibromyalgia focuses on the manner by which the CNS processes ascending neural input from the musculoskeletal structures. Perhaps future investigations will reveal that fibromyalgia has its origin in the brainstem with a poorly functioning descending inhibitory system (merely my opinion).

History. Patients experiencing fibromyalgia report chronic and generalized musculoskeletal pain complaints in numerous sites throughout the body. Patients often present with a sedentary lifestyle accompanied by some degree of clinical depression. They also commonly report a poor quality of sleep.

Clinical characteristics. Patients suffering with fibromyalgia reveal the following clinical characteristics:

1. *Structural dysfunction.* Patients with fibromyalgia reveal a decrease in the velocity and range of movement secondary to the inhibitory effect of pain.
2. *Pain at rest.* A common complaint of fibromyalgia is a global report of muscle pain. This pain appears in at least three of the four quadrants of the body and is present even when the muscles are at rest.
3. *Increased pain with function.* Fibromyalgia patients report an increase in pain with functional movements of the involved muscles.
4. *Weakness and fatigue.* Patients experiencing fibromyalgia report a general feeling of muscle weakness. They also commonly report chronic fatigue.
5. *Presence of tender points.* Fibromyalgia is characterized by numerous tender points throughout the various quadrants of the body (not to be confused with *trigger points* associated with myofascial pain). These tender points do not produce heterotopic pain when palpated. This finding represents a distinct clinical difference between fibromyalgia and myofascial pain. According to established criteria,[70] fibromyalgia patients must reveal tenderness in at least 11 of 18 predetermined sites throughout three of the four quadrants of the body.
6. *Sedentary physical condition.* Patients with fibromyalgia generally lack physical conditioning. Because muscle function increases pain, fibromyalgia patients often avoid exercise. This becomes a perpetuating condition because sedentary physical condition can be a predisposing factor in fibromyalgia.

TEMPOROMANDIBULAR JOINT DISORDERS

TMJ disorders have their chief symptoms and dysfunctions associated with altered condyle-disc function. Arthralgia is often reported, but dysfunction is the more common finding. Dysfunction symptoms are associated with condylar movement and reported as sensations of clicking and catching of the joint. They are usually constant, repeatable, and sometimes progressive. The presence of pain is not a reliable finding.

TMJ disorders can be subdivided into three major categories: derangements of the condyle-disc complex, structural incompatibilities of the articular surfaces, and inflammatory disorders of the joint.

Derangements of the Condyle-Disc Complex

Causes. Derangements of the condyle-disc complex arise from breakdown of the normal rotational function of the disc on the condyle. This loss of normal disc movement can occur when there is elongation of the discal collateral ligaments and the inferior retrodiscal lamina. Thinning of the posterior border of the disc also predisposes to these types of disorders.

The most common etiologic factor associated with breakdown of the condyle-disc complex is trauma.[72-77] This may be macrotrauma such as a blow to the jaw (open-mouth macrotrauma is usually seen with elongation of the ligaments) or microtrauma[78] as associated with chronic muscle hyperactivity and orthopedic instability (see Chapter 8).

The three types of derangements of the condyle-disc complex are disc displacement, disc dislocation with reduction, and disc dislocation without reduction. These conditions may represent a progression along a continuum and will be presented as such here.

Disc Displacement. If the inferior retrodiscal lamina and the discal collateral ligament become elongated, the disc can be positioned more anteriorly by the superior lateral pterygoid muscle. When this anterior pull is constant, a thinning of the posterior border of the disc may allow the disc to be displaced in a more anterior position (Fig. 10-18).

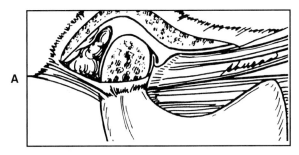

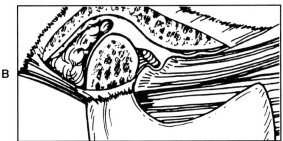

Fig. 10-18 FUNCTIONAL DISPLACEMENT OF THE DISC. A, Normal condyle-disc relationship in the resting closed joint. **B,** Anterior functional displacement of the disc. The posterior discal border has been thinned, and the discal and inferior retrodiscal lamina are sufficiently elongated to allow the disc to be anteromedially displaced.

With the condyle resting on a more posterior portion of the disc, an abnormal translatory shift of the condyle over the disc can occur during opening. Associated with the abnormal condyle-disc movement is a click, which may be felt just during opening (single click) or during both opening and closing (reciprocal clicking).

History. A history of trauma is commonly associated with the onset of joint sounds.[79] Accompanying pain may or may not exist. If pain is present, it is intracapsular and a concomitant of the dysfunction (the click).

Clinical characteristics. Examination reveals joint sounds during opening and closing. Disc displacement is characterized by a normal range of jaw movement during both opening and eccentric movements. Any limitation is caused by pain and not a true structural dysfunction. When reciprocal clicking is present, the two clicks normally occur at different degrees of opening, with the closing click occurring near the intercuspal position. Pain may or may not be present, but when present it is directly related to joint function.

Disc Dislocation with Reduction. If the inferior retrodiscal lamina and discal collateral ligaments become further elongated and the posterior border of the disc sufficiently thinned, the disc can slip or be forced completely through the discal space. Because the disc and condyle no longer articulate, this condition is referred to as a *disc dislocation* (Fig. 10-19). If the patient can so manipulate the jaw as to reposition the condyle onto the posterior border of the disc, the disc is said to be reduced.

History. Normally there is a long history of clicking in the joint and more recently some catching sensation. The patient reports that when it catches and gets stuck, he or she can move the jaw around a little and get it back to functioning normally. The catching may or may not be painful, but if pain is

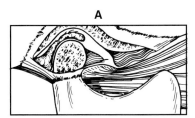

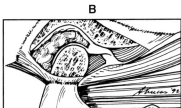

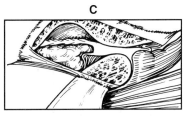

Fig. 10-19 ANTERIORLY DISLOCATED DISC WITH REDUCTION.
A, Resting closed joint position. **B,** During the early stages of translation, the condyle moves up onto the posterior border of the disc. This can be accompanied by a clicking sound. **C,** During the remainder of opening, the condyle assumes a more normal position on the intermediate zone of the disc as the disc is rotating posteriorly on the condyle. During closure the exact opposite occurs. In the final closure the disc is again functionally dislocated anteromedially. Sometimes this is accompanied by a second (reciprocal) click.

present it is directly associated with the dysfunctional symptoms.

Clinical characteristics. Unless the jaw is shifted to the point of reducing the disc, the patient presents with a limited range of opening. When opening reduces the disc, there is a noticeable deviation in the opening pathway. In some instances a sudden loud pop will be heard during the recapturing of the disc. After the disc is reduced, a normal range of mandibular movement is present. In many instances, keeping the mouth in a slightly protruded position after recapturing the disc will eliminate the catching sensations, even during opening and closing. The interincisal distance at which the

disc is reduced during opening is usually greater than when the disc is redislocated during closing.

Disc Dislocation without Reduction. As the ligament becomes more elongated and the elasticity of the superior retrodiscal lamina is lost, recapturing of the disc becomes more difficult. When the disc is not reduced, the forward translation of the condyle merely forces the disc in front of the condyle (Fig. 10-20).

History. Most patients with a history of disc dislocation without reduction know precisely when the dislocation occurred. They can readily relate it to an event (biting on a hard piece of meat or waking up with the condition). They report that the

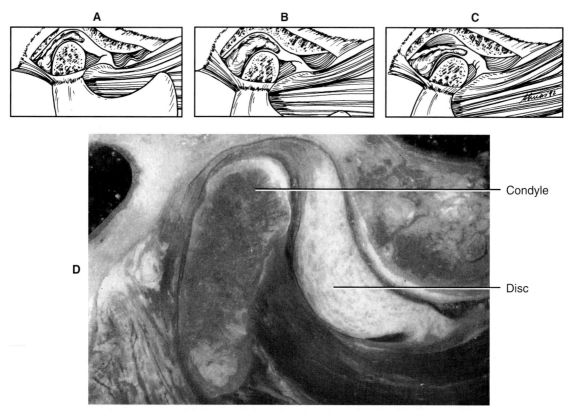

Fig. 10-20 ANTERIORLY DISLOCATED DISC WITHOUT REDUCTION. A, Resting closed joint position. **B,** During the early stages of translation, the condyle does not move onto the disc but instead pushes the disc forward. **C,** The disc becomes jammed forward in the joint, preventing the normal range of condylar translatory movement. This condition is referred to clinically as a *closed lock.* **D,** In this specimen the disc **(D)** is dislocated anterior to the condyle **(C).** *(Courtesy Dr. Per-Lennart Westesson, University of Rochester, NY.)*

jaw is locked closed, so normal opening cannot be achieved. Pain can be associated with dislocation without reduction, but not always. When pain is present, it usually accompanies attempts to open beyond the joint restriction. The history also reveals that the clicking occurred before the locking but not since the disc dislocation has occurred.

Clinical characteristics. The range of mandibular opening is 25 to 30 mm, and the mandible deflects to the involved joint. The maximum point of opening reveals a hard end feel. In other words, if mild, steady, downward force is applied to the lower incisors, there is little increase in mouth opening. Eccentric movements are relatively normal on the ipsilateral side but restricted on the contralateral side. Loading the joint with bilateral manual manipulation is often painful to the affected joint because the condyle is seated on the retrodiscal tissues.

The previous description of a disc dislocation without reduction is especially common when the condition is acute. However, when the condition becomes chronic, the clinical picture becomes less clear. The reason for this is related to the clinical characteristics of ligaments. Remember, ligaments are collagenous fibers that do not stretch. They act as guide wires to limit the border movements of the joint. With time, however, continued forces applied to ligaments cause them to become elongated. This elongation results in a greater range of jaw movement, making the differential diagnosis more difficult. In some patients the only definitive way to be certain that the disc is permanently dislocated is by soft tissue imaging (i.e., magnetic resonance imaging).

Structural Incompatibilities of the Articular Surfaces

Causes. Structurally incompatible articular surfaces can cause several types of disc derangement disorder. They result when normally smooth-sliding surfaces are so altered that friction and sticking inhibit normal joint movements.

A common causative factor is macrotrauma. A blow to the jaw with the teeth together causes impact loading of the articular surfaces, and this may lead to alterations in the joint surfaces. In addition, any trauma-producing hemarthrosis can create structural incompatibility. Hemarthrosis, likewise, may result from injury to the retrodiscal tissue (e.g., a blow to the side of the face) or even from surgical intervention.

The four types of structural incompatibilities of the articular surfaces are (1) deviation in form, (2) adhesions, (3) subluxation, and (4) spontaneous dislocation.

Deviation in Form

Causes. Deviations in form are caused by actual changes in the shape of the articular surfaces. They can occur to the condyle, the fossa, and/or the disc. Alterations in form of the bony surfaces may be a flattening of the condyle or fossa or even a bony protuberance on the condyle (Figs. 10-21 and 10-22). Changes in the form of the disc include both thinning of the borders and perforations.

History. The history associated with alterations in form is usually a long-term dysfunction that may not present as a painful condition. Often the patient has learned a pattern of mandibular movement (altered muscle engrams) that avoids the deviation in form and therefore avoids painful symptoms.

Clinical characteristics. Most deviations in form cause dysfunction at a particular point of movement. Therefore the dysfunction becomes a repeatable observation at the same point of opening (Fig. 10-23). During opening the dysfunction is

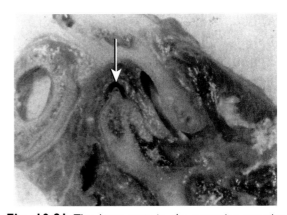

Fig. 10-21 The bony spur in the posterior superior aspect of the condyle *(arrow)* is demonstrated. This significant alteration in form appears to impinge on the retrodiscal tissues likely to lead to pain. *(Courtesy Dr. Terry Tanaka, Chula Vista, Calif.)*

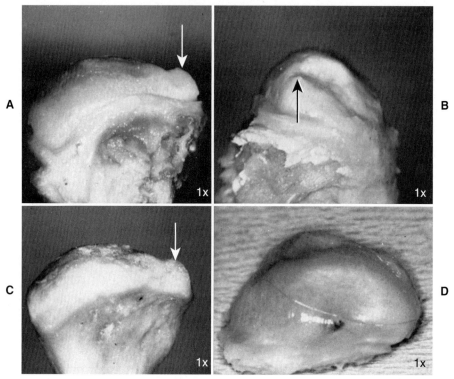

Fig. 10-22 STRUCTURAL INCOMPATIBILITY OF THE ARTICULAR SURFACE. A, Frontal view of a condyle with the fibrous articular surfaces present. The sharp projection *(arrow)* on the medial pole is demonstrated. This type of bony spicule is likely to create interferences during function. **B,** Medial view. The bony spicule *(arrow)* is demonstrated. **C,** The fibrous articular surface has been removed, revealing the sharp bony spicule. **D,** Inferior view of the articular disc. The bony irregularity of the condyle has created a perforation in the disc, an example of what incompatibilities of the structures can do to the joint. *(Courtesy Dr. L.R. Bean, University of Kentucky College of Dentistry, Lexington.)*

observed at the same degree of mandibular separation as during closing. This is a significant finding because disc displacements and dislocations do not present in this manner. Also with deviation in form, the speed and force of opening do not alter the point of dysfunction. With a displaced disc, changing the speed and force of opening can alter the interincisal distance of the click.

Adherences/Adhesions

Causes. An adherence represents a temporary sticking of the articular surfaces and may occur between the condyle and the disc (inferior joint space) or between the disc and the fossa (superior joint space). Adherences commonly result from prolonged static loading of the joint structures.

Adhesions may also arise from a loss of effective lubrication secondary to an hypoxia/reperfusion injury as described in Chapter 8.[80-85]

Although adherences are normally temporary, if they remain they may lead to the more permanent condition of adhesion. Adhesions are produced by the development of fibrosis connective tissue between the articular surfaces of the fossae or condyle and the disc or its surrounding tissues. Adhesions may develop secondary to hemarthrosis or inflammation caused by macrotrauma or surgery.

History. Adherences that develop occasionally but are broken or released during function can be diagnosed only through the history. Usually the patient will report a long period when the jaw was

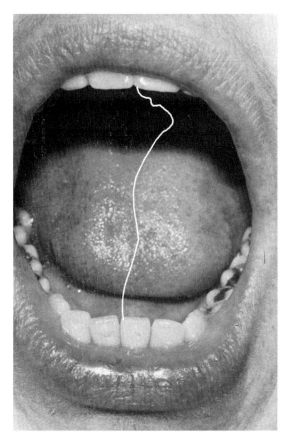

Fig. 10-23 MANDIBULAR DEVIATION ASSO-CIATED WITH INCOMPATIBILITIES OF THE ARTICULAR SURFACE OF THE TEMPORO-MANDIBULAR JOINT. A deviation in opening occurs at the point of structural incompatibility of the joint. Once the incompatibility has been negotiated (passed), the pathway assumes a more normal midline relationship.

statically loaded (such as clenching during sleep). This period was followed by a sensation of limited mouth opening. As the patient tried to open, a single click was felt and normal range of movement was immediately returned. The click or catching sensation does not return during opening and closing unless the joint is again statically loaded for a prolonged time. The adherence occurs because static loading of the joint exhausts weeping lubrication (see Chapter 1). As soon as enough energy is exerted through joint movement to break the adherence, boundary lubrication takes over and sticking does not recur unless the static loading is repeated. These patients typically report that in the morning the jaw appears "stiff" until they pop it once and normal movement is restored. It is believed that, if unattended, these adherences may develop into true adhesions.

When adhesions permanently fix the articular surfaces, the patient complains of reduced function usually associated with limited opening. The symptoms are constant and repeatable. Pain may or may not be present. If pain is a symptom, it is normally associated with attempts to increase opening that elongates ligaments.

Clinical characteristics. When adherences or adhesions occurs between the disc and fossa (superior joint space), normal translation of the condyle-disc complex is inhibited. Therefore movement of the condyle is limited only to rotation (Fig. 10-24). The patient presents with a mandibular opening of only 25 to 30 mm. This is similar to the finding of a disc dislocation without reduction. The major difference is that when the joint is loaded through bilateral manipulation, the intracapsular pain is not provoked. No pain is noted because the manual loading is applied to a disc that is still in

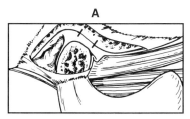
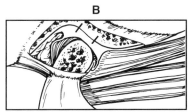
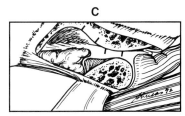

Fig. 10-24 A, Adherence in the superior joint space. **B,** The presence of the adherence limits the joint to only rotation. **C,** If the adherence is freed, normal translation can occur.

proper position for loading. With a disc dislocation without reduction, loading occurs on the retrodiscal tissues, which will likely produce pain.

If long-standing superior joint cavity adhesions are present, the discal collateral and anterior capsular ligaments can become elongated. With this the condyle begins to translate forward, leaving the disc behind. When the condyle is forward, it would appear as if the disc is posteriorly dislocated. In reality the condition is better described as a *fixed disc* (Fig. 10-25). A fixed disc or posterior disc dislocation is not nearly as common as an anterior disc dislocation but has certainly been reported.[86,87] Most posterior disc displacements

are likely the result of an adhesion problem in the superior joint space.

A chronic fixed disc is characterized by relatively normal opening movement with little or no restriction, but during closure the patient senses an inability to get the teeth back into occlusion. In most instances the patient can move the mandible slightly eccentrically and reestablish normal occlusion. The deviation during closure represents the condyle's movement over the anterior border of the disc and back to the intermediate zone.

Adherences or adhesions in the inferior joint space are often more difficult to diagnose. When sticking occurs between the condyle and disc,

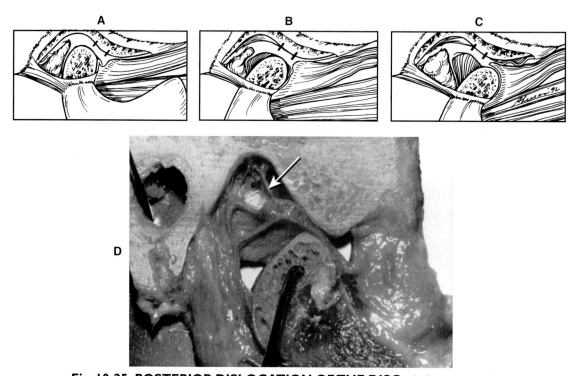

Fig. 10-25 POSTERIOR DISLOCATION OF THE DISC. A, Permanent adhesion between the disc and fossa. **B,** Continued movement of condyle causes elongation of the discal and anterior capsular ligaments, permitting the condyle to move onto the anterior border of the disc. **C,** Eventually the condyle passes over the anterior border of the disc, causing a posterior dislocation of the disc. **D,** In this specimen there appears to be a fibrous attachment from the disc to the superior aspect of the fossa *(arrow).* This attachment limits anterior movement of the disc from the fossa. If the condyle continues to move anteriorly, the disc will be held from moving with the condyle. The condyle will then move over the anterior border of the disc, causing a posterior disc dislocation. *(Courtesy Dr. Terry Tanaka, Chula Vista, Calif.)*

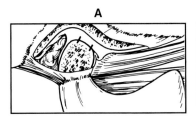 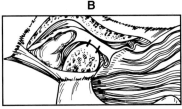 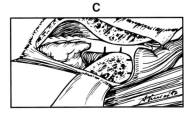

Fig. 10-26 A, Adherence in the inferior joint space. **B,** As the mouth opens, translation between the disc and fossa can occur, but rotation between the disc and condyle is inhibited. This can lead to a sensation of tightness and irregular movement. **C,** If the adherence is freed, normal disc movement returns.

normal rotational movement between them is lost but translation between the disc and fossa is normal (Fig. 10-26). The result is that the patient can open almost normally but senses a stiffness or catching on the way to maximum opening. It is best for the clinician to listen carefully to the patient as he or she describes this sensation because it may be difficult for the examiner to observe.

Subluxation (Hypermobility). Subluxation of the TMJ represents a sudden forward movement of the condyle during the latter phase of mouth opening. As the condyle moves beyond the crest of the eminence, it appears to jump forward to the wide-open position.

Causes. Subluxation occurs in the absence of any pathologic condition. It represents normal joint movement as a result of certain anatomic features. A TMJ whose articular eminence has a steep, short, posterior slope followed by a longer anterior slope that is often more superior than the crest tends to subluxate. This occurs because the steep eminence requires a great deal of rotational movement of the disc on the condyle as the condyle translates out of the fossa. Often the amount of rotational movement of the disc permitted by the anterior capsular ligament is fully utilized before complete translation of the condyle is reached. Because the disc cannot rotate any farther posteriorly, the remaining condylar translation occurs in the form of an anterior movement of the condyle and disc as a unit. This represents a sudden forward jump of the condyle and disc to the maximum translated position.

History. The patient who subluxates will often report that the jaw "goes out" any time he or she opens wide. Some patients report jaw clicking, but

when observed clinically the click is not similar to a disc displacement. The joint sound is best described as a "thud."

Clinical characteristics. Subluxation can be observed clinically merely by requesting the patient to open wide. At the latter stage of opening the condyle will jump forward, leaving a small depression in the face behind it. The lateral pole can be felt or observed during this movement. The midline pathway of mandibular opening will be seen to deviate and return as the condyle moves over the eminence. The deviation is much greater and much closer to the maximally open position than that seen with a disc derangement disorder. Usually no pain is associated with the movement unless it is repeated often (abuse). Subluxation is a repeatable clinical phenomenon that does not vary with changes in speed or force of opening.

Spontaneous Dislocation (Open Lock)

Causes. Spontaneous dislocation represents a hyperextension of the TMJ, resulting in a condition that fixes the joint in the open position and prevents any translation. This condition is clinically referred to as an *open lock* because the patient cannot close the mouth. Like subluxation, it can occur in any joint that is forced open beyond the normal restrictions provided by the ligaments. It occurs most often in joints with anatomic features that produce subluxation.

When the condyle is in the full forward translatory position, the disc is rotated to its fullest posterior extent on the condyle and firm contact exists among the disc, condyle, and articular eminence. In this position the strong retracting force of the superior retrodiscal lamina, along with the

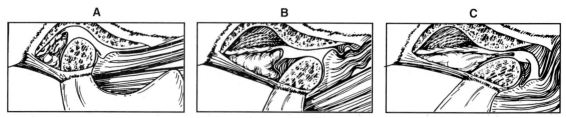

Fig. 10-27 SPONTANEOUS DISLOCATION (WITH DISC ANTERI-ORLY DISLOCATED). A, Normal condyle-disc relationship in the resting closed joint position. **B,** Maximum translated position. The disc has rotated posteriorly on the condyle as far as permitted by the anterior capsular ligament. **C,** If the mouth is forced open wider, the disc is pulled forward by the anterior capsular ligament through the disc space. As the condyle moves superiorly, the disc space collapses, trapping the disc forward.

lack of activity of the superior lateral pterygoid, prevents the disc from being anteriorly displaced. The superior lateral pterygoid normally does not become active until the turnaround phase of the closing cycle. If for some reason it becomes active early (during the most forward translatory position), its forward pull may overcome the superior retrodiscal lamina and the disc will be pulled through the anterior disc space, resulting in a spontaneous anterior dislocation (Fig. 10-27). This premature activity of the muscle can occur during a yawn or when the muscles are fatigued from maintaining the mouth open for a long time.

Spontaneous dislocation can also occur when, at the full extent of translation, force is applied that overextends the opening movement. Because the disc is already in its most posterior rotational position on the condyle, any further rotation tends to carry it into the anterior disc space. If the additional

movement is great enough (forced opening), a spontaneous anterior dislocation results. When this occurs, the condyle moves superiorly against the retrodiscal tissues, reducing the disc space and trapping the disc anterior to the condyle. The amount of anterior displacement is limited by the inferior retrodiscal lamina, which attaches the disc to the posterior aspect of the condyle. If force is applied to the mandible in an attempt to close the mouth without first reducing the dislocation, the inferior retrodiscal lamina will be painfully elongated. Because the superior retrodiscal lamina is fully extended during a spontaneous dislocation, as soon as the discal space becomes wide enough, the disc is drawn back on the condyle and the dislocation is reduced.

Imaging of the TMJ in the open lock position has demonstrated that the disc may also be found posterior to the condyle[88] (Fig. 10-28). The precise

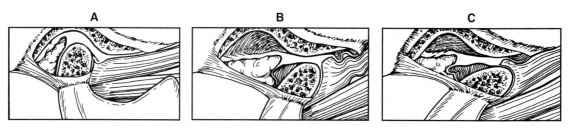

Fig. 10-28 SPONTANEOUS DISLOCATION (WITH DISC POSTERI-ORLY DISLOCATED). A, Normal condyle-disc relationship in the resting closed joint position. **B,** In the maximum translated position the disc has rotated posteriorly on the condyle as far as permitted by the anterior capsular ligament. **C,** If the mouth is forced open wider, the condyle is forced over the disc, dislocating it posterior to the condyle. As the condyle moves superiorly, the disc space collapses, trapping the disc posteriorly.

position of the disc may vary and certainly warrants further study, but in either case the condyle is found to be in front of the crest of the eminence with the discal space collapsed, disallowing normal return of the condyle to the fossa.

The previous description of a spontaneous dislocation reports the etiology to be an anatomic consideration accompanied with a forced opening. Although this is likely the most common cause, it is not the only cause. Some patients present with a history of spontaneous locking that is unrelated to a jaw-opening incidence. In this instance the clinician needs to be suspicious of a muscle etiology causing the open lock. Certain muscle dystonias that affect the jaw muscles can create a sudden, uncontrolled, and often unprovoked muscle contraction. If this dystonia affects the jaw-opening muscles, it causes a sudden and prolonged jaw opening. Specifically this is called a *jaw-opening oromandibular dystonia*. As described in later chapters, this can also affect jaw-closing muscles, disallowing the patient to open the mouth. Importantly, the clinician must appreciate if the spontaneous dislocation is caused by the anatomic structures of the joint or by dystonic activity of the muscles because the treatments are different.

History. Spontaneous dislocation is often associated with wide-open mouth procedures, such as a long dental appointment, but it may also follow an extended yawn. The patient reports that he or she cannot close the mouth. Pain is associated with the dislocation, and this usually causes great distress.

Clinical characteristics. Spontaneous dislocation is easy to diagnosis because it is sudden and the patient is locked in the wide-open mouth position (Fig. 10-29). Clinically the anterior teeth are usually separated, with the posterior teeth closed. The patient cannot verbalize the problem because his or her jaw is locked open but needs to make known the distress and pain felt.

Inflammatory Joint Disorders

Inflammatory disorders of the TMJ are characterized by continuous deep pain, usually accentuated by function. Because the pain is continuous, it can produce secondary central excitatory effects. These usually appear as referred pain, excessive sensitivity to touch (hyperalgesia), and/or increased protective

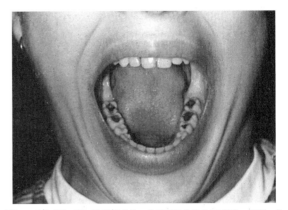

Fig. 10-29 CLINICAL APPEARANCE OF A SPONTANEOUS DISLOCATION (OPEN LOCK). The patient is unable to close the mouth.

co-contraction. Inflammatory joint disorders are classified according to the structures involved: synovitis, capsulitis, retrodiscitis and the arthritides. Several associated structures can also become inflamed.

Synovitis or Capsulitis. Inflammation of the synovial tissues (synovitis) and of the capsular ligament (capsulitis) presents clinically as one disorder; thus a differential diagnosis is difficult. The only way they can be differentiated is by using arthroscopy. Because treatment for each is identical, it becomes academic to separate the two conditions.

Causes. Synovitis and capsulitis usually follow trauma to the tissue, such as macrotrauma (e.g., a blow to the chin) or microtrauma (e.g., a slow impingement on these tissues by an anterior displacement of the disc). Trauma may also arise from wide-open mouth procedures or abusive movements. Sometimes inflammation may spread from adjacent structures.

History. The history often includes an incident of trauma or abuse. The continuous pain usually originates in the joint area, and any movement that elongates the capsular ligament increases it. Because it is a deep, constant pain, secondary central excitatory effects can be created.

Clinical characteristics. The capsular ligament can be palpated by finger pressure over the lateral pole of the condyle. Pain caused by this indicates a capsulitis (Fig. 10-30). Limited mandibular opening secondary to pain is common, and therefore a soft

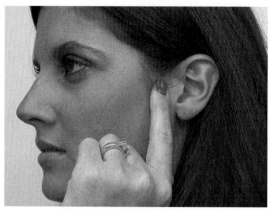

Fig. 10-30 INFLAMMATORY DISORDER OF THE JOINT WITH TENDERNESS TO PALPATION. Movement accentuates the pain.

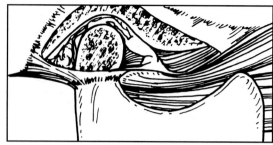

Fig. 10-31 BREAKDOWN OF THE RETRODISCAL TISSUES. Chronic anterior dislocation of the disc will lead to breakdown of the retrodiscal tissues. Once the elasticity of the superior retrodiscal lamina is lost, there is no mechanism to retract or reduce the dislocation. When this occurs, the dislocation is permanent.

end feel is noted. If edema from the inflammation is present, the condyle may be displaced inferiorly, which will create a disocclusion of the ipsilateral posterior teeth.

Retrodiscitis

Causes. Inflammation of the retrodiscal tissues (retrodiscitis) can result from macrotrauma such as a blow to the chin. This trauma can suddenly force the condyle posteriorly into the retrodiscal tissues. When trauma injures these tissues, a secondary inflammatory reaction may result. Microtrauma may also cause retrodiscitis such as in the progressive phases of disc displacement and dislocation. During these conditions the condyle gradually encroaches on the inferior retrodiscal lamina and retrodiscal tissues. This gradually insults these tissues, leading to retrodiscitis (Fig. 10-31).

History. An incident of trauma to the jaw or a progressive disc derangement disorder is the usual finding. The pain is constant, originating in the joint area, and jaw movement accentuates it. Clenching of the teeth increases pain, but clenching on an ipsilateral separator often reduces the pain. Because of the constant deep pain, secondary central excitatory effects are common.

Clinical characteristics. Limited jaw movement is caused by arthralgia. A soft end feel is present unless the inflammation is associated with a disc dislocation. If the retrodiscal tissues swell because of inflammation, the condyle can be forced slightly forward and down the eminence. This creates an acute malocclusion that is observed clinically as disocclusion of the ipsilateral posterior teeth and heavy contact of the contralateral anterior teeth.

Arthritides. *Arthritis* means inflammation of the articular surfaces of the joint. Several types of arthritides can affect the TMJ. The following categories will be used: osteoarthritis, osteoarthrosis, and polyarthritides.

Osteoarthritis and osteoarthrosis

Causes. Osteoarthritis represents a destructive process by which the bony articular surfaces of the condyle and fossa become altered. It is generally considered to be the body's response to increased loading of a joint.[89-91] As loading forces continue and the articular surface becomes softened (chondromalacia), the subarticular bone begins to resorb.[92] Progressive degeneration eventually results in loss of the subchondral cortical layer, bone erosion, and subsequent radiographic evidence of osteoarthritis.[90] Importantly, radiographic changes are only seen in later stages of osteoarthritis and may not reflect the disease accurately (see Chapter 9).

Osteoarthritis is often painful, and symptoms are accentuated by jaw movement. Crepitation (grating joint sounds) is a common finding with this disorder.[93,94] Osteoarthritis can occur any time the joint is overloaded but is most commonly associated with disc dislocation[95-97] or perforation.[98] Once the disc is dislocated and the retrodiscal tissues break down, the condyle begins to articulate directly with the fossa, accelerating the destructive process. In time the dense fibrous articular surfaces are destroyed and bony changes occur (Fig. 10-32). Radiographically, the surfaces seem to be eroded and flattened. Any movement of these surfaces creates pain, so jaw function usually becomes restricted. Although osteoarthritis is in the category of inflammatory disorders, it is not a true inflammatory condition. Often once loading is decreased, the arthritic condition can become adaptive yet the bony morphology remains altered. The adaptive stage has been referred to as *osteoarthrosis*.[89,99] (A more detailed description of osteoarthritis/osteoarthrosis appears in Chapter 13.)

Overloading of the articular surfaces may be caused by high levels of parafunctional activity, especially when the joint structures are not properly aligned to accept the force (orthopedic instability). This occurs particularly in disc dislocations,

when the disc is not interposed between the articular surfaces.

History. The patient with osteoarthritis usually reports unilateral joint pain that is aggravated by mandibular movement. The pain is usually constant but may worsen in the late afternoon or evening. Secondary central excitatory effects are often present. Because osteoarthrosis represents a stable adaptive phase, the patient does not report symptoms.

Clinical characteristics. Limited mandibular opening is characteristic because of the joint pain. A soft end feel is common unless the osteoarthritis is associated with an anteriorly dislocated disc. Crepitation can typically be felt or reported by the patient. The diagnosis is usually confirmed by TMJ radiographs, which will reveal evidence of structural changes in the subarticular bone of the condyle or fossa (i.e., flattening, osteophytes, erosions, which are discussed in Chapter 9) (Fig. 10-33). Osteoarthrosis is confirmed when structural changes in the subarticular bone are seen on radiographs but the patient reports no clinical symptoms of pain.

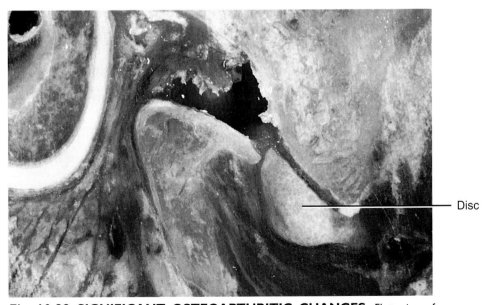

Disc

Fig. 10-32 SIGNIFICANT OSTEOARTHRITIC CHANGES. Flattening of the articular surface of the condyle and the osteophyte is demonstrated. The disc is anteriorly dislocated. *(Courtesy Dr. Per-Lennart Westesson, University of Rochester, NY.)*

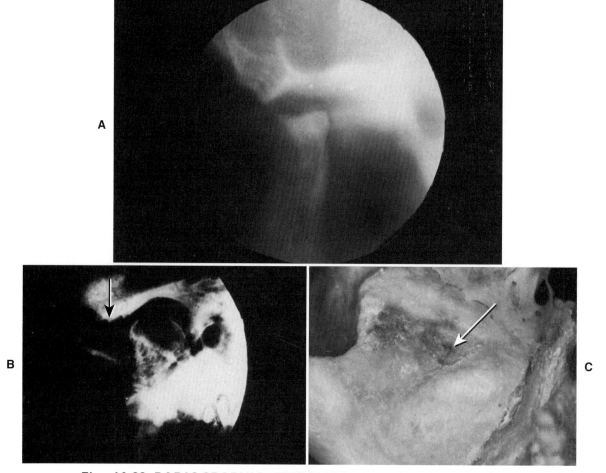

Fig. 10-33 RADIOGRAPHIC EVIDENCE OF OSTEOARTHRITIS.
A, Severely deformed condyle resulting from osteoarthritis (lateral tomogram). **B,** Condyle and fossa (transcranial projection). Irregular surfaces of the subarticular bone near the crest of the articular eminence *(arrow)* are shown. **C,** Mandibular fossa in the previous radiograph (inferior view). Degenerative changes in the articular eminence *(arrow)* are shown. *(Courtesy Dr. L.R. Bean, University of Kentucky College of Dentistry, Lexington.)*

Polyarthritides. Polyarthritides represent a group of disorders in which the articular surfaces of the joint become inflamed. Each is identified according to its causative factors.

Traumatic arthritis. Macrotrauma to the jaw can cause articular surface changes that are great enough to produce inflammation of these surfaces. A positive history of macrotrauma is usually found and can be closely related to the onset of symptoms.

The patient reports constant arthralgia accentuated with movement. There is limited mandibular opening secondary to pain. A soft end feel is common. Acute malocclusion may exist if swelling is present.

Infectious arthritis. A sterile inflammatory reaction of the articular surfaces can be associated with a systemic disease or immunologic response. A nonsterile, inflammatory arthritis may result from a bacterial invasion caused by a penetrating wound, spreading infection from adjacent structures, or even bacteremia following a systemic infection. The history reveals local infection of adjacent tissues or a penetrating wound to the joint. Constant pain is accentuated with movement. Joint swelling and elevated tissue temperature are present clinically. Blood studies and fluid aspirated from the joint cavity may assist in diagnosis.

Rheumatoid arthritis. The precise cause of this systemic disorder affecting multiple joints in the body is unknown. It is an inflammation of the synovial membranes[100-104] that extends into the surrounding connective tissues and articular surfaces, which then become thickened and tender. As force is placed on these surfaces, the synovial cells release enzymes that damage the joint tissues, especially the cartilage.[105] In severe cases even the osseous tissues can be resorbed, with significant loss of condylar support[106] (Fig. 10-34).

Although rheumatoid arthritis is more commonly associated with the joints of the hands, it also may occur in the TMJs and is then almost always bilateral.[107,108] A history of multiple joint complaints is a significant diagnostic finding. In severe cases, when condylar support has been lost, an acute malocclusion results, characterized by heavy posterior contacts and an anterior open bite (Fig. 10-35).[109-112] The diagnosis is confirmed by blood studies.

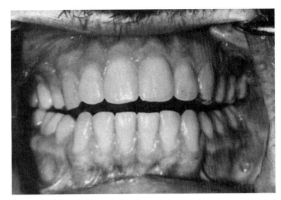

Fig. 10-35 Acute malocclusion from severe condylar bone loss associated with rheumatoid arthritis.

Hyperuricemia. Sometimes dietary changes can lead to hyperuricemia, commonly called *gout*.[113-117] When high levels of serum uric acid persist, urates can be precipitated in the synovial fluid of the TMJs and cause hyperuricemia in these joints. Although the great toe seems to be the joint most commonly involved, the TMJs can also be affected. The symptoms are usually seen in older persons and commonly recur in both joints. Dietary changes are often associated with an increase in symptoms. The pain may or may not be increased with movement. Blood studies or uric acid levels will confirm the diagnosis.

Inflammatory Disorders of Associated Structures. Although not directly related to joint disorders, a few associated structures can also become inflamed. Discussing these conditions in this category is most appropriate. Two structures that need to be considered are (1) temporalis tendonitis and (2) stylomandibular ligament inflammation.

Temporalis tendonitis

Causes. The temporal muscle is attached to the coronoid process by a relatively large tendon. This tendon is susceptible to inflammation, as are other tendons (i.e., elbow).[118,119] Constant and prolonged activity of the temporalis muscle can result in a temporal tendonitis. This muscle hyperactivity may be secondary to bruxism, increased emotional stress, or a constant source of deep pain such as intracapsular pain.

History. Patients with temporal tendonitis will often report a constant pain felt in the temple

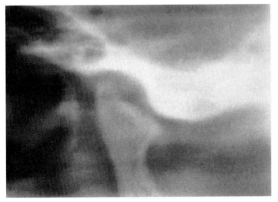

Fig. 10-34 Lateral tomogram of a temporomandibular joint affected by rheumatoid arthritis. (*Courtesy Dr. Jay Mackman, Radiology and Dental Imaging Center of Wisconsin, Milwaukee.*)

region and/or behind the eye. It is usually a unilateral complaint that is aggravated by jaw function.

Clinical characteristics. Temporal tendonitis will commonly produce pain whenever the temporalis muscle is activated (mandibular elevation). A restricted jaw opening is noted with a soft end feel. Intraoral palpation of the temporal tendon will produce extreme pain. This is accomplished by placing a finger on the ascending ramus and moving it up as high as possible to the most superior portion of the coronoid process.

Stylomandibular ligament inflammation. Some authors[120,121] have suggested that the stylomandibular ligament can become inflamed, producing pain at the angle of the mandibular and even radiating superiorly to the eye and temple. Although little scientific evidence has been found, it is not unrealistic to assume that on occasion this ligament may become inflamed. This condition can be identified by placing the finger at the angle of the mandible and attempting to move inward onto the medial aspect of the mandible where the stylomandibular ligament is attached.

CHRONIC MANDIBULAR HYPOMOBILITY

Chronic mandibular hypomobility is a long-term, painless restriction of the mandible. Pain is elicited only when force is used to attempt opening beyond the limitations. The condition can be classified according to the cause as ankylosis, muscle contracture, and coronoid process impedance.

Ankylosis

Sometimes the intracapsular surfaces of the joint develop adhesions that prohibit normal movements. This is called *ankylosis*. When ankylosis is present, the mandible cannot translate from the fossa, resulting in a restricted range of movement. Ankylosis can result from fibrous adhesions in the joint or fibrotic changes in the capsular ligament. On occasion a bony ankylosis can develop in which the condyle actually joins with the fossa.

Causes. The most common source of ankylosis is macrotrauma. This trauma causes tissue damage resulting in secondary inflammation. Trauma may also cause hemarthrosis or bleeding

within the joint that can set up a matrix for the development of fibrosis. Another common source of trauma is TMJ surgery. Surgery often produces fibrotic changes in the capsular ligament, restricting mandibular movement. Osseous ankylosis is more commonly associated with a previous infection.

History. Patients often report a previous injury or capsulitis along with an obvious limitation in mandibular movement. The limited opening has been present for a considerable period of time.

Clinical Characteristics. Movement is restricted in all positions (open, lateral, protrusive), and if the ankylosis is unilateral, midline pathway deflection will be to that side during opening. TMJ radiographs can be used to confirm this. The condyle will not move significantly in protrusion or laterotrusion to the contralateral side, and therefore no significant difference is apparent in these two films. Bony ankylosis can also be confirmed with radiographs.

Muscle Contracture

In this discussion, *muscle contracture* refers to the clinical shortening of the resting length of a muscle without interfering in its ability to contract further. Bell[122] has described two types of muscle contracture: (1) *myostatic* and (2) *myofibrotic*. It may be difficult to differentiate between these clinically, but differentiation is important because they respond differently to therapy. In fact, sometimes it is the therapy that confirms the diagnosis.

Myostatic Contracture

Causes. Myostatic contracture results when a muscle is kept from fully relaxing (stretching) for a prolonged time. The restriction may be caused by the fact that full relaxation causes pain in an associated structure. For example, if the mouth can open only 25 mm without pain in the TMJ, the elevator muscles will protectively restrict movement to within this range. If this situation continues, myostatic contraction will result.

History. The patient reports a long history of restricted jaw movement. It may have begun secondary to a pain condition that has now resolved.

Clinical characteristics. Myostatic contracture is characterized by painless limitation of mouth opening.

Myofibrotic Contracture

Causes. Myofibrotic contracture occurs as a result of tissue adhesions within the muscle or its sheath. It commonly follows a myositic condition or trauma to the muscle.

History. The history for myofibrotic contracture reveals a previous muscle injury or a long-term restriction in the range of movement. The patient has no pain complaints. Sometimes the patient will not even be aware of the limited range of opening because it has been present for so long.

Clinical characteristics. Myofibrotic contracture is characterized by painless limitation of mouth opening. Lateral condylar movement is unaffected (Fig. 10-36). Thus if the diagnosis is difficult, radiographs showing limited condylar movement during opening but normal movement during lateral excursions may help. No acute malocclusion occurs.

Coronoid Impedance

Causes. During opening the coronoid process passes anteroinferiorly between the zygomatic process and the posterior lateral surface of the maxilla. If the coronoid process is extremely long or if fibrosis has developed in this area, its movement will be inhibited and chronic hypomobility of the mandible may result.[123-127] Trauma to or an infection in the area just anterior to the coronoid process can lead to fibrotic adhesions or union of these tissues. Surgical intervention in the area can also cause coronoid impedance. Possibly in certain conditions the coronoid process becomes elongated, which would prevent its movement through this soft tissue area. These conditions may all be related to a chronically dislocated disc.[128]

History. Painless restriction of opening in many cases followed trauma to the area or an infection. A long-standing anterior disc dislocation may also have occurred.

Clinical Characteristics. Limitation is evident in all movements, but especially in protrusion. A straight midline opening path is commonly observed, unless one coronoid process is more free than the other. If the problem is unilateral, opening will deflect the mandible to the same side.

GROWTH DISORDERS

TMDs resulting from growth disturbances may be caused by a variety of etiologies. The growth disturbance may be in the bones or the muscles. Common growth disturbances of the bones are agenesis (no growth), hypoplasia (insufficient growth), hyperplasia (too much growth), or neoplasia (uncontrolled, destructive growth). Common growth disturbances of the muscles are hypotrophy (weakened muscle), hypertrophy (increased size and strength of the muscle), and neoplasia (uncontrolled, destructive growth).

Causes

Deficiency of or alterations in growth typically result from trauma and can induce major malocclusions. Neoplastic activity involving the TMJ is rare but, if left undiagnosed, can become aggressive.

History

A common characteristic of growth disorders is that the clinical symptoms reported by the patient are directly related to the structural changes present.

Clinical Characteristics

Any alteration of function or the presence of pain is secondary to structural changes. Clinical asymmetry may be noticed that is associated with and indicative of a growth or developmental interruption. Radiographs of the TMJ are extremely important in identifying structural (bony) changes that have taken place.

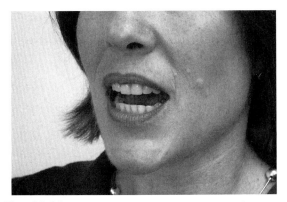

Fig. 10-36 Myofibrotic contracture has caused permanent restriction in mandibular opening. The restricted movement is not painful.

SUMMARY

A classification to aid in the identification and diagnosis of TMDs has been presented. It does not include all disorders that cause pain and dysfunction of the head and neck. Diseases of vascular origins (e.g., arteritis, migraine headache) and neural origin (e.g., trigeminal and glossopharyngeal neuralgia) have not been included. Likewise, craniocervical disorders, as well as ear and eye diseases, have not been addressed. This classification is useful, however, in identifying the common functional disturbances of the masticatory system that fall within the context of this book. When a patient's problems do not fit into one of these categories, more extensive examination procedures are indicated. The reader is encouraged to pursue other texts[129] on the subject.

References

1. Travell JG, Simons DG: *Myofascial pain and dysfunction. The trigger point manual,* Baltimore, 1983, Williams & Wilkins, pp 74-86.
2. Pizzolato P, Mannheimer W: *Histopathologic effects of local anesthetic drugs and related substances,* Springfield, Ill, 1961, Charles C Thomas.
3. Burke GWJ, Fedison JR, Jones CR: Muscle degeneration produced by local anesthetics, *Va Dent J* 49:33-37, 1972.
4. Travell JG, Simons DG: *Myofascial pain and dysfunction. The trigger point manual,* Baltimore, 1983, Williams & Wilkins, pp 165-332.
5. Yagiela JA, Benoit PW, Buoncristiani RD, Peters MP, Fort NF: Comparison of myotoxic effects of lidocaine with epinephrine in rats and humans, *Anesth Analg* 60:471-480, 1981.
6. Ernest EA: *Temporomandibular joint and craniofacial pain,* Montgomery, Ala, 1983, Ernest Publications, pp 105-113.
7. Laskin JL, Wallace WR, DeLeo B: Use of bupivacaine hydrochloride in oral surgery—a clinical study, *J Oral Surg* 35:25-29, 1977.
8. Guttu RL, Page DG, Laskin DM: Delayed healing of muscle after injection of bupivacaine and steroid, *Ann Dent* 49:5-8, 1990.
9. Simons DG, Travell JG, Simons LS: *Travell & Simons' myofascial pain and dysfunction: the trigger point manual,* ed 2, Baltimore, 1999, Lippincott Williams & Wilkins.
10. Fine PG, Milano R, Hare BD: The effects of myofascial trigger point injections are naloxone reversible, *Pain* 32:15-20, 1988.
11. Hameroff SR, Crago BR, Blitt CD, Womble J, Kanel J: Comparison of bupivacaine, etidocaine, and saline for trigger-point therapy, *Anesth Analg* 60:752-755, 1981.
12. Schmidt BL, Pogrel MA, Necoechea M, Kearns G: The distribution of the auriculotemporal nerve around the temporomandibular joint, *Oral Surg Oral Med Oral Pathol Oral Radiol Endod* 86:165-168, 1998.
13. Donlon WC, Truta MP, Eversole LR: A modified auriculotemporal nerve block for regional anesthesia of the temporomandibular joint, *J Oral Maxillofac Surg* 42:544-545, 1984.
14. Isacsson G, Linde C, Isberg A: Subjective symptoms in patients with temporomandibular joint disk displacement versus patients with myogenic craniomandibular disorders, *J Prosthet Dent* 61:70-77, 1989.
15. Bush FM, Whitehill JM, Martelli MF: Pain assessment in temporomandibular disorders, *Cranio* 7:137-143, 1989.
16. Bell WE: *Temporomandibular disorders: classification, diagnosis, management,* ed 2, Chicago, 1986, Year Book Medical.
17. Griffiths RH: Report of the President's Conference on examination, diagnosis and management or temporomandibular disorders, *J Am Dent Assoc* 106:75-77, 1983.
18. Lund JP, Olsson KA: The importance of reflexes and their control during jaw movements, *Trends Neuro Sci* 6:458-463, 1983.
19. Stohler C, Yamada Y, Ash MM: Antagonistic muscle stiffness and associated reflex behaviour in the pain-dysfunctional state, *Helv Odont Acta* 29:719-726, 1985.
20. Stohler CS, Ash MM: Excitatory response of jaw elevators associated with sudden discomfort during chewing, *J Oral Rehabil* 13:225-233, 1986.
21. Ashton-Miller JA, McGlashen KM, Herzenberg JE, Stohler CS: Cervical muscle myoelectric response to acute experimental sternocleidomastoid pain, *Spine* 15:1006-1012, 1990.
22. Lund JP, Donga R, Widmer CG, Stohler CS: The pain-adaptation model: a discussion of the relationship between chronic musculoskeletal pain and motor activity, *Can J Physiol Pharmacol* 69:683-694, 1991.
23. Smith AM: The coactivation of antagonist muscles, *Can J Physiol Pharmacol* 59:733-747, 1981.
24. Stohler CS: Clinical perspectives on masticatory and related muscle disorders. In Sessle BJ, Bryant PS, Dionne RA, editors: *Temporomandibular disorders and related pain conditions,* Seattle, 1995, IASP Press, pp 3-29.
25. Carlson CR, Okeson JP, Falace DA, Nitz AJ, Curran SL et al: Comparison of psychological and physiological functioning between patients with masticatory muscle pain and matched controls, *J Orofac Pain* 7:15-22, 1993.
26. Curran SL, Carlson CR, Okeson JP: Emotional and physiologic responses to laboratory challenges: patients with temporomandibular disorders versus matched control subjects, *J Orofac Pain* 10:141-150, 1996.
27. De Leeuw R, Bertoli E, Schmidt JE, Carlson CR: Prevalence of post-traumatic stress disorder symptoms in orofacial pain patients, *Oral Surg Oral Med Oral Pathol Oral Radiol Endod* 99:558-568, 2005.
28. Lindroth JE, Schmidt JE, Carlson CR: A comparison between masticatory muscle pain patients and intracapsular pain patients on behavioral and psychosocial domains, *J Orofac Pain* 16:277-283, 2002.

29. Sherman JJ, Carlson CR, Wilson JF, Okeson JP, McCubbin JA: Post-traumatic stress disorder among patients with orofacial pain, *J Orofac Pain* 19:309-317, 2005.

30. Lous I, Sheik-Ol-Eslam A, Moller E: Postural activity in subjects with functional disorders of the chewing apparatus, *Scand J Dent Res* 78:404-410, 1970.

31. Sheikholeslam A, Moller E, Lous I: Postural and maximal activity in elevators of mandible before and after treatment of functional disorders, *Scand J Dent Res* 90:37-46, 1982.

32. Schroeder H, Siegmund H, Santibanez G, Kluge A: Causes and signs of temporomandibular joint pain and dysfunction: an electromyographical investigation, *J Oral Rehabil* 18:301-310, 1991.

33. Lund JP, Widmer CG, Feine JS: Validity of diagnostic and monitoring tests used for temporomandibular disorders, *J Dent Res* 74:1133-1143, 1995.

34. Mao J, Stein RB, Osborn JW: Fatigue in human jaw muscles: a review, *J Orofac Pain* 7:135-142, 1993.

35. Watanabe M, Tabata T, Huh JI, Inai T, Tsuboi A et al: Possible involvement of histamine in muscular fatigue in temporomandibular disorders: animal and human studies, *J Dent Res* 78:769-775, 1999.

36. Hikida RS, Staron RS, Hagerman FC, Sherman WM, Costill DL: Muscle fiber necrosis associated with human marathon runners, *J Neurol Sci* 59:185-203, 1983.

37. Schmitt HP, Bersch W, Feustel HP: Acute abdominal rhabdomyolysis after body building exercise: is there a rectus abdominus syndrome? *Muscle Nerve* 6:228-232, 1983.

38. Byrnes WC, Clarkson PM: Delayed onset muscle soreness and training, *Clin Sports Med* 5:605-614, 1986.

39. Bobbert MF, Hollander AP, Huijing PA: Factors in delayed onset muscular soreness of man, *Med Sci Sports Exerc* 18:75-81, 1986.

40. Mense S: Nociception from skeletal muscle in relation to clinical muscle pain, *Pain* 54:241-289, 1993.

41. Mense S: Considerations concerning the neurobiological basis of muscle pain, *Can J Physiol Pharmacol* 69:610-616, 1991.

42. Sinn DP, de Assis EA, Throckmorton GS: Mandibular excursions and maximum bite forces in patients with temporomandibular joint disorders, *J Oral Maxillofac Surg* 54:671-679, 1996.

43. High AS, Macgregor AJ, Tomlinson GE, Salkouskis PM: A gnathodynanometer as an objective means of pain assessment following wisdom tooth removal, *Br J Oral Maxillofac Surg* 26:284-291, 1988.

44. Okeson JP: *Bell's orofacial pains*, ed 6, Chicago, 2005, Quintessence, pp 63-94.

45. Gonzales R, Coderre TJ, Sherbourne CD, Levine JD: Postnatal development of neurogenic inflammation in the rat, *Neurosci Lett* 127:25-27, 1991.

46. Levine JD, Dardick SJ, Basbaum AI, Scipio E: Reflex neurogenic inflammation. I. Contribution of the peripheral nervous system to spatially remote inflammatory responses that follow injury, *J Neurosci* 5:1380-1386, 1985.

47. Carlson CR, Okeson JP, Falace DA, Nitz AJ, Lindroth JE: Reduction of pain and EMG activity in the masseter region by trapezius trigger point injection, *Pain* 55:397-400, 1993.

48. Yemm R: A neurophysiological approach to the pathology and aetiology of temporomandibular dysfunction, *J Oral Rehabil* 12:343-353, 1985.

49. Lund JP, Widmer CG: Evaluation of the use of surface electromyography in the diagnosis, documentation, and treatment of dental patients, *J Craniomandib Disord* 3:125-137, 1989.

50. Kakulas BA, Adams RD: *Diseases of muscle*, Philadelphia, 1985, Harper & Row, pp 725-727.

51. Fricton JR, Kroening R, Haley D, Siegert R: Myofascial pain syndrome of the head and neck: a review of clinical characteristics of 164 patients, *Oral Surg Oral Med Oral Pathol* 60:615-623, 1985.

52. Travell JG, Rinzler SH: The myofascial genesis of pain, *Postgrad Med* 11:425-434, 1952.

53. Laskin DM: Etiology of the pain-dysfunction syndrome, *J Am Dent Assoc* 79:147-153, 1969.

54. Fischer AA: Documentation of myofascial trigger points, *Arch Phys Med Rehabil* 69:286-291, 1988.

55. Vecchiet L, Giamberardino MA, Saggini R: Myofascial pain syndromes: clinical and pathophysiological aspects, *Clin J Pain* 1:S16-22, 1991.

56. Hong CZ, Simons DG: Pathophysiologic and electrophysiologic mechanisms of myofascial trigger points, *Arch Phys Med Rehabil* 79:863-872, 1998.

57. Simons DG, Travell J: Myofascial trigger points, a possible explanation [letter], *Pain* 10:106-109, 1981.

58. Mense S, Meyer H: Bradykinin-induced sensitization of high-threshold muscle receptors with slowly conducting afferent fibers, *Pain* (suppl 1):S204, 1981.

59. Travell J: Introductory comments. In Ragan C, editor: *Connective tissues. Transactions of the fifth conference*, New York, 1954, Josiah Macy Jr, pp 12-22.

60. Simons DG, Travell JG, Simons LS: *Travell & Simons' myofascial pain and dysfunction: the trigger point manual*, ed 2, Baltimore, 1999, Lippincott Williams & Wilkins, pp. 19-44.

61. Hong CZ, Kuan TS, Chen JT, Chen SM: Referred pain elicited by palpation and by needling of myofascial trigger points: a comparison, *Arch Phys Med Rehabil* 78:957-960, 1997.

62. Simons DG, Travell JG, Simons LS: *Travell & Simons' myofascial pain and dysfunction: the trigger point manual*, ed 2, Baltimore, 1999, Lippincott Williams & Wilkins, pp 178-235.

63. Simons DG, Travell JG, Simons LS: *Travell & Simons' myofascial pain and dysfunction: the trigger point manual*, ed 2, Baltimore, 1999, Lippincott Williams & Wilkins, p 125.

64. Moldofsky H, Scarisbrick P: Induction of neurasthenic musculoskeletal pain syndrome by selective sleep stage deprivation, *Psychosom Med* 38:35-44, 1976.

65. Moldofsky H, Scarisbrick P, England R, Smythe H: Musculoskeletal symptoms and non-REM sleep disturbance in patients with "fibrositis" and healthy subjects, *Psychosom Med* 37:341, 1986.

66. Simons DG, Travell JG, Simons LS: *Travell & Simons' myofascial pain and dysfunction: the trigger point manual,* ed 2, Baltimore, 1999, Lippincott Williams & Wilkins, pp 445-471.

67. Simons DG, Travell JG, Simons LS: *Travell & Simons' myofascial pain and dysfunction: the trigger point manual,* ed 2, Baltimore, 1999, Lippincott Williams & Wilkins, pp 110-112.

68. Hoheisel U, Mense S, Simons DG, Yu XM: Appearance of new receptive fields in rat dorsal horn neurons following noxious stimulation of skeletal muscle: a model for referral of muscle pain? *Neurosci Lett* 153:9-12, 1993.

69. Mense S: The pathogenesis of muscle pain, *Curr Pain Headache Rep* 7:419-425, 2003.

70. Wolfe F, Smythe HA, Yunus MB, Bennett RM, Bombardier C et al: The American College of Rheumatology 1990 criteria for the classification of fibromyalgia. Report of the Multicenter Criteria Committee, *Arthritis Rheum* 33: 160-172, 1990.

71. Griep EN, Boersma JW, de Kloet ER: Altered reactivity of the hypothalamic-pituitary-asdrenal axis in the primary fibromyalgia syndrome, *J Rheumatol* 20:469-474, 1993.

72. Harkins SJ, Marteney JL: Extrinsic trauma: a significant precipitating factor in temporomandibular dysfunction, *J Prosthet Dent* 54:271-272, 1985.

73. Braun BL, DiGiovanna A, Schiffman E, Bonnema J, Fricton J: A cross-sectional study of temporomandibular joint dysfunction in post-cervical trauma patients, *J Craniomandib Disord* 6:24-31, 1992.

74. Pullinger AG, Seligman DA: TMJ osteoarthrosis: a differentiation of diagnostic subgroups by symptom history and demographics, *J Craniomandib Disord* 1:251-256, 1987.

75. Pullinger AG, Seligman DA: Trauma history in diagnostic groups of temporomandibular disorders, *Oral Surg Oral Med Oral Pathol* 71:529-534, 1991.

76. Skolnick J, Iranpour B, Westesson PL, Adair S: Prepubertal trauma and mandibular asymmetry in orthognathic surgery and orthodontic patients, *Am J Orthod Dentofacial Orthop* 105:73-77, 1994.

77. Yun PY, Kim YK: The role of facial trauma as a possible etiologic factor in temporomandibular joint disorder, *J Oral Maxillofac Surg* 63:1576-1583, 2005.

78. Zhang ZK, Ma XC, Gao S, Gu ZY, Fu KY: Studies on contributing factors in temporomandibular disorders, *Chin J Dent Res* 2:7-20, 1999.

79. Pullinger AG, Monteiro AA: History factors associated with symptoms of temporomandibular disorders, *J Oral Rehabil* 15:117-124, 1988.

80. Nitzan DW, Nitzan U, Dan P, Yedgar S: The role of hyaluronic acid in protecting surface-active phospholipids from lysis by exogenous phospholipase A(2), *Rheumatology (Oxford)* 40:336-340, 2001.

81. Nitzan DW: The process of lubrication impairment and its involvement in temporomandibular joint disc displacement: a theoretical concept, *J Oral Maxillofac Surg* 59: 36-45, 2001.

82. Nitzan DW, Marmary Y: The "anchored disc phenomenon": a proposed etiology for sudden-onset, severe, and persistent closed lock of the temporomandibular joint, *J Oral Maxillofac Surg* 55:797-802; discussion 802-803, 1997.

83. Zardeneta G, Milam SB, Schmitz JP: Iron-dependent generation of free radicals: plausible mechanisms in the progressive deterioration of the temporomandibular joint, *J Oral Maxillofac Surg* 58:302-308; discussion 309, 2000.

84. Dan P, Nitzan DW, Dagan A, Ginsburg I, Yedgar S: H2O2 renders cells accessible to lysis by exogenous phospholipase A2: a novel mechanism for cell damage in inflammatory processes, *FEBS Lett* 383:75-78, 1996.

85. Nitzan DW: 'Friction and adhesive forces'—possible underlying causes for temporomandibular joint internal derangement, *Cells Tissues Organs* 174:6-16, 2003.

86. Blankestijn J, Boering G: Posterior dislocation of the temporomandibular disc, *Int J Oral Surg* 14:437-443, 1985.

87. Gallagher DM: Posterior dislocation of the temporomandibular joint meniscus: report of three cases, *J Am Dent Assoc* 113:411-415, 1986.

88. Kai S, Kai H, Nakayama E, Tabata O, Tashiro H et al: Clinical symptoms of open lock position of the condyle. Relation to anterior dislocation of the temporomandibular joint, *Oral Surg Oral Med Oral Pathol* 74:143-148, 1992.

89. Stegenga B, de Bont LG, Boering G: Osteoarthrosis as the cause of craniomandibular pain and dysfunction: a unifying concept, *J Oral Maxillofac Surg* 47:249-256, 1989.

90. Stegenga B, de Bont LG, Boering G, van Willigen JD: Tissue responses to degenerative changes in the temporomandibular joint: a review, *J Oral Maxillofac Surg* 49: 1079-1088, 1991.

91. De Bont LG, Stegenga B: Pathology of temporomandibular joint internal derangement and osteoarthrosis, *Int J Oral Maxillofac Surg* 22:71-74, 1993.

92. Quinn JH, Stover JD: Arthroscopic management of temporomandibular joint disc perforations and associated advanced chondromalacia by discoplasty and abrasion arthroplasty: a supplemental report, *J Oral Maxillofac Surg* 56:1237-1239; discussion 1239-1240, 1998.

93. De Leeuw R, Boering G, Stegenga B, de Bont LG: Temporomandibular joint osteoarthrosis: clinical and radiographic characteristics 30 years after nonsurgical treatment: a preliminary report, *Cranio* 11:15-24, 1993.

94. De Leeuw R, Boering G, Stegenga B, de Bont LG: Clinical signs of TMJ osteoarthrosis and internal derangement 30 years after nonsurgical treatment, *J Orofac Pain* 8:18-24, 1994.

95. De Bont LGM, Boering G, Liem RSB, Eulderink F, Westesson PL: Osteoarthritis and internal derangement of the temporomandibular joint: a light microscopic study, *J Oral Maxillofac Surg* 44:634-643, 1986.

96. Mills DK, Daniel JC, Herzog S, Scapino RP: An animal model for studying mechanisms in human temporomandibular joint disc derangement, *J Oral Maxillofac Surg* 52:1279-1292, 1994.

97. Dimitroulis G: The prevalence of osteoarthrosis in cases of advanced internal derangement of the temporomandibular joint: a clinical, surgical and histological study, *Int J Oral Maxillofac Surg* 34:345-349, 2005.

98. Helmy E, Bays R, Sharawy M: Osteoarthrosis of the temporomandibular joint following experimental disc perforation in Macaca fascicularis, *J Oral Maxillofac Surg* 46:979-990, 1988.

99. Boering G: *Temporomandibular joint arthrosis: a clinical and radiographic investigation: thesis*, Groningen, The Netherlands, 1966, University of Groningen.

100. Carlsson GE: Arthritis and allied diseases of the temporomandibular joint. In Zarb GA, Carlsson GE, editors: *Temporomandibular joint; function and dysfunction*, St Louis, 1979, Mosby, pp 293-304.

101. Appelgren A, Appelgren B, Kopp S, Lundeberg T, Theodorsson E: Neuropeptide in arthritic TMJ and symptoms and signs from the stomatognathic system with special consideration to rheumatoid arthritis, *J Orofac Pain* 9:215-225, 1995.

102. Moore ME: Management of pain of rheumatologic origin in the head and neck, *Trans Pa Acad Ophthalmol Otolaryngol* 34:174-178, 1981.

103. Larheim TA, Johannessen S, Tveito L: Abnormalities of the temporomandibular joint in adults with rheumatic disease. A comparison of panoramic, transcranial and transpharyngeal radiography with tomography, *Dentomaxillofac Radiol* 17:109-113, 1988.

104. Donaldson KW: Rheumatoid diseases and the temporomandibular joint: a review, *Cranio* 13:264-269, 1995.

105. Kerby GP, Taylor SM: Enzymatic activity in human synovial fluid from rheumatoid and nonrheumatoid patients, *Proc Soc Exp Biol Med* 126:865-868, 1962.

106. Grinin VM, Smirnov AV: [The clinical x-ray variants of the osteolytic forms of rheumatoid arthritis of the temporomandibular joint], *Stomatologia* 75:40-43, 1996.

107. Celiker R, Gokce-Kutsal Y, Eryilmaz M: Temporomandibular joint involvement in rheumatoid arthritis. Relationship with disease activity, *Scand J Rheumatol* 24:22-25, 1995.

108. Chenitz JE: Rheumatoid arthritis and its implications in temporomandibular disorders, *Cranio* 10:59-69, 1992.

109. Guyuron B: Facial deformity of juvenile rheumatoid arthritis, *Plast Reconstr Surg* 81:948-951, 1988.

110. Nordahl S, Alstergren P, Eliasson S, Kopp S: Radiographic signs of bone destruction in the arthritic temporomandibular joint with special reference to markers of disease activity. A longitudinal study, *Rheumatology (Oxford)* 40:691-694, 2001.

111. Pedersen TK, Jensen JJ, Melsen B, Herlin T: Resorption of the temporomandibular condylar bone according to subtypes of juvenile chronic arthritis, *J Rheumatol* 28:2109-2115, 2001.

112. Kobayashi R, Utsunomiya T, Yamamoto H, Nagura H: Ankylosis of the temporomandibular joint caused by rheumatoid arthritis: a pathological study and review, *J Oral Sci* 43:97-101, 2001.

113. Wyngarden JB: Etiology and pathogenesis of gout. In Hollender JL, editor: *Arthritis and allied conditions*, Philadelphia, 1966, Lea & Febiger, pp 899-905.

114. Gross BD, Williams RB, DiCosimo CJ, Williams SV: Gout and pseudogout of the temporomandibular joint, *Oral Surg Oral Med Oral Pathol* 63:551-554, 1987.

115. Chun HH: Temporomandibular joint gout, *JAMA* 226:353, 1973.

116. Tanaka TT: A rational approach to the differential diagnosis of arthritic disorders, *J Prosthet Dent* 56:727-731, 1986.

117. Holmes EW: Clinical gout and the pathogenesis of hyperuricemia. In McCarty DJ, editor: *Arthritis and allied conditions*, Philadelphia, 1985, Lea & Febiger, pp 245-250.

118. Ernest EA, Martinez ME, Rydzewski DB, Salter EG: Photomicrographic evidence of insertion tendonosis: the etiologic factor in pain for temporal tendonitis, *J Prosthet Dent* 65:127-131, 1991.

119. Ernest EA: Temporal tendonitis: a painful disorder that mimics migraine headache, *J Neurol Orthop Surg* 8:160-167, 1987.

120. Ernest EA: Three disorders that frequently cause temporomandibular joint pain: internal derangement, temporal tendonitis, and Ernest syndrome, *J Neurol Orthop Surg* 7:189-195, 1987.

121. Shankland WE: Ernest syndrome as a consequence of stylomandibular ligament injury: a report of 68 patients, *J Prosthet Dent* 57:501-506, 1987.

122. Bell WE: *Temporomandibular disorders: classification, diagnosis, management*, ed 3, Chicago, 1990, Year Book Medical, p 173.

123. Shultz RE, Theisen FC: Bilateral coronoid hyperplasia. Report of a case, *Oral Surg Oral Med Oral Pathol* 68:23-26, 1989.

124. Hall RE, Orbach S, Landesberg R: Bilateral hyperplasia of the mandibular coronoid processes: a report of two cases, *Oral Surg Oral Med Oral Pathol* 67:141-145, 1989.

125. Munk PL, Helms CA: Coronoid process hyperplasia: CT studies, *Radiology* 171:783-784, 1989.

126. Loh HS, Ling SY, Lian CB, Shanmuhasuntharam P: Bilateral coronoid hyperplasia—a report with a view on its management, *J Oral Rehabil* 24:782-787, 1997.

127. Murakami K, Yokoe Y, Yasuda S, Tsuboi Y, Iizuka T: Prolonged mandibular hypomobility patient with a "square mandible" configuration with coronoid process and angle hyperplasia, *Cranio* 18:113-119, 2000.

128. Isberg A, Isacsson G, Nah KS: Mandibular coronoid process locking: a prospective study of frequency and association with internal derangement of the temporomandibular joint, *Oral Surg Oral Med Oral Pathol* 63:275-279, 1987.

129. Okeson JP: *Bell's orofacial pains*, ed 6, Chicago, 2005, Quintessence.

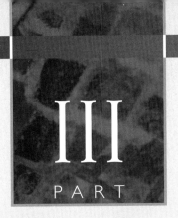

III
PART

Treatment of Functional Disturbances of the Masticatory System

Functional disturbances of the masticatory system can be as complicated as the system itself. Although numerous treatments have been advocated, none are universally effective for all patients all the time. Effective treatment selection begins with a thorough understanding of the disorder and its etiology. An appreciation of the various types of treatments is essential for effective management of the symptoms.

Part III consists of six chapters that discuss treatment methods used for each temporomandibular disorder presented in Part II. Treatment selection must be based on accurate diagnosis and understanding of the disorder.

General Considerations in the Treatment of Temporomandibular Disorders

11 CHAPTER

"TMD is a complex and multifactorial condition; so also are our patients."

—JPO

INTERRELATIONSHIPS OF VARIOUS TEMPOROMANDIBULAR DISORDERS

*A*ccurately diagnosing and treating temporomandibular disorders (TMDs) can be a difficult and confusing task. This is often true primarily because patients' symptoms do not always fit into one classification. In many instances several classifications seem to be appropriate because in reality the patient is suffering from more than one disorder. In many patients one disorder contributes to another. Therefore it is appropriate when more than one disorder appears to be present that an attempt be made to distinguish the primary from the secondary disorder. For example, a patient complains of right temporomandibular joint (TMJ) pain 2 weeks after a fall that traumatized the joint. The pain has been present for 12 days, but during the last week it has been aggravated by a decrease in mouth opening associated with muscle discomfort. The primary diagnosis is a traumatic injury to this joint, whereas the secondary diagnosis is protective co-contraction or local muscle soreness associated with restricted movement of the painful joint. During treatment both diagnoses must be considered and appropriately managed.

The interrelationship of the various TMDs must always be considered in the evaluation and treatment of patients. Sometimes it is nearly impossible to identify which disorder preceded the other. Often the evidence to determine such an order can be obtained only from a thorough history. The following examples demonstrate the complex interrelationship among several TMDs.

A patient suffering from a masticatory muscle disorder such as local muscle soreness or myofascial pain will commonly report a chief complaint of myalgia. These muscle conditions are likely to increase the tonicity of the elevator muscles, creating an increase in interarticular pressure of the joint. The condition may be further aggravated by hyperactivity of the superior lateral pterygoid muscle (bruxism), which can accentuate a subclinical disc derangement disorder.

Masticatory muscle $\rightarrow$ Disc derangement
disorder   disorder

Another patient complains of an early disc derangement disorder. If pain is associated with it, secondary muscle co-contraction can result in an attempt to prevent painful movements. If the muscle co-contraction becomes protracted, local muscle soreness can result. In this instance a disc derangement disorder has created a masticatory muscle disorder.

Disc derangement $\rightarrow$ Masticatory muscle
disorder   disorder

When some disc derangement disorders progress, the bony articular surfaces of the joint may undergo changes. In other words, disc derangement disorders can lead to inflammatory disorders of the joint.

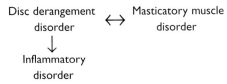

When masticatory muscle disorders persist, limited mandibular movement can become protracted and lead to chronic mandibular hypomobility disorders. Likewise, inflammatory disorders can also induce chronic mandibular hypomobility disorders.

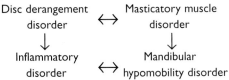

Trauma is another condition that affects all these disorders. Trauma to any structure of the masticatory system can either cause or contribute to most of the other TMDs.

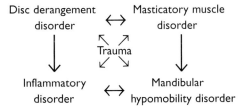

This diagram begins to depict the complicated interrelationships that may exist among the various TMDs. It demonstrates why many patients have symptoms that are associated with more than one disorder and how these relationships can make diagnosis and treatment decisions difficult.

TREATMENT OF TEMPOROMANDIBULAR DISORDERS

The treatments that have been suggested for TMDs vary enormously over a great spectrum of modalities. In order for the clinician to confidently select an appropriate treatment, he or she should demand adequate scientific evidence to support its use. This support should be found in evidence-based literature that documents the success and failure of a described treatment. Unfortunately, this is not always the case. Numerous published articles suggest success of a variety of treatment options that may not be soundly substantiated with scientific evidence. Perhaps this is why the profession is so confused regarding the management of TMD.

It is also interesting to note that the popularity of certain treatment methods can be found to be geographically regionalized. It is highly unlikely that this is appropriate because epidemiologic studies do not report regionalization of any particular TMD. It can also be noted that treatment selection correlates strongly with the specialty of the doctor whom the patient has consulted. If the patient comes to an orthodontist, orthodontic treatment is likely to be administered; if to an oral surgeon, a surgical procedure is likely; if to a prosthodontist, occlusal therapy. No rationale indicates why patients with similar problems should receive different treatments in different regions. Nor is there any reason why patients with similar problems should be treated differently by different specialties.

Another interesting observation is that some treatments that are presented as new and revolutionary were actually presented to the profession years earlier and found to have little to no value. It seems that once a generation has passed, someone rediscovers the treatment and introduces it as new. Then clinicians accept the idea and begin treating their patients. This is certainly unfortunate for patients because they must suffer and endure additional expense and sometimes irreversible dental procedures that are doomed to fail.

The question that must be asked is how so many different types of therapies can have publications that suggest they are helpful in managing TMDs. No simple answers to this question are available. However, certain considerations may help explain this controversy. Here are a few:

1. Adequate scientific evidence that soundly relates therapy to treatment effects is lacking. Although many published studies have investigated TMDs, most are methodologically flawed. Only recently has the dental profession begun to demand sound evidence-based research methodology. The controlled, double-blinded, clinical trial is the standard for clinical research, and these studies are rare in the field of TMD. The profession must encourage more of these studies to advance the body of knowledge in the field.[1]

2. Significant research efforts can only begin with agreement regarding the specific diagnostic categories of TMDs. As has been stressed in this text, the most important task of the clinician is in establishing the proper diagnosis. Different disorders respond differently to different treatments. Therefore only with proper diagnosis can proper therapy be selected. This fact makes diagnosis extremely important. In the past many studies describe their treatment group as "TMJ patients." This broad description does not increase the body of knowledge because the therapy investigated may affect one subcategory and not another. In order to evaluate the treatment effects of a particular treatment, these therapies must be tested in patient groups with specific common diagnoses. When the clinician is evaluating current research, he or she needs to be critical of the patient groups tested in the study.[1]

3. Some etiologic factors that contribute to TMDs are difficult to control or eliminate (e.g., emotional stress). When these factors are present, the effects of dental treatment are minimized. More effective treatment methods must be developed for these factors.

4. Some factors leading to TMDs have yet to be identified and may not be influenced by present treatment methods. Thus symptoms persist after treatment. As these additional factors are identified, treatment selection and effectiveness will be greatly improved.

5. Often the pain intensity of many musculoskeletal disorders vary greatly over time. In other words, some days may be very painful, and other days the patient has little to no pain. This variation may occur for months. As the symptoms vary, the patient's perceived need for treatment can change. The patient will most commonly seek treatment for the condition when the symptoms are most intense. At this time the dentist offers treatment and the symptoms begin to resolve. The question that must be asked is, "Did the patient's symptoms resolve because of the therapeutic effect of the treatment, or did they resolve merely because they returned to a lower level associated with the nature fluctuation of the symptoms?" This is

an important concept and is referred to as *regression to the mean.*[2] Once one appreciates this concept, it can be clearly seen that many treatments can appear to be successful when actually they have no real therapeutic value. In order to study the true therapeutic value of a treatment, it must be compared over time with no treatment at all. This is why control clinical trials are necessary. Unfortunately, these types of studies are rare in the field of TMD. The concept of regression to the mean is discussed in more detail in Chapter 15.

Tables 11-1 and 11-2 show the results of a group of long-term studies[3-43] for the treatment of various TMDs. Long-term treatment studies should give the most accurate information regarding effectiveness of treatment. The studies have been placed in one of two categories: those that provided basically conservative, reversible therapy and those that provided rather nonconservative, irreversible therapy.

When reviewing these studies, one must remember that the types of patients, criteria for diagnosis, and success rates vary and thus it is difficult to compare studies. An interesting general observation, however, is that conservative and nonconservative therapies seem to report similar success rates on a long-term basis (70% to 85%). Although it is likely that the patient population between these groups was quite different, both conservative and nonconservative treatments have been comparably successful on a long-term basis. Therefore it would appear that a logical approach to patient management is to attempt conservative (reversible) therapy first and to consider nonconservative (irreversible) therapy only when the reversible treatment has failed to resolve the disorder adequately.[44,45] This philosophy is the basis for managing TMDs, as well as any other type of disorder.

All the treatment methods being used for TMDs can be categorized generally into one of two types: definitive treatment or supportive therapy. *Definitive treatment* refers to methods that are directed toward controlling or eliminating the etiologic factors that have created the disorder. *Supportive therapy* refers to treatment methods that are directed toward altering patient symptoms.

TABLE 11-1

Long-Term Studies of Conservative (Reversible) Therapy

Author	Diagnosis*	Treatment	No. of Patients	Yrs Since Treatment	% Success Reported
Greene and Laskin	Muscle	Exercise, meds, PT, appliances	135	0.5-8.0	76.0
Greene and Markovic	Joint	Exercise, meds, PT, appliances	32	0.5-3.0	84.0
Carlsson and Gale	Muscle and joint	Biofeedback	11	0.4-1.3	73.0
Carraro and Caffesse	Muscle	Appliances	27	0.5-4.0	85.0
	Joint	Appliances	20	0.5-4.0	70.0
	Muscle and joint	Counsel, exercise, meds	40	0.5-12.0	76.0
Cohen	Muscle and joint	Counsel, exercise, meds	118	0.5-12.0	85.0
Dohrmann and Laskin	Muscle	Biofeedback	16	1.0	75.0
Nel	Muscle	Meds, exercise, SG, appliances	127	2.5	95.0
Heloe and Heiberg	Muscle	Counsel, meds, appliances, SG	108	1.5	81.0
Wessberg et al.	Muscle and joint	TENS, appliances	21	1.0	86.0
Green and Laskin	Muscle	Biofeedback, meds, relax, appliances	175	5.0	90.0
Magnusson and Carlsson	Muscle and joint	Counsel, exercise, appliances	52	2.5	76.0
Wedel and Carlsson	Muscle and joint	Exercise, appliances, SG	350	2.5	75.0
Strychalsky et al.	Muscle and joint	Exercise, appliances	31	2.0-3.0	72.0
Okeson and Hayes	Muscle and joint	Meds, relax, appliances, SG	110	4.0-5.0	85.5
Randolph et al.	Muscle and joint	Counsel, appliances, meds, TENS, PT	110	2.0	88.0
Okeson	Joint	Appliances	40	2.5	75.0
Williamson	Joint	Appliances	160	0.3	89.4
Kurita	Muscle and joint	Appliances	232	0.16	84.0
Sato	Joint	None	22	1.5	68.2

meds, Prescription medications; *PT*, physical therapy; *SG*, selective grinding; *TENS*, transcutaneous electrical nerve stimulation.
*The diagnosis established for each patient population is designated *muscle* for extracapsular muscle disorders or *joint* for intracapsular disorders.

DEFINITIVE TREATMENT

Definitive therapy is aimed directly at the elimination or alteration of the etiologic factors that are responsible for the disorder. For example, definitive treatment for an anterior dislocation of the articular disc will reestablish the proper condyle-disc relationship. Because it is directed toward the etiology, an accurate diagnosis is essential. An improper diagnosis leads to improper treatment selection. The specific definitive treatment for each TMD is discussed in future chapters. In this chapter the common etiologic and/or contributing factor will be considered.

As stated in Chapter 7, TMDs result when normal activity of the masticatory system is interrupted by an event (Fig. 11-1). The event therefore is the etiology. Definitive therapy would attempt to eliminate the event or its consequence. Common events may be local trauma to tissues or increased emotional stress. An event may also be anything that acutely alters sensory input to the masticatory structures (i.e., acute changes in the occlusion). As discussed in Chapter 7,

TABLE 11-2

Long-Term Studies of Nonconservative (Irreversible) Therapy

Author	Diagnosis*	Treatment	No. of Patients	Yrs Since Treatment	% Success Reported
Zarb and Thompson	Muscle and joint	Appliance, SG, reconstruction	56	2.5-3.0	79.0
Banks and Mackenzie	Joint	Condylotomy	174	1.0-20.0	91.0
Cherry and Frew	Joint	High condylectomy	55	0.4-4.0	70.0
Brown	Joint	Meniscectomy	214	0.3-15.0	80.0
Bjornland and Larheim	Joint	Discectomy	15	3.0	73.0
Marcianini and Ziegler	Joint	TMJ surgery	51	2.9	77.0
Merjesjo and Carlsson	Muscle and joint	Counsel, appliances, SG, reconstruction	154	7.0	80.0
Upton et al.	Joint	Ortho, ortho-surg	55	2.0-5.0	78.0
Benson and Keith	Joint	Plica, high condylotomy	84	2.0	88.0
Eriksson and Westesson	Joint	Discectomy	69	0.5-20.0	74.0
Silver	Joint	Meniscectomy	224	1.0-20.0	85.0
Holmlund et al.	Joint	Discectomy	21	1.0	86.0
	Joint	Plica, high condylectomy	68	2.5	90.0
Moses and Poker	Joint	Arthroscopy	237	0.0-9.0	92.0
Murakami et al.	Joint	Arthroscopy	15	3.0-5.0	93.3
Kirk	Joint	Arthrotomy and arthroplasty	210	4.0-9.0	90.1
Murakami	Joint	Arthroscopy	41	5.0	70.0
Gynther	Joint	Arthroscopy	23	1.0	74.0
Summer	Joint	Reconstruction	75	1.0-6.0	84.0-92.0
Sato	Joint	Arthrocentesis, HA acid	26	0.5	71.3
Nitzan	Joint	Arthrocentesis	39	1.4	95.0
Rosenberg	Joint	Arthrocentesis	90	2.5	82.0
Carvajal	Joint	Arthrocentesis	26	4.0	88.0
Hall	Joint	Condylotomy	22	3.0	94.0

HA, Hyaluronic; *ortho-surg*, orthodontic-surgical; *plica*, plication; *SG*, selective grinding; *TMJ*, temporomandibular joint.
*The diagnosis established for each patient population is designated *muscle* for extracapsular muscle disorders or *joint* for intracapsular disorders.

this represents one mechanism in which occlusion may lead to certain TMDs.

The second influencing effect of occlusion is through orthopedic instability. As previously discussed, orthopedic instability alone does not necessarily lead to TMDs. Problems arise when orthopedic instability is combined with forces associated with loading. Therefore orthopedic instability is considered to be one component that influences the patient's physiologic tolerance.

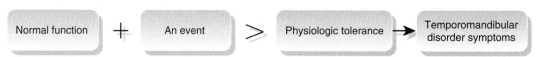

Fig. 11-1 RELATIONSHIP OF ETIOLOGIC AND CONTRIBUTING FACTORS THAT CREATE TEMPOROMANDIBULAR DISORDERS (as discussed in Chapter 7). Definitive treatments are those that alter the factors associated with the event that has interrupted normal function of the masticatory system.

Occlusion therefore can influence TMDs in two ways. The history and examination are extremely important in understanding the role of the occlusal condition in the TMD. One should always remember that the mere presence of occlusal interferences is not indicative of etiology. Almost all individuals have occlusal interferences. The occlusion condition is certainly not the etiology of all TMDs. The occlusal condition must have been acutely changed or represent significant orthopedic instability. When the occlusion does represent an etiologic factor, occlusal treatments become definitive therapies.

Another common etiology of TMDs is increased emotional stress. When this condition is suspected, therapies used to reduce stress are considered to be definitive.

Although trauma can also cause TMDs, often trauma represents a single event with the etiology no longer being present when the patient seeks treatment. Treatment to the tissues that have been affected by the trauma can only be supportive therapy. On the other hand, if the trauma is the result of repeated microtrauma—for example, functional activity in the presence of a disc displacement—then definitive treatment would be any therapy that would set up a more favorable environment for loading.

As discussed in Chapter 7, any source of deep pain may also be responsible for creating the TMD. Deep pain input can refer pain to the face and cause protective muscle co-contraction. When a source of deep pain input is present, it needs to be eliminated so that the secondary pain and muscle response will be resolved. Elimination of this pain is considered definitive therapy.

The last etiology that was discussed in Chapter 7 was parafunctional activity. Whether this be diurnal or nocturnal, bruxing or clenching, this type of muscle activity can be responsible for TMD symptoms. When this is present, definitive therapy is aimed at eliminating this muscle activity.

In this section each of the five types of etiologic considerations is discussed, and definitive treatments for each are listed. Ascertaining the most important etiologic factor causing the TMD is often difficult, especially on an initial visit. Therefore it is wise to move cautiously with treatment and avoid being too aggressive at first. With this rationale the

following statement is made: *All initial treatment should be conservative, reversible, and noninvasive.*

Definitive Therapy Considerations for Occlusal Factors

Occlusal therapy is considered to be any treatment that is directed toward altering the mandibular position and/or occlusal contact pattern of the teeth. It can be of two types: reversible and irreversible.

Reversible Occlusal Therapy. Reversible occlusal therapy alters the patient's occlusal condition only temporarily and is best accomplished with an occlusal appliance. This is an acrylic device worn over the teeth of one arch that has an opposing surface that creates and alters the mandibular position and contact pattern of the teeth (Fig. 11-2).

The exact mandibular position and occlusion will depend on the etiology of the disorder. When parafunctional activity is to be treated, the appliance provides a mandibular position and occlusion that fit the criteria for optimum occlusal relationships (see Chapter 5). Thus when the appliance is being worn, an occlusal contact pattern is established that is in harmony with the optimum condyle-disc-fossa relationship for the patient. The appliance therefore provides orthopedic stability. This type of appliance has been used to decrease symptoms associated with various TMDs,[6,46-48] as well as decrease parafunctional activity.[49-60] Of course, the orthopedic stability is maintained only while the appliance is being worn

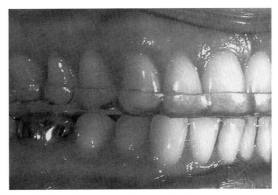

Fig. 11-2 Full-arch maxillary occlusal appliance, a type of reversible occlusal therapy.

and therefore it is considered to be a reversible treatment. When it is removed, the preexisting condition returns. An occlusal appliance that uses the musculoskeletally stable (centric relation) position of the condyles is referred to as a *stabilization appliance.*

Irreversible Occlusal Therapy. Irreversible occlusal therapy is any treatment that permanently alters the occlusal condition and/or mandibular position. Examples are selective grinding of teeth and restorative procedures that modify the occlusal condition (Fig. 11-3). Other examples are orthodontic treatment and surgical procedures aimed at altering the occlusion and/or mandibular position. Appliances that are designed to alter growth or permanently reposition the mandible are also considered irreversible occlusal therapies. These treatments are discussed in Part IV of this text.

When treating a patient, one should always be mindful of the complexity of many TMDs. Often, especially when dealing with muscle hyperactivity, it is impossible to be certain of the major etiologic factor. Therefore reversible therapy is always indicated as the initial treatment for patients with TMDs. The success or failure of this treatment may be helpful in determining the need for later irreversible occlusal therapy. When a patient responds successfully to reversible occlusal therapy (stabilization appliance), there appear to be indications that irreversible occlusal therapy may also be helpful. This correlation is sometimes true but certainly not always true. Occlusal appliances

can affect masticatory function in a variety of ways (see Chapter 15).

Definitive Therapy Considerations for Emotional Stress

Some TMDs are etiologically related to certain emotional states.[61,62] Emotional stress is certainly one of several psychologic factors that need to be considered.

Increased levels of emotional stress can affect muscle function by increasing the resting activity[63,64] (protective co-contraction), increasing bruxism, or both. Increased levels of emotional stress also activate the sympathetic nervous system, which may in itself be a source of muscle pain.[65,66] Activation of the autonomic nervous system may also be associated with other psychophysiologic disorders commonly associated with TMD, such as irritable bowel syndrome, premenstrual syndrome, and interstitial cystitis.[67] It is extremely important that the clinician recognizes this relationship and alters treatments appropriately. Unfortunately, the dental practitioner is not often trained well in this area of medicine and therefore can easily feel inept or uncertain. Nevertheless, dentists who treat TMDs must have an appreciation for these problems so that, if indicated, proper referrals can be made.

The following will serve as a brief review of the personality traits and emotional states that can influence TMD symptoms. A more extensive review is available in texts written specifically on the subject.

Common Personality Traits. Personality traits are considered to be a relatively permanent feature in individuals. It would be significant and helpful in establishing a diagnosis if particular traits were commonly found in TMDs. Numerous studies[68-75] have attempted to classify common personality traits. Some[74,75] have concluded that TMD patients are generally perfectionists, compulsive, and domineering. Another study[76] reports TMD patients as more introverted and more neurotic with more trait anxiety. One study suggests that type A personalities seem to be more common in TMD patients than type B personalities.[77] Others[68,69] have described these patients as responsible and generous. Still another[73] has suggested that they are generally unhappy, dissatisfied,

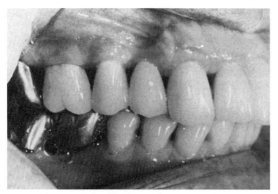

Fig. 11-3 Complete fixed reconstruction of the dentition, a type of irreversible occlusal therapy.

and self-destructive. Some authors[76] have suggested that TMD patients have personalities that are more vulnerable to life stressors than nonpatients. Yet other studies[78-80] report no differences among a TMD group, a group of other pain patients, and a control group in personality type, response to illness, and ways of coping with stress. As studies continue, they only seem to conflict more. Thus the conclusion that can be drawn is that the enormous variation in personality traits in this patient population prevents the common traits from being helpful in identifying the etiologic factors of TMDs.

Common Emotional States. Unlike personality traits, emotional states can have short-term effects on human behavior. When groups of TMD patients are studied for common emotional states, some consistent results are reported. In most studies[63,72,81-90] high levels of anxiety appeared to be common. It was not determined whether these high levels were the cause of symptoms or whether the presence of the symptoms increased the levels of anxiety. Quite likely both conditions existed. Other common emotional states reported were apprehension, frustration, hostility, anger, and fear.*

The combined input of these emotional states determines the level of stress experienced by the patient. Some evidence[49,50,81,93-95] exists to demonstrate that greater levels of emotional stress can create increased parafunctional activity in the masticatory system. This increased muscle activity may not only be associated with clinching and/or bruxing but may merely represent a generalized increase in muscle tonicity.[63] Thus a correlation may be drawn among increased levels of anxiety, fear, frustration, and anger and muscle hyperactivity. Therefore it is necessary to be mindful of these states when interviewing patients. Unfortunately, however, no psychologic tests can be given to determine whether these emotional states are contributing to muscle hyperactivity.[96,97] Importantly, not all studies find a clear relationship between increased levels of emotional stress and increased levels of parafunctional activity.[97,98]

The fact that a group of patients reveals higher levels of anxiety does not in itself mean that a given patient with a high anxiety score is necessarily experiencing muscle hyperactivity because of the anxiety. Being aware of this relationship between emotional stress and muscle hyperactivity is important so that it can be considered in selecting appropriate treatment. If increased levels of emotional stress and anxiety were related to increased muscle hyperactivity, one would expect to see more muscle disorders than intracapsular disorders associated with these emotional states. Clinicians do see more muscle disorders, so this is apparently true. Patients suffering from muscle disorders do report higher levels of emotional stress than do patients suffering from disc derangement disorders.[61,87,99-101]

Another emotional state that has been related to TMDs is depression.[61,73,96,102-107] Although some studies[108,109] suggest differently, depression may play a significant role in certain TMDs. Depression is unlikely to cause a TMD, but it is common that patients who suffer with chronic pain will experience depression.[104,110-115] When TMD symptoms and depression coexist, patients respond best to therapies that address both the dental and depressive factors.[116] This is true regardless of the cause-and-effect relationship. The suggestion has been made[117] that patients with masticatory muscle disorders who do not respond to conventional therapy may fit into the category of clinical depression and need to be treated for this disorder. If this is true, it would be helpful to predict in advance treatment outcome according to emotional health. At present, however, studies that have attempted to accomplish this have not been successful.[100,118-120] Therefore as with other emotional states, no test is available that will help determine in advance which treatment will be successful.[121]

Another psychologic consideration that appears to be significantly linked to chronic facial pain is a history of physical or sexual abuse. Studies[122-128] report that women who suffer from chronic, nonresponsive facial pain and headaches have a significantly higher incidence of past physical or sexual abuse. In some patients an abusive history leads to posttraumatic stress disorder, a psychologic condition that represents a generalized increase in the

---

*References 71, 72, 74, 82, 91, 92.

autonomic nervous system responsiveness. This upregulation of the autonomic nervous system seems to change the body's ability to overcome new challenges, whether physical or psychologic. If, in fact, these prior experiences are related to chronic facial pain, the dentist can be placed in a compromised position. Most patients presenting to a dental office for treatment of facial pain are not aware of any relationship with past traumatic emotional experiences and therefore do not report these experiences to the dentist. If past physical or sexual abuse is a significant part of the chronic pain problem, the dentist may fail to manage the pain with dental therapies. On the other hand, the dentist must be careful in approaching this subject because of its sensitivity and because the patient is not likely to be aware of the relationship of the abuse to the pain problem. When physical or sexual abuse is suspected, it is often best for the dentist to refer the patient to a qualified clinical psychologist or psychiatrist for evaluation and appropriate therapy. However, the dentist is capable of assisting in this patient's treatment by instructing the individual in techniques that will assist in downregulating the autonomic nervous system. These techniques are presented later in this chapter.

Still another emotional condition that sometimes must be addressed in treating a patient with chronic facial pain is known as *secondary gain*. For some patients, experiencing pain furnishes certain needed benefits. It can provide attention and consolation from a spouse or friends.[129,130] It also can be used as an excuse from work or other unpleasant obligations. Although not a major concern in the treatment of most TMD patients, secondary gain should be considered as a possible factor in chronic treatment failures.[131] When patients receive secondary gain from the pain, it is more likely that treatment efforts will fail.

When studies separate masticatory muscle disorder patients from those with intracapsular complaints, some differences seem to appear.[61,87,132] Muscle pain patients report a higher degree of pain and distress than intracapsular patients.[133] They also report greater concern for bodily function and illness. Another study shows no difference in muscle and joint pain patients when evaluating stress and anxiety but finds that the muscle pain

patients generally feel as if they have lost control of their life situations.[64,84] This is supported by still another study[134] that reveals no difference in self-reported depression and anxiety levels between TMD patients and controls; however, the patients felt less in control of their problem. Perhaps the feeling of being out of control will prove to be a significant factor in TMD. If this is correct, then teaching our patients better methods of controlling their life conditions should significantly affect the number of patients seeking care.

Summary of Personality Traits and Emotional States. The following conclusions can be made regarding patients who have an emotional factor contributing to their TMD:

1. No single personality trait appears to be common in this group of patients. Instead, a variety of traits is found. There is no research evidence, however, that suggests these patients are either neurotic or psychotic. In contrast, they generally have a normal range of personality traits. A significant number of TMD patients have personality characteristics or emotional conditions that make managing or coping with life situations difficult.[99,135-138] No personality trait test that will effectively aid in selecting appropriate treatment can be given to an individual.

2. It appears that TMD patients, especially chronic conditions, generally experience and report increased levels of anxiety, frustration, and anger. The presence of these emotional states tends to increase levels of emotional stress, which can contribute to the TMD.[139,140] Depression and anxiety related to major life events may alter the patient's perception and tolerance of symptoms, causing him or her to seek more care.[72,141-143] No evidence suggests, however, that testing an individual for levels of these emotional states will be useful in selecting an appropriate treatment.

Types of Emotional Stress Therapy. When treating a patient with TMD symptoms, especially a masticatory muscle disorder, one must always be aware of emotional stress as an etiologic factor. However, there is no way to be certain of the part that emotional stress plays in the disorder. As mentioned earlier, reversible occlusal therapy may be helpful in ruling out other etiologic factors and thereby assisting in the diagnosis of emotional stress factors. When high levels of emotional stress are suspected, treatment is directed toward the reduction of these levels.

Many dentists do not feel comfortable providing treatment for emotional stress. This is justifiable because dental education does not normally furnish adequate background for such treatment. After all, dentists are primarily responsible for the health of the mouth, not the psychologic welfare of the patient. However, TMDs are one area of dentistry that can be closely related to the emotional state of the patient. Dentists may not be able to provide psychologic therapy, but they must be aware of this relationship and be able to relate this information to the patient. When psychologic therapy is indicated, the patient should be referred to a properly trained therapist. In many cases, however, patients are merely experiencing high levels of emotional stress from their daily routines. When this is suspected, the following simple types of emotional stress therapy may be employed.

Patient awareness. Many persons who have orofacial pain and/or functional disturbance of the masticatory system are not aware of the possible relationship between their problem and emotional stress. It would be surprising to think any differently because their symptoms arise from structures in the masticatory system. Therefore when a patient comes to the dentist with symptoms that are closely related to muscle hyperactivity, the first treatment is to educate that person regarding the relationship between emotional stress, muscle hyperactivity, and the problem. An awareness of this relationship must be created before any treatment begins. Remember also that parafunctional activity occurs almost entirely at subconscious times and therefore patients are generally unaware of it. They commonly deny any clenching or bruxism. They also commonly deny the presence of high levels of stress in their life. Therefore one must be sure that the patient is aware that stress is a common everyday experience and not a neurotic or psychotic disorder. These concepts are often new to patients and sometimes are best appreciated only with time.

The patient should try to become aware of any time the teeth contact other than chewing, swallowing, and speaking. Often patients deny that any

of these nonfunctional tooth contacts occur until they have actively tried to identify them. Patients will frequently return for a second visit with a better appreciation for the amount of nonfunctional tooth contacts that occur during previously unaware times. Establishing an awareness of nonfunctional tooth contacts, muscle hyperactivity, and stress is essential to treatment.

Restrictive use. Pain present in the masticatory system often limits the functional range of mandibular movement. When possible, therefore, painful movements should be avoided because they often increase protective muscle co-contraction. In addition, these movements should be avoided because they can enhance the symptoms of the disorder through central excitatory effects and cyclic muscle pain.

The patient is instructed to function within a painless range of movement. A general rule is, "If it hurts, don't do it." This usually means that the diet should be altered. The patient is encouraged to eat softer foods, take smaller bites, and generally chew slowly. An awareness of any oral habits is developed, and attempts are made to discontinue them.

Although it may seem to be an obvious statement, all patients need instruction in voluntarily restricting use of their mandible to within painless ranges. Unless specifically trained, patients may continue to abuse their jaw with an existing diet and/or oral habit (e.g., chewing gum, clenching). In most cases prolonged fixation of the dental arch is contraindicated because myostatic contracture of the elevator muscles may result.

Voluntary avoidance. Once the patient is aware of nonfunctional tooth contacts, muscle hyperactivity treatment can begin. The patient should be instructed that any time the teeth contact, other than chewing, swallowing, and speaking, he or she should quickly disengage them. This can be easily accomplished by puffing a little air between the lips and teeth, which allows the jaw to assume a relaxed position. The lips can then be passively brought together, and the teeth remain slightly apart. This is the most relaxed position of the jaw and should be the position of the mandible whenever the patient is not chewing, swallowing, or speaking. This rest position not only decreases muscle activity and therefore muscle pain but also minimizes interarticular pressure promoting joint repair. This simple exercise should be repeated all day until a habit is achieved that maintains the mandible in this rest position throughout the day.

Other oral habits such as biting on objects (pencils) or cradling the telephone between the mandible and shoulder can further aggravate TMD symptoms. These habits need to be identified and discontinued.[144] Parafunctional activity that occurs at subconscious times, especially during sleep, is difficult to control voluntarily and therefore other therapy, such as an occlusal appliance, is often indicated.

Emotional stress can also be controlled to some extent voluntarily. Once the stressors are identified, the patient is encouraged when possible to avoid them. For example, if stress is increased by driving through heavy traffic, alternate routes should be developed that will avoid major traffic areas. When stress is caused by specific encounters at work, these should be avoided. Obviously, all stressors cannot and should not be avoided. As discussed in Chapter 7, some are positive and help motivate the individual toward particular goals. As Hans Selye[145] stated, "Complete freedom from stress is death." When stressors cannot be completely avoided, the frequency and duration of exposure to them should be reduced.

Relaxation therapy. Two types of relaxation therapy can be instituted to reduce levels of emotional stress: substitutive and active.

Substitutive relaxation therapy can be either a substitution for stressors or an interposition between them in an attempt to lessen their impact on the patient. It is more accurately described as behavioral modification, and it may be any activity enjoyed by the patient that removes him or her from a stressful situation. Patients are encouraged when possible to remove themselves from stressors and substitute other activities that they enjoy, such as allowing more time for sports, hobbies, or recreational activities. For some patients this may include some quiet time alone. It should be an enjoyable time and an opportunity to forget their stressors. Such activities are considered to be external stress-releasing mechanisms and to lead to an overall reduction of emotional stress experienced by the patient.[146]

Regular exercise may also be an active external stress-releasing mechanism. It is encouraged for patients who find it enjoyable. Obviously it will not be suitable for all patients, and general body condition and health must always be considered before advising patients to initiate an active exercise program.

Active relaxation therapy directly reduces muscle activity. One common complaint of patients with functional disturbances is muscle pain and tenderness. The pain of local muscle soreness originates from compromised muscle tissues following the increased demands of co-contraction. If a patient can be trained to relax the symptomatic muscles, establishment of normal function can be aided.

Training the patient to relax muscles effectively reduces symptoms in two different ways. First, it requires regular quiet periods of time away from the stressors. These training sessions are in themselves a substitutive relaxation therapy. Second, it aids in the establishment of normal function and health to compromised muscle tissues. Muscles that experience chronic and sometimes constant hyperactivity often become ischemic to fatigue. When a patient is trained to relax symptomatic muscles voluntarily, blood flow to these tissues is encouraged and the metabolic waste substances that stimulate the nociceptors (pain receptors) are eliminated. This then diminishes the pain. Therefore relaxation therapy is considered both a definitive treatment for the reduction of emotional stress and a supportive treatment for the reduction of muscle symptoms.

Training a patient to relax effectively can be accomplished by using several techniques. One that has been well researched is progressive relaxation. Many of these techniques are modifications of Jacobson's method,[147] developed in 1968. The patient tenses the muscles and then relaxes them until the relaxed state can be felt and maintained. The patient is instructed to concentrate on relaxing the peripheral areas (hands and feet) and to move progressively centrally to the abdomen, chest, and face. Results can be enhanced by having the patient relax, preferably by lying down[148] in a quiet comfortable environment with the eyes closed (Fig. 11-4). The relaxation procedures are slowly explained in a calm and soothing voice.

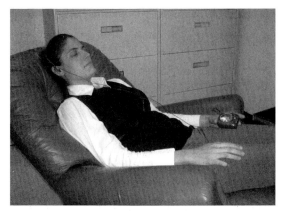

Fig. 11-4 RELAXATION PROCEDURES. For 20 minutes each day the patient is advised to lie back and relax in a comfortable, quiet setting. An audio recording of a progressive relaxation technique is provided and assists in achieving muscle relaxation. This can help many patients decrease their muscle symptoms.

An audio recording of the procedures can be developed to aid in the technique. The patient listens to the recording at the training session in the office and then, after understanding what is to be accomplished, takes the recording home with instructions to listen at least once a day to become proficient at relaxing the muscles. Muscle symptoms generally decrease as the individual becomes more skilled in the technique.

Relaxation techniques have been demonstrated to be effective in several studies.[149-158] They would appear to be best accomplished by well-trained therapists during frequent visits to help and encourage proper relaxation habits. Although it is not harmful to send the patient home to learn the technique alone, it is less likely that good results will be achieved by mere simple explanations of the relaxation procedures.[159] Also, the best results are achieved over months of training and not just days or weeks.

Another form of progressive relaxation uses a reverse approach. Instead of asking the patient to contract the muscle and then relax, the muscles are passively stretched and then relaxed.[160-162] It appears that this technique is also effective in teaching progressive relaxation and has one major inherent advantage over the Jacobson technique.

Patients with masticatory muscle disorders often report pain when asked to contract their muscles. This increase in pain makes relaxation more difficult. In contrast, gentle stretching of the muscle seems to assist in relaxation. Many patients find this technique more suitable than the Jacobson technique.

Progressive relaxation techniques are the most common method of promoting relaxation used in dentistry. Other training methods also encourage relaxation but are used to a lesser degree. Self-hypnosis, meditation, and yoga all promote relaxation and may help reduce levels of emotional stress, as well as the symptoms associated with muscle hyperactivity.[163-165] They likewise are best learned and applied with help from a trained therapist. Hypnosis provided by a trained therapist has also proved to be helpful in reducing TMD pain.[166-168]

Although the relaxation of muscles would appear to be a simple procedure, often it is not. Patients, especially those with muscle pain, frequently find it difficult to learn to relax their muscles effectively. They can sometimes benefit from immediate feedback regarding the success or failure of their efforts.

One method of achieving this is with biofeedback,[158,169-173] a technique that assists the patient in regulating bodily functions that are generally controlled unconsciously. It has been used to help patients alter such functions as blood pressure, blood flow, and brain wave activity, as well as muscle relaxation. It is accomplished by electromyographically monitoring the state of contraction or relaxation of the muscles through surface electrodes placed over the muscles to be monitored. Among facial muscles, the masseter is often selected (Fig. 11-5). When full-body relaxation is the goal, the frontalis muscle is commonly monitored.

The electrodes are connected to a monitoring system that lets the patient see the spontaneous electrical activity in the muscles being assessed. The monitor provides feedback by way of a scale or a digital readout or sometimes even a light bar mechanism. Most biofeedback units also give auditory feedback, which is beneficial for patients who relax best with their eyes closed. When a patient clenches, high readings appear

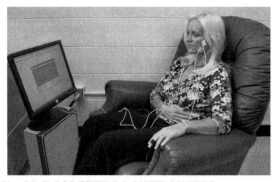

Fig. 11-5 BIOFEEDBACK TRAINING. The patient is encouraged to assume a relaxed position in a comfortable, quiet setting. The electromyographic sensors are attached to the masseter muscle. A finger sensor may also be used to monitor temperature and/or galvanic skin response. The patient is instructed to relax the muscles as much as possible. The computer monitor provides immediate feedback regarding the success in reducing the muscle activity. After several training sessions the patient becomes aware of effective relaxation and is encouraged to accomplish this without the biofeedback unit. Effective relaxation of muscle reduces muscle symptoms.

on the scale or an elevated tone is heard. When the muscles are relaxed, these signals are lowered. The patient attempts to lower the readings or the tone. This can be achieved by any relaxation technique, but progressive relaxation is encouraged because it is easily accomplished at a later date when the biofeedback instrument is not available.

Once the patient can achieve low levels of activity in the muscles, the next instruction is to become familiar with the sense or feeling of relaxation. When this has been accomplished and low levels of muscle activity have been adequately sensed, the patient can be more effective in regaining this state at a later time even without the aid of the biofeedback instrument and is encouraged to work toward achieving this goal. A progressive relaxation tape can aid in the training.

Another method of decreasing muscle hyperactivity is negative biofeedback. In this technique electrodes are placed on the masseter and lead to a monitoring instrument. The monitoring instrument is connected to a sounding device. The threshold for the feedback is adjusted such that the

functional activity of speech and swallowing can occur without eliciting any response. However, if clenching or bruxing occurs, the feedback mechanism is activated and a loud sound is heard. These devices are small and can be worn through the day and night. During the day the patient is told that any sound from the instrument indicates clenching or bruxism, and this activity should be discontinued immediately. The feedback unit brings parafunctional activity to a conscious level and therefore allows it to be more readily controlled. At night the volume of the sound is increased until it wakes the patient when the parafunctional activity begins. Again, the patient is told that if awakened by the sound, clenching or bruxing is occurring and an effort should be made to stop it. Although the negative biofeedback appears to decrease parafunctional activity successfully, it apparently has few long-term effects.[154,174,175] Once the feedback is discontinued, the parafunctional activity returns. This is especially true with nocturnal bruxing.

Therefore the most effective biofeedback for the treatment of symptoms associated with parafunctional activity appears to be feedback that helps the patient learn effective relaxation of the symptomatic muscles. It is important to remember that biofeedback is only an aid to assist the patient in learning a technique that helps alleviate the symptoms.

Important considerations in using emotional stress therapy. Before any discussion on emotional stress therapy concludes, four general considerations need to be mentioned:

1. Evaluation of the level of emotional stress in a patient's life is extremely difficult. Many variations exist from patient to patient, and often even the most thorough history fails to reveal all the significant factors. Even when many stressors are present, their significance may be unknown. Remember, it is not the number of stressors that a patient is experiencing that is significant but the impact that these stressors have on the patient's overall health and function.

2. When high levels of emotional stress are suspected as an etiologic factor contributing to a disorder, stress reduction therapy should be initiated. This should consist of the simple and noninvasive procedures just mentioned.

If a patient does not respond to this therapy, personnel more trained in behavioral modification and psychologic therapy should be consulted. Patients who do not respond may be suffering from disorders that are best managed by other health professionals.

3. One effective method of reducing stress is to establish a positive doctor-patient relationship. This begins with an appreciation of the fact that the patient has come into the office with pain and dysfunction. Pain, especially when chronic, induces stress, which potentiates the problem. The patient's uncertainty regarding the severity of the problem and the proper treatment can also increase the level of emotional stress. The doctor should communicate a warm, friendly, and reassuring attitude, which will promote confidence. The patient should be offered a thorough explanation of the disorder and be reassured (when indicated) that it is not as serious as might have been thought. The manner in which the doctor-patient relationship is developed is extremely important to the outcome of treatment (Fig. 11-6). Great effort should be taken by the doctor to minimize the patient's apprehension, frustration, hostility, anger, and fear.

4. Because emotional stress is a difficult factor to assess, it can easily become a scapegoat for unsuccessful treatment. Too often practitioners

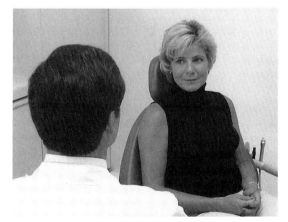

Fig. 11-6 Successful treatment of any temporomandibular disorder begins with a thorough explanation of the problem to the patient. The doctor-patient relationship can be extremely important to the success of treatment.

conclude that stress is a major contributing factor when their proposed treatment fails to resolve the patient's problem; actually either their treatment goals were not adequately met or they established an improper diagnosis. One cannot overemphasize the need for a thorough history and examination so that the proper diagnosis is established. Because of inherent difficulties in evaluating emotional stress, extensive emotional therapy should be seriously considered only after all other etiologies have been ruled out.

Definitive Therapy Considerations for Trauma

Trauma is one of the five etiologic factors that can lead to a TMD. As previously discussed, trauma can occur in two forms: macrotrauma and microtrauma. In the case of macrotrauma, definitive therapy has little meaning because the trauma is usually no longer present. Once macrotrauma has produced tissue injury, the only therapy that will help resolve the tissue response is supportive therapy. However, in the case of macrotrauma, preventive measures should always be considered. When macrotrauma is likely, such as when participating in a sporting event,[176] proper protection of the masticatory structures should be considered. A simple and effective manner to minimize injury associated with macrotrauma is to wear a soft occlusal appliance or mouth guard. When this appliance is in place, the mandible is stabilized with the maxilla, which minimizes injury to the masticatory structures during an episode of macrotrauma.[177,178] Athletes should protect themselves with a soft appliance whenever macrotrauma is possible. The unfortunate fact is that most patients who report to the dental office with a traumatic injury never expected to receive trauma. The most common example is a motor vehicle accident.

Sometimes injury is the result not of sudden macrotrauma but instead of small amounts of force that are repeated over a long period of time. This condition is referred to as *microtrauma* and, when present, definitive therapy is indicated to curtail the trauma. Microtrauma may result from repeated loading of the joint structures, such as with bruxing or clenching. In this condition, definitive therapy would consist of reducing or eliminating these parafunctional activities. In another situation the microtrauma may result from normal functional loading but the loading occurs on the retrodiscal tissues because of an anteriorly displaced disc. In this case, definitive therapy would be aimed at establishing a more favorable condyle/disc relationship that will unload the retrodiscal tissues and load the disc. This may be accomplished by an occlusal appliance (see Chapter 13).

Definitive Therapy Considerations for Deep Pain Input

Probably the most commonly overlooked etiologic factor associated with a TMD is another source of deep pain input. Too often the clinician is quick to assume that because the patient has facial pain the problem most be a TMD. This assumption leads to many treatment failures. As discussed in previous chapters, orofacial pain is complex. Many structures in the head and neck can produce pain complaints that mimic TMD. Adding to the confusion is pain referral (see Chapter 2). As has been emphasized in many previous chapters, the most critical task of the clinician is to establish the correct diagnosis. Without it, treatment is doomed to fail. Before ever beginning treatment for a TMD, the clinician should make sure that the thorough history and examination support the diagnosis of a specific type of TMD. If the clinician cannot find evidence that the orofacial pain has its source in the musculoskeletal structures of the masticatory system, the true source most be located before proper therapy can be selected. If the source of the pain is not obvious, a referral to another dentist or another health professional may be indicated to assist in establishing the diagnosis.

The clinician must also remember that some TMDs may actually be secondary to another source of deep pain (see Chapter 2). In these patients a TMD is identified during the history and examination, but if the TMD is treated without also managing the deep pain input, the treatment will fail. The example that has already been discussed is the patient who sustains a cervical injury, and the deep pain input from cervical structures produce referred pain to the face and secondary masticatory muscle protective co-contraction. If the clinician only recognizes the masticatory muscle disorder and treats it without regard to the cervical pain, the treatment will fail. However, if the clinician does recognize the cervical pain and its relationship to the masticatory muscle pain and manages it appropriately (i.e., referral to a physical therapist), appropriate treatment to the masticatory muscles will be successful. Both treatments provided at the same time will provide the best success for the patient.

Importantly, when a TMD secondary to another source of pain has been successfully managed, there is normally no need for any follow-up dental therapy. The reason for this is that the cause of the TMD was not occlusal but secondary to a deep source of pain. Once the deep source of pain is resolved, the TMD will also resolve. In the past many dentists would have gone on to change the patient's occlusion. Understanding of TMD is far better now, and the clinician should be able to recognize that the TMD was simply secondary to the deep pain input.[181]

Definitive Therapy Considerations for Parafunctional Activity

For many years dentists were convinced that bruxing and clinching the teeth were the major causative factors leading to TMDs. Although this is certainly true for some patients, it is not the case for many individuals. In fact, sleep studies reveal that tooth contacts during sleep in healthy, pain-free subjects are not only common but in fact normal. Tooth contacts seem to occur during arousal periods of sleep[179-181] and in fact can be initiated by shining lights in the sleep subject's face or making a sound that partially arouses him or her.[182] Bruxing certainly occurs in many individuals without TMD symptoms, as reflected in patients with significant tooth wear but no pain. The dental profession has had to reevaluate the relationship between bruxing and TMD. Yet even today with our present research it is obvious that bruxing and clenching the teeth are related etiologies in some TMD patients.

The exact mechanism that activates muscle hyperactivity has yet to be clearly described. As discussed in Chapter 7, many factors including emotional stress may affect the level of activity. The influence of these factors, however, may vary greatly not only among patients but also among the types of parafunctional activity. As stated in Chapter 7, there are several types of parafunctional activities but clenching and bruxism (grinding) seem to be the most significant. They can be either diurnal or nocturnal.[183] The characteristics and controlling factors of each are likely to be different. Diurnal activity may be more closely related to an acute alteration in the occlusal condition, increased levels of emotional stress, or both. Because diurnal activity can usually be brought to the patient's level of awareness, it is often managed well with patient education and cognitive awareness strategies.

Patient education should begin by informing the patient that the teeth should only contact during chewing, speaking, and swallowing. During all other times the jaw should be positioned with the teeth apart. Most patients are quite unaware of their tooth contacts, and making them aware is the first step in controlling excessive tooth contacts during unnecessary times. Once the patient becomes aware of tooth contacts, he or she should be asked to make a conscious effort to keep the teeth apart during all waking moments.[184] More patient education information is reviewed in Chapter 12.

Nocturnal bruxism, however, seems to be different. It appears to be influenced less by tooth contacts[183] and more by emotional stress levels[77,93,185,186] and sleep patterns.[179-182,187-190] Because of these differences, nocturnal bruxism responds poorly to patient education, relaxation and biofeedback techniques, and occlusal alterations.[191] In many cases it can be effectively reduced (for at least for short periods of time) with occlusal appliance therapy.[50-52,81] The mechanism by which occlusal appliances reduce bruxism is not clear. (A more thorough explanation is given in Chapter 15.)

Because diurnal and nocturnal parafunctional activities may be different in character and origin, it is important that they be identified and separated. Often this differentiation can be made through a careful history regarding the timing of symptoms (i.e., morning pain with nocturnal bruxism). Identifying the type of parafunctional activity present allows for more effective treatment selection.

SUPPORTIVE THERAPY

Supportive therapy is directed toward altering the patient's symptoms and often has no effect on the cause of the disorder. A simple example is giving a patient aspirin for a headache that is caused by hunger. The patient may feel relief from the headache, but there is no change in the causative factor (hunger) that created the symptom. Because many patients suffer greatly from TMDs, supportive therapy is often extremely helpful in providing immediate relief of the symptoms. Always remember, however, that supportive therapy is only symptomatic and not a replacement for definitive therapy. Etiologic factors need to be addressed and eliminated so that long-term treatment success can be achieved. Supportive therapy is directed toward the reduction of pain and dysfunction. The two general types of supportive therapies are pharmacologic therapy and physical therapy.

Pharmacologic Therapy

Pharmacologic therapy can be an effective method of managing symptoms associated with many TMDs. Patients should be aware that medication does not usually offer a solution or cure to their problems. However, medication in conjunction with appropriate physical therapy and definitive treatment can offer the most complete approach to many problems.

Care must be taken with the type and manner in which drugs are prescribed. Because many TMDs present symptoms that are periodic or cyclic, there is a tendency to prescribe drugs on a "take as needed" (or prn) basis. This type of management encourages patient drug abuse,[192-195] which may lead to physical or psychologic dependency. The drugs most commonly abused by patients are the narcotic analgesics and tranquilizers. These provide a brief period of euphoria or feeling of well-being and can sometimes become an unconscious reward for having suffered pain. Continued prn use of drugs tends to lead to more frequent pain cycles and less drug effectiveness. The general suggestion is that when drugs are indicated for TMDs, they should be prescribed at regular intervals for a specific period (e.g., three times a day [tid] for 10 days). At the end of this time it is hoped that the definitive treatment will be providing relief of the symptoms and the medication will no longer be necessary. This is especially true for the narcotic analgesics and tranquilizing agents.

The most common pharmacologic agents used for the management of TMD include analgesics, nonsteroidal antiinflammatory drugs (NSAIDs), corticosteroids, anxiolytics, muscle relaxants, antidepressants, and local anesthetics. Analgesics, corticosteroids, and anxiolytics are indicated for acute TMD pain; NSAIDs, muscle relaxants, and local anesthetics may be used for both acute and chronic conditions; and the tricyclic antidepressants are primarily indicated for chronic orofacial pain management.

Analgesics. Analgesic medications can often be an important part of supportive therapy for many TMDs. In disorders in which deep pain input is actually the cause of the disorder (cyclic muscle pain), analgesics represent a definitive treatment. Analgesics are either opiate or nonopiate preparations. The nonopiate analgesics are a heterogeneous group of compounds that share certain therapeutic actions and side effects. They are effective for mild to moderate pain associated with TMD. One of the first medications of choice for moderate pain relief is Tylenol (acetaminophen).[196] This medication is usually tolerated well by the patient with minimal side effects. Aspirin (salicylate), which inhibits prostaglandin synthesis, is the prototype for analgesic compounds. All salicylate drugs are antipyretic, analgesic, and antiinflammatory, but there are important differences in their effects. If the patient is sensitive to aspirin, a nonacetylated aspirin, choline magnesium trisalicylate (Trilisate), or salsalate (Disalcid) may be effective. The therapeutic effect of opioid narcotics acts on specific opiate receptor sites in the central and peripheral nervous systems. These drugs have central nervous system depressive qualities and addiction liabilities. They may be considered for short-term use for moderate to severe acute pain.[197]

On rare occasions stronger analgesics may be necessary. In these cases, codeine or hydrocodone combined with either a salicylate or acetaminophen can be helpful. The therapeutic effect of opioid narcotics acts on specific opiate receptor sites in the central and peripheral nervous systems. These drugs have central nervous system depressive qualities and addiction liabilities. They may be considered for short-term use for moderate to severe acute pain.[197] If these drugs are necessary, they should be prescribed in regular dosages over a short period so as to minimize abuse. The strongly addictive drugs (e.g., morphine) are generally contraindicated for musculoskeletal pain.

Nonsteroidal Antiinflammatory Drugs. NSAIDs are helpful with most TMD pains. These drugs are effective for mild to moderate inflammatory conditions and acute postoperative pain.[197] For a more through review of NSAIDs, other, more complete pharmacologic sources should be pursued.[197-199] NSAIDs can offer good management for the musculoskeletal pains associated with TMD. However, as with other medications, these drugs provide only symptomatic relief and do not arrest the progression of pathologic tissue injury with the possible exception of active inflammatory joint disease.

In the presence of tissue injury, certain chemical mediators are released into the injured site. One such important chemical mediator is prostaglandin. This chemical mediator excites local nociceptors resulting in pain. NSAIDs work by inhibiting the action of cyclooxygenase (COX), which is an enzyme used to synthesize prostaglandins from arachidonic acid.

NSAIDs can be divided into two groups of compounds: (1) the indoles (of which indomethacin [Indocin] is the prototype), which include sulindac (Clinoril) and Tolmetin sodium (Tolectin); and (2) propionic acid derivatives with a shorter half-life (e.g., ibuprofen [Motrin], naproxen [Naprosyn], and fenoprofen [Nalfon]). These agents, when prescribed for antiinflammatory effect, should be taken for a minimum of 2 weeks on a rigid time schedule.

Ibuprofen (e.g., Motrin, Advil, Nuprin) has proved to be effective in reducing musculoskeletal pains. A common dosage of 600 to 800 mg three times a day will often reduce pain and stop the cyclic effects of the deep pain input. Numerous other NSAIDs are available, and if ibuprofen does not reduce the pain, another should be tried.

Individual patients may respond differently to these medications. Continued use may result in stomach irritation or even ulceration,[200,201] so the patient should be questioned for prior stomach problems before use and monitored closely during treatment. These medications should be taken with meals to lessen the likelihood of stomach irritation.

A relatively new class of NSAID drugs is the COX-2 inhibitors. As mentioned earlier, cyclooxygenase (COX) is an enzyme used to synthesize prostaglandins from arachidonic acid. COX inhibits the synthesis of prostaglandin by way of two distinct pathways. These are known as COX-1 and COX-2. The COX-1 pathway is involved in maintaining homeostatic functions including the maintenance of gastric and renal integrity. The COX-2 pathway has greater effects on the inflammatory response. Most NSAIDs inhibit both pathways, therefore reducing inflammation but at the same time diminishing gastric secretions that protect the stomach wall. The results are often pain reduction but also stomach irritation. The new COX-2 inhibitors predominantly affect only the COX-2 pathway, which reduces the inflammatory response without greatly affecting gastric and renal function.[202]

An available COX-2 inhibitor at the time of this writing is celecoxib (Celebrex). This medication has not only the advantage of less gastric side effects but also needs to be taken only once or twice a day. Early studies suggest that this medication can assist in managing TMD pain[203] but perhaps no more so than naproxen.[204]

Another method of administering an NSAID is by way of a topical gel or ointment. Some studies report that the topical application of an NSAID, such as ketoprofen, has a greater effect on pain reduction than a placebo gel.[205,206] Unfortunately, at this time the data are still mixed regarding the true effectiveness of topical NSAIDs.

Antiinflammatory Agents. When inflammatory conditions are present, antiinflammatories can be helpful in altering the course of the disorder. These agents suppress the body's overall response to the irritation. Antiinflammatory agents can be administered orally or by injection.

Oral NSAIDs have already been discussed under the category of analgesics. When taken on a regular basis, these medications are quite useful in the management of inflammatory joint disorders, as well as chronic centrally mediated myalgia. Aspirin or ibuprofen can serve in this capacity while providing an analgesic effect. Many other oral antiinflammatories exist (e.g., naproxen, flurbiprofen, nabumetone, ketoprofen). Remember, however,

that these drugs often do not immediately achieve good blood levels and therefore should be taken on a regular schedule for a minimum of 3 weeks. The general health and condition of the patient must always be considered before these (or any) medications are prescribed; and, as is often the case, it may be necessary to consult the patient's physician regarding the advisability of such drug therapy. If stomach irritation becomes a problem, a COX-2 inhibitor might be considered.

Corticosteroids. Corticosteroids are potent antiinflammatories not commonly prescribed for systemic use in the treatment of TMDs because of their side effects. The exception is for acute, generalized muscle and joint inflammation associated with the polyarthritides. Corticosteroids can be administered either orally or by injection.

Oral corticosteroids can be provided in a convenient package that provides the patient with a significant dose earlier in the treatment period and is later followed by a gradual reduction in dosing until the medication is stopped. This is the safest way to use a corticosteroid to prevent a secondary infection.

Injecting an antiinflammatory such as hydrocortisone into the joint has been advocated[207-211] for the relief of pain and restricted movements. A single intraarticular injection seems to be most helpful in older patients; however, less success has been observed[209] in patients younger than age 25. Although a single injection is occasionally helpful, some studies[212-214] reported that multiple injections may be harmful to the structures of the joint and should be avoided. A long-term follow-up to intraarticular corticosteroid injection for TMJ osteoarthritis, however, was encouraging.[211] Injection of corticosteroids has also been reported to improve acute TMJ symptoms caused by rheumatoid arthritis with no long-term adverse sequelae.[211]

Another injectable solution that is used for intracapsular injections is sodium hyaluronate. Although this is not a local anesthetic, sodium hyaluronate has been suggested for the treatment of TMJ articular disease.[215,210] Studies in the treatment of disc displacements and disc dislocations without reduction are promising.[216-218] Some studies[39,219,220] have found that the use of sodium hyaluronate following arthrocentesis of the TMJ can be helpful in reducing pain (see Chapter 13). The use of sodium hyaluronate in the TMJ is limited at this time because it has not yet received approval for this use in the United States.

Anxiolytic Agents. When high levels of emotional stress are thought to be contributing to a TMD, anxiolytic agents (antianxiety) may be helpful in managing the symptoms.[221,222] Remember that anxiolytic agents do not eliminate stress but merely alter the patient's perception or reaction to the stress. Use of anxiolytic agents therefore is supportive therapy. A commonly used group of anxiolytics are the benzodiazepines, of which diazepam (Valium) has received the most attention. It can be prescribed on a daily basis but, because of potential dependency, should not be used for more than 7 days consecutively. A single dose (2.5 to 5 mg) of diazepam is often helpful at bedtime to relax the muscles and perhaps lessen nocturnal parafunctional activity.[183,223] When only this single dose is prescribed, the duration of its use can be extended to 2 weeks.

Two other benzodiazepines that have been used with certain masticatory muscle disorders are clonazepam (Klonopin)[224-226] and alprazolam (Xanax).[227] These agents can be useful in the management of acute symptoms, especially related to anxiety and perhaps nocturnal bruxism, but as with Valium, the addictive potential and sedating effects contraindicate long-term use with more chronic conditions.[221]

Muscle Relaxants. For many years muscle relaxants have been prescribed for TMD patients, although most clinicians would agree that their effect on symptoms is minimal. Perhaps this is understandable when one appreciates that most muscle pain conditions are not associated with a significant increase in muscle activity (see Chapter 8). Most muscle relaxants have a central effect that sedates the patient. Perhaps this sedation is the main explanation for the positive response of some patients.

Mephenesin is the prototype for the majority of the oral skeletal muscle relaxants, which include the propanediols (e.g., carisoprodol [Soma], methocarbamol [Robaxin], and chemically related chloraxazome [Paraflex, Parafon]).[228] Experimentally, muscle relaxants depress spinal polysynaptic reflexes preferentially over monosynaptic reflexes. These compounds affect neuronal activity associated with muscle stretch reflexes, primarily in the lateral reticular area of the brainstem. The oral doses of all of these drugs are well below the levels required to elicit experimental muscle relaxant activity.[229] A muscle relaxant that has fewer central effects is metaxalone [Skelaxin]. This medication may be more appropriate for the patient who must work while taking a muscle relaxant.

It should be noted that in order for some muscle relaxants to reach therapeutic effects on the muscles of mastication, the dosage must often be raised to a level that does not allow the patient to carry out normal activities. Patients who take muscle relaxants should be warned of the sedation and told not to drive or use heavy equipment.

Some central skeletal muscle relaxants are available in combination with analgesics (e.g., carisoprodol with phenacetin and caffeine [Soma Compound], chlorzoxazone with acetaminophen [Parafon Forte], orphenadrine citrate with aspirin and caffeine [Norgesic Forte], methocarbamol with aspirin [Robaxisal]).

A muscle relaxant that seems to provide a positive effect on a variety of muscle pain, as well as TMDs, is cyclobenzaprine [Flexeril].[230-233] This medication is a compound similar to the tricyclic antidepressants and therefore may work in a similar manner. A single dose of 5 to 10 mg before sleep can reduce muscle pain, especially in the morning. Another dose of 5 to 10 mg during the day may be helpful for pain, but often patients find that it makes them too drowsy to function.

Antidepressants. Although the tricyclic antidepressants were originally developed for the management of depression, the more recent development of the selective serotonin reuptake inhibitors (SSRIs) has proved to be far more effective. At this time tricyclic antidepressants are rarely used for depression. However, the tricyclics have found new value in the management of a variety of chronic pain conditions.[222,234-242] This is especially the case with neuropathic pain.[243] It has been demonstrated[244-251] that a low dose of amitriptyline (10 mg) just before sleep can have an analgesic effect on chronic pain but has little effect on acute pain.[252,253] This clinical effect is not related to any antidepressive action because antidepressive dosages are from 10 to 20 times higher. The therapeutic effect of these drugs is thought to be related to their ability to increase the availability of the biogenic amines serotonin and norepinephrine at the synaptic junction in the central nervous system. The tricyclic antidepressants are beneficial in dosages as low as 10 mg in the treatment of tension-type headache and musculoskeletal pain.[234,254] They decrease the number of awakenings, increase stage IV (delta) sleep, and markedly decrease time spent in rapid eye movement (REM) sleep. For these reasons, they may have potential in the treatment of certain types of nocturnal bruxism, as well as for improving the quality of sleep.[255] Amitriptyline can be helpful in the management of certain sleep disorders associated with musculoskeletal pains.[256-259] Amitriptyline can be an important part of the management of fibromyalgia[260-264] (see Chapter 12).

When used as antidepressants, which require an increase in therapeutic dosage, these drugs should only be prescribed by clinicians who have had special training in the diagnosis and treatment of depression.

Local Anesthetics. Local anesthetics can be useful in the diagnosis and even management of a variety of TMDs. One of the most important uses is for establishing the correct diagnosis. Local anesthetic can be used to differentiate a true source of pain from a site of pain (see Chapter 10). When a source of pain is present in a muscle or joint, injecting local anesthetic into the source will eliminate the pain, confirming the diagnosis.[265]

Local anesthetics can also be used for certain disorders as actual therapy.[266] For example, the injection of local anesthetic into a myofascial trigger point can result in significant pain reduction long after the anesthetic has been metabolized.[267-271] The concept and rationale for using trigger point injections in the management of myofascial pain is discussed in Chapter 12.

Another use of local anesthetics in the management of some chronic TMDs is related to pain management.[272] The therapeutic effect is achieved by breaking the pain cycle. Once a source of deep pain input is eliminated (even temporarily), sensitized central neurons have an opportunity to return to a more normal state.[273] If the pain can be eliminated for a significant period of time, when the nociceptive input returns the patient will often report a significant reduction in pain intensity.[274] This pain reduction may last for hours or even days. In this sense the local anesthetic has a therapeutic effect on the pain experience.

The two most common local anesthetic drugs used for short-duration pain reduction in TMDs are 2% lidocaine (Xylocaine) and 3% mepivacaine (Carbocaine).[275] Although procaine has been suggested for myofascial trigger point injections,[276] it is no longer packaged in dental carpules and thus is less convenient for use in standard dental syringes. For muscle injections a solution without a vasoconstrictor should be used.[277] When a longer-acting anesthetic is indicated, 0.5% bupivacaine (Marcaine) may be used.[278] Although bupivacaine is sometimes indicated for joint pain (auriculotemporal nerve block), it should not be routinely used with muscle injections because of its myotoxicity.[279]

Another injectable solution that is used for intracapsular injections is sodium hyaluronate. Although this is not a local anesthetic, sodium hyaluronate has been suggested for the treatment of TMJ articular disease.[215,210] Studies in the treatment of disc displacements and disc dislocations without reduction are promising.[216-218,280] Some studies[39,219,220] have found that the use of sodium hyaluronate following arthrocentesis of the TMJ can be helpful in reducing pain (see Chapter 13). The use of sodium hyaluronate in the TMJ is limited at this time but seems promising.[281]

Physical Therapy

Physical therapy represents a group of supportive actions that is usually instituted in conjunction with definitive treatment. It can be an important part of the successful management of many TMDs.[282-284] Although physical therapy has been used to reduce the symptoms associated with TMD, the evidence that supports each specific type of treatment has yet to be established.[285] Because physical therapy techniques are normally quite conservative, the profession feels relatively comfortable using them without evidence-based data.

Most physical therapy fits into one of two general categories: modalities and manual techniques. Although these categories are discussed separately, they often work best when appropriately selected and combined to the individual needs of the patient. Selection of the most appropriate modality or manual technique for each patient may be difficult for the dentist because dentists are not often trained in this area of management. Clinicians who frequently treat TMD patients should establish a working relationship with a physical therapist who also has interest in TMD. Establishing this relationship will be most rewarding for both the patient and the clinician.

Physical Therapy Modalities. Physical therapy modalities represent the physical treatments that can be applied to the patient.[286-288] They can be divided into the following types: thermotherapy, coolant therapy, ultrasound, phonophoresis, iontophoresis, electrogalvanic stimulation (EGS) therapy, transcutaneous electrical nerve stimulation (TENS), acupuncture, and laser.

Thermotherapy. Thermotherapy uses heat as a prime mechanism and is based on the premise that heat increases circulation to the applied area. Although the origin of muscle pain is unclear and complex, most theories contend that the initial condition of decreased blood flow to the tissues is responsible for myalgia associated with local muscle soreness. Thermotherapy counteracts this by creating vasodilation in the compromised tissues, leading to reduction of the symptoms.

Surface heat is applied by laying a hot, moist towel over the symptomatic area (Fig. 11-7).[289] A hot water bottle over the towel will help maintain the heat. This combination should remain in place for 10 to 15 minutes, not to exceed 30 minutes. An electrical heating pad may be used, but care must be taken not to leave it unattended. Falling asleep on a heating pad can lead to a serious burn.

Coolant therapy. Like thermotherapy, coolant therapy has proved to be a simple and often effective method of reducing pain (Fig. 11-8).[290] The suggestion has been made[291,292] that cold encourages the relaxation of muscles that are in spasm and thus relieves the associated pain. Ice should be applied directly to the affected area and moved in a circular motion without pressure to the tissues.

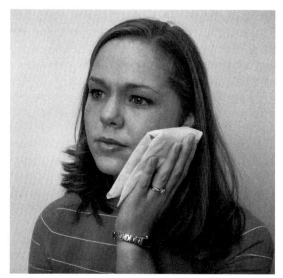

Fig. 11-7 Moist heat applied to the symptomatic muscle can often reduce levels of pain and discomfort. A commercially available moist heat pad can be moistened and heated in a microwave. A warm, moist towel can also be used.

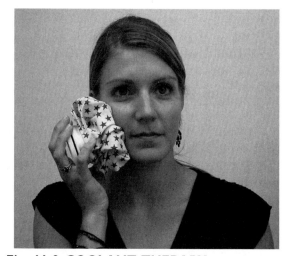

Fig. 11-8 COOLANT THERAPY. An ice pack is applied to the painful area for 2 to 4 minutes or until the tissue feels numb. Then the tissue is allowed to slowly warm again. This can be repeated as needed. Ice should not be left on the face for longer than 5 to 7 minutes or tissue injury may result.

The patient will initially experience an uncomfortable feeling that will quickly turn into a burning sensation. Continued icing will result in a mild aching and then numbness.[293] When numbness begins, the ice should be removed. The ice should not be left on the tissues for longer than 5 to 7 minutes. After a period of warming a second application may be desirable. It is thought that during warming there is an increase in blood flow to the tissues that assists tissue repair.

A simple method of providing ice therapy is to have the patient place a Styrofoam cup filled with water in the freezer. Once it is frozen it can be removed and the bottom of the cup torn away, exposing the ice. The rest of the cup can be used as a convenient holder so that the patient's fingers do not get too cold. The cup can also be placed in a plastic bag so that as the ice melts, the water is contained in the bag and not all over the patient. Another convenient method of coolant therapy is using a bag of frozen vegetables (corn or peas). The bag can be easily molded to the surface that is to be chilled and held there. As it warms, it can be refrozen and used again.

A common coolant therapy uses a vapor spray. Two of the most common sprays used are ethyl chloride and fluoromethane. In early studies[291,292] ethyl chloride was generally used, but it was found to be both flammable and a cardiac depressant if inhaled. Thus fluoromethane has been more recently suggested[267] because it does not pose these risks. Vapocoolant spray is applied to the desired area from a distance of 1 or 2 feet (Fig. 11-9) for approximately 5 seconds. After the tissue has been rewarmed, the procedure can be repeated. Care must be taken not to allow the spray to contact the eyes, ears, nose, or mouth. A towel can be used to protect these areas. Vapocoolant sprays do not penetrate tissue as does ice, and therefore it is likely that the reduction in pain is more associated with the stimulation of cutaneous nerve fibers that in turn shut down the smaller pain fibers (the C fibers), as discussed in Chapter 2. This type of pain reduction is likely to be of short duration.

When myofascial (trigger point) pain is present, a technique described as "spray and stretch" is used.[267,294,295] This involves spraying the tissue over a muscle with a trigger point and then immediately passively stretching the muscle. The technique is

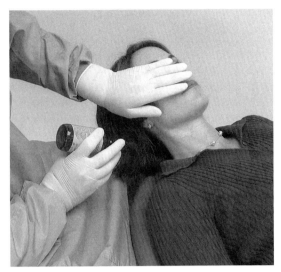

Fig. 11-9 COOLANT THERAPY. Fluoromethane spray is applied to the painful areas for approximately 5 seconds. The muscle is then gently stretched. This is repeated several times during each visit. The eyes, nose, and ears are protected from the spray.

discussed more fully later in this chapter and in Chapter 12.

Ultrasound therapy. Ultrasound is a method of producing an increase in temperature at the interface of the tissues and therefore affects deeper tissues than does surface heat (Fig. 11-10).[296]

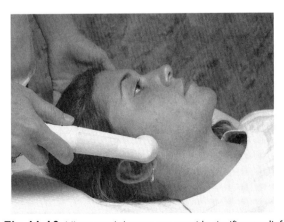

Fig. 11-10 Ultrasound therapy can provide significant relief of symptoms for many patients. It increases the temperature of the interface of the tissues and thus provides a deep heat.

Not only does ultrasound increase the blood flow in deep tissues, it also seems to separate collagen fibers. This improves the flexibility and extensibility of connective tissues.[297] Some experts have suggested[298,299] that surface heat and ultrasound be used together, especially when treating post-trauma patients. Although this modality has been used for years with apparent clinical success, the data regarding its effectiveness are mixed.[300]

Phonophoresis. Ultrasound has also been used[301-304] to administer drugs through the skin by a process known as *phonophoresis.* For example, 10% hydrocortisone cream is applied to an inflamed joint and the ultrasound transducer is then directed at the joint. The effects of salicylates and other topical anesthetics can also be enhanced in this manner.

Iontophoresis. Iontophoresis, like phonophoresis, is a technique by which certain medications can be introduced into the tissues without affecting any other organs.[305,306] With iontophoresis the medication is placed in a pad and the pad is placed on the desired tissue area (Fig. 11-11). Then a low electrical current is passed through the pad, driving the medication into the tissue.[307] Local anesthetics and antiinflammatories are common medications used with iontophoresis.[288,298,308-310] Not all studies show the efficacy of this modality.[311]

Electrogalvanic stimulation therapy. EGS[312,313] uses the principle that electrical stimulation of a muscle

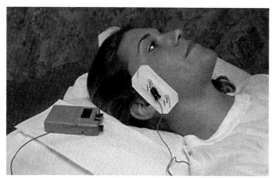

Fig. 11-11 IONTOPHORESIS TREATMENT. Medication is placed in a pad, and then a low electrical current is passed through the pad, driving the medication into the tissue. Local anesthetics and antiinflammatories are common medications used with iontophoresis.

causes it to contract. EGS uses a high-voltage, low-amperage, monophasic current of varied frequency. A rhythmic electrical impulse is applied to the muscle, creating repeated involuntary contractions and relaxations. The intensity and frequency of these can be varied according to the desired effect, and they may help to break up myospasms, as well as increase blood flow to the muscles. Both effects lead to a reduction of pain in compromised muscle tissues. If, however, significant motor stimulation occurs concurrently, this may impair the analgesic effect and actually exacerbate acute muscle pain.[314] Microcurrent electrical stimulation is reputed to apply a microvoltage in a range similar to that which occurs at the synaptic junction. It has been used primarily for pain control. At present, only anecdotal clinical evidence supports the use of EGS in the treatment of painful TMDs of muscle origin. Some clinicians go on to believe that once the pain is reduced, the ideal mandibular position can be located with this stimulation and dental changes are in order. This concept is highly suspect to error and totally unfounded by scientific evidence (see Chapter 5). This area of study needs considerable investigation.

Transcutaneous electrical nerve stimulation. TENS,[315-317] as described in Chapter 2, is produced by a continuous stimulation of cutaneous nerve fibers at a sub-painful level.[318] When a TENS unit is placed over the tissues of a painful area, the electrical activity decreases pain perception. TENS uses a low-voltage, low-amperage, biphasic current of varied frequency and is designed primarily for sensory counterstimulation in painful disorders.[319-321]

When the intensity of a TENS unit is increased to the point that motor fibers are activated, the TENS unit becomes an EGS unit that is no longer used for pain control but instead for muscle relaxation, as mentioned earlier. Frequent interchange of these terms confuses some professionals.

Portable TENS units have been developed for long-term use by patients with chronic pain[322] (Fig. 11-12) and can be effective with various TMDs.[11,56,299,320,323-327]

Acupuncture. Another technique of modulating pain, acupuncture (see Chapter 2), uses the body's own antinociceptive system to reduce the levels of pain felt. Stimulation of certain areas

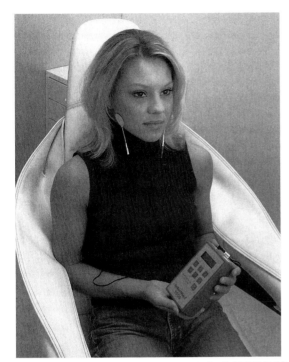

Fig. 11-12 TRANSCUTANEOUS ELECTRICAL NERVE STIMULATION (TENS). A portable TENS unit placed over the painful areas can provide relief of symptoms. This is accomplished by mild electrical stimulation of cutaneous sensory nerves.

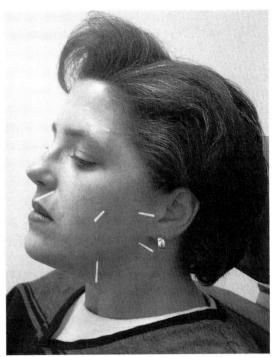

Fig. 11-13 Acupuncture needles placed in the face help reduce pain in these areas. These needles are maintained in place for approximately 30 minutes, during which they are twirled (stimulated) every 5 to 10 minutes.

(or acupuncture points) appears to cause the release of endorphins, which reduce painful sensations by flooding the afferent interneurons with subthreshold stimuli (Fig. 11-13). These effectively block the transmission of noxious impulses and thus reduce the sensations of pain. Intermittent stimulation of about two pulses per second seems to be most effective in reducing the discomfort connected with masticatory dysfunction.[328] Acupuncture has been successfully used with some TMD symptoms,[54,329-332] although patients seem to prefer the more traditional treatments.[333] Acupuncture appears to be a promising modality, although its mechanism of action is not well understood. Further investigation is certainly indicated.[334]

Although acupuncture and TENS seem to involve similar mechanisms, some evidence suggests they are physiologically different. Acupuncture seems to

use endorphins for pain modulation, whereas TENS may not.[335]

Cold laser. In recent years the cold or soft laser has been investigated for wound healing and pain relief. Currently, it is not considered to be a routine physical therapy modality but is included in this section for completeness. Most studies on the cold laser report on its use in chronic musculoskeletal, rheumatic, and neurologic pain conditions.[336-345] A cold laser is thought to accelerate collagen synthesis, increase vascularity of healing tissues, decrease the number of microorganisms, and decrease pain.

Several case studies in which cold laser therapy has been used on persistent TMJ pain have been published.[282,330,346-349] Although the results of these studies have been favorable, the studies lack controls and adequate sample size. More investigations will be necessary before laser therapy becomes a routine modality in dentistry.

Manual Techniques. Manual techniques are the "hands-on" therapies provided by the physical therapist for the reduction of pain and dysfunction. Manual techniques are divided into three categories: soft tissue mobilization, joint mobilization, and muscle conditioning.

Soft tissue mobilization. Physical therapy can be helpful in regaining normal function and mobility of injured or painful tissues. Soft tissue mobilization is useful for muscle pain conditions and is accomplished by superficial and deep massage. As discussed previously, mild stimulation of cutaneous sensory nerves exerts an inhibitory influence on pain.[318,350] Thus gentle massage of the tissues overlying a painful area can often reduce pain perception. The patient can be taught gentle self-massage techniques and is encouraged to do this as needed for reduction of pain. This technique along with painless stretching of the muscles can be quite helpful in reducing pain. These techniques also get the patient actively involved in the treatment, which can give the patient an important feeling of control (Fig. 11-14).

Deep massage can be more helpful than gentle massage in reestablishing normal muscle function.

Deep massage, however, must be provided by another individual such as a physical therapist. Deep massage can assist in mobilizing tissues, increasing blood flow to the area and eliminating trigger points.[351] In order to enhance the effectiveness of deep massage, the patients should receive 10 to 15 minutes of moist heat before beginning the massage. The deep heat tends to relax the muscle tissues, decreasing pain and enhancing the effectiveness of the deep massage.

Joint mobilization. Mobilization of the TMJ is useful in decreasing interarticular pressure, as well as increasing range of joint movement. Gentle distraction of the joint can assist in reducing temporary adhesions and perhaps even mobilize the disc. In some instances distraction of the joint is useful in managing an acute disc dislocation without reduction (see Chapter 13). Passive distraction is thought to inhibit the activity of muscles that pull across the joint. Distraction of the TMJ is accomplished by placing the thumb in the patient's mouth over the lower second molar area on the side to be distracted. With the cranium stabilized by the other hand, the thumb places downward force on the molar as the rest of the same hand pulls up on the anterior portion of the mandible (chin) (Fig. 11-15). Distraction for relaxing muscles does not require translation of the joint but merely

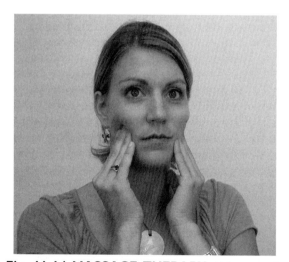

Fig. 11-14 MASSAGE THERAPY. When muscle pain is the major complaint, massage can be helpful. The patient is encouraged to apply gentle massage to the painful areas regularly throughout the day. This can stimulate cutaneous sensory nerves to exert an inhibitory influence on the pain. If it increases the pain, it should be stopped.

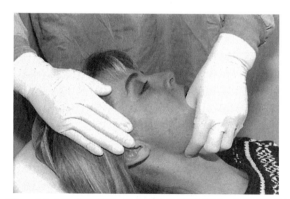

Fig. 11-15 JOINT DISTRACTION OF THE TEMPOROMANDIBULAR JOINT. This can be accomplished by placing the thumb in the patient's mouth over the mandibular second molar area on the side to be distracted. While the cranium is stabilized with the other hand, the thumb exerts downward force on the molar.

unloading in the closed joint position. The distraction is maintained for several seconds and then released. It can be repeated several times. When joint immobility is the problem, distraction is combined with manual translation of the joint.

Of important note is that mild distraction of a normal joint does not produce pain. If pain is elicited, the therapist should be suspicious of an inflammatory joint disorder and discontinue the distraction procedure.

Distraction of the cervical spine may also be helpful in some patients with orofacial pain complaints. It should be instituted and monitored by a specialist trained in cervicospinal function. Dentists are not normally training in cervical traction therapy and therefore do not recommend this type of therapy. However, the dentist treating orofacial pain may encounter patients who are using cervical traction as recommended by their physician for a cervical disorder.

When cervical traction is used, care must be taken not to place too much force on the TMJs. Some cervicospinal traction devices tend to retrude the mandible, increasing the likelihood of disc derangement disorders. Patients who are actively undergoing cervical traction should be educated to the potential risks of injury to the TMJs. They should be told to always keep their teeth together while undergoing traction. This tends to stabilize and control loading to the joint structures. Clinicians should also recommend that the patient purchase a soft athletic appliance that can be worn during the traction period. This type of appliance can provide more stability, minimizing potential injury to the TMJs.

Muscle conditioning. Patients who experience TMD symptoms often decrease the use of their jaw because of pain. If this is prolonged, the muscles can become shorted and atrophied. The patient should be instructed in self-administering exercises that can help restore normal function and range of movement. Four types of exercises programs can be instituted by the physical therapist or the dentist: passive muscle stretching, assisted muscle stretching, resistance exercises, and postural training.

Passive muscle stretching. Passive muscle stretching of painful, shortened muscles can be effective in managing some TMDs.[352,353] This muscle stretching counteracts the shortened muscle length that contributes to decreased blood flow and the accumulation of algogenic substances that may be responsible for muscle pain. Often gentle passive stretching of a muscle can assist in reestablishing normal muscle length and function. The patient should be instructed to slowly and deliberately open the mouth until pain is felt. Pain should be avoided because it can lead to cyclic muscle pain. Sometimes it is helpful for patients experiencing muscle pain to observe their mouth opening in a mirror so that they can make the pathway straight, without defect or deviation (Fig. 11-16). Lateral eccentric movements and protrusive moves should also be encouraged within the painless ranges.

With intracapsular disorders a straight mouth opening may not be possible or desirable. Asking a patient with a disc dislocation or structural incompatibility to open on a straight pathway may actually aggravate the pain condition. These patients should be instructed to open as wide as is comfortable in a manner that causes the least resistance to the disc interference disorder. Sometimes deflections

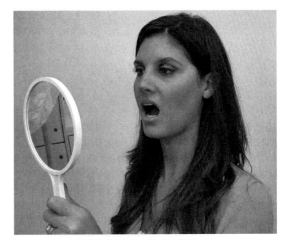

Fig. 11-16 PASSIVE EXERCISES. Patients with dysfunctional jaw movements can often be trained to avoid these movements by simply watching themselves in a mirror. The patient is encouraged to open on a straight opening pathway. In many instances, if this can be accomplished following a more rotational path with less translation, disc derangement disorders will be avoided.

in the opening pathway have been learned by the patient (muscle engrams), and attempts to correct this may actually aggravate the condition.

Passive muscle stretching can actually be helpful in training patients to perform movements that will overcome certain intracapsular dysfunctions.[354] For example, during an opening movement, patients with a joint sound often translate the condyle forward before it is rotated. Patients with these types of problems are encouraged to visualize their mandibular movement in a mirror and to rotate open before translation. Again, diagnosis is the key to proper treatment selection.

Sometimes passive stretching of the muscle can be assisted by the use of a vapocoolant spray. The vapocoolant spray can reduce pain, allowing the patient to achieve a greater mouth opening without pain. This may be especially helpful in treating trigger points associated with myofascial pain (more details in the next section).

Assisted muscle stretching. Assisted muscle stretching is used when there is a need to regain muscle length. Stretching should never be sudden or forceful. Instead, it should be performed with gentle intermittent force that is gradually increased. Patients can help in providing their own stretching because they are not likely to overstretch or traumatize the involved tissues (Fig. 11-17). When someone else assists with the stretching exercises, the patient must be advised to communicate any discomfort. If pain is elicited, the amount of force is decreased.

Assisted muscle stretching is an important treatment regimen in the management of myofascial pain.[352] Simons and Travell[351] have described a spray-and-stretch technique that is the most commonly used treatment for the elimination of trigger points. The technique uses fluoromethane spray as a counterirritant before stretching the muscle. The fluoromethane spray is applied over the area of the trigger point and then directed toward the area of the referred pain. The spray is then stopped, and another sweep of the spray is repeated in the same manner. After three or four sweeps of the spray, the muscle is actively stretched to its maximum functional length.

Once the muscle has been stretched, it is warmed with the hand and the procedure is repeated two to

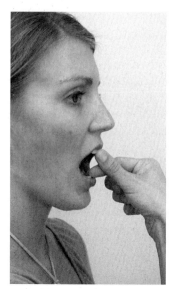

Fig. 11-17 Stretching exercises can often be used to regain normal opening movement. The patient is instructed to apply stretching force gently and intermittently to the elevator muscle with the fingers. Pain should not be elicited. If it is, then the force should be decreased or the exercises stopped completely.

three times. It is assumed that the trigger points are eliminated by the active stretching of the muscle. The spray is used merely as a counterirritant that temporarily reduces pain so that the muscle can be stretched without pain (gate control theory[350]). If pain is produced during the stretch, the muscle will likely contract, reducing the effectiveness of the technique. Producing pain can also encourage a cyclic muscle pain condition.

Another use of assisted exercises is following TMJ surgery. Often after surgery the TMJ can develop adhesions or the capsular ligament can fibrose and tighten. This can greatly restrict mouth opening. Studies[355,356] suggest that active exercises following arthroscopy and arthrotomy assist in achieving better range of mandibular movements. Assisted exercises are also helpful in achieving increased range of movement in patients experiencing permanent disc dislocation without reducing.[357-360]

Resistance exercises. Resistance exercises[361] use the concept of reflex relaxation or reciprocal inhibition. When the patient attempts to open, the mandibular depressors are active. The elevator muscles, which normally relax slowly, keep the mandible from dropping suddenly. If the depressor muscles meet resistance, the neurologic message sent to the antagonistic muscles (the elevators) is to relax more fully. This concept can be used by instructing the patient to place the fist under the chin and open the mouth gently against the resistance (Fig. 11-18, A). If eccentric movements are restricted, the patient can be asked to move the mandible in an eccentric position against slight resistance (Fig. 11-18, B). These exercises are repeated 10 times each session, six sessions a day. If they elicit pain, they are discontinued. These exercises are only useful if the restricted opening is secondary to a muscle condition and should not be used for painful intracapsular restrictions. It is also important that these resisted movements do not produce pain, which could lead to cyclic muscle pain.

Isometric exercises (resistance exercises) may be helpful in young adults with painless early clicking. It has been suggested that loading the joint structures at this age assists in strengthening the ligaments and the articular surfaces.[362] Isometric

exercises also strengthen the muscles that support the joint, improving function and resistance to displacements.

Postural training. Although there is evidence that cervical disorders are closely related to TMD symptoms, the exact relationship is not completely clear. Certainly the referred pain effects caused by central excitation are a major contributor (see Chapter 2). Some clinicians[363,364] have also suggested that the posture of the head, neck, and shoulders can contribute to TMD symptoms. Although this may be logical, the scientific evidence is weak[365,366] and in some cases unsupportive.[367-369] A forward head posture has drawn the most attention. It has been described that if the head is in the forward position, the patient must rotate the head upward in order to see adequately. This forward and rotated head position produces elongation of the suprahyoid and infrahyoid muscles and also closes the posterior space between the atlas and axis. It has been suggested that maintaining this position often leads to muscular and cervical symptoms. In TMD patients with muscle pain who also have forward head posture, training the

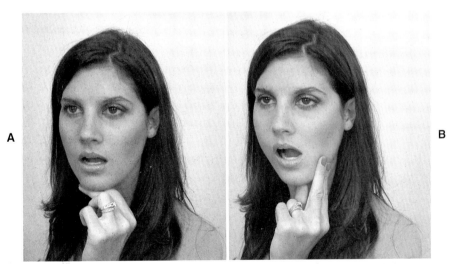

Fig. 11-18 Resistance exercises use the concept of reflex relaxation to provide an increase in mandibular opening. **A,** The patient is instructed to open against gentle resistance provided by the fingers. This will promote relaxation in the elevator muscles, thus allowing increased mandibular opening. **B,** When eccentric movement is limited, the patient can be asked to move in the eccentric position with gentle resistance from the fingers. These exercises are repeated 10 times each session, six sessions a day. If they elicit pain, they are discontinued.

patient to keep the head in a more normal relationship with the shoulders may be helpful in reducing TMD symptoms.[370]

Exercises have been suggested to assist patients in improving cervical and head posture.[367,370] Because these exercises are simple and noninvasive, they can be presented to all patients with a forward head position and TMD pain. The effectiveness of these exercises, however, has not been established. Sound scientific studies in this area are necessary.

Of note is that the effectiveness of physical therapy modalities and techniques needs to be more thoroughly evaluated in controlled clinical trials. Most of these management styles have developed antidotally, with little evidence-based science.[285,300,357,371,372] Because most of these therapies are conservative, it is likely that no harm is done. On the other hand, in a financially conscious society, cost effectiveness needs to be considered.

THE CONCEPT OF PHYSICAL SELF-REGULATION

When a TMD is acute, immediate therapy directed to an obvious etiology is normally sufficient to reduce and often eliminate symptoms. However, when symptoms are prolonged, management becomes far more difficult. Chronic TMD is often not resolved by simple dental procedures (i.e., an occlusal appliance). This is likely because of the presence of other significant factors that are not strongly linked to the dental condition. Some of these factors may be psychosocial issues that are associated with characteristic changes in brain-controlled physiology. In an interesting study by Phillips et al.,[140] patients with acute TMD symptoms were evaluated psychosocially but not offered any formal treatment. These individuals were then recalled in 6 months to determine the status of their TMD symptoms. Phillips reported that individuals who continued to experience TMD symptoms were different in several psychosocial considerations from those who no longer experienced symptoms. Chronic TMD individuals had more anxiety disorders and depressive disorders than those who had recovered. Differences were

also reported between men and women. Men who develop chronic TMD were more likely to demonstrate a personality disorder, whereas women were more likely to demonstrate a significant degree of a major of psychopathology. The important thought here is that some individuals may have certain psychosocial issues and altered physiologic responses to innocuous stimuli that make them more prone to becoming chronic TMD suffers. As mentioned in an earlier section of this chapter, prior emotional traumas experienced by an individual can chronically upregulate the autonomic nervous system. This upregulation and disturbed physiology may make it more difficult for an individual to recover from a recent injury or onset of symptoms, thus leading to a chronic condition. This is why as TMD becomes chronic a team approach should be considered. The minimal team for chronic TMD is a dentist, a psychologist, and a physical therapist or practitioners who have a combination of skills from each of these disciplines.

A reasonable treatment approach in managing chronic TMD and orofacial pains is to develop interventions that address the specific characteristics commonly found in chronic TMD patients. The research laboratory at the University of Kentucky has developed a program of research[85,373] that suggests persons with chronic muscle-related orofacial pains are distinguished by five characteristics:

1. These individuals report significant pain intensity when compared with other pain patients, and they are also more sensitive to painful stimuli in the trigeminal region. This sensitivity to painful stimuli is consistent with research findings in other orofacial pain settings.[374,375]
2. Pain patients report significant levels of fatigue that impair normal functioning. This fatigue may be closely related to the third important characteristic, depression.
3. Depression is common among patients with chronic muscle-related orofacial pains. However, a significant component of the fatigue is not linked to depression itself.
4. Breathing patterns are disrupted so that end-tidal carbon dioxide levels are lower in these patients than in comparable controls. This finding

suggests that altered breathing patterns may be contributing to the overall "physical dysregulation" reported by these patients.

5. Pain patients report significant sleep disturbances involving either sleep-onset difficulties or disruptive awakenings.

These five characteristics represent a constellation of symptoms indicative of "autonomic dysregulation" and provide direction for the application of specific intervention strategies to address the underlying physiologic disturbances that may be contributing to the maintenance of the pain disorder.

The following is a treatment approach for chronic orofacial pains that is based on the interpretations of research findings developed by Drs. Peter Bertrand and Charles Carlson in 1993. The focus of this treatment is on (1) addressing the pain and fatigue as a physiologic disturbance in need of correction, (2) managing autonomic dysregulation, (3) altering dysfunctional breathing patterns, and (4) improving sleep. Because this approach involves entrainment of specific skills to alter physiologic parameters, the approach has been called *physical self-regulation* (PSR) training. A training manual for PSR was developed by Drs. Carlson and Bertrand in 1995 to codify and standardize the procedures.[376] In 1997 Drs. Bertrand and Carlson conducted a randomized, controlled clinical trial of the PSR approach in a clinical sample of orofacial pain patients at the National Naval Dental Center in Bethesda, Maryland.[377] The clinical trial included randomization of 44 patients with an average age of 34.6 years and with pain lasting for 52 months into either a group receiving PSR or a group receiving standard dental care (SDC) that included a stabilization appliance. Both treatments resulted in significant decreases in pain intensity and life interference from the pains 6 weeks after treatment was initiated. At 6 months' follow-up, however, the PSR group reported less pain than the SDC group. Comfortable and maximum mouth opening improved for both groups initially as well. At the 6-month follow-up, the PSR group had greater comfortable and maximum mouth opening than did the SDC group. These results provide support for the use and continued evaluation of the PSR approach for managing orofacial pains.

The PSR approach consists of eight areas of education and training. First, patients are provided with an explanation of their condition and an opportunity to develop personal ownership of the problem. Second, the patients are given instructions regarding the rest positions for structures in the orofacial region[378] and the importance of diminishing muscle activation by recognizing whether head and neck muscle responses are relevant for specific tasks. Third, specific skills are provided for improving awareness of postural positioning, especially of the head and neck regions. This is termed *proprioceptive reeducation*, and the rationale for this is further elaborated by Carlson et al.[377] Fourth, a skill for relaxing upper back tension is also imparted to patients through an exercise involving gentle movement of the rhomboid muscle groups. Fifth, a brief progressive relaxation procedure involving the positioning of body structures is given to patients, along with instructions to take at least two periods during daily activities to deeply relax muscles and reduce tension. This training is followed by specific diaphragmatic breathing entrainment instructions so that patients regularly take time to breathe with the diaphragm at a slow, relaxed pace when the body's major skeletal muscles are not being employed in response to stimuli. Seventh, patients are given instructions for beginning sleep in a relaxed position, along with other sleep hygiene recommendations. Finally, patients are provided with instructions on the role of fluid intake, nutrition, and exercise for the restoration of normal functioning. The entire PSR program is presented within a framework that focuses on understanding pain as a physiologic disturbance that is best managed by addressing those disturbances through rest, nutrition, tissue repair, behavioral regulation of autonomic functioning, and appropriate activity. The PSR approach focuses on limiting any activity that increases the sense of discomfort or pain to promote return of pain-free function.

Clinical experience in working with PSR over the past 13 years suggests it is a valuable treatment for a variety of orofacial pain conditions. Although it was initially designed predominately for masticatory muscle pain disorders, it has also been helpful in managing many intracapsular disorders.

PSR assists in managing intracapsular disorders by enabling recognition of inappropriate muscle activity that can lead to co-contraction and inhibition of synovial fluid diffusion efficiency into previously overloaded joints. By reducing muscle loading, PSR helps reestablish normal function with pain-free range of motion. In fact, PSR is helpful in most pain conditions because it enables the patient to gain control of many physiologic functions and reverse "dysregulation" of their physiologic systems. For those interested in adding this approach to their clinical practices, a more detailed description of the PSR approach can be obtained elsewhere.[376,377,379] Although more clinical trials are necessary to further evaluate the PSR approach, current data from controlled scientific study and clinical practice indicate that patients can receive substantial benefits from PSR training.

References

1. Albino JEN, Committee Chairperson: The National Institutes of Health Technology Assessment Conference Statement on the Management of Temporomandibular Disorders, *J Am Dent Assoc* 127:1595-1599, 1996.
2. Whitney CW, Von Korff M: Regression to the mean in treated versus untreated chronic pain, *Pain* 50:281-285, 1992.
3. Greene CS, Laskin DM: Long-term evaluation of conservative treatment for myofascial pain-dysfunction syndrome, *J Am Dent Assoc* 89:1365-1368, 1974.
4. Greene CS, Markovic MA: Response to nonsurgical treatment of patients with positive radiographic findings in the temporomandibular joint, *J Oral Surg* 34:692-697, 1976.
5. Carlsson SG, Gale EN: Biofeedback in the treatment of long-term temporomandibular joint pain: an outcome study, *Biofeedback Self Regul* 2:161-171, 1977.
6. Carraro JJ, Caffesse RG: Effect of occlusal splints on TMJ symptomatology, *J Prosthet Dent* 40:563-566, 1978.
7. Cohen SR: Follow-up evaluation of 105 patients with myofascial pain-dysfunction syndrome, *J Am Dent Assoc* 97:825-828, 1978.
8. Dohrmann RJ, Laskin DM: An evaluation of electromyographic biofeedback in the treatment of myofascial pain-dysfunction syndrome, *J Am Dent Assoc* 96:656-662, 1978.
9. Nel H: Myofascial pain-dysfunction syndrome, *J Prosthet Dent* 40:438-441, 1978.
10. Heloe B, Heiberg AN: A follow-up study of a group of female patients with myofascial pain-dysfunction syndrome, *Acta Odontol Scand* 38:129-134, 1980.
11. Wessberg GA, Carroll WL, Dinham R, Wolford LM: Transcutaneous electrical stimulation as an adjunct in the management of myofascial pain-dysfunction syndrome, *J Prosthet Dent* 45:307-314, 1981.
12. Greene CS, Laskin DM: Long-term evaluation of treatment for myofascial pain-dysfunction syndrome: a comparative analysis, *J Am Dent Assoc* 107:235-238, 1983.
13. Magnusson T, Carlsson GE: A 2½-year follow-up of changes in headache and mandibular dysfunction after stomatognathic treatment, *J Prosthet Dent* 49:398-402, 1983.
14. Wedel A, Carlsson GE: Retrospective review of 350 patients referred to a TMJ clinic, *Community Dent Oral Epidemiol* 11:69-73, 1983.
15. Strychalski ID, Mohl ND, McCall WD Jr, Uthman AA: Three year follow-up TMJ patients: success rates and silent periods, *J Oral Rehabil* 11:71-78, 1984.
16. Okeson JP, Hayes DK: Long-term results of treatment for temporomandibular disorders: an evaluation by patients, *J Am Dent Assoc* 112:473-478, 1986.
17. Randolph CS, Greene CS, Moretti R, Forbes D, Perry HT: Conservative management of temporomandibular disorders: a posttreatment comparison between patients from a university clinic and from private practice, *Am J Orthod Dentofacial Orthop* 98:77-82, 1990.
18. Okeson JP: Long-term treatment of disk-interference disorders of the temporomandibular joint with anterior repositioning occlusal splints, *J Prosthet Dent* 60:611-616, 1988.
19. Williamson EH, Rosenzweig BJ: The treatment of temporomandibular disorders through repositioning splint therapy: a follow-up study, *Cranio* 16:222-225, 1998.
20. Kurita H, Kurashina K, Kotani A: Clinical effect of full coverage occlusal splint therapy for specific temporomandibular disorder conditions and symptoms, *J Prosthet Dent* 78:506-510, 1997.
21. Sato S, Kawamura H, Nagasaka H, Motegi K: The natural course of anterior disc displacement without reduction in the temporomandibular joint: follow-up at 6, 12, and 18 months, *J Oral Maxillofac Surg* 55:234-238; discussion 238-239, 1997.
22. Zarb GA, Thompson GW: Assessment of clinical treatment of patients with temporomandibular joint dysfunction, *J Prosthet Dent* 24:542-554, 1970.
23. Banks P, Mackenzie I: Condylotomy. A clinical and experimental appraisal of a surgical technique, *J Maxillofac Surg* 3:170-181, 1975.
24. Cherry CQ, Frew A Jr: High condylectomy for treatment of arthritis of the temporomandibular joint, *J Oral Surg* 35:285-288, 1977.
25. Brown WA: Internal derangement of the temporomandibular joint: review of 214 patients following meniscectomy, *Can J Surg* 23:30-32, 1980.
26. Bjornland T, Larheim TA: Synovectomy and diskectomy of the temporomandibular joint in patients with chronic arthritic disease compared with diskectomies in patients with internal derangement. A 3-year follow-up study, *Eur J Oral Sci* 103:2-7, 1995.

27. Marciani RD, Ziegler RC: Temporomandibular joint surgery: a review of fifty-one operations, *Oral Surg Oral Med Oral Pathol* 56:472-476, 1983.

28. Mejersjo C, Carlsson GE: Analysis of factors influencing the long-term effect of treatment of TMJ-pain dysfunction, *J Oral Rehabil* 11:289-297, 1984.

29. Upton LG, Scott RF, Hayward JR: Major maxillomandibular malrelations and temporomandibular joint pain-dysfunction, *J Prosthet Dent* 51:686-690, 1984.

30. Benson BJ, Keith DA: Patient response to surgical and non-surgical treatment for internal derangement of the temporomandibular joint, *J Oral Maxillofac Surg* 43:770-777, 1985.

31. Eriksson L, Westesson PL: Results of temporomandibular joint diskectomies in Sweden 1965-85, *Swed Dent J* 11:1-9, 1987.

32. Silver CM: Long-term results of meniscectomy of the temporomandibular joint, *Cranio* 3:46-57, 1984.

33. Holmlund A, Gynther G, Axelsson S: Efficacy of arthroscopic lysis and lavage in patients with chronic locking of the temporomandibular joint, *Int J Oral Maxillofac Surg* 23:262-265, 1994.

34. Moses JJ, Poker ID: TMJ arthroscopic surgery: an analysis of 237 patients, *J Oral Maxillofac Surg* 47:790-794, 1989.

35. Murakami K, Moriya Y, Goto K, Segami N: Four-year follow-up study of temporomandibular joint arthroscopic surgery for advanced stage internal derangements, *J Oral Maxillofac Surg* 54:285-290, 1996.

36. Kirk WS Jr: Risk factors and initial surgical failures of TMJ arthrotomy and arthroplasty: a four to nine year evaluation of 303 surgical procedures, *Cranio* 16:154-161, 1998.

37. Murakami KI, Tsuboi Y, Bessho K, Yokoe Y, Nishida M et al: Outcome of arthroscopic surgery to the temporomandibular joint correlates with stage of internal derangement: five-year follow-up study, *Br J Oral Maxillofac Surg* 36:30-34, 1998.

38. Summer JD, Westesson PL: Mandibular repositioning can be effective in treatment of reducing TMJ disk displacement. A long-term clinical and MR imaging follow-up, *Cranio* 15:107-120, 1997.

39. Sato S, Ohta M, Ohki H, Kawamura H, Motegi K: Effect of lavage with injection of sodium hyaluronate for patients with nonreducing disk displacement of the temporomandibular joint, *Oral Surg Oral Med Oral Pathol Oral Radiol Endod* 84:241-244, 1997.

40. Nitzan DW, Samson B, Better H: Long-term outcome of arthrocentesis for sudden-onset, persistent, severe closed lock of the temporomandibular joint, *J Oral Maxillofac Surg* 55:151-157; discussion 157-158, 1997.

41. Rosenberg I, Goss AN: The outcome of arthroscopic treatment of temporomandibular joint arthropathy, *Aust Dent J* 44:106-111, 1999.

42. Carvajal WA, Laskin DM: Long-term evaluation of arthrocentesis for the treatment of internal derangements of the temporomandibular joint, *J Oral Maxillofac Surg* 58:852-855; discussion 856-857, 2000.

43. Hall HD, Navarro EZ, Gibbs SJ: One- and three-year prospective outcome study of modified condylotomy for treatment of reducing disc displacement, *J Oral Maxillofac Surg* 58:7-17, 2000.

44. De Boever JA, Carlsson GE, Klineberg IJ: Need for occlusal therapy and prosthodontic treatment in the management of temporomandibular disorders. Part II: tooth loss and prosthodontic treatment, *J Oral Rehabil* 27:647-659, 2000.

45. Yatani H, Minakuchi H, Matsuka Y, Fujisawa T, Yamashita A: The long-term effect of occlusal therapy on self-administered treatment outcomes of TMD, *J Orofac Pain* 12:75-88, 1998.

46. Ramfjord SP, Ash MM: *Occlusion*, ed 3, Philadelphia, 1983, Saunders, p 500.

47. Franks AST: Conservative treatment of temporomandibular joint dysfunction: a comparative study, *Dent Pract Dent Rec* 15:205-210, 1965.

48. Okeson JP, Kemper JT, Moody PM: A study of the use of occlusion splints in the treatment of acute and chronic patients with craniomandibular disorders, *J Prosthet Dent* 48:708-712, 1982.

49. Clark GT, Beemsterboer PL, Solberg WK, Rugh JD: Nocturnal electromyographic evaluation of myofascial pain dysfunction in patients undergoing occlusal splint therapy, *J Am Dent Assoc* 99:607-611, 1979.

50. Solberg WK, Clark GT, Rugh JD: Nocturnal electromyographic evaluation of bruxism patients undergoing short term splint therapy, *J Oral Rehabil* 2:215-223, 1975.

51. Fuchs P: The muscular activity of the chewing apparatus during night sleep. An examination of healthy subjects and patients with functional disturbances, *J Oral Rehabil* 2:35-48, 1975.

52. Okeson JP: The effects of hard and soft occlusal splints on nocturnal bruxism, *J Am Dent Assoc* 114:788-791, 1987.

53. Brown DT, Gaudet EL Jr: Outcome measurement for treated and untreated TMD patients using the TMJ scale, *Cranio* 12:216-222, 1994.

54. Dahlstrom L: Conservative treatment methods in craniomandibular disorder, *Swed Dent J* 16:217-230, 1992.

55. Yustin D, Neff P, Rieger MR, Hurst T: Characterization of 86 bruxing patients with long-term study of their management with occlusal devices and other forms of therapy, *J Orofac Pain* 7:54-60, 1993.

56. Linde C, Isacsson G, Jonsson BG: Outcome of 6-week treatment with transcutaneous electric nerve stimulation compared with splint on symptomatic temporomandibular joint disk displacement without reduction, *Acta Odontol Scand* 53:92-98, 1995.

57. Garefis P, Grigoriadou E, Zarifi A, Koidis PT: Effectiveness of conservative treatment for craniomandibular disorders: a 2-year longitudinal study, *J Orofac Pain* 8:309-314, 1994.

58. Wright E, Anderson G, Schulte J: A randomized clinical trial of intraoral soft splints and palliative treatment for masticatory muscle pain, *J Orofac Pain* 9:192-199, 1995.

59. Yap AU: Effects of stabilization appliances on nocturnal parafunctional activities in patients with and without signs of temporomandibular disorders, *J Oral Rehabil* 25:64-68, 1998.

60. Ekberg EC, Vallon D, Nilner M: Occlusal appliance therapy in patients with temporomandibular disorders. A double-blind controlled study in a short-term perspective, *Acta Odontol Scand* 56:122-128, 1998.

61. Kight M, Gatchel RJ, Wesley L: Temporomandibular disorders: evidence for significant overlap with psychopathology, *Health Psychol* 18:177-182, 1999.

62. Wexler GB, Steed PA: Psychological factors and temporomandibular outcomes, *Cranio* 16:72-77, 1998.

63. Carlson CR, Okeson JP, Falace DA, Nitz AJ, Curran SL et al: Comparison of psychologic and physiologic functioning between patients with masticatory muscle pain and matched controls, *J Orofac Pain* 7:15-22, 1993.

64. De Leeuw J, Steenks MH, Ros WJ, Bosman F, Winnubst JA et al: Psychosocial aspects of craniomandibular dysfunction. An assessment of clinical and community findings, *J Oral Rehabil* 21:127-143, 1994.

65. Grassi C, Passatore M: Action of the sympathetic system on skeletal muscle, *Ital J Neurol Sci* 9:23-28, 1988.

66. Passatore M, Grassi C, Filippi GM: Sympathetically-induced development of tension in jaw muscles: the possible contraction of intrafusal muscle fibres, *Pflugers Arch* 405:297-304, 1985.

67. Korszun A, Papadopoulos E, Demitrack M, Engleberg C, Crofford L: The relationship between temporomandibular disorders and stress-associated syndromes, *Oral Surg Oral Med Oral Pathol Oral Radiol Endod* 86:416-420, 1998.

68. Lupton DE: A preliminary investigation of the personality of female temporomandibular joint dysfunction patients, *Psychother Psychosom* 14:199-216, 1966.

69. Grieder A: Psychologic aspects of prosthodontics, *J Prosthet Dent* 30:736-744, 1973.

70. Solberg WK, Flint RT, Brantner JP: Temporomandibular joint pain and dysfunction: a clinical study of emotional and occlusal components, *J Prosthet Dent* 28:412-422, 1972.

71. Gross SM, Vacchiano RB: Personality correlates of patients with temporomandibular joint dysfunction, *J Prosthet Dent* 30:326-329, 1973.

72. Molin C, Edman G, Schalling D: Psychological studies of patients with mandibular pain dysfunction syndrome. 2. Tolerance for experimentally induced pain, *Sven Tandlak Tidskr* 66:15-23, 1973.

73. Engle GL: Primary atypical facial neuralgia, *Psychosom Med* 13:375-396, 1951.

74. Moulton R: Psychiatric considerations in maxillofacial pain, *J Am Dent Assoc* 51:408-414, 1955.

75. Lesse S: Atypical facial pain syndrome of psychogenic origin, *J Nerv Ment Dis* 124:346-351, 1956.

76. Southwell J, Deary IJ, Geissler P: Personality and anxiety in temporomandibular joint syndrome patients, *J Oral Rehabil* 17:239-243, 1990.

77. Pingitore G, Chrobak V, Petrie J: The social and psychologic factors of bruxism, *J Prosthet Dent* 65:443-446, 1991.

78. Schnurr RF, Brooke RI, Rollman GB: Psychosocial correlates of temporomandibular joint pain and dysfunction [see comments], *Pain* 42:153-165, 1990.

79. Marbach JJ: The 'temporomandibular pain dysfunction syndrome' personality: fact or fiction? *J Oral Rehabil* 19:545-560, 1992.

80. Michelotti A, Martina R, Russo M, Romeo R: Personality characteristics of temporomandibular disorder patients using M.M.P.I., *Cranio* 16:119-125, 1998.

81. Solberg WK, Rugh JD: The use of bio-feedback devices in the treatment of bruxism, *J South Calif Dent Assoc* 40:852-853, 1972.

82. Kydd WL: Psychosomatic aspects of temporomandibular joint dysfunction, *J Am Dent Assoc* 59:31-44, 1959.

83. McCal CMJ, Szmyd L, Ritter RM: Personality characteristics in patients with temporomandibular pain and dysfunction syndrome: psychosocial, health behavior, physical illness and injury, *J Am Dent Assoc* 62:694-698, 1961.

84. Marbach JJ, Lennon MC, Dohrenwend BP: Candidate risk factors for temporomandibular pain and dysfunction syndrome: psychosocial, health behavior, physical illness and injury, *Pain* 34:139-151, 1988.

85. Carlson CR, Reid KI, Curran SL, Studts J, Okeson JP et al: Psychological and physiological parameters of masticatory muscle pain, *Pain* 76:297-307, 1998.

86. Madland G, Feinmann C, Newman S: Factors associated with anxiety and depression in facial arthromyalgia, *Pain* 84:225-232, 2000.

87. Glaros AG: Emotional factors in temporomandibular joint disorders, *J Indiana Dent Assoc* 79:20-23, 2000.

88. Mongini F, Ciccone G, Ibertis F, Negro C: Personality characteristics and accompanying symptoms in temporomandibular joint dysfunction, headache, and facial pain, *J Orofac Pain* 14:52-58, 2000.

89. De Leeuw R, Bertoli E, Schmidt JE, Carlson CR: Prevalence of post-traumatic stress disorder symptoms in orofacial pain patients, *Oral Surg Oral Med Oral Pathol Oral Radiol Endod* 99:558-568, 2005.

90. Sherman JJ, Carlson CR, Wilson JF, Okeson JP, McCubbin JA: Post-traumatic stress disorder among patients with orofacial pain, *J Orofac Pain* 19:309-317, 2005.

91. Kinney RK, Gatchel RJ, Ellis E, Holt C: Major psychological disorders in chronic TMD patients: implications for successful management [see comments], *J Am Dent Assoc* 123:49-54, 1992.

92. Meldolesi G, Picardi A, Accivile E, Toraldo di Francia R, Biondi M: Personality and psychopathology in patients with temporomandibular joint pain-dysfunction syndrome. A controlled investigation, *Psychother Psychosom* 69:322-328, 2000.

93. Rugh JD, Solberg WK: Electromyographic studies of bruxist behavior before and during treatment, *J Calif Dent Assoc* 3:56-59, 1975.

94. Rugh JD, Solberg WK: Psychological implications in temporomandibular pain and dysfunction, *Oral Sci Rev* 7:3-30, 1976.

95. Van Selms MK, Lobbezoo F, Wicks DJ, Hamburger HL, Naeije M: Craniomandibular pain, oral parafunctions, and psychological stress in a longitudinal case study, *J Oral Rehabil* 31:738-745, 2004.

96. Moss RA, Adams HE: The assessment of personality, anxiety and depression in mandibular pain dysfunction subjects, *J Oral Rehabil* 11:233-235, 1984.

97. Pierce CJ, Chrisman K, Bennett ME, Close JM: Stress, anticipatory stress, and psychologic measures related to sleep bruxism, *J Orofac Pain* 9:51-56, 1995.

98. Watanabe T, Ichikawa K, Clark GT: Bruxism levels and daily behaviors: 3 weeks of measurement and correlation, *J Orofac Pain* 17:65-73, 2003.

99. Eversole LR, Stone CE, Matheson D, Kaplan H: Psychometric profiles and facial pain, *Oral Surg Oral Med Oral Pathol* 60:269-274, 1985.

100. Pierce CJ, Gale EN: Prediction of outcome for bruxing treatment, *J Dent Res* 65:233, 1986 (abstract).

101. Lindroth JE, Schmidt JE, Carlson CR: A comparison between masticatory muscle pain patients and intracapsular pain patients on behavioral and psychosocial domains, *J Orofac Pain* 16:277-283, 2002.

102. Fine EW: Psychological factors associated with nonorganic temporomandibular joint pain dysfunction syndrome, *Br Dent J* 131:402-404, 1971.

103. Haley WE, Turner JA, Romano JM: Depression in chronic pain patients: relation to pain, activity, and sex differences, *Pain* 23:337-343, 1985.

104. Bassett DL, Gerke DC, Goss AN: Psychological factors in temporomandibular joint dysfunction: depression, *Aust Prosthodont J* 4:41-45, 1990.

105. Rugh JD, Woods BJ, Dahlstrom L: Temporomandibular disorders: assessment of psychological factors, *Adv Dent Res* 7:127-136, 1993.

106. Magni G, Moreschi C, Rigatti-Luchini S, Merskey H: Prospective study on the relationship between depressive symptoms and chronic musculoskeletal pain, *Pain* 56:289-297, 1994.

107. Auerbach SM, Laskin DM, Frantsve LM, Orr T: Depression, pain, exposure to stressful life events, and long-term outcomes in temporomandibular disorder patients, *J Oral Maxillofac Surg* 59:628-633, 2001.

108. Marbach JJ, Lund P: Depression, anhedonia and anxiety in temporomandibular joint and other facial pain syndromes, *Pain* 11:73-84, 1981.

109. Olson RE, Schwartz RA: Depression in patients with myofascial pain-dysfunction syndrome, *J Dent Res* 56:160, 1977 (abstract).

110. Tauschke E, Merskey H, Helmes E: Psychological defense mechanisms in patients with pain, *Pain* 40:161-170, 1990.

111. Gamsa A: Is emotional disturbance a precipitator or a consequence of chronic pain? *Pain* 42:183-195, 1990.

112. Magni G, Marchetti M, Moreschi C, Merskey H, Luchini SR: Chronic musculoskeletal pain and depressive symptoms in the National Health and Nutrition Examination I. Epidemiologic follow-up study, *Pain* 53:163-168, 1993.

113. Von Korff M, Le Reschle L, Dworkin SF: First onset of common pain symptoms: a prospective study of depression as a risk factor, *Pain* 55:251-258, 1993.

114. Yap AU, Dworkin SF, Chua EK, List T, Tan KB et al: Prevalence of temporomandibular disorder subtypes, psychologic distress, and psychosocial dysfunction in Asian patients, *J Orofac Pain* 17:21-28, 2003.

115. Manfredini D, di Poggio AB, Romagnoli M, Dell'Osso L, Bosco M: Mood spectrum in patients with different painful temporomandibular disorders, *Cranio* 22:234-240, 2004.

116. Tversky J, Reade PC, Gerschman JA, Holwill BJ, Wright J: Role of depressive illness in the outcome of treatment of temporomandibular joint pain-dysfunction syndrome, *Oral Surg Oral Med Oral Pathol* 71:696-699, 1991.

117. Gessel AH: Electromyographic biofeedback and tricyclic antidepressants in myofascial pain-dysfunction syndrome: psychological predictors of outcome, *J Am Dent Assoc* 91:1048-1052, 1975.

118. Schwartz RA, Greene CS, Laskin DM: Personality characteristics of patients with myofascial pain-dysfunction (MPD) syndrome unresponsive to conventional therapy, *J Dent Res* 58:1435-1439, 1979.

119. Millstein-Prentky S, Olson RE: Predictability of treatment outcome in patients with myofascial pain-dysfunction (MPD) syndrome, *J Dent Res* 58:1341-1346, 1979.

120. Dworkin SF: Benign chronic orofacial pain. Clinical criteria and therapeutic approaches, *Postgrad Med* 74:239-242, 245, 247-248, 1983.

121. Schulte J, Anderson G, Hathaway KM: Psychometric profile and related pain characteristics of temporomandibular disorders patients, *J Orofac Pain* 7:247-253, 1993.

122. Wurtele SK, Kaplan GM, Keairnes M: Childhood sexual abuse among chronic pain patients, *Clin J Pain* 6:110-113, 1990.

123. Domino JV, Haber JD: Prior physical and sexual abuse in women with chronic headache: clinical correlates, *Headache* 27:310-314, 1987.

124. Curran SL, Sherman JJ, Cunningham LL, Okeson JP, Reid KI et al: Physical and sexual abuse among orofacial pain patients: linkages with pain and psychologic distress, *J Orofac Pain* 9:340-346, 1995.

125. Toomey TC, Hernandez JT, Gittelman DF, Hulka JF: Relationship of sexual and physical abuse to pain and psychological assessment variables in chronic pelvic pain patients, *Pain* 53:105-109, 1993.

126. Haber JD, Roos C: Effects of spouse abuse and/or sexual abuse in the development and maintenance of chronic pain in women, *Adv Pain Res Ther* 9:889-894, 1985.

127. Riley JL III, Robinson ME, Kvaal SA, Gremillion HA: Effects of physical and sexual abuse in facial pain: direct or mediated? *Cranio* 16:259-266, 1998.

128. Campbell LC, Riley JL III, Kashikar Zuck S, Gremillion H, Robinson ME: Somatic, affective, and pain characteristics of chronic TMD patients with sexual versus physical abuse histories, *J Orofac Pain* 14:112-119, 2000.

129. Romano JM, Turner JA, Friedman LS, Bulcroft RA, Jensen MP et al: Sequential analysis of chronic pain behaviors and spouse responses, *J Consult Clin Psychol* 60:777-782, 1992.

130. Stenger EM: Chronic back pain: view from a psychiatrist's office, *Clin J Pain* 8:242-246, 1992.

131. Burgess JA, Dworkin SF: Litigation and post-traumatic TMD: how patients report treatment outcome, *J Am Dent Assoc* 124:105-110, 1993.

132. De Leeuw J, Ros WJ, Steenks MH, Lobbezoo-Scholte AM, Bosman F et al: Multidimensional evaluation of craniomandibular dysfunction. II: pain assessment, *J Oral Rehabil* 21:515-532, 1994.

133. McCreary CP, Clark GT, Merril RL, Flack V, Oakley ME: Psychological distress and diagnostic subgroups of temporomandibular disorder patients, *Pain* 44:29-34, 1991.

134. Stockstill JW, Callahan CD: Personality hardiness, anxiety, and depression as constructs of interest in the study of temporomandibular disorders, *J Craniomandib Disord* 5:129-134, 1991.

135. Rugh JD, Solberg WK: Psychological implications in temporomandibular pain and dysfunction. In Zarb GA, Carlsson GE, editor: *Temporomandibular joint function and dysfunction*, Copenhagen, 1979, Munksgard, pp 239-268.

136. Duinkerke AS, Luteijn F, Bouman TK, de Jong HP: Relations between TMJ pain dysfunction syndrome (PDS) and some psychologic and biographic variables, *Community Dent Oral Epidemiol* 13:185-189, 1985.

137. Suvinen TI, Hanes KR, Reade PC: Outcome of therapy in the conservative management of temporomandibular pain dysfunction disorder, *J Oral Rehabil* 24:718-724, 1997.

138. Epker J, Gatchel RJ: Coping profile differences in the biopsychosocial functioning of patients with temporomandibular disorder, *Psychosom Med* 62:69-75, 2000.

139. Hagberg C, Hagberg M, Kopp S: Musculoskeletal symptoms and psychosocial factors among patients with craniomandibular disorders, *Acta Odontol Scand* 52:170-177, 1994.

140. Phillips JM, Gatchel RJ, Wesley AL, Ellis E III: Clinical implications of sex in acute temporomandibular disorders, *J Am Dent Assoc* 132:49-57, 2001.

141. Malow RM, Olson RE, Greene CS: Myofascial pain dysfunction syndrome: a psychophysiological disorder. In Golden C, Alcaparras S, Strider F, Graber B, editors: *Applied techniques in behavioral medicine*, New York, 1981, Grune & Stratton, pp 101-133.

142. Melzack R: Neurophysiological foundations of pain. In Sternback RA, editor: *The psychology of pain*, New York, 1986, Raven, pp 1-25.

143. Rugh JD: Psychological components of pain, *Dent Clin North Am* 31:579-594, 1987.

144. Gramling SE, Neblett J, Grayson R, Townsend D: Temporomandibular disorder: efficacy of an oral habit reversal treatment program, *J Behav Ther Exp Psychiatry* 27:245-255, 1996.

145. Selye H: *Stress without distress*, Philadelphia, 1974, JB Lippincott, p 32.

146. Oakley ME, McCreary CP, Clark GT, Holston S, Glover D et al: A cognitive-behavioral approach to temporomandibular dysfunction treatment failures: a controlled comparison, *J Orofac Pain* 8:397-401, 1994.

147. Jacobson E: *Progressive relaxation*, Chicago, 1968, University of Chicago Press, pp 69-87.

148. Moller E, Sheik-Ol-Eslam A, Lous I: Deliberate relaxation of the temporal and masseter muscles in subjects with functional disorders of the chewing apparatus, *Scand J Dent Res* 79:478-482, 1971.

149. Gessel AH, Alderman MM: Management of myofascial pain dysfunction syndrome of the temporomandibular joint by tension control training, *Psychosomatics* 12:302-309, 1971.

150. Goldberg G: The psychological, physiological and hypnotic approach to bruxism in the treatment of periodontal disease, *J Am Soc Psychosom Dent Med* 20:75-91, 1973.

151. Reading A, Raw M: The treatment of mandibular dysfunction pain. Possible application of psychological methods, *Br Dent J* 140:201-205, 1976.

152. Blanchard F, Andrasik F, Evans D, Neff D, Applebaum K et al: Behavioral treatment of 250 chronic headache patients: a clinical replication series, *Behavior Ther* 16:308-327, 1985.

153. Larsson B, Melin L: Chronic headaches in adolescents: treatment in a school setting with relaxation training as compared with information-contact and self-registration, *Pain* 25:325-336, 1986.

154. Dahlstrom L, Carlsson SG: Treatment of mandibular dysfunction: the clinical usefulness of biofeedback in relation to splint therapy, *J Oral Rehabil* 11:277-284, 1984.

155. Lacroix JM, Clarke MA, Bock JC, Doxey NC: Muscle-contraction headaches in multiple-pain patients: treatment under worsening baseline conditions, *Arch Phys Med Rehabil* 67:14-18, 1986.

156. Hijzen TH, Slangen JL, van Houweligen HC: Subjective, clinical and EMG effects of biofeedback and splint treatment, *J Oral Rehabil* 13:529-539, 1986.

157. Raft D, Toomey T, Gregg JM: Behavior modification and haloperidol in chronic facial pain, *South Med J* 72:155-159, 1979.

158. Erlandson PM Jr, Poppen R: Electromyographic biofeedback and rest position training of masticatory muscles in myofascial pain-dysfunction patients, *J Prosthet Dent* 62:335-338, 1989.

159. Okeson JP, Moody PM, Kemper JT, Haley JV: Evaluation of occlusal splint therapy and relaxation procedures in patients with temporomandibular disorders, *J Am Dent Assoc* 107:420-424, 1983.

160. Carlson CR, Ventrella MA, Sturgis ET: Relaxation training through muscle stretching procedures: a pilot case, *J Behav Ther Exp Psychiatry* 18:121-126, 1987.

161. Carlson CR, Collins FL Jr, Nitz AJ, Sturgis ET, Rogers JL: Muscle stretching as an alternative relaxation training procedure, *J Behav Ther Exp Psychiatry* 21:29-38, 1990.

162. Carlson CR, Okeson JP, Falace DA, Nitz AJ, Anderson D: Stretch-based relaxation and the reduction of EMG activity among masticatory muscle pain patients, *J Craniomandib Disord* 5:205-212, 1991.

163. Shaw RM, Dettmar DM: Monitoring behavioural stress control using a craniomandibular index, *Aust Dent J* 35:147-151, 1990.

164. Manns A, Zuazola RV, Sirhan RM, Quiroz M, Rocabado M: Relationship between the tonic elevator mandibular activity and the vertical dimension during the states of vigilance and hypnosis, *Cranio* 8:163-170, 1990.

165. Gerschman J, Burrows G, Reade P: Hypnotherapy in the treatment of oro-facial pain, *Aust Dent J* 23:492-496, 1978.

166. Simon EP, Lewis DM: Medical hypnosis for temporomandibular disorders: treatment efficacy and medical utilization outcome, *Oral Surg Oral Med Oral Pathol Oral Radiol Endod* 90:54-63, 2000.

167. Stam HJ, McGrath PA, Brooke RI, Cosier F: Hypnotizability and the treatment of chronic facial pain, *Int J Clin Exp Hypn* 34:182-191, 1986.

168. Dubin LL: The use of hypnosis for temporomandibular joint (TMJ), *Psychiatr Med* 10:99-103, 1992.

169. Flor H, Birbaumer N: Comparison of the efficacy of electromyographic biofeedback, cognitive-behavioral therapy, and conservative medical interventions in the treatment of chronic musculoskeletal pain, *J Consult Clin Psychol* 61:653-658, 1993.

170. Santoro F, Maiorana C, Campiotti A: [Neuromuscular relaxation and CCMDP. Biofeedback and TENS. 4], *Dent Cadmos* 57:88-89, 1989.

171. Crider AB, Glaros AG: A meta-analysis of EMG biofeedback treatment of temporomandibular disorders, *J Orofac Pain* 13:29-37, 1999.

172. Mishra KD, Gatchel RJ, Gardea MA: The relative efficacy of three cognitive-behavioral treatment approaches to temporomandibular disorders, *J Behav Med* 23:293-309, 2000.

173. Grazzi L, Bussone G: Effect of biofeedback treatment on sympathetic function in common migraine and tension-type headache, *Cephalalgia* 13:197-200, 1993.

174. Funch DP, Gale EN: Factors associated with nocturnal bruxism and its treatment, *J Behav Med* 3:385-397, 1980.

175. Cassisi JE, McGlynn FD, Belles DR: EMG-activated feedback alarms for the treatment of nocturnal bruxism: current status and future directions, *Biofeedback Self Reg* 12:13-30, 1987.

176. Lee-Knight CT, Harrison EL, Price CJ: Dental injuries at the 1989 Canada games: an epidemiological study, *J Can Dent Assoc* 58:810-815, 1992.

177. Garon MW, Merkle A, Wright JT: Mouth protectors and oral trauma: a study of adolescent football players, *J Am Dent Assoc* 112:663-665, 1986.

178. Seals RR Jr, Morrow RM, Kuebker WA, Farney WD: An evaluation of mouthguard programs in Texas high school football, *J Am Dent Assoc* 110:904-909, 1985.

179. Okeson JP, Phillips BA, Berry DT, Cook Y, Paesani D et al: Nocturnal bruxing events in healthy geriatric subjects, *J Oral Rehabil* 17:411-418, 1990.

180. Okeson JP, Phillips BA, Berry DT, Cook YR, Cabelka JF: Nocturnal bruxing events in subjects with sleep-disordered

breathing and control subjects, *J Craniomandib Disord* 5:258-264, 1991.

181. Okeson JP, Phillips BA, Berry DT, Baldwin RM: Nocturnal bruxing events: a report of normative data and cardiovascular response, *J Oral Rehabil* 21:623-630, 1994.

182. Satoh T, Harada Y: Electrophysiological study on tooth-grinding during sleep, *Electroencephalogr Clin Neurophysiol* 35:267-275, 1973.

183. Rugh JD, Robbins JW: Oral habits disorders. In Ingersoll B, editor: *Behavioral aspects in dentistry*, New York, 1982, Appleton-Century-Crofts, 1982, pp 179-202.

184. Turk DC, Rudy TE, Kubinski JA, Zaki HS, Greco CM: Dysfunctional patients with temporomandibular disorders: evaluating the efficacy of a tailored treatment protocol, *J Consult Clin Psychol* 64:139-146, 1996.

185. Clarke NG: Occlusion and myofascial pain dysfunction: is there a relationship? *J Am Dent Assoc* 104:443-446, 1982.

186. Hicks RA, Conti P: Nocturnal bruxism and self reports of stress-related symptoms, *Percept Mot Skills* 72:1182, 1991.

187. Clarke NG, Townsend GC: Distribution of nocturnal bruxing patterns in man, *J Oral Rehabil* 11:529-534, 1984.

188. Lavigne GJ, Montplaisir JY: Bruxism: epidemiology, diagnosis, pathophysiology, and pharmacology. In Fricton JR, Dubner RB, editors: *Orofacial pain and temporomandibular disorders*, New York, 1995, Raven, pp 387-404.

189. Miguel AV, Montplaisir J, Rompre PH, Lund JP, Lavigne GJ: Bruxism and other orofacial movements during sleep, *J Craniomandib Disord* 6:71-81, 1992.

190. Westrup DA, Keller SR, Nellis TA, Hicks RA: Arousability and bruxism in male and female college students, *Percept Mot Skills* 75:796-798, 1992.

191. Bailey JO, Rugh JD: Effects of occlusal adjustment on bruxism as monitored by nocturnal EMG recordings, *J Dent Res* 59:317, 1980.

192. Fordyce WE: *Behavior methods for chronic pain and illness*, St Louis, 1976, Mosby, p 500.

193. Black RG: The chronic pain syndrome, *Surg Clin North Am* 55:999-1011, 1975.

194. Turk DC, Brody MC: Chronic opioid therapy for persistent noncancer pain: panacea or oxymoron? *Am Pain Soc Bull* 1:4-7, 1993.

195. Fordyce WE: On opioids and treatment targets, *Am Pain Society Bull* 1:1-13, 1991.

196. Abbadie C, Besson JM: Chronic treatments with aspirin or acetaminophen reduce both the development of polyarthritis and Fos-like immunoreactivity in rat lumbar spinal cord, *Pain* 57:45-54, 1994.

197. Hargreaves KM, Troullos ES, Dionne RA: Pharmacologic rationale for the treatment of acute pain, *Dent Clin North Am* 31:675-694, 1987.

198. Ekberg EC, Kopp S, Akerman S: Diclofenac sodium as an alternative treatment of temporomandibular joint pain, *Acta Odontol Scand* 54:154-159, 1996.

199. Dionne RA, Berthold CW: Therapeutic uses of nonsteroidal anti-inflammatory drugs in dentistry, *Crit Rev Oral Biol Med* 12:315-330, 2001.

200. Garcia RLA, Jick H: Risk of upper gastrointestinal bleeding and perforation associated with individual non-steroidal anti-inflammatory drugs [published erratum appears in *Lancet* 343:1048, 1994], *Lancet* 343:769-772, 1994.

201. Langman MJ, Weil J, Wainwright P, Lawson DH, Rawlins MD et al: Risks of bleeding peptic ulcer associated with individual non-steroidal anti-inflammatory drugs [see comments] [published erratum appears in *Lancet* 343:1302, 1994], *Lancet* 343:1075-1078, 1994.

202. Cicconetti A, Bartoli A, Ripari F, Ripari A: COX-2 selective inhibitors: a literature review of analgesic efficacy and safety in oral-maxillofacial surgery, *Oral Surg Oral Med Oral Pathol Oral Radiol Endod* 97:139-146, 2004.

203. Quinn JH, Kent JH, Moise A, Lukiw WJ: Cyclooxygenase-2 in synovial tissue and fluid of dysfunctional temporomandibular joints with internal derangement, *J Oral Maxillofac Surg* 58:1229-1232, 2000.

204. Ta LE, Dionne RA: Treatment of painful temporomandibular joints with a cyclooxygenase-2 inhibitor: a randomized placebo-controlled comparison of celecoxib to naproxen, *Pain* 111:13-21, 2004.

205. Svensson P, Houe L, Arendt-Nielsen L: Effect of systemic versus topical nonsteroidal anti-inflammatory drugs on postexercise jaw-muscle soreness: a placebo-controlled study, *J Orofac Pain* 11:353-362, 1997.

206. Airaksinen O, Venalainen J, Pietilainen T: Ketoprofen 2.5% gel versus placebo gel in the treatment of acute soft tissue injuries, *Int J Clin Pharmacol Ther Toxicol* 31:561-563, 1993.

207. Henny FA: Intra-articular injection of hydrocortisone into the temporomandibular joint, *J Oral Surg* 12:314-319, 1954.

208. Toller PA: Osteoarthrosis of the mandibular condyle, *Br Dent J* 134:223-231, 1973.

209. Toller P: Non-surgical treatment of dysfunctions of the temporo-mandibular joint, *Oral Sci Rev* 7:70-85, 1976.

210. Kopp S, Carlsson GE, Haraldson T, Wenneberg B: Long-term effect of intra-articular injections of sodium hyaluronate and corticosteroid on temporomandibular joint arthritis, *J Oral Maxillofac Surg* 45:929-935, 1987.

211. Wenneberg B, Kopp S, Grondahl HG: Long-term effect of intra-articular injections of a glucocorticosteroid into the TMJ: a clinical and radiographic 8-year follow-up, *J Craniomandib Disord* 5:11-18, 1991.

212. Poswillo D: Experimental investigation of the effects of intra-articular hydrocortisone and high condylectomy on the mandibular condyle, *Oral Surg Oral Med Oral Pathol* 30:161-173, 1970.

213. Zarb GA, Spech JE: The treatment of mandibular dysfunction. In Zarb GA, Carlsson GE, editors: *Temporomandibular joint: function and dysfunction*, St Louis, 1979, Mosby.

214. Schindler C, Paessler L, Eckelt U, Kirch W: Severe temporomandibular dysfunction and joint destruction after intra-articular injection of triamcinolone, *J Oral Pathol Med* 34:184-186, 2005.

215. Kopp S, Wenneberg B, Haraldson T, Carlsson GE: The short-term effect of intra-articular injections of sodium hyaluronate and corticosteroid on temporomandibular joint pain and dysfunction, *J Oral Maxillofac Surg* 43:429-435, 1985.

216. Bertolami CN, Gay T, Clark GT, Rendell J, Shetty V et al: Use of sodium hyaluronate in treating temporomandibular joint disorders: a randomized, double-blind, placebo-controlled clinical trial, *J Oral Maxillofac Surg* 51:232-242, 1993.

217. Alpaslan C, Bilgihan A, Alpaslan GH, Guner B, Ozgur Yis M et al: Effect of arthrocentesis and sodium hyaluronate injection on nitrite, nitrate, and thiobarbituric acid-reactive substance levels in the synovial fluid, *Oral Surg Oral Med Oral Pathol Oral Radiol Endod* 89:686-690, 2000.

218. Hirota W: Intra-articular injection of hyaluronic acid reduces total amounts of leukotriene C4, 6-keto-prostaglandin F1alpha, prostaglandin F2alpha and interleukin-1beta in synovial fluid of patients with internal derangement in disorders of the temporomandibular joint, *Br J Oral Maxillofac Surg* 36:35-38, 1998.

219. Sato S, Sakamoto M, Kawamura H, Motegi K: Disc position and morphology in patients with nonreducing disc displacement treated by injection of sodium hyaluronate, *Int J Oral Maxillofac Surg* 28:253-257, 1999.

220. Alpaslan GH, Alpaslan C: Efficacy of temporomandibular joint arthrocentesis with and without injection of sodium hyaluronate in treatment of internal derangements, *J Oral Maxillofac Surg* 59:613-618, 2001.

221. Dellemijn PL, Fields HL: Do benzodiazepines have a role in chronic pain management? *Pain* 57:137-152, 1994.

222. Denucci DJ, Dionne RA, Dubner R: Identifying a neurobiologic basis for drug therapy in TMDs, *J Am Dent Assoc* 127:581-593, 1996.

223. Rugh JD, Harlan J: Nocturnal bruxism and temporomandibular disorders. In Jankovic J, Tolosa E, editors: *Facial dyskinesias*, New York, 1988, Raven, pp 329-341.

224. Harkins S, Linford J, Cohen J, Kramer T, Cueva L: Administration of clonazepam in the treatment of TMD and associated myofascial pain: a double-blind pilot study, *J Craniomandib Disord* 5:179-186, 1991.

225. McQuay H, Carroll D, Jadad AR, Wiffen P, Moore A: Anticonvulsant drugs for management of pain: a systematic review, *Br Med J* 311:1047-1052, 1995.

226. Wiffen P, McQuay H, Carroll D, Jadad A, Moore A: Anticonvulsant drugs for acute and chronic pain, *Cochrane Database Syst Rev* CD001133, 2000.

227. Nemcovsky CE, Gross MD: A comparative study of the stereognathic ability between patients with myofascial pain dysfunction syndrome and a control group, *Cranio* 9:35-38, 1991.

228. Stanko JR: Review of oral skeletal muscle relaxants for the craniomandibular disorder (CMD) practitioner, *Cranio* 8:234-243, 1990.

229. Tseng TC, Wang SC: Locus of action of centrally acting muscle relaxants, diazepam and tybamate, *J Pharmacol Exp Ther* 178:350-360, 1971.

230. Borenstein DG, Lacks S, Wiesel SW: Cyclobenzaprine and naproxen versus naproxen alone in the treatment of

acute low back pain and muscle spasm, *Clin Ther* 12:125-131, 1990.

231. Reynolds WJ, Moldofsky H, Saskin P, Lue FA: The effects of cyclobenzaprine on sleep physiology and symptoms in patients with fibromyalgia, *J Rheumatol* 18:452-454, 1991.

232. Hamaty D, Valentine JL, Howard R, Howard CW, Wakefield V et al: The plasma endorphin, prostaglandin and catecholamine profile of patients with fibrositis treated with cyclobenzaprine and placebo: a 5-month study, *J Rheumatol Suppl* 19:164-168, 1989.

233. Herman CR, Schiffman EL, Look JO, Rindal DB: The effectiveness of adding pharmacologic treatment with clonazepam or cyclobenzaprine to patient education and self-care for the treatment of jaw pain upon awakening: a randomized clinical trial, *J Orofac Pain* 16:64-70, 2002.

234. Kreisberg MK: Tricyclic antidepressants: analgesic effect and indications in orofacial pain, *J Craniomandib Disord* 2:171-177, 1988.

235. Lascelles RG: Atypical facial pain and depression, *Br J Psychiatry* 112:651-659, 1966.

236. Brown RS, Bottomley WK: Utilization and mechanism of action of tricyclic antidepressants in the treatment of chronic facial pain: a review of the literature, *Anesth Prog* 37:223-229, 1990.

237. Philipp M, Fickinger M: Psychotropic drugs in the management of chronic pain syndromes, *Pharmacopsychiatry* 26:221-234, 1993.

238. Ward N, Bokan JA, Phillips M, Benedetti C, Butler S et al: Antidepressants in concomitant chronic back pain and depression: doxepin and desipramine compared, *J Clin Psychiatry* 45:54-59, 1984.

239. Dionne RA: Pharmacologic treatments for temporomandibular disorders, *Oral Surg Oral Med Oral Pathol Oral Radiol Endod* 83:134-142, 1997.

240. Brazeau GA, Gremillion HA, Widmer CG, Mahan PE, Benson MB et al: The role of pharmacy in the management of patients with temporomandibular disorders and orofacial pain, *J Am Pharm Assoc (Wash)* 38:354-361, 1998.

241. Pettengill CA, Reisner-Keller L: The use of tricyclic antidepressants for the control of chronic orofacial pain, *Cranio* 15:53-56, 1997.

242. Plesh O, Curtis D, Levine J, McCall WD Jr: Amitriptyline treatment of chronic pain in patients with temporomandibular disorders, *J Oral Rehabil* 27:834-841, 2000.

243. Saarto T, Wiffen PJ: Antidepressants for neuropathic pain, *Cochrane Database Syst Rev* CD005454, 2005.

244. Sharav Y, Singer E, Schmidt R, Dionne RA, Dubner R: The analgesic effect of amitriptyline on chronic facial pain, *Pain* 31:199-209, 1987.

245. Fields HL: Pain II: new approaches to management, *Ann Neurol* 9:101-106, 1981.

246. Spiegel K, Kalb R, Pasternak GW: Analgesic activity of tricyclic antidepressants, *Ann Neurol* 13:462-465, 1983.

247. Zitman FG, Linssen AC, Edelbroek PM, Stijnen T: Low dose amitriptyline in chronic pain: the gain is modest, *Pain* 42:35-42, 1990.

248. Benoliel R, Eliav E, Elishoov H, Sharav Y: Diagnosis and treatment of persistent pain after trauma to the head and neck, *J Oral Maxillofac Surg* 52:1138-1147, 1994.

249. Egbunike IG, Chaffee BJ: Antidepressants in the management of chronic pain syndromes, *Adv Pain Res Ther* 10:262-270, 1990.

250. Tura B, Tura SM: The analgesic effect of tricyclic antidepressants, *Brain Res* 518:19-22, 1990.

251. Rizzatti-Barbosa CM, Nogueira MT, de Andrade ED, Ambrosano GM, de Barbosa JR: Clinical evaluation of amitriptyline for the control of chronic pain caused by temporomandibular joint disorders, *Cranio* 21:221-225, 2003.

252. Kerrick JM, Fine PG, Lipman AG, Love G: Low-dose amitriptyline as an adjunct to opioids for postoperative orthopedic pain: a placebo-controlled trial, *Pain* 52:325-330, 1993.

253. Harris M: Medical versus surgical management of temporomandibular joint pain and dysfunction, *Br J Oral Maxillofac Surg* 25:113-120, 1987.

254. Moja PL, Cusi C, Sterzi RR, Canepari C: Selective serotonin re-uptake inhibitors (SSRIs) for preventing migraine and tension-type headaches, *Cochrane Database Syst Rev* CD002919, 2005.

255. Ware JC: Tricyclic antidepressants in the treatment of insomnia, *J Clin Psychiatry* 44:25-28, 1983.

256. Wilke WS, Mackenzie AH: Proposed pathogenesis of fibrositis, *Cleve Clin Q* 52:147-154, 1985.

257. Treadwell BL: Fibromyalgia or the fibrositis syndrome: a new look, *N Z Med J* 94:457-459, 1981.

258. Moldofsky H, Scarisbrick P, England R, Smythe H: Musculoskeletal symptoms and non-REM sleep disturbance in patients with fibrositis syndrome and healthy subjects, *Psychosom Med* 37:341-351, 1975.

259. Moldofsky H, Scarisbrick P: Induction of neurasthenic musculoskeletal pain syndrome by selective sleep stage deprivation, *Psychosom Med* 38:35-44, 1976.

260. Carette S, McCain GA, Bell DA, Fam AG: Evaluation of amitriptyline in primary fibrositis. A double-blind, placebo-controlled study, *Arthritis Rheum* 29:655-659, 1986.

261. Goldenberg DL, Felson DT, Dinerman H: A randomized, controlled trial of amitriptyline and naproxen in the treatment of patients with fibromyalgia, *Arthritis Rheum* 29:1371-1377, 1986.

262. Wolfe F: The clinical syndrome of fibrositis, *Am J Med* 81:7-14, 1986.

263. Goldenberg DL: A review of the role of tricyclic medications in the treatment of fibromyalgia syndrome, *J Rheumatol Suppl* 19:137-139, 1989.

264. Gendreau RM, Thorn MD, Gendreau JF, Kranzler JD, Ribeiro S et al: Efficacy of milnacipran in patients with fibromyalgia, *J Rheumatol* 32:1975-1985, 2005.

265. Okeson JP: *Bell's orofacial pains*, ed 6, Chicago, 2005, Quintessence, pp 141-196.

266. Tremont-Lukats IW, Challapalli V, McNicol ED, Lau J, Carr DB: Systemic administration of local anesthetics to

relieve neuropathic pain: a systematic review and meta-analysis, *Anesth Analg* 101:1738-1749, 2005.

267. Simons DG, Travell JG, Simons LS: *Travell & Simons' myofascial pain and dysfunction: the trigger point manual*, ed 2, Baltimore, 1999, Lippincott Williams & Wilkins.

268. Fine PG, Milano R, Hare BD: The effects of myofascial trigger point injections are naloxone reversible, *Pain* 32:15-20, 1988.

269. Hameroff SR, Crago BR, Blitt CD, Womble J, Kanel J: Comparison of bupivacaine, etidocaine, and saline for trigger-point therapy, *Anesth Analg* 60:752-755, 1981.

270. Graboski CL, Gray DS, Burnham RS: Botulinum toxin A versus bupivacaine trigger point injections for the treatment of myofascial pain syndrome: a randomised double blind crossover study, *Pain* 118:170-175, 2005.

271. Kamanli A, Kaya A, Ardicoglu O, Ozgocmen S, Zengin FO et al: Comparison of lidocaine injection, botulinum toxin injection, and dry needling to trigger points in myofascial pain syndrome, *Rheumatol Int* 25:604-611, 2005.

272. Danzig W, May S, McNeill C, Miller A: Effect of an anesthetic injected into the temporomandibular joint space in patients with TMD, *J Craniomandib Disord* 6:288-295, 1992.

273. Gracely RH, Lynch SA, Bennett GJ: Painful neuropathy: altered central processing maintained dynamically by peripheral input [published erratum appears in *Pain* 52:251-253, 1993] [see comments], *Pain* 51:175-194, 1992.

274. Black RG, Bonica JJ: Analgesic blocks, *Postgrad Med* 53:105-110, 1973.

275. Ernest EA: *Temporomandibular joint and craniofacial pain*, Montgomery, Ala, 1983, Ernest Publications, pp 105-113.

276. Travell J: Temporomandibular joint pain referred from muscles of the head and neck, *J Prosthet Dent* 10:745-763, 1960.

277. Bell WE: *Temporomandibular disorders: classification, diagnosis, management*, ed 3, Chicago, 1990, Year Book Medical, pp 215-218.

278. Laskin JL, Wallace WR, DeLeo B: Use of bupivacaine hydrochloride in oral surgery—a clinical study, *J Oral Surg* 35:25-29, 1977.

279. Guttu RL, Page DG, Laskin DM: Delayed healing of muscle after injection of bupivacaine and steroid, *Ann Dent* 49:5-8, 1990.

280. Hepguler S, Akkoc YS, Pehlivan M, Ozturk C, Celebi G et al: The efficacy of intra-articular sodium hyaluronate in patients with reducing displaced disc of the temporomandibular joint, *J Oral Rehabil* 29:80-86, 2002.

281. Guarda-Nardini L, Tito R, Staffieri A, Beltrame A: Treatment of patients with arthrosis of the temporomandibular joint by infiltration of sodium hyaluronate: a preliminary study, *Eur Arch Otorhinolaryngol* 259:279-284, 2002.

282. Gray RJ, Quayle AA, Hall CA, Schofield MA: Physiotherapy in the treatment of temporomandibular joint disorders: a comparative study of four treatment methods, *Br Dent J* 176:257-261, 1994.

283. Heinrich SD, Sharps CH: Lower extremity torsional deformities in children: a prospective comparison of two treatment modalities, *Orthopedics* 14:655-659, 1991.

284. Di Fabio RP: Physical therapy for patients with TMD: a descriptive study of treatment, disability, and health status, *J Orofac Pain* 12:124-135, 1998.

285. McNeely ML, Armijo Olivo S, Magee DJ: A systematic review of the effectiveness of physical therapy interventions for temporomandibular disorders, *Phys Ther* 86:710-725, 2006.

286. Hall LJ: Physical therapy treatment results for 178 patients with temporomandibular joint syndrome, *Am J Otol* 5:183-196, 1984.

287. Heinrich S: The role of physical therapy in craniofacial pain disorders: an adjunct to dental pain management, *Cranio* 9:71-75, 1991.

288. Murphy GJ: Physical medicine modalities and trigger point injections in the management of temporomandibular disorders and assessing treatment outcome, *Oral Surg Oral Med Oral Pathol Oral Radiol Endod* 83:118-122, 1997.

289. Nelson SJ, Ash MM Jr: An evaluation of a moist heating pad for the treatment of TMJ/muscle pain dysfunction, *Cranio* 6:355-359, 1988.

290. Burgess JA, Sommers EE, Truelove EL, Dworkin SF: Short-term effect of two therapeutic methods on myofascial pain and dysfunction of the masticatory system, *J Prosthet Dent* 60:606-610, 1988.

291. Schwartz LL: Ethyl chloride treatment of limited painful mandibular movement, *J Am Dent Assoc* 48:497-507, 1954.

292. Travell J: Ethyl chloride spray for painful muscle spasms, *Arch Phys Med Rehabil* 33:291-298, 1952.

293. Satlerthwaite JR: Ice massage, *Pain Management* 2:116, 1989.

294. Travell JG, Rinzler SH: The myofascial genesis of pain, *Postgrad Med* 11:425-434, 1952.

295. Jaeger B, Reeves JL: Quantification of changes in myofascial trigger point sensitivity with the pressure algometer following passive stretch, *Pain* 27:203-210, 1986.

296. Esposito CJ, Veal SJ, Farman AG: Alleviation of myofascial pain with ultrasonic therapy, *J Prosthet Dent* 51:106-108, 1984.

297. Griffin JE, Karselis TC: *Physical agents for physical therapists*, ed 2, Springfield, Ill, 1982, Charles C Thomas, pp 279-312.

298. Kahn J: Iontophoresis and ultrasound for postsurgical temporomandibular trismus and paresthesia, *Phys Ther* 60:307-308, 1980.

299. Phero JC, Raj PP, McDonald JS: Transcutaneous electrical nerve stimulation and myoneural injection therapy for management of chronic myofascial pain, *Dent Clin North Am* 31:703-723, 1987.

300. Van der Windt DA, van der Heijden GJ, van den Berg SG, ter Riet G, de Winter AF et al: Ultrasound therapy for musculoskeletal disorders: a systematic review, *Pain* 81:257-271, 1999.

301. Kleinkort JA, Wood F: Phonophoresis with 1 percent versus 10 percent hydrocortisone, *Phys Ther* 55:1320-1324, 1975.

302. Cameron MH, Monroe LG: Relative transmission of ultrasound by media customarily used for phonophoresis [see comments], *Phys Ther* 72:142-148, 1992.

303. Shin SM, Choi JK: Effect of indomethacin phonophoresis on the relief of temporomandibular joint pain, *Cranio* 15:345-348, 1997.

304. Klaiman MD, Shrader JA, Danoff JV, Hicks JE, Pesce WJ et al: Phonophoresis versus ultrasound in the treatment of common musculoskeletal conditions, *Med Sci Sports Exerc* 30:1349-1355, 1998.

305. Banta CA: A prospective, nonrandomized study of iontophoresis, wrist splinting, and antiinflammatory medication in the treatment of early-mild carpal tunnel syndrome, *J Occup Med* 36:166-168, 1994.

306. Kahn J: Iontophoresis and ultrasound for postsurgical temporomandibular tissues and paresthesias, *Phys Ther* 60:307-308, 1980.

307. Lark MR, Gangarosa LP Sr: Iontophoresis: an effective modality for the treatment of inflammatory disorders of the temporomandibular joint and myofascial pain, *Cranio* 8:108-119, 1990.

308. Gangarosa LP: *Iontophoresis in dental practice*, Chicago, 1983, Quintessence, pp 35-39.

309. Braun BL: Treatment of an acute anterior disk displacement in the temporomandibular joint. A case report, *Phys Ther* 67:1234-1236, 1987.

310. Schiffman EL, Braun BL, Lindgren BR: Temporomandibular joint iontophoresis: a double-blind randomized clinical trial, *J Orofac Pain* 10:157-165, 1996.

311. Reid KI, Dionne RA, Sicard-Rosenbaum L, Lord D, Dubner RA: Evaluation of iontophoretically applied dexamethasone for painful pathologic temporomandibular joints, *Oral Surg Oral Med Oral Pathol* 77:605-609, 1994.

312. Jankelson B, Swain CW: Physiological aspects of masticatory muscle stimulation: the myomonitor, *Quintessence Int* 3:57-62, 1972.

313. Murphy GJ: Electrical physical therapy in treating TMJ patients, *J Craniomandib Pract* 1:67-73, 1983.

314. Mohl ND, Ohrbach RK, Crow HC, Gross AJ: Devices for the diagnosis and treatment of temporomandibular disorders. Part III: thermography, ultrasound, electrical stimulation, and electromyographic biofeedback, *J Prosthet Dent* 63:472-477, 1990.

315. Kane K, Taub A: A history of local electrical analgesia, *Pain* 1:125-138, 1975.

316. Long DM, Hagfors N: Electrical stimulation in the nervous system: the current status of electrical stimulation of the nervous system for relief of pain, *Pain* 1:109-123, 1975.

317. Sternback RH, Ignelzi RJ, Deems LM, Timmermans G: Transcutaneous electrical analgesia: a follow-up analysis, *Pain* 2:35-41, 1976.

318. Wall PD: The gate control theory of pain mechanisms: a reexamination and restatement, *Brain* 101:1-18, 1978.

319. Dubner R: Neurophysiology of pain, *Dent Clin North Am* 22:11-30, 1978.

320. Moystad A, Krogstad BS, Larheim TA: Transcutaneous nerve stimulation in a group of patients with rheumatic disease involving the temporomandibular joint, *J Prosthet Dent* 64:596-600, 1990.

321. Marchand S, Charest J, Jinxue L, Chenard JR, Lavignolle B et al: Is TENS purely a placebo effect? A controlled study on chronic low back pain, *Pain* 54:99-106, 1993.

322. Jay GW, Brunson J, Branson SJ: The effectiveness of physical therapy in the treatment of chronic daily headaches, *Headache* 29:156-162, 1989.

323. Lapeer GL: High-intensity transcutaneous nerve stimulation at the Hoku acupuncture point for relief of muscular headache pain. Literature review and clinical trial, *Cranio* 4:164-171, 1986.

324. Black RR: Use of transcutaneous electrical nerve stimulation in dentistry, *J Am Dent Assoc* 113:649-652, 1986.

325. Ghia JN, Mao W, Toomey TC, Gregg JM: Acupuncture and chronic pain mechanisms, *Pain* 2:285-299, 1976.

326. Graff-Radford SB, Reeves JL, Baker RL, Chiu D: Effects of transcutaneous electrical nerve stimulation on myofascial pain and trigger point sensitivity, *Pain* 37:1-5, 1989.

327. Dos Santos J Jr: Supportive conservative therapies for temporomandibular disorders, *Dent Clin North Am* 39:459-477, 1995.

328. Raustia AM, Pohjola RT: Acupuncture compared with stomatognathic treatment for TMJ dysfunction. Part III: effect of treatment on mobility, *J Prosthet Dent* 56:616-623, 1986.

329. Johansson A, Wenneberg B, Wagersten C, Haraldson T: Acupuncture in treatment of facial muscular pain, *Acta Odontol Scand* 49:153-158, 1991.

330. Wang K: A report of 22 cases of temporomandibular joint dysfunction syndrome treated with acupuncture and laser radiation, *J Tradit Chin Med* 12:116-118, 1992.

331. Elsharkawy TM, Ali NM: Evaluation of acupuncture and occlusal splint therapy in the treatment of temporomandibular joint disorders, *Egypt Dent J* 41:1227-1232, 1995.

332. Goddard G: Short term pain reduction with acupuncture treatment for chronic orofacial pain patients, *Med Sci Monit* 11:CR71-74, 2005.

333. List T, Helkimo M, Karlsson R: Pressure pain thresholds in patients with craniomandibular disorders before and after treatment with acupuncture and occlusal splint therapy: a controlled clinical study, *J Orofac Pain* 7:275-282, 1993.

334. Rosted P: The use of acupuncture in dentistry: a review of the scientific validity of published papers, *Oral Dis* 4:100-104, 1998.

335. Hansson P, Ekblom A, Thomsson M, Fjellner B: Influence of naloxone on relief of acute oro-facial pain by transcutaneous electrical nerve stimulation (TENS) or vibration, *Pain* 24:323-329, 1986.

336. Kleinkort JA, Foley R: Laser acupuncture. Its use in physical therapy, *Am J Acupunct* 12:51-55, 1984.

337. Snyder-Mackler L, Bork CE: Effect of helium-neon laser irradiation on peripheral sensory nerve latency, *Phys Ther* 68:223-225, 1988.

338. Walker J: Relief from chronic pain by low power laser irradiation, *Neurosci Lett* 43:339-344, 1983.

339. Bliddal H, Hellesen C, Ditlevsen P, Asselberghs J, Lyager L: Soft-laser therapy of rheumatoid arthritis, *Scand J Rheumatol* 16:225-228, 1987.

340. Roynesdal AK, Bjornland T, Barkvoll P, Haanaes HR: The effect of soft-laser application on postoperative pain and swelling. A double-blind, crossover study, *Int J Oral Maxillofac Surg* 22:242-245, 1993.

341. Hall G, Anneroth G, Schennings T, Zetterqvist L, Ryden H: Effect of low level energy laser irradiation on wound healing. An experimental study in rats, *Swed Dent J* 18: 29-34, 1994.

342. Gam AN, Thorsen H, Lonnberg F: The effect of low-level laser therapy on musculoskeletal pain: a meta-analysis, *Pain* 52:63-66, 1993.

343. Bertolucci LE, Grey T: Clinical analysis of mid-laser versus placebo treatment of arthralgic TMJ degenerative joints, *Cranio* 13:26-29, 1995.

344. Bertolucci LE, Grey T: Clinical comparative study of microcurrent electrical stimulation to mid-laser and placebo treatment in degenerative joint disease of the temporomandibular joint, *Cranio* 13:116-120, 1995.

345. Nunez SC, Garcez AS, Suzuki SS, Ribeiro MS: Management of mouth opening in patients with temporomandibular disorders through low-level laser therapy and transcutaneous electrical neural stimulation, *Photomed Laser Surg* 24:45-49, 2006.

346. Hanson TL: Infrared laser in the treatment of craniomandibular arthrogenous pain, *J Prosthet Dent* 61:614-617, 1989.

347. Palano D, Martelli M: A clinical statistical investigation of laser effect in the treatment of pain and dysfunction of the temporomandibular joint (TMJ), *Med Laser Rep* 2:21-29, 1985.

348. Bezuur NJ, Habets LL, Hansson TL: The effect of therapeutic laser treatment in patients with craniomandibular disorders, *J Craniomandib Disord* 2:83-86, 1988.

349. Conti PC: Low level laser therapy in the treatment of temporomandibular disorders (TMD): a double-blind pilot study, *Cranio* 15:144-149, 1997.

350. Melzack R, Wall PD: Pain mechanisms: a new theory, *Science* 150:971-979, 1965.

351. Simons DG, Travell JG, Simons LS: *Travell & Simons' myofascial pain and dysfunction: the trigger point manual*, ed 2, Baltimore, 1999, Lippincott Williams & Wilkins, pp 126-173.

352. Magnusson T, Syren M: Therapeutic jaw exercises and interocclusal appliance therapy. A comparison between two common treatments of temporomandibular disorders, *Swed Dent J* 23:27-37, 1999.

353. Maloney GE, Mehta N, Forgione AG, Zawawi KH, Al-Badawi EA et al: Effect of a passive jaw motion device on pain and range of motion in TMD patients not responding to flat plane intraoral appliances, *Cranio* 20:55-66, 2002.

354. Nicolakis P, Erdogmus B, Kopf A, Djaber Ansari A, Piehslinger E et al: Exercise therapy for craniomandibular disorders, *Arch Phys Med Rehabil* 81:1137-1142, 2000.

355. Wilk BR, McCain JP: Rehabilitation of the temporomandibular joint after arthroscopic surgery, *Oral Surg Oral Med Oral Pathol Oral Radiol Endod* 73:531-536, 1992.

356. Austin BD, Shupe SM: The role of physical therapy in recovery after temporomandibular joint surgery, *J Oral Maxillofac Surg* 51:495-498, 1993.

357. Kropmans TJ, Dijkstra PU, Stegenga B, de Bont LG: Therapeutic outcome assessment in permanent temporomandibular joint disc displacement, *J Oral Rehabil* 26:357-363, 1999.

358. Casares G, Benito C, de la Hoz JL: Treatment of TMJ static disk with arthroscopic lysis and lavage: a comparison between MRI arthroscopic findings and clinical results, *Cranio* 17:49-57, 1999.

359. Chung SC, Kim HS: The effect of the stabilization splint on the TMJ closed lock, *Cranio* 11:95-101, 1993.

360. Nicolakis P, Erdogmus B, Kopf A, Ebenbichler G, Kollmitzer J et al: Effectiveness of exercise therapy in patients with internal derangement of the temporomandibular joint, *J Oral Rehabil* 28:1158-1164, 2001.

361. Chayes CM, Schwartz LL: Management of mandibular dysfunction: general and specific considerations. In Schwartz LL, Chayes CM, editors: *Facial pain and mandibular dysfunction*, Philadelphia, 1968, Saunders.

362. Gage JP: Collagen biosynthesis related to temporomandibular joint clicking in childhood, *J Prosthet Dent* 53:714-717, 1985.

363. Rocabado M: Diagnosis and treatment of abnormal craniocervical and craniomandibular mechanics. In Solberg WK, Clark GT, editors: *Abnormal jaw mechanics*, Chicago, 1984, Quintessence, pp 141-159.

364. Darnell MW: A proposed chronology of events for forward head posture, *J Craniomandib Pract* 1:49-54, 1983.

365. Lee WY, Okeson JP, Lindroth J: The relationship between forward head posture and temporomandibular disorders, *J Orofac Pain* 9:161-167, 1995.

366. Komiyama O, Kawara M, Arai M, Asano T, Kobayashi K: Posture correction as part of behavioural therapy in treatment of myofascial pain with limited opening, *J Oral Rehabil* 26:428-435, 1999.

367. Clark GT, Green EM, Dornan MR, Flack VF: Craniocervical dysfunction levels in a patient sample from a temporomandibular joint clinic, *J Am Dent Assoc* 115:251-256, 1987.

368. Darlow LA, Pesco J, Greenberg MS: The relationship of posture to myofascial pain dysfunction syndrome, *J Am Dent Assoc* 114:73-75, 1987.

369. Munhoz WC, Marques AP, de Siqueira JT: Evaluation of body posture in individuals with internal temporomandibular joint derangement, *Cranio* 23:269-277, 2005.

370. Wright EF, Domenech MA, Fischer JR Jr: Usefulness of posture training for patients with temporomandibular disorders [see comments], *J Am Dent Assoc* 131:202-210, 2000.

371. Feine JS, Lund JP: An assessment of the efficacy of physical therapy and physical modalities for the control of chronic musculoskeletal pain, *Pain* 71:5-23, 1997.

372. Feine JS, Widmer CG, Lund JP: Physical therapy: a critique [see comments], *Oral Surg Oral Med Oral Pathol Oral Radiol Endod* 83:123-127, 1997.

373. Curran SL, Carlson CR, Okeson JP: Emotional and physiologic responses to laboratory challenges: patients with temporomandibular disorders versus matched control subjects, *J Orofac Pain* 10:141-150, 1996.

374. Maixner W, Fillingim R, Booker D, Sigurdsson A: Sensitivity of patients with painful temporomandibular disorders to experimentally evoked pain, *Pain* 63:341-351, 1995.

375. Svensson P, Arendt-Nielsen L, Nielsen H, Larsen JK: Effect of chronic and experimental jaw muscle pain on pain-pressure thresholds and stimulus-response curves, *J Orofac Pain* 9:347-356, 1995.

376. Carlson CR, Bertrand P: *Self-regulation training manual*, Lexington, Ky, 1995, University Press.

377. Carlson C, Bertrand P, Ehrlich A, Maxwell A, Burton RG: Physical self-regulation training for the management of temporomandibular disorders, *J Orofac Pain* 15:47-55, 2001.

378. Carlson CR, Sherman JJ, Studts JL, Bertrand PM: The effects of tongue position on mandibular muscle activity, *J Orofac Pain* 11:291-297, 1997.

379. Bertrand PM: *The management of facial pain, American Association of Oral and Maxillofacial Surgery Knowledge Update Series*, Bethesda, Md, 2002, Bethesda Press.

Classification System Used for Diagnosing Temporomandibular Disorders

Bolded type indicates the disorders discussed in this chapter.

I. Masticatory muscle disorders (Chapter 12)
- **A. Protective co-contraction**
- **B. Local muscle soreness**
- **C. Myospasm**
- **D. Myofascial pain**
- **E. Centrally mediated myalgia**
- **F. Fibromyalgia**
- **G. Centrally mediated motor disorders**

II. Temporomandibular joint (TMJ) disorders (Chapter 13)
- A. Derangements of the condyle-disc complex
  1. Disc displacements
  2. Disc dislocations with reduction
  3. Disc dislocation without reduction
- B. Structural incompatibility of the articular surfaces
  1. Deviation in form
     a. Disc
     b. Condyle
     c. Fossa
  2. Adherences and adhesions
     a. Disc to condyle
     b. Disc to fossa
  3. Subluxation
  4. Spontaneous dislocation
- C. Inflammatory disorders of the TMJ
  1. Synovitis and capsulitis
  2. Retrodiscitis
  3. Arthritides
     a. Osteoarthritis
     b. Osteoarthrosis
     c. Polyarthritides
        i. Traumatic arthritis
        ii. Infectious arthritis
        iii. Rheumatoid arthritis
        iv. Hyperuricemia
        v. Psoriatic arthritis
        vi. Ankylosing spondylitis
  4. Inflammatory disorders of associated structures
     a. Temporal tendonitis
     b. Stylomandibular ligament inflammation
- D. General considerations when treating acute trauma to the TMJ

III. Chronic mandibular hypomobility (Chapter 14)
- A. Ankylosis
  1. Capsular fibrosis
  2. Bony
- B. Muscle contracture
  1. Myositis
     a. Passive stretching
     b. Resistant-opening exercises
  2. Myofibrotic
- C. Coronoid process impedance

IV. Growth disorders (Chapter 14)
- A. Congenital and developmental bone disorders
  1. Agenesis
  2. Hypoplasia
  3. Hyperplasia
  4. Neoplasia
- B. Congenital and developmental muscle disorders
  1. Hypotrophy
  2. Hypertrophy
  3. Neoplasia

Treatment of Masticatory Muscle Disorders

12 CHAPTER

"Masticatory muscle pain is the most common symptom of TMD. So why do so many clinicians call this 'TMJ'?"

—JPO

his is the first of three chapters that will address the treatment of the various temporomandibular disorders (TMDs). A chapter is devoted to each of the major disorders. In each chapter the individual subclasses are briefly outlined according to cause, history, and clinical findings. (A more detailed description has already been presented in Chapters 8 and 10.) Following this review, appropriate definitive and supportive therapy is discussed. Finally, at the end of each chapter, several clinical case reports are presented.

The predominant complaint of patients with masticatory muscle disorders is myalgia. This is often reported as having a sudden onset and being recurrent. The pain originates in the muscles, and therefore any restriction of mandibular movement is caused by the extracapsular muscular pain. All masticatory muscle disorders are not the same clinically. As discussed in Chapter 8, there are at least five different types, and being able to distinguish among them is important because the treatment of each is quite different. The five types are (1) protective co-contraction (muscle splinting), (2) local muscle soreness, (3) myofascial (trigger point) pain, (4) myospasm, and (5) chronic centrally mediated myalgia. Two other types will be discussed

in this chapter. They are centrally mediated motor disorders and fibromyalgia. The first three conditions (protective co-contraction, local muscle soreness, and myofascial pain) are commonly seen in the dental office. The other three are seen less frequently.

Some muscle disorders occur and resolve in a relatively short period of time (co-contraction and local muscle soreness). When these conditions are not resolved, more chronic pain disorders may result. Chronic masticatory muscle disorders become more complicated, and treatment is generally oriented differently than for acute problems. With time, the central nervous system (CNS) can play an important role in maintaining the muscle disorder (myofascial pain, myospasm, chronic centrally mediated myalgia, and centrally mediated motor disorders). Therefore it becomes important that the clinician be able to identify acute muscle disorders from chronic disorders so that proper therapy can be applied. Fibromyalgia is a chronic myalgic disorder that presents as a systemic musculoskeletal pain problem that must be recognized by the dentist and best managed by referral to appropriate medical personnel.

PROTECTIVE CO-CONTRACTION (MUSCLE SPLINTING)

Protective co-contraction is the initial response of a muscle to altered sensory or proprioceptive input or injury (or threat of injury). This response has been called *protective muscle splinting*[1] or *coactivation*.[2] This condition has been demonstrated by several researchers.[3-7] Co-contraction is a common phenomenon and can be observed during many normal functional activities such as bracing the arm when attempting a task with the fingers.[2] In the presence of altered sensory input or pain, antagonistic muscle groups seem to fire during movement in an attempt to protect the injured part. Therefore pain felt in the masticatory system can produce protective co-contraction of masticatory muscles.[3] Clinically this results in an increased activity of the jaw-opening muscles during closure of the mouth, as well as an increase in closing muscle activity during mouth opening. One should remember that protective co-contraction is not a pathologic condition but a normal physiologic response of the musculoskeletal system.[7]

CAUSE

The following events are responsible for protective co-contraction:
1. Altered sensory or proprioceptive input
2. The presence of constant deep pain input
3. Increased emotional stress

HISTORY

The key to identifying protective co-contraction is that it immediately follows an event, and therefore the history is important. Protective co-contraction only remains a few days. If it is not resolved, local muscle soreness is likely to follow. The history will reveal one of the following:
1. A recent alteration in local structures
2. A recent source of constant deep pain
3. A recent increase in emotional stress

CLINICAL CHARACTERISTICS

The following clinical characteristics are present with protective co-contraction:
1. Structural dysfunction: decreased range of movement, but the patient can achieve a relatively normal range when requested to do so

2. Minimal pain at rest
3. Increased pain with function
4. A feeling of muscle weakness

DEFINITIVE TREATMENT

Importantly, the clinician must remember that protective co-contraction is a normal CNS response and therefore there is no indication to treat the muscle condition itself. Treatment should instead be directed toward the reason for the co-contraction. When co-contraction results from trauma, definitive treatment is not indicated because the cause is no longer present.

When co-contraction results from the introduction of a poorly fitting restoration, definitive treatment consists of altering the restoration to harmonize with the existing occlusion. Altering the occlusal condition to eliminate co-contraction is directed only at the offending restoration and not the entire dentition. Once the offending restoration has been eliminated, the occlusal condition is returned to its preexisting state, which resolves the symptoms (Fig. 12-1).

If the co-contraction is the result of a source of deep pain, the pain must be appropriately addressed. If an increase in emotional stress is the cause, appropriate stress management such as physical self-regulation (PSR) techniques should be instituted.

SUPPORTIVE THERAPY

When the cause of protective co-contraction is tissue injury, supportive therapy is often the only type of treatment rendered. It begins with instructing the patient to restrict use of the mandible to within painless limits. A soft diet may be recommended until the pain subsides. Short-term pain medication (nonsteroidal antiinflammatory drugs [NSAIDs]) may be indicated. Simple PSR techniques (see Chapter 11) can also be initiated. Generally, however, muscle exercises and other physical therapies are not indicated. Co-contraction is usually of short duration; if the causes are controlled, symptoms will resolve in several days (Fig. 12-2).

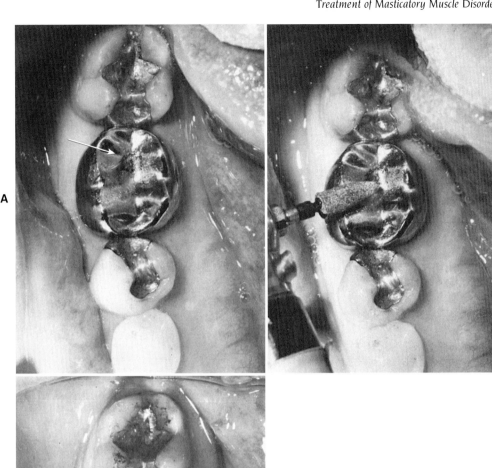

Fig. 12-1 Introduction of a heavy occlusal contact can initiate protective co-contraction. **A,** A heavy occlusal contact exists in the central fossa of this crown *(arrow)*. **B,** The contact is carefully altered to occlude simultaneously with the adjacent teeth in the arch. **C,** After the adjustment, occlusal contacts are equal on all teeth.

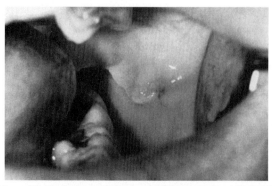

Fig. 12-2 AN ACUTE APHTHOUS ULCER THAT ELICITED PAIN WHEN RUBBED AGAINST THE ADJACENT MOLARS. This pain led to protective co-contraction. Proper supportive therapy was initiated to minimize the pain and thus reduce the co-contraction symptoms.

LOCAL MUSCLE SORENESS (NONINFLAMMATORY MYALGIA)

Local muscle soreness is a primary, noninflammatory, myogenous pain disorder. It is often the first response of the muscle tissue to continued protective co-contraction. Although co-contraction represents a CNS-induced muscle response, local muscle soreness represents a change in the local environment of the muscle tissues. It represents the initial response to overuse, which we think of as fatigue.

CAUSE

The following conditions lead to local muscle soreness:
1. Protracted protective co-contraction secondary to a recent alteration in local structures or a continued source of constant deep pain
2. Local tissue trauma or unaccustomed use of the muscle
3. Increased levels of emotional stress

HISTORY

The history reported by a patient with local muscle soreness will include one of the following:
1. Pain began several hours/days following an event associated with protective co-contraction.

2. Pain began associated with tissue injury (injection, opening wide, or unaccustomed muscle use in which the pain may be delayed).
3. Pain began secondary to another source of deep pain.
4. There was a recent episode of increased emotional stress.

CLINICAL CHARACTERISTICS

Local muscle soreness presents with the following clinical characteristics:
1. Structural dysfunction: marked decrease in the velocity and range of mandibular movement (full range of movement cannot be achieved by patient)
2. Minimum pain at rest
3. Pain increased with function
4. Actual muscle weakness present[8]
5. Local tenderness when the involved muscles are palpated

DEFINITIVE TREATMENT

Because local muscle soreness produces deep pain that often creates secondary protective co-contraction, with time cyclic muscle pain is common. Therefore the primary goal in treating local muscle soreness is to decrease sensory input (such as pain) to the CNS. The following steps decrease sensory input:
1. Eliminate any ongoing altered sensory or proprioceptive input.
2. Eliminate any ongoing source of deep pain input (whether dental or other).
3. Provide patient education and information on self-management (PSR). The following four areas should be emphasized:
   a. Advise the patient to restrict mandibular use to within painless limits. Any time that use of the mandible causes pain, co-contraction can be reestablished. Therefore the patient should be instructed not to open to the point of pain. A soft diet should be encouraged, along with smaller bites and slower chewing.
   b. The patient should be encouraged to use the jaw within the painless limits so that the proprioceptors and mechanoceptors in the

musculoskeletal system are stimulated. This activity seems to encourage return to normal muscle function.[9] Therefore careful and deliberate use of the muscle can promote resolution of local muscle soreness. The patient should be encouraged to use the muscles but only within painless limits. Complete lack of muscle use is not appropriate for patients experiencing local muscle soreness.

c. The patient should be encouraged to reduce any nonfunctional tooth contacts. This begins by asking the patient to become more aware of those subconscious times when the teeth are in contact and then developing techniques to eliminate these contacts (cognitive awareness).[10,11] The patient is instructed to keep the lips together and the teeth apart. Most patients can develop the skills necessary to voluntarily disengage the teeth during the waking hours.

d. The patient should be made aware of the relationship between increased levels of emotional stress and the muscle pain condition. When emotional stress appears to be a significant contributor to the local muscle soreness, techniques that reduce stress and promote relaxation should be encouraged.[12]

4. Although patients can often control daytime tooth contacts, most have little control over nocturnal tooth contacts.[13] When nighttime clenching or bruxing is suspected (early morning pain), it is appropriate to fabricate an occlusal appliance for nighttime use.[14-19] An occlusal appliance is an acrylic device that fits over the teeth of one arch and provides precise occlusal contact with the opposing arch (Fig. 12-3). A stabilization (i.e., centric relation [CR]) appliance will provide even occlusal contacts when the condyles are in their anterosuperior position resting on the articular discs against the posterior slopes of the articular eminences (musculoskeletally stable). Eccentric guidance is developed on the canines only. The patient is instructed to wear the appliance at night during sleep and only occasionally during the day if it helps reduce the pain. The part-time use of this type of appliance for local muscle soreness has been demonstrated to be more effective in reducing muscle pain than full-time use.[20] Its fabrication is discussed in Chapter 15.

The occlusal appliance has been advocated by the dental profession for years, and data suggest it can be helpful in reducing masticatory muscle pain disorders.[19,21-24] However, because the profession demands more evidence-based studies, the occlusal appliance may not be as helpful as clinicians first thought.[25,26] We need to encourage more controlled clinical trials to better understand the

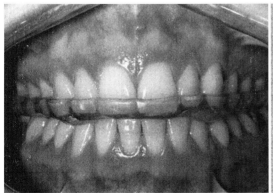
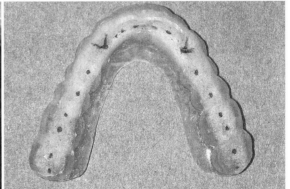

Fig. 12-3 A, Stabilization appliance. **B,** Occlusal contacts have been marked. Note that in the musculoskeletally stable position of the condyles (centric relation) there are even and simultaneous contacts of all posterior teeth (cusp tips contacting flat surfaces). Eccentric guidance is provided by the canines.

effects of appliances on TMD symptoms. However, because a well-fabricated stabilization appliance is a reversible therapy with few negative side effects, it can be considered in the management of local muscle soreness.

5. If the previously mentioned therapies fail to resolve the pain condition, the clinician may consider the use of a mild analgesic and/or possibly a muscle relaxant.[27] These pharmacotherapies will help reduce the constant deep pain input that may result in cyclic muscle pain and therefore may be considered both definitive and supportive therapy.

SUPPORTIVE THERAPY

Supportive therapy for local muscle soreness is directed toward reducing pain and restoring normal muscle function. In most cases, pain can be easily controlled by the definitive treatments discussed earlier. However, if pain continues, it can usually be controlled with a mild analgesic such as aspirin, acetaminophen, or an NSAID (e.g., ibuprofen). The patient should be encouraged to take the medication regularly so that all pain will be controlled. If the patient takes the medication only occasionally, the cyclic effect of the deep pain input may not be stopped. The patient should be instructed to take the medication every 4 to 6 hours for 5 to 7 days so that the pain is eliminated and the cycle is broken. After this, the patient should no longer need medication.

Manual physical therapy techniques such as passive muscle stretching and gentle massage may also be helpful. Relaxation therapy may also be helpful if increased emotional stress is suspected.

Local muscle soreness should respond to therapy in 1 to 3 weeks. When this therapy is not effective, the clinician should consider the possibility of a misdiagnosis. If a reevaluation of the pain condition reinforces a masticatory muscle disorder, one of the more complicated myalgic disorders should be considered.

Of particular note is that activities within the CNS influence the following four muscle conditions: myospasm, myofascial pain, chronic centrally mediated myalgia, and fibromyalgia. The clinician's appreciation of the role of the CNS is therapeutically important. Myospasm is an acute local disorder, whereas myofascial pain and chronic centrally mediated myalgia are more chronic regional disorders. Fibromyalgia is a chronic systemic (global) pain disorder.

MYOSPASMS (TONIC CONTRACTION MYALGIA)

Myospasm is an involuntary, CNS-induced, tonic muscle contraction often associated with local metabolic conditions within the muscle tissues. Although this condition can certainly affect the muscles of mastication, it is not as common as once thought.

CAUSE

The following conditions can cause myospasm:
1. Continued deep pain input
2. Local metabolic factors within the muscle tissues associated with fatigue or overuse[28]
3. Idiopathic myospasm mechanisms

HISTORY

The patient reports a sudden onset of restricted jaw movement usually accompanied by muscle rigidity.

CLINICAL CHARACTERISTICS

The following clinical characteristics are associated with myospasms:
1. Structural dysfunction: marked restriction in range of mandibular movement according to the muscle(s) involved; acute malocclusion common
2. Pain at rest
3. Pain increased with function
4. Affected muscle is firm and painful when palpated.
5. Generalized feeling of significant muscle tightness

DEFINITIVE TREATMENT

Two treatments are suggested for acute myospasms. The first is directed toward immediately reducing the spasm itself, whereas the other addresses the cause:

1. Myospasms are best treated by reducing the pain and then passively lengthening or stretching the involved muscle. Reduction of the pain can be achieved by manual massage (Fig. 12-4), vapo-coolant spray, ice, or even an injection of local anesthetic into the muscle in spasm. Once the pain is reduced, the muscle is passively stretched to its full length. If an injection is used (often it is the most effective manner to stop a persistent spasm), 2% lidocaine without a vaso-constrictor is recommended.
2. When obvious causes are present (i.e., deep pain input), attempts should be directed toward elimination of these factors so as to lessen the likelihood of recurrent myospasms. When the myospasms are secondary to fatigue and overuse (prolonged exercise), the patient is advised to rest the muscle(s) and reestablish normal electrolyte balance.

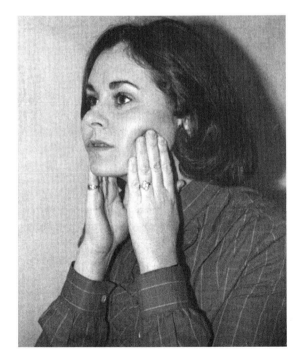

Fig. 12-4 Pain resulting from acute myospasms can often be reduced by gentle massaging of the muscles. This effect is produced primarily by an alteration of sensory input.

Occasionally myospasms occur repeatedly with no identifiable causes. When this occurs in the same muscle, the condition may actually represent an oromandibular dystonia. Dystonias are repeated, uncontrolled spastic contraction of muscles often thought to have central etiologies. Dystonias are managed differently than acute and occasional myospasms and are discussed in a separate section at the end of this chapter.

SUPPORTIVE THERAPY

Often physical therapy techniques are the key to managing myospasms. Soft tissue mobilization such as deep massage and passive stretching are the two most important immediate treatments. Once the myospasm is reduced, other physical therapies can be helpful in addressing local and systemic factors such as muscle conditioning exercises and relaxation techniques. Pharmacologic therapy is not usually indicated because of the acuteness of the condition.

MYOFASCIAL PAIN (TRIGGER POINT MYALGIA)

Myofascial pain is a regional myogenous pain condition characterized by local areas of firm, hypersensitive bands of muscle tissue known as *trigger points*.[29] This condition is also called *myofascial trigger point pain*. The presence of central excitatory effects is common with this myalgic disorder. The most common effect is referred pain, often described by the patient as a tension-type headache.

CAUSE

Although a complete understanding of this disorder is lacking, the following causes have been related to myofascial pain:

1. Continued source of deep pain input[30,31]
2. Increased levels of emotional stress[32]
3. Presence of sleep disturbances[33,34]
4. Local factors that influence muscle activity such as habits, posture, muscle strains, or even chilling

5. Systemic factors such as nutritional inadequacies,[35] poor physical conditioning, fatigue,[30] and viral infections[36]
6. Idiopathic trigger point mechanism

HISTORY

The patient's chief complaint is often the heterotopic pain and not the actual source of pain (the trigger points). Therefore the patient will direct the clinician to the headache (tension-type) or protective co-contraction. If the clinician is not careful, he or she will likely direct treatment to the secondary pains, which, of course, will fail. The clinician must have the knowledge and diagnostic skills necessary to identify the primary source of pain so that proper treatment can be selected.

CLINICAL CHARACTERISTICS

An individual suffering with myofascial pain will commonly reveal the following clinical characteristics:

1. Structural dysfunction: A slight decrease in the velocity and range of mandibular movement may exist depending on the location and intensity of the trigger points. This mild structural dysfunction is secondary to the inhibitory effects of pain (protective co-contraction).
2. The heterotopic pain is felt even at rest.
3. Pain may increase pain with function.
4. When provoked, tight muscle bands with trigger points increase the heterotopic pain.

DEFINITIVE TREATMENT

The treatment of myofascial pain is directed toward the elimination or reduction of causes. The clinician can accomplish this with the following treatment protocol:

1. Eliminate any source of ongoing deep pain input in an appropriate manner according to the cause.
2. Reduce the local and systemic factors that contribute to myofascial pain. This treatment is individualized to the patient's needs. For example, if emotional stress is an important part of the disorder, stress management techniques are indicated. When posture or work position

contributes to myofascial pain, attempts should be made to improve these conditions. PSR techniques (see Chapter 11) are useful in managing myofascial pain.
3. If a sleep disorder is suspected, proper evaluation and referral should be made. Often low dosages of a tricyclic antidepressant, such as 10 to 20 mg of amitriptyline before bedtime, can be helpful (see Chapter 11).
4. One of the most important considerations in the management of myofascial pain is the treatment and elimination of the trigger points. This is accomplished by painlessly stretching the muscle containing the trigger points. The following techniques can be used to achieve this.

Spray and Stretch

One of the most common and conservative methods of eliminating trigger points is with a spray-and-stretch technique.[37,38] This technique consists of spraying a vapocoolant spray (e.g., fluoromethane) on the tissue overlying the muscle with a trigger point and then actively stretching the muscle. The vapocoolant spray provides a burst of cutaneous nerve stimulation that temporarily reduces pain perception in the area (see Chapter 2). Once the tissue has been sprayed, the muscle is stretched to its full length painlessly (Fig. 12-5). The vapocoolant spray is applied from a distance of approximately 18 inches and in the direction of the referred symptoms. Importantly, the passive stretching of the muscle is performed without producing pain. If pain is elicited, the muscle will likely protectively co-contract, resulting in more muscle activity (cyclic muscle pain). The precise technique for each muscle has been described by Simons and Travell.[39] This text should be an essential part of the armamentarium of any clinician treating myofascial pain.

Pressure and Massage

In some instances massage or manipulation of a trigger point can cause it to be eliminated. Care must be taken, however, not to produce pain. Some experts have suggested[37] that increased pressure applied to a trigger point is also an effective eliminating technique. The pressure is increased to approximately 20 lb and is

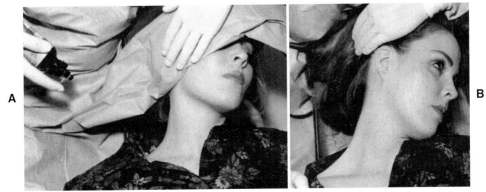

Fig. 12-5 SPRAY-AND-STRETCH TECHNIQUE. A, Vapocoolant spray is applied to the upper trapezius and to the cervical muscles to eliminate myofascial trigger points. The eyes, nose, mouth, and ear are protected from the spray. **B,** Immediately following the spray, the muscles are painlessly stretched.

maintained for 30 to 60 seconds. If this technique produces pain, it must be stopped because the pain can reinforce cyclic muscle pain.

Ultrasound and Electrogalvanic Stimulation

Physical therapy modalities such as ultrasound and electrogalvanic stimulation (EGS) can sometimes be useful in managing trigger points. Ultrasound produces deep heat to the area of the trigger point, causing local muscle relaxation.[40] Low-voltage EGS can be used to rhythmically stimulate or pulse the muscles. This therapy leads to reduced muscle activity and encourages muscle relaxation.[41,42] Although there is little research to verify the efficacy of these techniques, they are generally conservative and may be useful.

Injection and Stretch

Another effective method of eliminating a trigger point is by using injection techniques (Fig. 12-6). Most commonly, local anesthetic is injected and the muscle is painlessly stretched.[43,44] Although the anesthetic is useful in reducing pain,[45] it is apparently not the most critical factor in eliminating the trigger point.[46,47] Rather, the mechanical disruption of the trigger point by the needle seems to provide the therapeutic effect.

Local anesthetic is used for two reasons: (1) It eliminates the immediate pain, allowing full painless stretching of the muscle, and (2) it is diagnostic

(i.e., once a trigger point is anesthetized, not only is the local pain reduced but the referred pain is also eliminated). Thus the clinician can gain valuable information regarding the source of referred pain. For example, the anesthetic injection of a

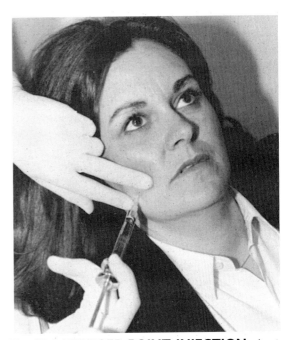

Fig. 12-6 TRIGGER POINT INJECTION. A trigger point in the right masseter is located, trapped between the fingers, and injected (with a short 27-gauge needle).

trigger point in the sternocleidomastoid will immediately eliminate a referred temporal headache and enable the true source of the headache pain to be identified. The immediate shutdown of pain relates to the interruption of the central excitatory effects produced by the deep pain (the trigger point). This suppression of pain may be in part related to the endorphin system.[48]

When local anesthetic injections are indicated, 1% procaine appears to be the least myotoxic. However, this medication is no longer packaged for use in dental syringes; thus when a dental syringe is used, 2% lidocaine is appropriate. A vasoconstrictor should not be used for muscle injections. A long-acting anesthetic such as bupivacaine (Marcaine) is not indicated for muscle injections because of increased myotoxicity, especially when used with steroids.[49] Only a small amount of lidocaine is necessary to treat a trigger point. One dental carpule is adequate for two or even three trigger point injections depending on the size of the muscle being injected. A half carpule is indicated for a trapezius trigger point; less than a third is adequate for a temporalis trigger point.

Trigger point injections may be an appropriate treatment for myofascial pain when it is found that the injections provide the patient with prolonged relief, even after the anesthetic effect has resolved. Repeated injections may be indicated if the period of pain relief continues to become longer between each injection. If trigger point injections fail to provide any prolonged pain relief, there is no indication to repeat the procedure.

As with any injection, the four rules described in Chapter 10 should always be followed. The anatomic considerations and injection technique for each muscle are described by Simons and Travell,[43] and their text should be consulted by clinicians interested in treating myofascial pain with trigger point injections.

SUPPORTIVE THERAPY

As already discussed, various physical therapy modalities and manual techniques are used to treat myofascial pain. These techniques are listed under Definitive Treatment because they address the actual elimination of trigger points. The most important are the soft tissue mobilization and muscle conditioning techniques.

Pharmacologic therapy such as a muscle relaxant can be helpful, but it will not usually eliminate the trigger points. A medication such as cyclobenzaprine (Flexeril), 10 mg before sleep, can often reduce pain, but the trigger points still need to be treated, as discussed earlier. Muscle relaxants help convert an active trigger point into a latent or dormant trigger point but may not necessarily eliminate it. Analgesics may also be helpful in interrupting the cyclic effect of pain.

Posture is another possible contributor in some patients to myofascial pain.[29] Muscles that are maintained at shortened length tend to develop trigger points more than others. Daily stretching to full length can be beneficial in maintaining them as pain free. This is especially true in the neck and shoulder region. Regular exercise should always be encouraged.[30,50,51]

CENTRALLY MEDIATED MYALGIA (CHRONIC MYOSITIS)

Centrally mediated myalgia is a chronic, continuous muscle pain disorder originating predominantly from CNS effects that are felt peripherally in the muscle tissues. This disorder clinically presents with symptoms similar to an inflammatory condition of the muscle tissue and therefore is sometimes referred to as *myositis*.

CAUSE

The cause of centrally mediated myalgia is, as the name suggests, the CNS and not the more commonly associated structures of the masticatory system. As the CNS becomes exposed to prolonged nociceptive input, brainstem pathways can functionally change. This can result in an antidromic effect on afferent peripheral neurons. In other words, neurons that normally only carry information from the periphery into the CNS can now be reversed to carry information from the CNS out to the peripheral tissues. This is likely to occur through the axon transport system.[52] When this occurs, the afferent neurons in the periphery can release nociceptive neurotransmitters such as substance P and bradykinin, which in turn causes peripheral tissue pain. This process is called *neurogenic inflammation*.[53-57]

The important concept to remember is that the muscle pain expressed by the patient with chronic centrally mediated myalgia cannot be treated by managing the painful muscle tissue itself. Management must be directed to the central mechanisms, a thought process that can be foreign to dentists.

Chronic centrally mediated myalgia may be caused by the prolonged input of muscle pain associated with local muscle soreness or myofascial pain. In other words, the longer the patient complains of myogenous pain, the greater the likelihood of chronic centrally mediated myalgia. However, it is also possible that other central mechanisms may play a significant role in the cause of centrally mediated myalgia, such as chronic upregulation of the autonomic nervous system, chronic exposure to emotional stress, or other sources of deep pain input (Fig. 12-7).

HISTORY

The patient reports a constant, primary, myogenous pain condition usually associated with a prolonged history of muscle complaints (months and even years).

CLINICAL CHARACTERISTICS

The following six clinical characteristics are common with centrally mediated myalgia:
1. Structural dysfunction: Patients experiencing centrally mediated myalgia present with a significant decrease in the velocity and range of mandibular movement.
2. Significant pain at rest
3. Pain increased with function
4. Generalized feeling of muscle tightness
5. Significant pain to muscle palpation
6. As chronic centrally mediated myalgia becomes protracted, it may induce muscle atrophy and/or myostatic or myofibrotic contracture.

DEFINITIVE TREATMENT

The clinician should recognize the condition of chronic centrally mediated myalgia because the outcome of therapy will not be as immediate as with treating local muscle soreness. Neurogenic inflammation of muscle tissue, as well as the chronic central sensitization that has produced it, often takes time to resolve. When the diagnosis of chronic centrally mediated myalgia is established, the clinician should discuss with the patient the expected results and timetable. The patient should be informed that reduction of symptoms is initially slow and not dramatic. Patients need to be aware

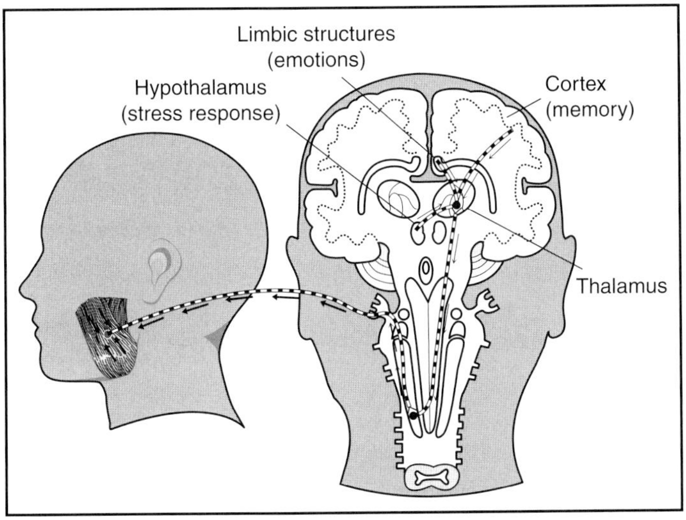

Fig. 12-7 CENTRALLY MEDIATED MYALGIA. Some muscle disorders have their origin in the central nervous system, even though the pain is felt peripherally in the muscles. This illustration depicts how central activation of the hypothalamus, limbic structures, and cortex can combine to produce an antidromic effect to the muscle tissues. When this occurs, the key to successful management of this pain lies in quieting the central mechanisms and not changing the peripheral structures (teeth, muscles, or joints).

of this so as to minimize disappointment in treatment results. As causes are controlled, neurogenic inflammation will resolve and symptoms will slowly decrease.

As is true with local muscle soreness, four general treatment strategies are followed in the patient with chronic centrally mediated myalgia. However, although somewhat similar, they are not identical. In fact, therapy for local muscle soreness will often aggravate chronic centrally mediated myalgia. Therefore if the clinician is treating local muscle soreness and the symptoms become greater, it is likely that the condition is actually chronic centrally mediated myalgia. The following regimen should then be used:

1. Restrict mandibular use to within painless limits. Using painful muscles only aggravates the condition. The patient should maintain the jaw as immobile as needed to reduce pain. A soft diet is initiated, along with slower chewing and smaller bites. If functional pain cannot be controlled, a liquid diet may be necessary. The liquid diet should be maintained long enough to allow pain reduction so that the patient can return to a soft diet without pain.

2. Avoid exercise and/or injections. Because the muscle tissue is neurogenically inflamed, any use initiates pain. The patient should rest the muscles as much as possible. Local anesthetic injections should be avoided because they traumatize already inflamed tissues. Local anesthetic blocking in chronic centrally mediated myalgia will often cause a marked increase in pain after the anesthetic has been metabolized. This clinical feature may help establish the diagnosis.

3. Disengage the teeth. As with local muscle soreness, the management of chronic centrally mediated myalgia is assisted by disengaging the teeth both voluntarily and involuntarily. Voluntary disengagement is accomplished by the PSR techniques discussed in Chapter 11. Involuntary disengagement of the teeth (nocturnal bruxism) is achieved by a stabilization appliance in the same manner as with local muscle soreness.

4. Begin taking an antiinflammatory medication. Because local muscle tissue is inflamed, it is quite appropriate to prescribe an antiinflammatory. An NSAID such as ibuprofen is a good choice and should be given on a regular basis (600 mg four times a day) for 2 weeks so that blood levels are sufficiently elevated to achieve a clinical effect. Irregular doses as needed will not achieve the desired effect. Ibuprofen is also analgesic, and it can thus help reduce cyclic muscle pain that can propagate chronic centrally mediated myalgia. As previously discussed, the patient should be questioned for any history of stomach complaints and monitored for any gastric irritation symptoms during the course of the medication. If these symptoms are present, a cyclooxygenase-2 (COX-2) inhibitor should be considered (see Chapter 11).

SUPPORTIVE THERAPY

Early in the treatment of chronic centrally mediated myalgia, physical therapy modalities should be used cautiously because any manipulation can increase the pain. Sometimes moist heat can be helpful (Fig. 12-8). For other patients, ice seems to be more helpful. The patients will clearly relate which is best for them. As the symptoms begin to resolve, ultrasound therapy and gentle stretching can begin. If pain is increased by the therapy, the intensity should be decreased.

Because the treatment of chronic centrally mediated myalgia often takes time, two distinct conditions can develop: hypotrophic changes and myostatic contracture. These occur as a result of the lack of use of the elevator muscles (temporalis, masseter, medial pterygoid). Once the acute symptoms have resolved, activity of the muscles should slowly begin. Some gentle isometric jaw exercise will be effective for increasing the strength and use of the muscles (Fig. 12-9). Passive stretching is also helpful in regaining the original length of the elevators (see Chapter 11). Remember, treating chronic centrally mediated myalgia is a slow process and it cannot be rushed. If physical therapy is introduced too quickly, the chronic centrally mediated myalgia can worsen.

FIBROMYALGIA (FIBROSITIS)

Fibromyalgia is a chronic, global, musculoskeletal pain disorder.[58] According to an earlier consensus

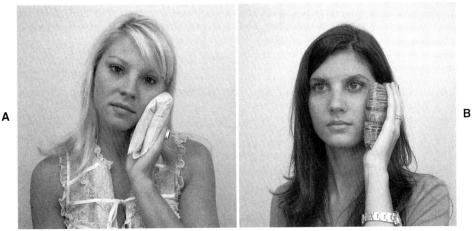

Fig. 12-8 Application of moist heat or cold can be helpful for chronic centrally mediated myalgia. **A,** A moist heat pack is applied to the masseter muscle for 15 to 20 minutes and repeated as often as needed throughout the day. **B,** When heat is not effective, cold may be tried. A frozen ice pack is placed on the symptomatic muscle until the tissue feels numb (no longer than 5 to 7 minutes). The muscle is allowed to gradually rewarm. If this results in less pain, the procedure can be repeated.

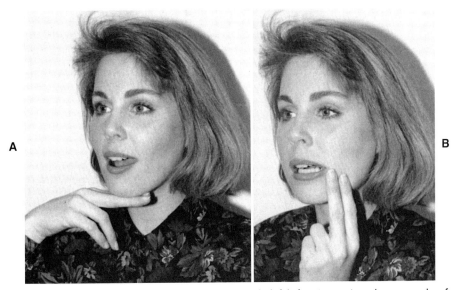

Fig. 12-9 Gentle isometric jaw exercises are helpful for increasing the strength of hypotrophic muscles. **A,** The objective is to resist slightly mouth-opening movement. **B,** The patient moves the jaw laterally while resisting the movement with the fingers. This is done for 3 to 5 seconds in an opening, a right, and a left lateral movement as well as in a protrusive movement. The exercises are repeated throughout the day.

report,[59] fibromyalgia is a widespread musculoskeletal pain disorder in which there is tenderness at 11 or more of 18 specific predetermined sites throughout the body. Fibromyalgia is not a masticatory pain disorder and therefore needs to be recognized and referred to appropriate medical personnel.

CAUSE

The etiology of fibromyalgia has not been well documented. It is likely related to an alteration in the processing of peripheral (musculoskeletal) input by the CNS. The descending inhibitory system, the hypothalamic-pituitary-adrenal (HPA) axis and immune systems, have been implicated.[60-64] Certainly other unidentified conditions that also lead to fibromyalgia exist.[58] Although the cause of fibromyalgia is likely different than masticatory muscle pain disorders, these two conditions coexist in many chronic patients.[65-74]

HISTORY

Patients experiencing fibromyalgia report chronic and generalized musculoskeletal pain complaints in three of the four quadrants of the body that has been present for 3 months or longer. The patient complains of arthralgic pain with no evidence of any articular disorder. Sleep disturbances are a common finding along with a sedentary physical condition and clinical depression.

CLINICAL CHARACTERISTICS

Fibromyalgia involves the presence of at least 11 of 18 designated tender points that do not produce heterotopic pain. Patients usually present with a sedentary physical condition.

Patients suffering with fibromyalgia reveal the following clinical characteristics:

1. Structural dysfunction: If the masticatory muscles are involved, there is significant decrease in the velocity and range of mandibular movement.
2. Generalized myogenous pain at rest fluctuates over time with other fibromyalgic complaints.
3. Pain is increased with function of the involved muscles.

4. Patients experiencing fibromyalgia report a general feeling of muscle weakness. They also commonly report generalized chronic fatigue.
5. Fibromyalgia is characterized by numerous tender points throughout the various quadrants of the body. These tender points do not produce heterotopic pain when palpated. This finding represents a distinct clinical difference between fibromyalgia and myofascial pain. According to established criteria,[59] fibromyalgia patients must reveal tenderness in at least 11 of 18 predetermined sites throughout three of the four quadrants of the body.
6. Patients with fibromyalgia generally lack physical conditioning. Because muscle function increases pain, fibromyalgia patients often avoid exercise. This becomes a perpetuating condition because sedentary physical condition can be a predisposing factor in fibromyalgia.

DEFINITIVE TREATMENT

Because knowledge of fibromyalgia is limited, treatment should be conservative and directed toward the causative and perpetuating factors. The clinician should remember that fibromyalgia is not a primary masticatory muscle disorder. Therefore the dentist should not assume the role of primary therapist. Instead, the dentist needs to be able to recognize fibromyalgia and make the proper referral. When significant masticatory symptoms are present, the dentist should manage these symptoms along with a team of health professionals. Other health professionals who can help manage this problem are from the fields of rheumatology, rehabilitative medicine, psychology, and physical therapy.[75] The following general treatments should be considered:

1. When other masticatory muscle disorders also exist, therapy should be directed toward these disorders.
2. When the perpetuating conditions discussed in Chapter 8 are present, they should be properly addressed.
3. NSAIDs seem to be of some benefit with fibromyalgic symptoms and should be administered in the same manner as with chronic centrally mediated myalgia.

4. If a sleep disturbance is identified, it should be addressed. Low dosages of a tricyclic antidepressant such as 10 to 50 mg of amitriptyline at bedtime can be helpful in reducing symptoms associated with fibromyalgia.[76-78] The mechanism is thought to be related to either an improvement in the quality of sleep[76,77,79] or a positive effect on the descending inhibitory system. Cyclobenzaprine (Flexril), 10 mg at bedtime, may also be helpful to assist in sleep and reduce pain.[80-82]

5. If depression is present, it should be managed by appropriate health professionals.

SUPPORTIVE THERAPY

Physical therapy modalities and manual techniques can be helpful for the patient with fibromyalgia. Techniques such as moist heat, gentle massage, passive stretching, and relaxation training can be the most helpful. In addition, muscle conditioning can be an important part of treatment. A mild and well-controlled general exercise program such as walking or light swimming can be helpful in lessening the muscle pain associated with fibromyalgia.[50,83] Care should be taken to develop an individual program for each patient.

CENTRALLY MEDIATED MOTOR DISORDERS

There are two conditions that can affect motor function of the masticatory muscles. Both are strongly influenced by the CNS. They are nocturnal bruxism and oromandibular dystonia. Nocturnal bruxism is a common phenomenon, whereas oromandibular dystonia is relatively rare. Both are discussed in this section.

NOCTURNAL BRUXISM

A factor that may lead or contribute to a masticatory muscle disorder is muscle hyperactivity, and that of greatest concern to the dentist is nocturnal bruxism and clenching. These activities are extremely difficult to control. At one time a widely held belief in dentistry was that malocclusion caused nocturnal bruxism.[84-91] However, well-controlled studies[92,93] have suggested that the occlusal condition exerts little influence on nocturnal muscle activity. Levels of emotional stress appear to have greater influence.[94,95] Yet it has been repeatedly demonstrated[14,15,94-101] that occlusal appliances decrease the level of nocturnal muscle activity, at least in the short term.

Originally experts thought that occlusal appliances were effective because they instantly introduced an ideal occlusal condition and, when worn, removed the malocclusion as a cause. This logic suggested that when an occlusal appliance led to a decrease in muscle symptoms, the malocclusion factors were the cause and selective grinding of the teeth was indicated to correct the condition permanently. Selective grinding, however, does *not* decrease bruxism.[93,102] The reason why occlusal appliances reduce TMD symptoms is far more complicated then merely how they may alter the occlusal condition. At least six other factors may be responsible for this symptom reduction (see Chapter 15 for a detailed discussion).

One of these factors is that the occlusal appliance provides an altered peripheral sensory input to the CNS, which activates a negative feedback mechanism that shuts down heavy muscle activity. In other words, the appliance may help maintain a more normal threshold for the protective reflex activity of the neuromuscular system. When normal reflex activity is present, the forces of bruxism are less likely to increase to levels of structural breakdown and symptoms.

Management Considerations for Nocturnal Bruxism
Currently no known treatment method exists that permanently eliminates bruxism. Although occlusal appliances can reduce the harmful effects of tooth wear and can help reduce musculoskeletal pains, they do not cure a patient of bruxing.[103] In most instances when the appliance is removed, even after long-term occlusal appliance therapy, the bruxism returns.[13]

In one study[104] it was demonstrated that 1 mg of clonazepam before sleep reduced the level of bruxing greater than a placebo drug. Some research[105] indicates that a low dosage of a tricyclic antidepressant (10 to 20 mg of amitriptyline per night) before sleep can alter the sleep cycle and decrease early morning muscle pain. Amitriptyline[106,107] and cyclobenzaprine[108] seem to reduce TMD symptoms, but the effect may not be directly related to a reduction in bruxing activity.

Because a cure for bruxism is unknown, the dentist should always select conservative reversible therapy. The stabilization appliance is such a modality. (Its specific effects on the masticatory system are considered in greater detail in Chapter 15.)

OROMANDIBULAR DYSTONIAS

By definition, *dystonia* means a "disordered tonicity of muscle."[109] Clinically this is observed as a sudden and uncontrolled contraction of a muscle. A single, sustained contraction is referred to as a *myospasm* (discussed earlier in this chapter). However, when the myospasm uncontrollably repeats itself, it is considered to be a dystonia. Some patients suffer with generalized dystonias involving many muscle groups. When the dystonia only involves specific muscles or muscle groups, the condition is referred to as a *focal dystonia*. Oromandibular dystonia is a focal dystonia whereby repetitive or sustained spasms occur in the masticatory, facial, or lingual muscles. These spasms result in involuntary and often painful jaw opening, closing, deflecting, retruding, or a combination of these actions.[110-112]

Oromandibular dystonia affects approximately 6.9/100,000 persons in the United States.[113] Some studies suggest that oromandibular dystonia affects more women than men with a mean age of symptom onset between 31 and 58 years.[114-116] Although evidence indicates that genetic predisposition may be a factor in some oromandibular dystonia patients,[111,117] in most cases the cause is unknown. Oromandibular dystonia is likely caused by a central brain/brainstem mechanism that causes the involved muscles to contract. Patients commonly report a precise onset of the first oromandibular dystonia episode. In studies by Tan and Jankovic,[114] the majority of cases are idiopathic in cause, accounting for 63% of cases reported. Other possible causes include drug induced (22.8%), peripheral induced (9.3%), postanoxia (2.5%), neurodegenerative disorder associated (1.8%), and head injury associated (0.8%).[114]

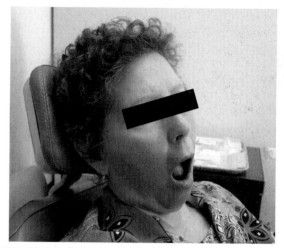

Fig. 12-10 This patient has a jaw opening oromandibular dystonia. She presented to the clinic with her mouth opened wide, and she cannot close it. She had been in this position for the past 36 hours.

The clinical characteristics of oromandibular dystonia are classified according to the affected muscles. The muscles involved may be the muscles of mastication, facial expression,[118] or tongue. Patients may present with jaw opening, jaw closing, jaw deflecting, jaw retruding, or a combination of any of these dystonias (Fig. 12-10). The uncontrolled or involuntary mandibular movements may be repetitive and/or sustained.[114] Similarly, dystonic spasms may result in nasal contractions, facial grimacing, lip pursing, lip sucking or smacking, chewing, bruxism, tongue dyskinesias, retractions of corners of mouth, and platysma contractions.[111,119,120] Other associated symptoms may include chewing difficulties, dysarthria, dysphagia, dysphonia, breathing difficulties, and alteration in vocalization depending on the muscles involved. Patients often report triggers or exacerbating factors such as emotional stress, depression, glaring light, watching television, driving, reading, talking, praying, fatigue, and chewing.[110-112,116,121] Patients frequently report that they have learned certain "sensory tricks" that help reduce the dystonia, such as sleeping, relaxing, talking, singing, humming, lip biting, tongue posturing, swallowing, chewing gum, and drinking alcohol.[116,122]

Management Consideration of Oromandibular Dystonias

No known cure for oromandibular dystonia exists. Treatment strategies are varied and are most effective when focused on the underlying cause and/or triggers.[123] Various drugs are usually tried as a first-line therapy for oromandibular dystonia. Although some drugs benefit some individuals, none are universally effective.[124] No evidence-based information exists regarding the efficacy of the different methods of pharmacologic therapeutic options currently being applied in dystonias.[125] Medications are prescribed in early stages and may have some effects in controlling the dystonic movements. The current lack of knowledge of the exact pathophysiology of dystonias has made specific pharmacologic therapies difficult. Systemic pharmacologic therapy benefits about one third of patients and consists of a wide variety of medications including cholinergics, benzodiazepams, antiparkinsonism drugs, anticonvulsants, baclofen, carbamazepine, and lithium.[126] In addition to these drugs, gabapentin has been reported to reduce symptoms in more than one third of patients.[127] Although most oral medications have low success rates, anticholinergic medications have been found to be the most effective oral medication for the treatment of dystonia.[128]

Botulinum toxin injections are currently the mainstay of treatment for most focal dystonias.[114,118,129,130] The neurotoxin botulinum toxin A, when injected into a muscle, causes a presynaptic blockade of the release of acetylcholine at the motor end plates.[131] The end result is a muscle that can no longer contract (paralysis). This process normally takes 1 to 2 weeks for the effect to be clinically noticeable. Once this has occurred, the neuromuscular end plates react with a collateral sprouting of axons that restores the preexisting condition. Normally, activity of the motor end plate is totally restored in 3 to 4 months. In other words, evidence suggests that effects of botulinum toxin A on muscles are completely reversible.

Numerous studies have confirmed a 90% to 95% response rate to botulinum toxin injection in oromandibular dystonia patients.[131] However, because the effect of botulinum toxin only lasts 3 to 4 months, it must be repeated for the oromandibular dystonia patient. On occasion this may lead to a problem because botulinum neurotoxins may be immunogenic.[132] The incidence of antibody-mediated resistance to botulinum toxin A, as determined by the mouse lethality assay, is reported to be between 3% and 10% and is generally accepted to be about 5%.[133] The only apparent symptom of the development of antibodies is lack of response to further injections. The use of other serotypes (F or B) may benefit those who have developed antibody resistance. Nevertheless, there have been only rare reports of patients with oromandibular dystonia treated with botulinum toxin A becoming immunoresistant. In one series of 86 patients with cervical and cranial dystonia, one patient with oromandibular dystonia had a positive botulinum toxin A serum antibody test.[133]

When treating a focal oromandibular dystonia patient, the first consideration is to identify the specific muscle or muscles guilty of producing the condition. In jaw-closing dystonias the muscles of concern are the elevator muscles such as the masseter and temporalis. These are normally easy to identify by simple palpation. The medial pterygoid may also be guilty in jaw-closing dystonias and is more difficult to identify. In jaw-opening dystonias the inferior lateral pterygoid muscles are often the offending muscles. In patients with a unilateral lateral pterygoid muscle dystonia, the jaw will be displaced laterally to the opposite side. Identifying the precise muscle or muscles involved is important to ensure that the botulinum toxin is injected into the correct muscle for maximum effect.

Once the specific dystonic muscles have been identified, they can be injected with the botulinum toxin. The same rules for injecting local anesthetic discussed in Chapter 10 are appropriate for injecting botulinum toxin. Botulinum toxin is injected using a short 30-gauge needle such as that used with a tuberculin syringe. The location and ease of access makes the masseter and temporalis muscles easy to inject.[134] Approximately 25 U of botulinum toxin A is normally appropriate for each of these muscles. The greatest number of motor end plates is found in the midbody of the muscle (halfway between the insertion and origin). Therefore this area should receive approximately 50% of the designated units of botulinum toxin A in several injections, and the remaining botulinum toxin A should be distributed throughout the remaining body of the muscle.

Sometimes the target muscles are difficult to locate and palpate (e.g., the inferior lateral pterygoid and medial pterygoid muscles). Although the dentist should know precisely where these muscles are located, when performing the injection it is difficult to confidently know the exact location of the needle tip. Therefore when these muscles need to be injected, electromyogram-guided needles should be used. This technique can verify that the botulinum toxin is delivered to the correct muscle (Fig. 12-11).

Other Uses of Botulinum Toxin Injections

Botulinum toxin can certainly provide excellent therapy for the oromandibular dystonia patient. However, as the clinician more broadly observes its clinical effects, it becomes obvious that other

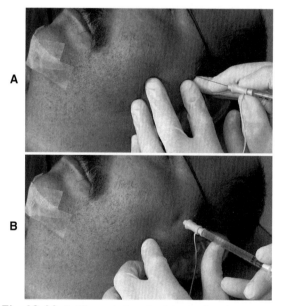

Fig. 12-11 A, The technique for injecting botulinum toxin into the inferior lateral pterygoid muscle. Note that there is an electrode on the chin and a wire attached to the needle so that the electromyographic activity can be monitored at the needle tip. **B,** Once the needle is placed to the proper depth, the patient is asked to push against resistance provided by the operator. If the needle is properly placed in the inferior lateral pterygoid muscle, the electromyogram will increase on the monitor. Once the proper position has been verified, the botulinum toxin is injected.

disorders may also benefit from botulinum toxin. In the area of TMD, some of the chronic muscle pain disorders may be good candidates for botulinum toxic injections. However, botulinum toxin is certainly not the first choice of treatment for most masticatory muscle pain disorders. One must always remember that botulinum toxin does not permanently relax muscles and therefore is not considered definitive therapy. Any time the clinician can eliminate the etiology of the pain disorder, it should be done. This is the most appropriate and effective manner to manage any disorders. Therefore the acute myalgic conditions such as protective co-contraction and local muscle soreness are not candidates for botulinum toxin. Even myofascial pain should be managed first by the techniques described early in this chapter. However, in cases in which muscle pain persists even after initial therapies have been tried, botulinum toxic may be considered. The management of chronic myofascial pain with botulinum toxic injections has growing support.[135-149] Some studies, however, reveal that botulinum toxin injections are no more effective than placebo injections.[150,151]

Support is also growing for the use of botulinum toxin for the management of refractory headache.[152-155] In fact, the evidence supports the use of botulinum toxic for both migraine[156-158] and tension-type headaches.[159] Yet not all studies are so positive.[160] One might wonder how relaxing muscles would have a positive effect on headache. Recent evidence suggests the botulinum toxin has greater biologic effects then merely muscle relaxation. It has been suggested that botulinum toxin can reduce neurogenic inflammation[161,162] in the peripheral tissues, as well as have some CNS effects in the dorsal root ganglion and brainstem. With this evidence, botulinum toxin is having an impact on neuropathic pain disorders.[163]

In summary, the injection of botulinum toxin into muscles shows some promising results. It is not the first line of treatment because it is not definitive therapy. Also, botulinum toxin is relatively expensive and may not be a suitable treatment option for all patients. However, in cases of chronic, repeated, muscle pain conditions, refractory headaches, and some neuropathic pain disorders, it should be considered.

Case Reports

Case 1

A 41-year-old salesman came to the dental office complaining of right masseter and temporalis pain that had been present for 2 days and had begun shortly after an amalgam restoration was placed. The pain was increased with jaw use and almost eliminated by simply not moving his mouth.

The clinical examination revealed tenderness in the right temporalis (score, 1) and pain in the right masseter (score, 2). The maximum comfortable interincisal opening was 32 mm, with maximum opening of 52 mm. The temporomandibular joint (TMJ) examination revealed no pain or tenderness. A click in the right jaw was noted at 24 mm of opening. It was asymptomatic, and the patient reported it had been present for 15 years. The occlusal examination revealed a complete natural dentition, in a good state of repair. Aside from a bright shiny mark on a recent restoration, no other significant clinical findings were noted.

DIAGNOSIS. Protective co-contraction secondary to placement of a high restoration.

TREATMENT. The amalgam restoration was adjusted to contact evenly and simultaneously with the adjacent and surrounding teeth. The patient was instructed to limit movement to within painless ranges until the pain subsided. He was also instructed to return to the office in 3 days and, if the pain became worse, to call immediately. When he returned, the pain had subsided and no symptoms were present. ▪

Case 2

A 19-year-old female college student reported to the dental office complaining of a generalized muscle soreness on the left side of her face. The pain was accentuated with chewing. It had been present for approximately 1 week. In discussing the problem, she revealed that this type of pain had been present on several other occasions, 2, 6, and 8 months ago. She did not report any noticeable change in her occlusion but felt that the pain did limit her mandibular opening. Further questioning revealed that each of the three episodes of pain, as well as this episode, accompanied her college examinations.

The clinical examination revealed tenderness of the right and left masseters (score, 1) and the left temporalis (score, 1) muscles. Functional manipulation of the left inferior lateral pterygoid provoked significant discomfort (score, 3). Her comfortable interincisal opening was measured at 22 mm. She could open maximally to 33 mm, but this was painful. Passive opening by the clinician reached 45 mm (soft end feel). The TMJ examination was negative for

pain or sounds. No other significant findings occurred during the clinical examination.

DIAGNOSIS. Local muscle soreness secondary to increased emotional stress associated with college examinations.

TREATMENT. The patient was made aware of the relationship among emotional stress, parafunctional activity, and the symptoms she was experiencing. She was instructed to restrict jaw movement to within painless limits and, when possible, to control parafunctional activity. Instructions were provided for PSR techniques to be employed during the day. A stabilization appliance was fabricated, and she was instructed to wear this at night while sleeping. The patient returned in 1 week for reevaluation, and significant pain reduction was reported. The PSR techniques were reinforced, and the appliance was slightly adjusted to provide sound occlusal contacts in an orthopedic stable relationship. When she returned in 3 weeks, the symptoms were no longer present. This problem had no indications for any dental therapy. ▪

Case 3

A 38-year-old male teacher came to the dental office complaining of limited mandibular opening and left-side facial pain. This condition had been present for 10 days. The history revealed that symptoms had begun shortly after a dental visit during which he received an injection of local anesthetic. Six hours after the injection the site had become sore, which limited his ability to open his mouth comfortably. He did not pursue treatment at that time, and since then the symptoms had slowly worsened. The pain was greatest in the early morning.

The clinical examination revealed a painful left medial pterygoid (score, 2). The left and right temporalis were tender to palpation (score, 1). The maximum comfortable opening was measured at 26 mm. The TMJ examination was negative for pain or dysfunction. No signs of any unusual findings were seen at the site of the local anesthetic injection. A panoramic radiograph was unremarkable. There were no other significant clinical findings.

DIAGNOSIS. Local muscle soreness secondary to protracted co-contraction associated with postinjection trauma.

TREATMENT. Because there was no evidence of inflammation at the site of the injection, no treatment was indicated for that area. Apparently the postinjection trauma had resolved, and the local muscle soreness had become self-perpetuating (cyclic muscle pain). The local muscle soreness was treated with a stabilization appliance during sleep for bruxism accompanied by instructions in restricting mandibular use. Clock-regulated ibuprofen was instituted

(600 mg three times a day). Massage and thermotherapy were also begun. After 1 week the patient returned and reported 60% relief of the symptoms. The same therapy was continued, and in 1 more week the symptoms were no longer present. ▪

Case 4

A 36-year-old female homemaker came to the dental office with a history of 3 weeks of pain originating in the muscles on the right side of her face. The pain was relatively constant. She reported that she had recurrent episodes of similar pain, but it had never been this bad or lasted this long. The history revealed no trauma, but the symptoms were commonly correlated to stresses associated with raising her two young children. The pain was greatest on awakening.

The clinical examination revealed generalized tenderness to palpation of the right temporalis and sternocleidomastoideus (score, 1) muscles and severe pain in the right masseter muscle (score, 3). The maximum comfortable mandibular opening was only 18 mm with significant pain when attempting to open wider. The TMJ examination failed to disclose any pain or dysfunction. During the occlusal examination it was noted that both mandibular first molars had been extracted and the second molars had drifted into the existing space, causing a lateral shifting of the mandible from the musculoskeletally stable position (CR) of the condyles to the maximum intercuspal position (ICP). The clinical examination revealed no other significant findings.

DIAGNOSIS. Chronic centrally mediated myalgia secondary to protracted local muscle soreness. Parafunctional activity is a contributing factor likely associated with emotional stress.

TREATMENT. The patient was made aware of the relationship among her emotional stress, parafunctional activity, and symptoms. She was also informed that her occlusal condition was not stable and might be contributing to her complaints. Instructions in PSR techniques were provided. A stabilization appliance was fabricated for nighttime use, and she was given instructions on keeping her teeth apart during the day. Emotional stress therapy was instituted by a clinical psychologist. She was referred to physical therapy for ultrasound treatments three times a week. After 2 weeks the symptoms were about 50% resolved. By the third week passive exercises were instituted to regain maximum comfortable mandibular opening. By the sixth week almost all the symptoms had resolved, and assisted stretching exercises were added to aid in regaining a normal range of movement. After 10 weeks the patient was completely free of symptoms. Passive and assisted stretching exercises were continued until normal range of opening was achieved.

After all symptoms had resolved, the significance of the occlusal condition was discussed with the patient. She was advised that replacement of the missing molars should be considered so that the dental arches could be stabilized and the occlusal condition improved. The clinician pointed out that completion of this treatment could not guarantee that the symptoms would not return, but the improved stability would hopefully decrease the likelihood of such recurrence. The patient was reminded about emotional stress factors and how stress alone can create the return of these symptoms. Other advantages regarding tooth replacement were discussed, and the patient elected to accept the treatment. The left and right second molars were both orthodontically uprighted, and posterior implants were placed with crowns to replace the missing first molars. The occlusal condition was developed to provide even and simultaneous contact on the fixed prostheses when the condyles were in the most musculoskeletally stable position (CR). Adequate laterotrusive contacts existed on the anterior teeth to disocclude the posterior teeth during eccentric movement. The 1- and 2-year recall appointments revealed no recurrence of the symptoms. ▪

Case 5

A 27-year-old female secretary reported to the dental office complaining of tightness in her jaw muscles and a constant headache. The headache was located bilaterally in her temple areas. The headache had been present for 4 months and appeared to be worse in the late afternoon after she had been typing all day. The tightness in the jaw muscles was increased by chewing but did not seem to aggravate her headache. However, neck movements and shoulder tightness did seem to increase her headache pain.

The clinical examination revealed a comfortable mandibular opening of 24 mm, with a maximum of 39 mm. A normal range of eccentric movements also existed. No joint pain or sound was noted. Bilateral masseter tenderness (score, 1) was present. Although the headache was felt in the temporal regions, the temporalis muscles were not tender to palpation. Palpation of the posterior neck and trapezius muscles revealed multiple trigger points. Pressure applied to those in the trapezius accentuated the headache in the temporal area. The clinical examination revealed no other significant findings.

DIAGNOSIS. Myofascial pain in the posterior cervical and trapezius muscles with referred pain (tension-type headache) to the temporal region along with secondary co-contraction and local muscle soreness in the masseter muscles.

TREATMENT. An explanation was given to the patient regarding myofascial pain and its common causes. The patient was informed regarding the relationship of myofascial pain and emotional stress. The possible effects of posture while typing were also discussed, and suggestions were given to improve her ergonomics while typing. Instructions in PSR techniques were provided. The trigger points in the trapezius and posterior neck muscles were sprayed and stretched. She was then sent home with recommendations for moist heat and passive stretching of the neck and shoulder muscles. She returned 1 week later and reported significant reduction in her headache. Her comfortable mandibular opening was now 35 mm, with a maximum range of 44 mm. Although most of the trigger points had resolved, there was an active trigger point found in the left trapezius that, when palpated, increased her headache pain. This trigger point was injected with 1 mL of 2% lidocaine (no vasoconstrictor), and the muscle was stretched. The injection immediately eliminated the residual headache complaint. The patient returned to the dental office after 1 more week and reported no headache pain. The patient was encouraged to continue to monitor her typing ergonomics and continue her PSR techniques. ■

Case 6

A 27-year-old man reported to the dental office on an emergency basis complaining that he "could not bite his teeth together." He reported that he could not open wide and his jaw seemed to be pulling to the left. This condition had been present since he woke up 2 hours earlier. He reported only mild pain when he rested the jaw, but when he tried to force his teeth together, the pain increased greatly on the right side. No history of trauma existed.

Examination revealed a significant acute malocclusion in which the mandible was positioning to the left approximately 10 mm. A 2- to 3-mm posterior open bite was on the right side with heavy contact during closure on the left canine. He could comfortably open his mouth only 30 mm, and a deflection was noted to the left. Functional manipulation revealed right-side pain to push against resistance. No significant joint sounds or pain was noted. A panoramic radiograph was unremarkable. No other significant clinical findings existed.

DIAGNOSIS. Acute myospasm of the right inferior lateral pterygoid muscle.

TREATMENT. Ice was applied to the right side of the face over the area of the lateral pterygoid muscle, followed by gentle manipulation of the mandible into proper occlusion (gentle stretching of the right inferior lateral pterygoid muscle). This did not seem to improve the condition. The right lateral pterygoid muscle was then injected with 1 mL of 2% lidocaine (no epinephrine). Within 5 minutes the condition resolved, and normal occlusion was reestablished. The patient was instructed to minimize jaw function for 2 to 3 days and institute a soft diet. The patient was asked

to call immediately if there was any return of the condition. The patient was seen for routine dental care 2 months later and reported no return of symptoms. ■

Case 7

A 45-year-old woman reported to the dental office with a complaint of headache. This pain was felt throughout the head and had been present for more than 2 months. She was able to work, but the pain reduced her effectiveness. The pain was bilateral and radiated up and down the neck.

Further questioning of the patient revealed muscle complaints in her shoulders, back, and legs. She reported poor sleep quality and a low energy level. The pain problem had greatly decreased her quality of life, and she was depressed. No history of trauma or recent dental changes existed.

The clinical examination revealed numerous sites of muscle tenderness throughout the head and neck. Palpation of the most tender areas did not aggravate or increase the headache pain. The mandibular range of movement was only mildly limited (38 mm), and no joint pain or sounds were noted. Her occlusal condition was stable in a musculoskeletally stable position of the mandible. A panoramic radiograph was unremarkable.

DIAGNOSIS. Tentative diagnosis of fibromyalgia with secondary masticatory symptoms.

TREATMENT. The tentative diagnosis was explained to the patient. The patient was referred to a rheumatologist, who confirmed the diagnosis of fibromyalgia. No masticatory treatments were indicated at the time. The patient was managed under the care of the rheumatologist with NSAIDs, amitriptyline (25 mg at night), and physical therapy. The patient was encouraged to increase her level of exercise slowly and was counseled for the psychologic management of this chronic pain condition. Because her history related increased masticatory pain in the morning secondary to bruxism, a stabilization appliance was fabricated for nighttime use. Within 4 weeks the patient reported a 50% reduction in symptoms. Over the next 6 months the patient continued with the same treatments and reported a gradual decrease of symptoms. She related periods of remissions as well as exacerbations. The patient's continued care was monitored by the rheumatologist. ■

Case 8

A 37-year-old woman reported to the clinic with a complaint of repeated spontaneous jaw-opening episodes. These episodes began 4 years ago and became more frequent over the past 6 months. During an episode she reports being "locked open" for hours at a time. She must routinely go to the hospital emergency department to be sedated and have her mouth forced closed. She has been to several dentists about this problem and received bilateral TMJ surgeries (eminectomies) 2 years ago. This surgery provided relief for only 2 months, and then the problem returned. Presently the episodes are reccurring every 2 to 3 weeks and are associated with significant pain. Between episodes she functions normally without pain. Most recently her dentist has been treating her with valium and wiring her teeth together for 2 to 3 weeks during the episodes. She has been referred by her dentist for evaluation.

The patient's initial visit occurred between episodes of her locking complaint. Therefore the examination revealed no unusual findings. The cranial nerve examination was within normal limits, as was the cervical evaluation. Palpation of the head and neck muscles failed to reveal any pain or tenderness. A normal range of jaw movement existed, although the patient was reluctant to open the mouth fully because this elicited a jaw-opening episode in the past. A sound occlusal relationship was found in a musculoskeletally stable position. A panoramic radiograph was unremarkable with the exception of shallow articular eminences that were likely secondary to the prior surgery. Orthodontic brackets were present on the posterior teeth that were being used to wire the mouth closed during the episodes.

DIAGNOSIS. Jaw-opening oromandibular dystonia (by history).

TREATMENT. The patient was informed of the diagnosis, and an explanation of the etiology and management options were provided. The patient was placed on gabapentin as a trial in an attempt to prevent any further episodes. The patient was instructed to return to the clinic if an episode reoccurred. The patient had no episodes for 1 month and then reported to the clinic in distress and pain with her mouth locked open. The patient was immediately given right and left lateral pterygoid muscle injections with 2% lidocaine (no vasoconstrictor). Within 5 minutes the pain reduced by 75%. At that time the mouth could be forced closed, and the teeth were wired together using the orthodontic brackets. The patient was dismissed with a prescription for cyclobenzaprine and pain medication. One week later the patient returned and reported that the "pulling" had almost resolved and she was relatively comfortable. During that visit 40 U of botulinum toxin A were injected into each of the right and left lateral pterygoid muscles using an electromyogram-guided needle. The patient was dismissed with the teeth still wired together. The patient returned in 1 week, and the interarch wires were removed. The patient was asked to return in 3 months for reevaluation or if the locking sensation returned. In 3 months the patient returned and reported no episodes of locking. She was pleased because this was the longest episode-free period she had experienced in more than a year. She did note that during the past week she felt some "twitching or pulling" return in the area of the lateral

pterygoid muscles. The botulinum toxin A injections were repeated at that time. The patient was dismissed and rescheduled for a reevaluation appointment in 4 months. The patient was asked to immediately report to the clinic if any symptoms returned. Presently she returns to the clinic every 4 to 5 months for repeated botulinum toxin A injections. ■

References

1. Bell WE: *Temporomandibular disorders: classification, diagnosis, management,* ed 3, Chicago, 1990, Year Book Medical, pp 60-61.
2. Smith AM: The coactivation of antagonist muscles, *Can J Physiol Pharmacol* 59:733, 1981.
3. Lund JP, Olsson KA: The importance of reflexes and their control during jaw movements, *Trends Neurosci* 6:458-463, 1983.
4. Finger M, Stohler CS, Ash MM Jr: The effect of acrylic bite plane splints and their vertical dimension on jaw muscle silent period in healthy young adults, *J Oral Rehabil* 12:381-388, 1985.
5. Ashton-Miller JA, McGlashen KM, Herzenberg JE, Stohler CS: Cervical muscle myoelectric response to acute experimental sternocleidomastoid pain, *Spine* 15:1006-1012, 1990.
6. Stohler CS: Clinical perspectives on masticatory and related muscle disorders. In Sessle BJ, Bryant PS, Dionne RA, editors: *Temporomandibular disorders and related pain conditions,* Seattle, 1995, IASP Press, pp 3-29.
7. Lund JP, Donga R, Widmer CG, Stohler CS: The pain-adaptation model: a discussion of the relationship between chronic musculoskeletal pain and motor activity, *Can J Physiol Pharmacol* 69:683-694, 1991.
8. Tzakis MG, Dahlstrom L, Haraldson T: Evaluation of masticatory function before and after treatment in patients with craniomandibular disorders, *J Craniomandib Disord* 6:267-272, 1992.
9. Bell WE: *Temporomandibular disorders: classification, diagnosis, management,* ed 3, Chicago, 1990, Year Book Medical, p 280.
10. Rosen JC: Self-monitoring in the treatment of diurnal bruxism, *J Behav Ther Exp Psychiatry* 12:347-350, 1981.
11. Bornstein PH, Hamilton SB, Bornstein MT: Self-monitoring procedures. In Ciminero AR, Calhoun KS, Adams HE, editors: *Handbook of behavioral assessment,* ed 2, New York, 1986, Wiley, pp 176-222.
12. Turk DC, Zaki HS, Rudy TE: Effects of intraoral appliance and biofeedback/stress management alone and in combination in treating pain and depression in patients with temporomandibular disorders, *J Prosthet Dent* 70:158-164, 1993.
13. Pierce CJ, Gale EN: A comparison of different treatments for nocturnal bruxism, *J Dent Res* 67:597-601, 1988.

14. Solberg WK, Clark GT, Rugh JD: Nocturnal electromyographic evaluation of bruxism patients undergoing short term splint therapy, *J Oral Rehabil* 2:215-223, 1975.

15. Clark GT, Beemsterboer PL, Solberg WK, Rugh JD: Nocturnal electromyographic evaluation of myofascial pain dysfunction in patients undergoing occlusal splint therapy, *J Am Dent Assoc* 99:607-611, 1979.

16. Yap AU: Effects of stabilization appliances on nocturnal parafunctional activities in patients with and without signs of temporomandibular disorders, *J Oral Rehabil* 25:64-68, 1998.

17. Kurita H, Kurashina K, Kotani A: Clinical effect of full coverage occlusal splint therapy for specific temporomandibular disorder conditions and symptoms, *J Prosthet Dent* 78:506-510, 1997.

18. Kreiner M, Betancor E, Clark G: Occlusal stabilization appliances: evidence of their efficacy, *J Am Dent Assoc* 132:700-717, 2001.

19. Ekberg E, Nilner M: Treatment outcome of appliance therapy in temporomandibular disorder patients with myofascial pain after 6 and 12 months, *Acta Odontol Scand* 62:343-349, 2004.

20. Wilkinson T, Hansson TL, McNeill C, Marcel T: A comparison of the success of 24-hour occlusal splint therapy versus nocturnal occlusal splint therapy in reducing craniomandibular disorders, *J Craniomandib Disord* 6:64-73, 1992.

21. Kuttila M, Le Bell Y, Savolainen-Niemi E, Kuttila S, Alanen P: Efficiency of occlusal appliance therapy in secondary otalgia and temporomandibular disorders, *Acta Odontol Scand* 60:248-254, 2002.

22. Ekberg E, Nilner M: A 6- and 12-month follow-up of appliance therapy in TMD patients: a follow-up of a controlled trial, *Int J Prosthodont* 15:564-570, 2002.

23. Ekberg E, Vallon D, Nilner M: The efficacy of appliance therapy in patients with temporomandibular disorders of mainly myogenous origin. A randomized, controlled, short-term trial, *J Orofac Pain* 17:133-139, 2003.

24. Forssell H, Kalso E, Koskela P, Vehmanen R, Puukka P et al: Occlusal treatments in temporomandibular disorders: a qualitative systematic review of randomized controlled trials, *Pain* 83:549-560, 1999.

25. Al-Ani MZ, Davies SJ, Gray RJ, Sloan P, Glenny AM: Stabilization splint therapy for temporomandibular pain dysfunction syndrome, *Cochrane Database Syst Rev* CD002778, 2004.

26. Wassell RW, Adams N, Kelly PJ: Treatment of temporomandibular disorders by stabilising splints in general dental practice: results after initial treatment, *Br Dent J* 197:35-41; discussion 31; quiz 50-51, 2004.

27. VanHelder WP: Medical treatment of muscle soreness [editorial; comment], *Can J Sport Sci* 17:74-79, 1992.

28. Kakulas BA, Adams RD: *Diseases of muscle*, Philadelphia, 1985, Harper & Row, pp 725-727.

29. Simons DG, Travell JG, Simons LS: *Travell & Simons' myofascial pain and dysfunction: the trigger point manual*, ed 2, Baltimore, 1999, Lippincott Williams & Wilkins, pp 19-30.

30. Simons DG, Travell JG, Simons LS: *Travell & Simons' myofascial pain and dysfunction: the trigger point manual*, ed 2, Baltimore, 1999, Lippincott Williams & Wilkins, pp 178-186.

31. Sarlani E, Grace EG, Reynolds MA, Greenspan JD: Evidence for up-regulated central nociceptive processing in patients with masticatory myofascial pain, *J Orofac Pain* 18:41-55, 2004.

32. Simons DG, Travell JG, Simons LS: *Travell & Simons' myofascial pain and dysfunction: the trigger point manual*, ed 2, Baltimore, 1999, Lippincott Williams & Wilkins, pp 220-222.

33. Simons DG, Travell JG, Simons LS: *Travell & Simons' myofascial pain and dysfunction: the trigger point manual*, ed 2, Baltimore, 1999, Lippincott Williams & Wilkins, pp 226-227.

34. Moldofsky H, Scarisbrick P: Induction of neurasthenic musculoskeletal pain syndrome by selective sleep stage deprivation, *Psychosom Med* 38:35-44, 1976.

35. Simons DG, Travell JG, Simons LS: *Travell & Simons' myofascial pain and dysfunction: the trigger point manual*, ed 2, Baltimore, 1999, Lippincott Williams & Wilkins, pp 186-220.

36. Simons DG, Travell JG, Simons LS: *Travell & Simons' myofascial pain and dysfunction: the trigger point manual*, ed 2, Baltimore, 1999, Lippincott Williams & Wilkins, pp 223-226.

37. Simons DG, Travell JG, Simons LS: *Travell & Simons' myofascial pain and dysfunction: the trigger point manual*, ed 2, Baltimore, 1999, Lippincott Williams & Wilkins, pp 127-142.

38. Jaeger B, Reeves JL: Quantification of changes in myofascial trigger point sensitivity with the pressure algometer following passive stretch, *Pain* 27:203-210, 1986.

39. Simons DG, Travell JG, Simons LS: *Travell & Simons' myofascial pain and dysfunction: the trigger point manual*, ed 2, Baltimore, 1999, Lippincott Williams & Wilkins, pp 138-142.

40. Zohn DA, Mennell JM: *Musculoskeletal pain: diagnosis and physical treatment*, Boston, 1976, Little, Brown, pp 126-137.

41. Bonica JJ: Management of myofascial pain syndromes in general practice, *JAMA* 164:732-738, 1957.

42. Kamyszek G, Ketcham R, Garcia R Jr, Radke J: Electromyographic evidence of reduced muscle activity when ULF-TENS is applied to the 5th and 7th cranial nerves, *Cranio* 19:162-168, 2001.

43. Simons DG, Travell JG, Simons LS: *Travell & Simons' myofascial pain and dysfunction: the trigger point manual*, ed 2, Baltimore, 1999, Lippincott Williams & Wilkins, pp 150-173.

44. Pippa P, Allegra A, Cirillo L, Doni L, Rivituso C: Fibromyalgia and trigger points, *Minerva Anestesiol* 60:281-283, 1994.

45. Carlson CR, Okeson JP, Falace DA, Nitz AJ, Lindroth JE: Reduction of pain and EMG activity in the masseter region by trapezius trigger point injection, *Pain* 55:397-400, 1993.

46. Hong CZ: Lidocaine injection versus dry needling to myofascial trigger point. The importance of the local twitch response, *Am J Phys Med Rehabil* 73:256-263, 1994.

47. Scicchitano J, Rounsefell B, Pilowsky I: Baseline correlates of the response to the treatment of chronic localized myofascial pain syndrome by injection of local anaesthetic, *J Psychosom Res* 40:75-85, 1996.

48. Fine PG, Milano R, Hare BD: The effects of myofascial trigger point injections are naloxone reversible, *Pain* 32:15-20, 1988.

49. Guttu RL, Page DG, Laskin DM: Delayed healing of muscle after injection of bupivacaine and steroid, *Ann Dent* 49:5-8, 1990.

50. McCain GA: Role of physical fitness training in fibrosis/fibromyalgia syndromes, *Am J Med* 81(suppl 3A): 73-77, 1986.

51. Zeno E, Griffin J, Boyd C, Oladehin A, Kasser R: The effects of a home exercise program on pain and perceived dysfunction in a woman with TMD: a case study, *Cranio* 19:279-288, 2001.

52. Okeson JP: *Bell's orofacial pains*, ed 6, Chicago, 2005, Quintessence, pp 45-62.

53. Bowsher D: Neurogenic pain syndromes and their management, *Br Med Bull* 47:644-666, 1991.

54. LaMotte RH, Shain CN, Simone DA, Tsai EF: Neurogenic hyperalgesia: psychophysical studies of underlying mechanisms, *J Neurophysiol* 66:190-211, 1991.

55. Sessle BJ: The neural basis of temporomandibular joint and masticatory muscle pain, *J Orofac Pain* 13:238-245, 1999.

56. Simone DA, Sorkin LS, Oh U, Chung JM, Owens C et al: Neurogenic hyperalgesia: central neural correlates in responses of spinothalamic tract neurons, *J Neurophysiol* 66:228-246, 1991.

57. Wong JK, Haas DA, Hu JW: Local anesthesia does not block mustard-oil-induced temporomandibular inflammation, *Anesth Analg* 92:1035-1040, 2001.

58. McCain GA, Scudds RA: The concept of primary fibromyalgia (fibrositis): clinical value, relation and significance to other chronic musculoskeletal pain syndromes, *Pain* 33:273-287, 1988.

59. Wolfe F, Smythe HA, Yunus MB, Bennett RM, Bombardier C et al: The American College of Rheumatology 1990 Criteria for the Classification of Fibromyalgia. Report of the Multicenter Criteria Committee [see comments], *Arthritis Rheum* 33:160-172, 1990.

60. Korszun A, Young EA, Singer K, Carlson NE, Brown MB et al: Basal circadian cortisol secretion in women with temporomandibular disorders, *J Dent Res* 81:279-283, 2002.

61. McLean SA, Williams DA, Harris RE, Kop WJ, Groner KH et al: Momentary relationship between cortisol secretion and symptoms in patients with fibromyalgia, *Arthritis Rheum* 52:3660-3669, 2005.

62. Crofford LJ, Demitrack MA: Evidence that abnormalities of central neurohormonal systems are key to understanding fibromyalgia and chronic fatigue syndrome, *Rheum Dis Clin North Am* 22:267-284, 1996.

63. Crofford LJ, Pillemer SR, Kalogeras KT, Cash JM, Michelson D et al: Hypothalamic-pituitary-adrenal axis perturbations in patients with fibromyalgia, *Arthritis Rheum* 37:1583-1592, 1994.

64. McBeth J, Chiu YH, Silman AJ, Ray D, Morriss R et al: Hypothalamic-pituitary-adrenal stress axis function and the relationship with chronic widespread pain and its antecedents, *Arthritis Res Ther* 7:R992-R1000, 2005.

65. Cimino R, Michelotti A, Stradi R, Farinaro C: Comparison of clinical and psychologic features of fibromyalgia and masticatory myofascial pain, *J Orofac Pain* 12:35-41, 1998.

66. Dao TT, Reynolds WJ, Tenenbaum HC: Comorbidity between myofascial pain of the masticatory muscles and fibromyalgia, *J Orofac Pain* 11:232-241, 1997.

67. Goldenberg DL: Fibromyalgia, chronic fatigue syndrome, and myofascial pain syndrome, *Curr Opin Rheumatol* 5:199-208, 1993.

68. Hedenberg Magnusson B, Ernberg M, Kopp S: Symptoms and signs of temporomandibular disorders in patients with fibromyalgia and local myalgia of the temporomandibular system. A comparative study, *Acta Odontol Scand* 55:344-349, 1997.

69. Hedenberg-Magnusson B, Ernberg M, Kopp S: Presence of orofacial pain and temporomandibular disorder in fibromyalgia. A study by questionnaire, *Swed Dent J* 23:185-192, 1999.

70. Hedenberg-Magnusson B, Ernberg M, Kopp S: Symptoms and signs of temporomandibular disorders in patients with fibromyalgia and local myalgia of the temporomandibular system. A comparative study, *Acta Odontol Scand* 55:344-349, 1997.

71. Plesh O, Wolfe F, Lane N: The relationship between fibromyalgia and temporomandibular disorders: prevalence and symptom severity, *J Rheumatol* 23:1948-1952, 1996.

72. Yunus MB, Kalyan-Raman UP, Kalyan-Raman K: Primary fibromyalgia syndrome and myofascial pain syndrome: clinical features and muscle pathology, *Arch Phys Med Rehabil* 69:451-454, 1989.

73. Rhodus NL, Fricton J, Carlson P, Messner R: Oral symptoms associated with fibromyalgia syndrome, *J Rheumatol* 30:1841-1845, 2003.

74. Manfredini D, Tognini F, Montagnani G, Bazzichi L, Bombardieri S et al: Comparison of masticatory dysfunction in temporomandibular disorders and fibromyalgia, *Minerva Stomatol* 53:641-650, 2004.

75. Bennett R, Campbell S, Burckhardt C, Clark S, O'Reilly C et al: A multidisciplinary approach to fibromyalgia management, *J Musculoskel Med* 8:21-32, 1991.

76. Carette S, McCain GA, Bell DA, Fam AG: Evaluation of amitriptyline in primary fibrositis. A double-blind, placebo-controlled study, *Arthritis Rheum* 29:655-659, 1986.

77. Goldenberg DL, Felson DT, Dinerman H: A randomized, controlled trial of amitriptyline and naproxen in the treatment of patients with fibromyalgia, *Arthritis Rheum* 29:1371-1377, 1986.

78. Crofford LJ: Meta-analysis of antidepressants in fibromyalgia, *Curr Rheumatol Rep* 3:115-122, 2001.

79. Goldenberg DL: A review of the role of tricyclic medications in the treatment of fibromyalgia syndrome, *J Rheumatol Suppl* 19:137-139, 1989.

80. Reynolds WJ, Moldofsky H, Saskin P, Lue FA: The effects of cyclobenzaprine on sleep physiology and symptoms in patients with fibromyalgia, *J Rheumatol* 18:452-454, 1991.

81. Hamaty D, Valentine JL, Howard R, Howard CW, Wakefield V et al: The plasma endorphin, prostaglandin and catecholamine profile of patients with fibrositis treated with cyclobenzaprine and placebo: a 5-month study, *J Rheumatol Suppl* 19:164-68, 1989.

82. Tofferi JK, Jackson JL, O'Malley PG: Treatment of fibromyalgia with cyclobenzaprine: a meta-analysis, *Arthritis Rheum* 51:9-13, 2004.

83. Granges G, Littlejohn GO: A comparative study of clinical signs in fibromyalgia/fibrositis syndrome, healthy and exercising subjects, *J Rheumatol* 20:344-351, 1993.

84. Ramfjord SP: Dysfunctional temporomandibular joint and muscle pain, *J Prosthet Dent* 11:353-362, 1961.

85. Ramfjord S: Bruxism: a clinical and electromyographic study, *J Am Dent Assoc* 62:21-28, 1961.

86. Randow K, Carlsson K, Edlund J, Oberg T: The effect of an occlusal interference on the masticatory system. An experimental investigation, *Odontol Rev* 27:245-256, 1976.

87. Arnold M: Bruxism and the occlusion, *Dent Clin North Am* 25:395-407, 1981.

88. Ramfjord SP, Ash MM: *Occlusion*, ed 3, Philadelphia, 1983, Saunders, p 342.

89. Graf H: Bruxism, *Dent Clin North Am* 13:659-665, 1969.

90. Shore NA: *Occlusal equilibration and temporomandibular joint dysfunction*, Philadelphia, 1959, Lippincott, p 500.

91. Posselt U: The temporomandibular joint syndrome and occlusion, *J Prosthet Dent* 25:432-438, 1971.

92. Rugh JD, Barghi N, Drago CJ: Experimental occlusal discrepancies and nocturnal bruxism, *J Prosthet Dent* 51: 548-553, 1984.

93. Bailey JO, Rugh JD: Effects of occlusal adjustment on bruxism as monitored by nocturnal EMG recordings, *J Dent Res* 59(special issue):317, 1980.

94. Rugh JD, Solberg WK: Electromyographic studies of bruxist behavior before and during treatment, *J Calif Dent Assoc* 3:56-59, 1975.

95. Solberg WK, Flint RT, Brantner JP: Temporomandibular joint pain and dysfunction: a clinical study of emotional and occlusal components, *J Prosthet Dent* 28:412-422, 1972.

96. Franks AST: Conservative treatment of temporomandibular joint dysfunction: a comparative study, *Dent Pract Dent Rec* 15:205-210, 1965.

97. Okeson JP, Moody PM, Kemper JT, Haley JV: Evaluation of occlusal splint therapy and relaxation procedures in patients with temporomandibular disorders, *J Am Dent Assoc* 107:420-424, 1983.

98. Okeson JP, Kemper JT, Moody PM: A study of the use of occlusion splints in the treatment of acute and chronic patients with craniomandibular disorders, *J Prosthet Dent* 48:708-712, 1982.

99. Okeson JP: The effects of hard and soft occlusal splints on nocturnal bruxism, *J Am Dent Assoc* 114:788-791, 1987.

100. Fuchs P: The muscular activity of the chewing apparatus during night sleep. An examination of healthy subjects and patients with functional disturbances, *J Oral Rehabil* 2:35-48, 1975.

101. Sheikholeslam A, Holmgren K, Riise C: A clinical and electromyographic study of the long-term effects of an occlusal splint on the temporal and masseter muscles in patients with functional disorders and nocturnal bruxism, *J Oral Rehabil* 13:137-145, 1986.

102. Tsukiyama Y, Baba K, Clark GT: An evidence-based assessment of occlusal adjustment as a treatment for temporomandibular disorders, *J Prosthet Dent* 86:57-66, 2001.

103. Holmgren K, Sheikholeslam A, Riise C: Effect of a full-arch maxillary occlusal splint on parafunctional activity during sleep in patients with nocturnal bruxisn and signs and symptoms of craniomandibular disorders, *J Prosthet Dent* 69:293-297, 1993.

104. Saletu A, Parapatics S, Saletu B, Anderer P, Prause W et al: On the pharmacotherapy of sleep bruxism: placebo-controlled polysomnographic and psychometric studies with clonazepam, *Neuropsychobiology* 51:214-225, 2005.

105. Ware JC: Tricyclic antidepressants in the treatment of insomnia, *J Clin Psychiatry* 44:25-28, 1983.

106. Rizzatti-Barbosa CM, Nogueira MT, de Andrade ED, Ambrosano GM, de Barbosa JR: Clinical evaluation of amitriptyline for the control of chronic pain caused by temporomandibular joint disorders, *Cranio* 21:221-225, 2003.

107. Plesh O, Curtis D, Levine J, McCall WD Jr: Amitriptyline treatment of chronic pain in patients with temporomandibular disorders, *J Oral Rehabil* 27:834-841, 2000.

108. Herman CR, Schiffman EL, Look JO, Rindal DB: The effectiveness of adding pharmacologic treatment with clonazepam or cyclobenzaprine to patient education and self-care for the treatment of jaw pain upon awakening: a randomized clinical trial, *J Orofac Pain* 16:64-70, 2002.

109. *Dorland's illustrated medical dictionary*, ed 30, Philadelphia, 2003, Saunders, p 579.

110. Tolosa E, Marti MJ: Blepharospasm-oromandibular dystonia syndrome (Meige's syndrome): clinical aspects, *Adv Neurol* 49:73-84, 1988.

111. Jankovic J: Etiology and differential diagnosis of blepharospasm and oromandibular dystonia, *Adv Neurol* 49:103-116, 1988.

112. Cardoso F, Jankovic J: Peripherally induced tremor and parkinsonism, *Arch Neurol* 52:263-270, 1995.

113. Nutt JG, Muenter MD, Aronson A, Kurland LT, Melton LJ III: Epidemiology of focal and generalized dystonia in Rochester, Minnesota, *Mov Disord* 3:188-194, 1988.

114. Tan EK, Jankovic J: Botulinum toxin A in patients with oromandibular dystonia: long-term follow-up, *Neurology* 53:2102-2107, 1999.

115. Bakke M, Werdelin LM, Dalager T, Fuglsang-Frederiksen A, Prytz S et al: Reduced jaw opening from paradoxical activity of mandibular elevator muscles treated with botulinum toxin, *Eur J Neurol* 10:695-699, 2003.

116. Sankhla C, Jankovic J, Duane D: Variability of the immunologic and clinical response in dystonic patients immunoresistant to botulinum toxin injections, *Mov Disord* 13:150-154, 1998.

117. Waddy HM, Fletcher NA, Harding AE, Marsden CD: A genetic study of idiopathic focal dystonias, *Ann Neurol* 29:320-324, 1991.

118. Behari M, Singh KK, Seshadri S, Prasad K, Ahuja GK: Botulinum toxin A in blepharospasm and hemifacial spasm, *J Assoc Physicians India* 42:205-208, 1994.

119. Tan EK, Jankovic J: Tardive and idiopathic oromandibular dystonia: a clinical comparison, *J Neurol Neurosurg Psychiatry* 68:186-190, 2000.

120. Singer C, Papapetropoulos S: A comparison of jaw-closing and jaw-opening idiopathic oromandibular dystonia, *Parkinsonism Relat Disord* 12:115-118, 2006.

121. Gray AR, Barker GR: Idiopathic blepharospasm-oromandibular dystonia syndrome (Meige's syndrome) presenting as chronic temporomandibular joint disloca-tion, *Br J Oral Maxillofac Surg* 29:97-99, 1991.

122. Evans BK, Jankovic J: Tuberous sclerosis and chorea, *Ann Neurol* 13:106-107, 1983.

123. Goetz CG, Horn SS: Treatment of tremor and dystonia, *Neurol Clin* 19:129-144, vi-vii, 2001.

124. Vazquez-Delgado E, Okeson JP: Treatment of inferior lateral pterygoid muscle dystonia with zolpidem tartrate, botulinum toxin injections, and physical self-regulation procedures: a case report, *Cranio* 22:325-329, 2004.

125. Balash Y, Giladi N: Efficacy of pharmacological treatment of dystonia: evidence-based review including meta-analysis of the effect of botulinum toxin and other cure options, *Eur J Neurol* 11:361-370, 2004.

126. Goldman JG, Comella CL: Treatment of dystonia, *Clin Neuropharmacol* 26:102-108, 2003.

127. Wessberg G: Management of oromandibular dystonia, *Hawaii Dent J* 34:15-16, 2003.

128. Bressman SB: Dystonia update, *Clin Neuropharmacol* 23:239-251, 2000.

129. Jankovic J, Orman J: Botulinum A toxin for cranial-cervical dystonia: a double-blind, placebo-controlled study, *Neurology* 37:616-623, 1987.

130. Poungvarin N, Devahastin V, Chaisevikul R, Prayoonwiwat N, Viriyavejakul A: Botulinum A toxin treatment for ble-pharospasm and Meige syndrome: report of 100 patients, *J Med Assoc Thai* 80:1-8, 1997.

131. Jankovic J, Brin MF: Therapeutic uses of botulinum toxin, *N Engl J Med* 324:1186-1194, 1991.

132. Zuber M, Sebald M, Bathien N, de Recondo J, Rondot P: Botulinum antibodies in dystonic patients treated with type A botulinum toxin: frequency and significance, *Neurology* 43:1715-1718, 1993.

133. Jankovic J, Schwartz K: Response and immunoresistance to botulinum toxin injections, *Neurology* 45:1743-1746, 1995.

134. Clark GT: The management of oromandibular motor disorders and facial spasms with injections of botulinum toxin, *Phys Med Rehabil Clin N Am* 14:727-748, 2003.

135. Gobel H, Heinze A, Reichel G, Hefter H, Benecke R: Efficacy and safety of a single botulinum type A toxin complex treatment (Dysport) for the relief of upper back myofascial pain syndrome: results from a randomized

136. Kamanli A, Kaya A, Ardicoglu O, Ozgocmen S, Zengin FO et al: Comparison of lidocaine injection, botulinum toxin injection, and dry needling to trigger points in myofascial pain syndrome, *Rheumatol Int* 25:604-611, 2005.

137. Royal MA: Botulinum toxins in pain management, *Phys Med Rehabil Clin N Am* 14:805-820, 2003.

138. Lang AM: A preliminary comparison of the efficacy and tolerability of botulinum toxin serotypes A and B in the treatment of myofascial pain syndrome: a retrospec-tive, open-label chart review, *Clin Ther* 25:2268-2278, 2003.

139. De Andres J, Cerda-Olmedo G, Valia JC, Monsalve V, Lopez A et al: Use of botulinum toxin in the treatment of chronic myofascial pain, *Clin J Pain* 19:269-275, 2003.

140. Lang AM: Botulinum toxin type A therapy in chronic pain disorders, *Arch Phys Med Rehabil* 84:S69-73; quiz S74-75, 2003.

141. Porta M: A comparative trial of botulinum toxin type A and methylprednisolone for the treatment of myofascial pain syndrome and pain from chronic muscle spasm, *Pain* 85:101-105, 2000.

142. Cheshire WP, Abashian SW, Mann JD: Botulinum toxin in the treatment of myofascial pain syndrome, *Pain* 59:65-69, 1994.

143. Freund B, Schwartz M, Symington JM: The use of botu-linum toxin for the treatment of temporomandibular disorders: preliminary findings, *J Oral Maxillofac Surg* 57:916-920, 1999.

144. Freund B, Schwartz M, Symington JM: Botulinum toxin: new treatment for temporomandibular disorders, *Br J Oral Maxillofac Surg* 38:466-471, 2000.

145. Daelen B, Thorwirth V, Koch A: Treatment of recurrent dislocation of the temporomandibular joint with type A botulinum toxin, *Int J Oral Maxillofac Surg* 26:458-460, 1997.

146. Ivanhoe CB, Lai JM, Francisco GE: Bruxism after brain injury: successful treatment with botulinum toxin-A, *Arch Phys Med Rehabil* 78:1272-1273, 1997.

147. Moore AP, Wood GD: The medical management of masseteric hypertrophy with botulinum toxin type A, *Br J Maxillofac Surg* 32:26-28, 1994.

148. Moore AP, Wood GD: Medical treatment of recurrent temporomandibular joint dislocation using botulinum toxin A, *Br Dent J* 183:415-417, 1997.

149. Sankhla C, Lai EC, Jankovic J: Peripherally induced oro-mandibular dystonia, *J Neurol Neurosurg Psychiatry* 65:722-728, 1998.

150. Ojala T, Arokoski JP, Partanen J: The effect of small doses of botulinum toxin A on neck-shoulder myofascial pain syndrome: a double-blind, randomized, and controlled crossover trial, *Clin J Pain* 22:90-96, 2006.

151. Graboski CL, Gray DS, Burnham RS: Botulinum toxin A versus bupivacaine trigger point injections for the treat-ment of myofascial pain syndrome: a randomized double blind crossover study, *Pain* 118:170-175, 2005.

double-blind placebo-controlled multicentre study, *Pain* 125:82-88, 2006.

152. Raj PP: Botulinum toxin therapy in pain management, *Anesthesiol Clin North America* 21:715-731, 2003.

153. Aoki KR: Evidence for antinociceptive activity of botulinum toxin type A in pain management, *Headache* 43(suppl 1):S9-15, 2003.

154. Gobel H: Botulinum toxin in migraine prophylaxis, *J Neurol* 251(suppl 1):I8-11, 2004.

155. Gobel H, Heinze A, Heinze-Kuhn K, Jost WH: Evidence-based medicine: botulinum toxin A in migraine and tension-type headache, *J Neurol* 248(suppl 1):34-38, 2001.

156. Binder WJ, Brin MF, Blitzer A, Schoenrock LD, Pogoda JM: Botulinum toxin type A (BOTOX) for treatment of migraine headaches: an open-label study, *Otolaryngol Head Neck Surg* 123:669-676, 2000.

157. Silberstein S, Mathew N, Saper J, Jenkins S: Botulinum toxin type A as a migraine preventive treatment. For the BOTOX Migraine Clinical Research Group, *Headache* 40:445-450, 2000.

158. Smuts JA, Schultz D, Barnard A: Mechanism of action of botulinum toxin type A in migraine prevention: a pilot study, *Headache* 44:801-805, 2004.

159. Dodick DW, Mauskop A, Elkind AH, DeGryse R, Brin MF et al: Botulinum toxin type A for the prophylaxis of chronic daily headache: subgroup analysis of patients not receiving other prophylactic medications: a randomized double-blind, placebo-controlled study, *Headache* 45:315-324, 2005.

160. Rollnik JD, Dengler R: Botulinum toxin (DYSPORT) in tension-type headaches, *Acta Neurochir Suppl* 79:123-126, 2002.

161. Mense S: Neurobiological basis for the use of botulinum toxin in pain therapy, *J Neurol* 251(suppl 1):1-7, 2004.

162. Argoff CE: A focused review on the use of botulinum toxins for neuropathic pain, *Clin J Pain* 18:S177-181, 2002.

163. Liu HT, Tsai SK, Kao MC, Hu JS: Botulinum toxin A relieved neuropathic pain in a case of post-herpetic neuralgia, *Pain Med* 7:89-91, 2006.

Classification System Used for Diagnosing Temporomandibular Disorders

Bolded type indicates the disorders discussed in this chapter.

I. Masticatory muscle disorders *(Chapter 12)*
   A. Protective co-contraction
   B. Local muscle soreness
   C. Myospasm
   D. Myofascial pain
   E. Centrally mediated myalgia
   F. Fibromyalgia
   G. Centrally mediated motor disorders

II. **Temporomandibular joint (TMJ) disorders**
   (Chapter 13)
   A. Derangements of the condyle-disc complex
      1. Disc displacements
      2. Disc dislocations with reduction
      3. Disc dislocation without reduction
   B. Structural incompatibility of the articular
      surfaces
      1. Deviation in form
         a. Disc
         b. Condyle
         c. Fossa
      2. Adherences and adhesions
         a. Disc to condyle
         b. Disc to fossa
      3. Subluxation
      4. Spontaneous dislocation
   C. Inflammatory disorders of the TMJ
      1. Synovitis and capsulitis
      2. Retrodiscitis
      3. Arthritides
         a. Osteoarthritis
         b. Osteoarthrosis
         c. Polyarthritides
            i. Traumatic arthritis
            ii. Infectious arthritis
            iii. Rheumatoid arthritis
            iv. Hyperuricemia
            v. Psoriatic arthritis
            vi. Ankylosing spondylitis
      4. Inflammatory disorders of associated
         structures
         a. Temporal tendonitis
         b. Stylomandibular ligament
            inflammation
   D. General considerations when treating
      acute trauma to the TMJ

III. Chronic mandibular hypomobility
   (Chapter 14)
   A. Ankylosis
      1. Capsular fibrosis
      2. Bony
   B. Muscle contracture
      1. Myositis
         a. Passive stretching
         b. Resistant-opening exercises
      2. Myofibrotic
   C. Coronoid process impedance

IV. Growth disorders *(Chapter 14)*
   A. Congenital and developmental bone
      disorders
      1. Agenesis
      2. Hypoplasia
      3. Hyperplasia
      4. Neoplasia
   B. Congenital and developmental muscle
      disorders
      1. Hypotrophy
      2. Hypertrophy
      3. Neoplasia

Treatment of Temporomandibular Joint Disorders

13 CHAPTER

"Intracapsular joint disorder: the mechanical part of TMD."

—JPO

This chapter discusses the management of capsular and intracapsular temporomandibular joint (TMJ) disorders. Each subdivision of this category is discussed from the early mild symptoms of disc displacements to the more severe and more difficult to manage inflammatory disorders. The correct management of disc derangement disorders is predicated on two factors: (1) making a correct diagnosis and (2) understanding the natural course of the disorder. Emphasis has already been placed on establishing a correct diagnosis. Each of the categories of TMJ disorders represents a clinical condition that is treated in a particular manner. An incorrect diagnosis only leads to mismanagement and ultimate treatment failure.

Successful management of intracapsular joint disorders is also based on the clinician's understanding of the natural course of the disorder. In Chapter 8 a progressive description of disc derangement disorders was presented. As the morphology of the disc becomes more altered and ligaments more elongated, the disc becomes progressively displaced and eventually dislocated. Once the disc is dislocated, the condyle begins to function on the retrodiscal tissues. These tissues begin to break down, leading to osteoarthritis or degenerative joint disease. Although this sequence is often clinically evident, it does

not account for the outcome of all intracapsular disorders.

Epidemiologic studies reveal that asymptomatic joint sounds are common. Many studies[1-11] reveal that TMJ sounds are detected in 25% to 35% of the general population. This poses an interesting question: If all joint sounds are not progressive, which sounds should be treated? In my opinion, only joint sounds associated with pain should be considered for treatment. The pain in this instance must be intracapsular in origin. In other words, patients who report with extracapsular muscle pain and a painless clicking point should not be managed for the disc derangement disorder. This approach will lead to treatment failure because it does not address the source of the pain. This concept is further discussed with literature support later in this chapter.

TMJ disorders are a broad category of temporomandibular disorders that arise from capsular and intracapsular structures. This category is divided into three subcategories: derangements of the condyle-disc complex, structural incompatibility of the articular surfaces, and inflammatory disorders.

DERANGEMENTS OF THE CONDYLE-DISC COMPLEX

This category is divided into two subcategories for the purpose of treatment: disc displacements/disc dislocations with reduction and disc dislocations without reduction.

DISC DISPLACEMENTS AND DISC DISLOCATIONS WITH REDUCTION

Disc displacements and disc dislocations with reduction represent the early stages of disc derangement disorders (Figs. 13-1 and 13-2). The clinical signs and symptoms relate to alterations or derangements in the condyle-disc complex.

Cause

Disc derangement disorders result from elongation of the capsular and discal ligaments coupled with thinning of the articular disc. These changes commonly result from either macrotrauma or microtrauma. Macrotrauma is often reported in the history, whereas microtrauma may go unnoticed by

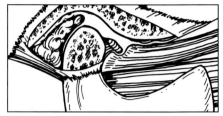

Fig. 13-1 ANTERIORLY DISPLACED DISC. The posterior border of the disc has been thinned and the inferior retrodiscal lamina (as well as the lateral collateral ligament, not shown) has been elongated. The disc is anteriorly displaced, resulting in the condyle articulating on the posterior border of the disc instead of the intermediate zone.

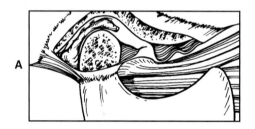

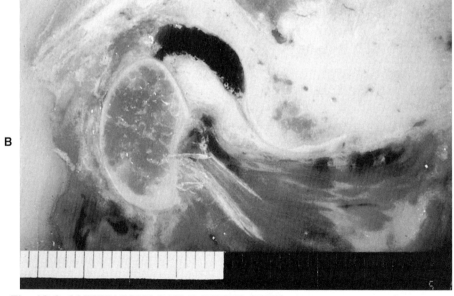

Fig. 13-2 ANTERIORLY DISLOCATED DISC. A, The posterior border of the disc has been thinned and ligaments have been elongated, allowing the disc to be dislocated through the discal space. The condyle now articulates on the retrodiscal tissues. **B,** Anterior dislocated disc. *(Courtesy Dr. Per-Lennart Westesson, University of Rochester, Rochester, NY.)*

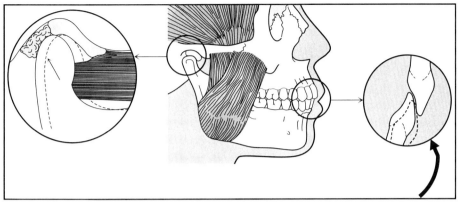

Fig. 13-3 When orthopedic instability exists, loading of the masticatory structures by the elevator muscles can displace a condyle from its musculoskeletally stable position in the fossa. This drawing depicts heavy anterior occlusal contacts that disallow posterior teeth to occlude in the alert feeding position. When the structures are loaded, the elevator muscles force the posterior teeth into occlusion, resulting in a posterior deflection of the condyle from the musculoskeletally stable position. The presence of this condition is considered a risk factor for the development of a disc displacement because it can lead to elongation of the inferior retrodiscal lamina and discal ligament, as well as thinning of the posterior border of the disc.

the patient. Common sources of microtrauma are hypoxia-reperfusion injuries,[12-16] bruxism,[17] and orthopedic instability (Fig. 13-3). Some studies[18-21] suggest that the Class II, division 2 malocclusion is commonly associated with orthopedic instability and therefore a causative factor related to disc derangement disorders (Fig. 13-4). Because not all studies[22-33] support this relationship (see Chapter 7),

other factors must be considered. As previously discussed, orthopedic instability plus joint loading seem to combine as causative factors in many disc derangement disorders.

Another concept that must be appreciated is that perhaps the disorder actually begins at the cellular level and then progresses to the macro changes seen clinically. In other words, unusually

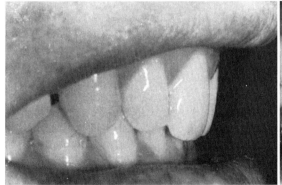

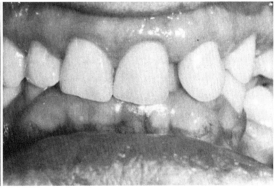

A   B

Fig. 13-4 In some patients the Class II, division 2, anterior tooth relationships may contribute to certain disc derangements especially if this occlusal condition is heavily loaded (i.e., bruxism, macrotrauma). **A,** Lingual inclination of the maxillary central incisors. **B,** Deep bite and tight anterior tooth relationship.

heavy and prolonged loading of the articular tissues exceed the functional capacity of the articular tissues and breakdown begins (hypoxia-reperfusion injury). When the functional limitation has been exceeded, the collagen fibrils become fragmented, resulting in a decrease in the stiffness of the collagen network. This allows the proteoglycan-water gel to swell and flow out into the joint space, leading to a softening of the articular surface. This softening is called *chondromalacia*.[34] The early stages of chondromalacia are reversible if the excessive loading is reduced. If, however, the loading continues to exceed the capacity of the articular tissues, irreversible changes can occur. Regions of fibrillation can begin to develop, resulting in focal roughening of the articular surfaces.[35] This alters the frictional characteristics of the surface and may lead to sticking of the articular surfaces, causing changes in the mechanics of condyle-disc movement. Continued sticking (adherences) and/or roughening leads to strains on the discal ligaments during movements and eventually disc displacements.[36] In this situation microtrauma is the responsible cause for the disc displacement.

History

When macrotrauma is the cause, the patient will often relate an event that precipitated the disorder.[37-46] Taking a good history from the patient may frequently reveal the more subtle findings of bruxism. The patient will also report the presence of joint sounds and may even report a catching sensation during mouth opening. The presence of pain associated with this dysfunction is important.

Clinical Characteristics

The clinical examination reveals a relatively normal range of movement with restriction only associated with the pain. Discal movement can be felt by palpation of the joints during opening and closing. Deviations in the opening pathway are common.

Definitive Treatment

Definitive treatment for a disc displacement is to reestablish a normal condyle-disc relationship. Although this may sound relatively easy, it has not proved to be so. During the past 35 years the

dental profession's attitude toward management of disc derangement disorders has changed greatly. In the early 1970s Farrar[47] introduced the concept of the anterior positioning appliance (Fig. 13-5). This appliance provides an occlusal relationship that requires the mandible to be maintained in a forward position. The position selected for the appliance is one that positions the mandible in a slightly protruded position in an attempt to reestablish the more normal condyle-disc relationship. This is usually achieved clinically by monitoring the clicking joint. The least amount of anterior positioning of the mandible that will eliminate the joint sound is selected.

Although eliminating the click does not always denote successful reduction of the disc,[48] it is a good clinical reference point for beginning therapy. Earlier authors recommended using arthrography,[48] computed tomography scan,[49] and more recently magnetic resonance imaging[50] to assist in establishing the optimum condyle-disc relationship for appliance fabrication. Although there is little doubt that these are more precise techniques, most clinicians cannot practically use them on a routine basis.

The idea behind the anterior positioning appliance was to reposition to condyle back on the disc ("recapture the disc"). It was originally suggested that this appliance be worn 24 hours a day for as long as 3 to 6 months. Although this appliance is still helpful in managing certain disc derangement disorders, its use has changed considerably once studies had the opportunity to evaluate its long-term effectiveness. The precise use of this appliance is discussed later in this section, and its fabrication is described in Chapter 15.

It was immediately discovered that the anterior positioning appliance was useful in quickly reducing painful joint symptoms by improving the condyle-disc relationship, which reduced loading on the retrodiscal tissues. When this appliance successfully reduced symptoms, a major treatment question was asked: What next? Some clinicians believed that the mandible needed to be permanently maintained in this forward position. Dental procedures were suggested to create an occlusal condition that maintained the mandible in this therapeutic position.[51,52] Accomplishing this task

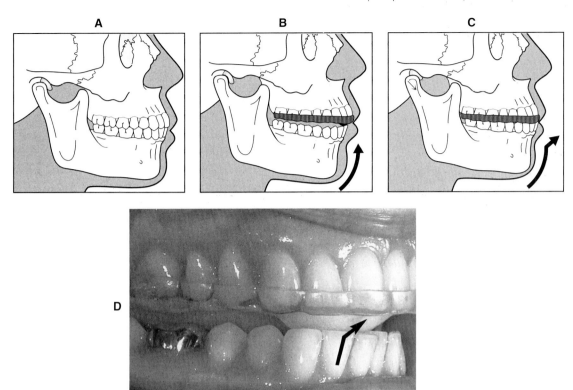

Fig. 13-5 A, In the resting closed joint position the disc has been anteriorly displaced from the condyle. **B,** A maxillary occlusal appliance has been fabricated to create an occlusal condition that requires the mandible to shift slightly forward. **C,** When the appliance is in place and the teeth are occluding, the condyle is repositioned on the disc in a more normal condyle-disc relationship. **D,** When the mouth is closed, the anterior teeth contact on the guiding ramp and the mandible is brought forward *(arrow)* to the therapeutic position that keeps the disc in a more normal relationship with the condyle. This device is called an *anterior positioning appliance.*

was never a simple dental procedure, and questions arose regarding joint stability at this position.[53] Others believed that once the discal ligaments were repaired, the mandible should be returned to the musculoskeletally stable position and the disc would remain in proper position (recaptured). Although one approach is more conservative than the other, neither can be supported with long-term data.

In early short-term studies[38,50,54-60] the anterior positioning appliance proved to be much more effective in reducing intracapsular symptoms than the more traditional stabilization appliance.

This, of course, led the profession to believe that returning the disc to its proper relationship with the condyle was an essential part of treatment. The greatest insight regarding the appropriateness of a treatment modality, however, is gained from long-term studies. Forty patients with various derangements of the condyle-disc complex were evaluated[56] 2.5 years after anterior positioning therapy and step-back procedures. None received any occlusal alterations. It was reported that 66% of the patients were found to still have joint sounds, yet only 25% were still experiencing any pain. If in this study the criterion for success was the elimination of pain and joint sounds, then success was achieved in only 28%. Other long-term studies[38,61] have reported similar findings. If the presence of asymptomatic joint sounds is not a rationale for treatment failure, however, then the success rate for anterior positioning appliances rises to 75%. The issue that must be addressed therefore is the relative clinical significance of asymptomatic joint sounds.

As already stated, joint sounds are common in the general population. In most cases[10,62-68] they do not appear to be related to pain or decreased joint mobility. If all clicking joints always progressed to more serious disorders, then this would be a good indication that each and every joint that clicked should be treated. The presence of unchanging joint sounds over time, however, indicates that some structures can adapt to less than optimum functional relationships. To understand the need for treatment, one needs to compare long-term studies of untreated joint sounds.

Greene et al.[69] reported on 100 patients with clicking joints who were reevaluated 5.2 years after receiving conservative therapy for masticatory muscle disorders. Thirty-eight percent no longer had joint sounds and, of these patients, only one (1%) had increased joint pain. In a similar study Okeson and Hayes[70] reported on 84 patients with TMJ sounds who were reevaluated 4.5 years after receiving conservative therapy for masticatory muscle disorders. None of these patients were treated for their joint sounds. In the study a similar 38% no longer had joint sounds, whereas 7.1% believed that their symptoms were increased. In a study by Bush and Carter,[71] 35 students entering dental school had joint sounds, but only 11 (31%) had them 3.2 years later at graduation. It was also noted in this study that of 65 dental students entering without joint sounds, 43 (or 66%) graduated with sounds.

In another interesting study by Magnusson et al.,[72] joint sounds were reported in a 15-year-old population and then again in the same population at age 20. Of the 35 subjects who had sounds at age 15, sixteen (or 46%) did not have them at age 20. The subjects were not given any treatment. Interestingly, in this study, of the 38 15-year-olds who did not have joint sounds, 19 (50%) did have them at age 20, which implies that a 15-year-old

with TMJ sounds has a 46% chance of losing them by age 20. The study also suggests, however, that if a 15-year-old does not have TMJ sounds there is a 50% chance he or she will by age 20. The authors concluded that joint sounds come and go and are often unrelated to major masticatory symptoms. Ten- and twenty-year follow-up examinations of this same population by Magnusson et al. continue to reveal the lack of a significant relationship between joint sounds and pain or dysfunction.[67,73]

In a similar study Kononen et al.[11] observed 128 young adults longitudinally over 9 years at ages 14, 15, 18, and 23 years of age. They reported that although clicking did increase significantly with age from 11% to 34%, there was no predictable pattern and only 2% of subjects showed consistent findings during the periods of evaluation. They found no relationship between clicking and the progression to locking.

A significant long-term study by de Leeuw et al.[74] found that 30 years after nonsurgical management of intracapsular disorders, joint sounds persisted in 54% of the patients. Although these findings reveal that joint sounds remain in many patients, it is important to note that none of these patients were experiencing any discomfort or even dysfunction from their joint condition. This study and the others referenced here suggest that joint sounds are often not associated with pain or even major TMJ dysfunction. This research group[75,76] also found that long-term osseous changes in the condyle were commonly associated with disc dislocation without reduction and not so commonly associated with disc dislocation with reduction. Yet even in the patients with significant alterations in condylar morphology (osteoarthrosis), little pain and dysfunction were noted.

Studies such as these bring into question the idea that not all joint sounds are progressive and need to be treated. Several studies[9,11,61,77-79] report that progression of intracapsular disorders as determined by joint sounds only occurs in 7% to 9% of the patients with sounds. It appears, however, that if the disc derangement disorder results in significant catching or locking, the chance that the disorder will progress is much greater.[80]

In order for a clinician to confidently recommend that TMJ sounds should be treated, he or she should first understand the rate of success for such treatment. Long-term studies reveal some enlightening information. Adler[81] gave 10 patients with disc derangement disorders an anterior positioning appliance and found that it eliminated their joint sounds. After a time, five received fixed prostheses in the therapeutic position and five were stepped back to their original occlusion. Both groups showed a 40% recurrence of joint sounds. In the Moloney and Howard study,[38] 43% of the patients who received fixed prostheses experienced a return of joint sounds. Tallents et al.[82] found similar results with fixed overlays. When orthodontic therapy was used, 50% of the patients experienced a return of the click.[38,83] Even with surgical procedures it has been found[84,85] that between 30% and 58% of the time clicking returns within 2 to 4 years. These studies all suggest that even when treatment is directed toward the elimination of TMJ sounds, success is not great.

The long-term studies reveal that anterior positioning appliances are not as effective as once thought for joint dysfunction. However, they appear to be helpful in reducing painful symptoms associated with disc displacements and dislocations with reduction in 75% of the patients. Joint sounds appear to be much more resistant to therapy and do not always indicate a progressive disorder. These studies give us insight as to how the joint responds to anterior positioning therapy. In many patients advancing the mandible forward for a therapeutic period of time prevents the condyle from articulating with the highly vascularized, well-innervated retrodiscal tissues. This is the likely explanation for an almost immediate reduction of intracapsular pain. During the forward positioning the retrodiscal tissues undergo adaptive and reparative changes. These tissues can become fibrotic and avascular.[20,86-96] These findings are demonstrated in the gross specimens depicted in Figs. 13-6 and 13-7, as well as the histologic findings in Fig. 13-8.

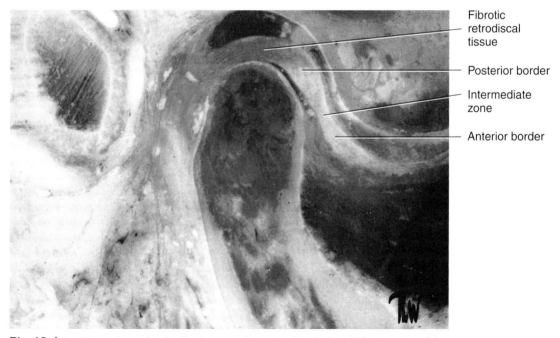

Fibrotic retrodiscal tissue

Posterior border

Intermediate zone

Anterior border

Fig. 13-6 In this specimen the disc has become thinned and is displaced. The location of the anterior border, intermediate zone, and posterior border of the disc are shown. Because the disc is anteriorly displaced, the condyle has been articulating on the retrodiscal tissues. This retrodiscal tissue appears to have become fibrotic, allowing function without pain. *(Courtesy Dr. Per-Lennart Westesson, University of Rochester, Rochester, NY.)*

FT   DISC

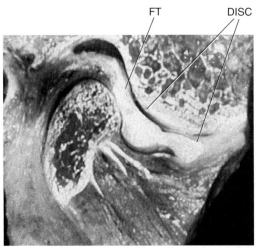

Fig. 13-7 A 28-YEAR-OLD FEMALE AUTOPSY SPECIMEN WITH A TOTALLY DISLOCATED DISC *(DISC).* This retrodiscal tissue has become fibrotic *(FT),* allowing function without pain. *(Courtesy Dr. William Solberg, UCLA, Los Angeles.)*

FT   DISC

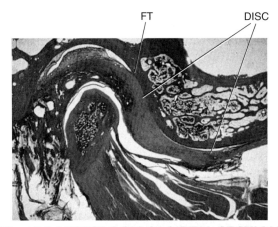

Fig. 13-8 HISTOLOGIC SAGITTAL SECTION OF A TEMPOROMANDIBULAR JOINT WITH AN ANTERIORLY DISLOCATED DISC *(DISC).* Note also that the tissue of the retrodiscal tissue, especially at the superior border has become fibrotic *(FT).* This represents the natural adaption of this tissue secondary to loading. *(Courtesy Dr. Carol Bibb, UCLA, Los Angeles.)*

Clinicians now know that discs are not permanently recaptured by anterior positioning appliances.[97-99] Instead, as the condyle returns to the fossa it moves posteriorly to articulate on the adaptive retrodiscal tissues. If these tissues have adequately adapted, loading can occur without pain. The condyle now functions on the newly adapted retrodiscal tissues, although the disc is still anteriorly displaced. The result is a painless joint that may continue to click with condylar movement (Fig. 13-9). At one time the dental profession believed that the presence of joint sounds indicated treatment failure. Studies have given the profession new insight regarding success and failure. Dentists, like their orthopedic colleagues, have learned to accept that some dysfunction is likely to persist once joint structures have been altered. Controlling pain while allowing joint structures to adapt appears to be the most important role of the therapist.

A few long-term studies[52,82,100] support the concept that permanent alteration of the occlusal condition can be successful in controlling most major symptoms. This treatment, however, requires a considerable amount of dental therapy and one must question the need when natural adaptation appears to work well for most patients. Dental reconstruction of the mouth or orthodontic therapy should be reserved *only* for those patients who present with a significant orthopedic instability.

The continuous use of anterior positioning appliance therapy is not without consequence. A certain percentage of patients who wear these appliances may develop a posterior open bite. A posterior open bite is usually the result of a reversible, myostatic contracture of the inferior lateral pterygoid muscle. When this condition occurs a gradual relengthening of the muscle can be accomplished by converting the anterior positioning appliance to a stabilization appliance that allows the condyles to assume the musculoskeletally stable position. This can also be accomplished by slowly decreasing use of the appliance. A treatment sequence to accomplish this is discussed next and can be found as a treatment flow chart in Chapter 16.

The degree of myostatic contracture that develops is likely to be proportional to the length of time the appliance has been worn. As already mentioned,

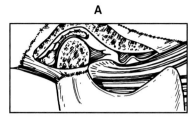 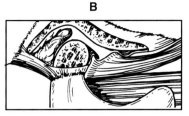 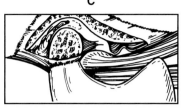

Fig. 13-9 A, Anteriorly displaced disc with the condyle articulating on the retrodiscal tissues, producing pain. **B,** An anterior positioning appliance is placed in the mouth to bring the condyle forward off the retrodiscal tissues onto the disc. This relationship lessens the loading of the retrodiscal tissues, which decreases the pain. **C,** Once the tissues have adapted, the appliance is removed, allowing the condyle to assume the original musculoskeletally stable position. The condyle now functions on adaptive fibrotic tissues, resulting in a painless functioning joint, but because the disc is still displaced, clicking can be present.

when these appliances were first introduced, it was suggested that they be worn 24 hours a day for 3 to 6 months. With this 24-hour use, the development of a posterior open bite was common. The present philosophy is to reduce the time the appliance is being worn so as to limit the adverse effects on the occlusal condition. For most patients full-time use is not necessary to reduce symptoms. The patient should be encouraged to wear the appliance only at night to protect the retrodiscal tissues from heavy loading (bruxism). During the day the patient should not wear the appliance so that the mandible will be allowed to return to its normal position. In most instances this will allow a mild loading of the retrodiscal tissue during the day, which will enhance the fibrotic response of the retrodiscal tissues. If the symptoms can be adequately controlled without daytime use, myostatic contracture is avoided. This technique is appropriate for most patients; however, if significant orthopedic instability exists, symptoms may not be controlled.

If the symptoms do persist with only nighttime use, the patient may need to wear the appliance more often. Daytime use may be necessary for a few weeks. As soon as the patient becomes symptom free, the use of the appliance should be gradually reduced. If reduction of use creates a return of symptoms, then the time allowed for tissue repair has not been adequate or orthopedic instability is present. It is best to assume that inadequate time for tissue repair is the reason for return

of symptoms. The anterior positioning appliance should therefore be reinstituted and more time given for tissue adaptation.

When repeated attempts to eliminate the appliance fail to control symptoms, orthopedic instability should be suspected. When this occurs the anterior positioning appliance should be converted to a stabilization appliance, which allows the condyle to return to the musculoskeletally stable position. Once the condyles are in the musculoskeletally stable position the occlusal condition should be assessed for orthopedic stability. This evaluation process is discussed more completely in later chapters.

Numerous factors determine the length of time an appliance needs to be worn. These factors often relate to the amount of time necessary for the retrodiscal tissues to adapt adequately. When the main etiologic factor is macrotrauma, the length and success of appliance therapy depend on four conditions:

1. *Acuteness of the injury:* Treatment rendered immediately after the injury is more likely to succeed than if it is delayed until the injury is months old.
2. *Extent of the injury:* Obviously, small injuries will repair more successfully and quickly than extensive ones. The clinician can use this information to prepare the patient for the length of time needed for treatment.
3. *Age and health of the patient:* The TMJ structures are relatively slow to repair, especially when

compared with more vascularized tissues. In general, younger patients will heal more quickly and completely than older patients.

4. *General health of the patient:* Patients who are compromised by other health conditions may not be good candidates for repair. The presences of conditions such as systemic arthritis (e.g., rheumatoid arthritis), diabetes, or immunodeficiencies often compromise the patient's ability to repair and adapt and therefore may require more time for the therapy to be successful.

Patients need to be treated individually according to their unique circumstances. As a general rule the therapist should keep in mind that fewer complications occur when the appliance is used for shorter periods of time.

In some patients posterior open bites may result even after careful use of the appliance. For these patients the condyle does not return to its pretreatment position in the fossa. The reason for this phenomenon is not well documented. One explanation is the development of a myofibrotic contracture of the inferior lateral pterygoid muscle. This condition creates a permanent shortening of the muscle length. Myofibrotic contracture may occur secondary to either inflammation or actual trauma to muscle tissues. A second possible explanation is the formation of thickened retrodiscal tissues, which disallows complete seating of the condyle in the fossa.

A third explanation for the development of a posterior open bite is a preexisting orthopedic instability that has just been discovered. Perhaps before therapy the occlusal position did not allow the condyle to be seated into the musculoskeletally stable position. Once the appliance was placed, the teeth contacting the appliance determined the condylar position. The appliance initially positions the condyle forward and then later steps it back to a stable condylar position in the fossa. For a patient who presents with a preexisting unstable relationship between the occlusal position and the condylar position, removal of the appliance may allow the condyle to be seated into a more musculoskeletally stable position. In this position the teeth may not occlude soundly in the preappliance position. For this patient, stepping back the appliance allows the relationship between the condyle

and fossa to determine the mandibular position and not the occlusion. If the patient were allowed to immediately function without the appliance, the elevator muscles would likely drive the teeth together, redisplacing the condyle from the stable relationship in the fossa, and the disc derangement disorder would return. When this condition exists, dental therapy is indicated to secure a stable occlusal position in the stable joint position (orthopedic stability). In this condition the condyle is not located down the articular eminence but in a stable position in the fossae.

None of the previous three explanations is supported with scientific documentation. Studies are necessary to determine the cause of a posterior open bite secondary to long-term anterior positioning therapy. Also important to note is that a posterior open bite is not the rule but the exception and is usually only a problem if the patient has used an anterior positioning appliance continuously and for a prolonged period of time. In my experience, the majority of patients can be successfully returned to their original occlusal position.

Clearly, anterior positioning appliance therapy can be effective in reducing symptoms associated with certain disc derangement disorders; however, dental instability can be a consequence. This type of therapy should therefore be used with discretion. For some patients with these disorders a stabilization appliance can reduce symptoms,[55,101] probably because a decrease in muscle activity (i.e., bruxism, clenching) reduces forces applied to the retrodiscal tissues. When a stabilization appliance reduces symptoms, it should be used instead of an anterior positioning appliance because this appliance rarely leads to irreversible occlusal changes. When an anterior positioning appliance is necessary, the patient should be advised that dental therapy may be necessary following the appliance. Although this is not common, the patient should be well informed of the possible complications.

Summary of Definitive Treatment of Disc Displacements and Disc Dislocations with Reduction. The reasonable goal of definitive therapy for disc displacements and disc dislocations with reduction is to reduce intracapsular pain, not to recapture the disc. A stabilization appliance should be used whenever possible because adverse long-term effects are minimized. When this appliance is not effective, an anterior positioning appliance should be fabricated. The patient should be initially instructed to wear the appliance always at night during sleep and during the day only when needed to reduce symptoms. This part-time use will minimize adverse occlusal changes. The patient should only be encouraged to wear the appliance more if it is the only way the pain can be controlled. As symptoms resolve, the patient is encouraged to decrease use of the appliance. With adaptive changes, most patients can gradually reduce use of the appliance with no need for any dental changes. These adaptive changes may take 8 to 10 weeks or even longer.

When elimination of the appliance produces a return of symptoms, two conditions should be evaluated. First, the adaptive process is not complete enough to allow the altered retrodiscal tissues to accept the functional forces of the condyle. When this is the case, the patient should be given more time with the appliance for adaptation. The second reason for a return of pain is that there is a lack of orthopedic stability, and removal of the appliance brings the patient back to his or her preexisting orthopedic instability. When orthopedic instability is present, dental therapy to correct this condition may be considered. This is the only condition that requires dental therapy. A sequence of this treatment is presented in Chapter 16.

Supportive Therapy

The patient should be informed and educated to the mechanics of the disorder and the adaptive process that is essential for successful treatment. The patient needs to be encouraged to decrease loading of the joint whenever possible. Softer foods, slower chewing, and smaller bites should be promoted. The patient should be told, when possible, not to allow the joint to click. If inflammation is suspected, a nonsteroidal antiinflammatory drug (NSAID) should be prescribed. Moist heat or ice can be used if the patient finds either helpful. Active exercises are not usually helpful because they cause joint movements that often increase pain. Passive jaw movements may be helpful, and, on occasion, distractive

manipulation by a physical therapist may assist in healing.

Even though this is an intracapsular disorder, physical self-regulation techniques should be provided to the patient. These techniques reduce loading to the joint and generally downregulate the central nervous system. These techniques help decrease pain and improve the patient's coping skills.

DISC DISLOCATION WITHOUT REDUCTION

Disc dislocation without reduction is a clinical condition in which the disc is dislocated, most frequently anteromedially, from the condyle and does not return to normal position with condylar movement.

Cause

Macrotrauma and microtrauma are the most common causes of disc dislocation without reduction.

History

Patients most often report the exact onset of this disorder. A sudden change in range of mandibular movement occurs that is apparent to the patient. The history may reveal a gradual increase in intracapsular symptoms (clicking and catching) before the dislocation. Most often joint sounds are no longer present immediately following the disc dislocation.

Clinical Characteristics

Examination reveals limited mandibular opening (25 to 30 mm) with normal eccentric movement to the ipsilateral side and restricted eccentric movement to the contralateral side.

Definitive Treatment

In both displacements and dislocations with reduction, the anterior positioning appliance therapeutically reestablishes the normal condyle-disc relationship. Fabricating an anterior positioning appliance for a patient with a disc dislocation without reduction, however, will only aggravate the condition by forcing the disc even more forward. Therefore fabricating an anterior positioning

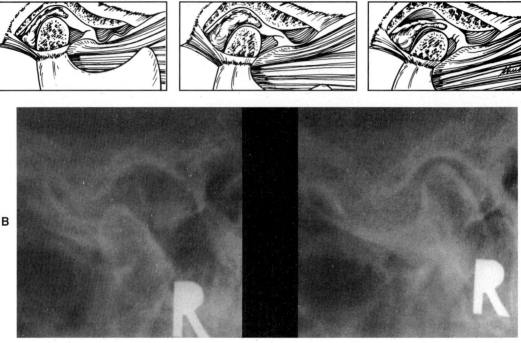

Fig. 13-10 A, Anterior disc dislocation without reduction. **B,** Radiographic evidence of an anteriorly dislocated disc without reduction. Right condyle in the closed joint *(left image)* and the maximally open position *(right image)*. The condyle reveals a restricted pattern of movement by not translating completely down the eminence. The anterior joint space in the closed position is much narrower than in the opened position. As the condyle translates forward, it jams onto the posterior border of the disc and becomes separated slightly from the eminence. This increases the anterior joint space, which is a meaningful finding only when corroborated by clinical evidence of a disc dislocation.

appliance is contraindicated for this patient. Patients who present with a disc dislocation without reduction (Fig. 13-10) need to be managed differently.

When the condition of disc dislocation without reduction is acute, the initial therapy should include an attempt to reduce or recapture the disc by manual manipulation. This manipulation can be successful with patients who are experiencing their first episode of locking. In these patients there is a great likelihood that tissues are healthy and not morphologically changed. Patients with a long history of locking are likely to present with discs and ligaments that have undergone changes that will not allow reduction of the disc. As a general rule, when patients report a history of being locked for 1 week or less, manipulation is usually successful. In patients with a longer history, success begins to decrease rapidly.

Technique for Manual Manipulation. The success of manual manipulation for the reduction of a dislocated disc will depend on three factors. The first is the level of activity in the superior lateral pterygoid muscle. This muscle must be *relaxed* to permit successful reduction. If it remains active because of pain, it may need to be injected with local anesthetic before any attempt to reduce the disc. Second, the disc space must be *increased* so that the disc can be repositioned on the condyle. When increased activity of the elevator muscles is present, the interarticular pressure is increased, making it more difficult to reduce the disc. The patient needs to be encouraged to relax and avoid forcefully closing the mouth. The third factor is that the condyle must be in the *maximum forward translatory position*. The only structure that can produce a posterior or retractive force on the disc is the superior retrodiscal lamina, and if this tissue is to be effective the condyle must be in the forward-most position.

The first attempt to reduce the disc should begin by having the patient attempt to self-reduce the dislocation. With the teeth slightly apart the patient is asked to move the mandible to the contralateral side of the dislocation as far as possible. From this eccentric position the mouth is opened maximally. If this is not successful at first, the patient should attempt this several times. If the patient is unable to reduce the disc, assistance with manual manipulating is indicated. The thumb is placed intraorally over the mandibular second molar on the affected side. The fingers are placed on the inferior border of the mandible anterior to the thumb position (Fig. 13-11). Firm but controlled downward force is then exerted on the molar at the same time that upward force is placed by the fingers on the outer inferior broader of the mandible. The opposite hand helps stabilize the cranium above the joint that is being distracted. While the joint is being distracted, the patient is asked to assist by slowly protruding the mandible, which translates the condyle downward and forward out of the fossa. It may also be helpful to bring the mandible to the contralateral side during the distraction procedure because the disc is likely to be dislocated anteriorly and medially and a contralateral movement will move the condyle into it better.

Once the full range of laterotrusive excursion has been reached, the patient is asked to relax while 20 to 30 seconds of constant distractive force is applied to the joint. The clinician needs to be sure that unusual heavy forces are not placed on the uninvolved joint. One would certainly not want to injure a healthy joint while trying to improve the condition of the other joint. The clinician should always ask the patient if he or she is feeling any discomfort in the uninvolved joint. If there is discomfort, the procedure should be immediately stopped and begun again with the proper directional force placed. A correctly performed manual manipulation to distract a TMJ should not jeopardize the healthy joint.

Once the distractive force has been applied for 20 to 30 seconds, the force is discontinued, and the fingers are removed from the mouth. The patient is then asked to lightly close the mouth to the incisal end-to-end position on the anterior teeth. After relaxing for a few seconds, the patient is asked to open wide and immediately return to this anterior position (not maximum intercuspation). If the disc has been successfully reduced, the patient should be able to open to the full range (no restrictions). When this occurs, the disc has likely been recaptured and an anterior positioning appliance is immediately placed to prevent clenching on the posterior teeth, which would likely redislocate the disc. At this point, the patient has a normal condyle-disc relationship and should be managed in the same manner as discussed for the patient with a disc dislocation with reduction with one exception.

When an acute disc dislocation has been reduced, it is advisable to have the patient wear the anterior positioning appliance continuously for the first 2 to 4 days before beginning only nighttime use. The rationale for this is that the dislocated disc may have become distorted during the dislocation, which may allow it to redislocate more easily. Maintaining the anterior positioning appliance in place constantly for a few days may help the disc reassume its more normal shape (thinnest in the intermediate band and thicker anterior and posterior). If the normal morphology is present, the disc will more likely maintain its normal position. However, if this disc has permanently lost its normal morphology, it will be difficult to maintain its position. This is why manual manipulations for disc dislocations are only attempted in acute conditions when the likelihood of normal disc morphology exists.

If the disc is not successfully reduced, a second and possibly third attempt can be made. Failure to reduce the disc may indicate a dysfunctional superior retrodiscal lamina or a general loss of disc morphology. Once these tissues have changed, the disc dislocation is most often permanent.

If the disc is permanently dislocated, what types of treatments are indicated? This question has been asked for many years. At one time it was felt that the disc needed to be in its proper position for

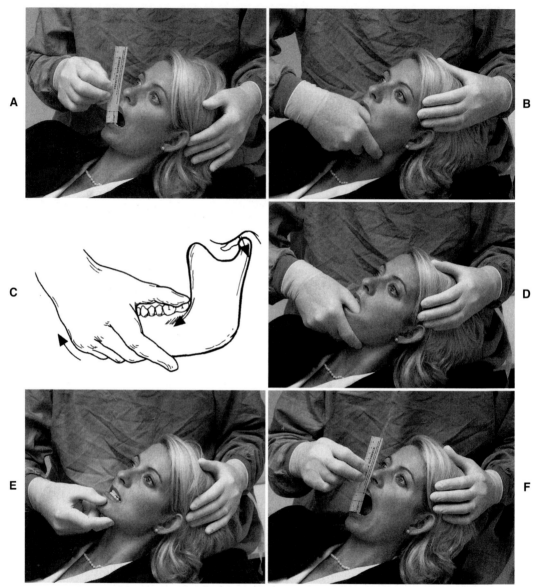

Fig. 13-11 MANUAL DISC REDUCTION TECHNIQUE. A, The patient presents with an acute disc dislocation without reduction in the left temporomandibular joint (closed lock). The maximum opening is only 23 mm. **B,** The clinician's right thumb is placed intraorally over the patient's left mandibular second molar, and the mandible is grasped. With the left hand stabilizing the cranium, gentle but firm force is applied downward on the molar and upward on the chin to distract the joint. **C,** Arrows depict the proper force vectors for effective joint distraction. **D,** Once the joint is distracted, the mandible is brought forward and to the right, enabling the condyle to move into the area of the dislocated disc. When this position is achieved, constant distractive force is applied for 30 to 40 seconds while the patient relaxes. **E,** After the distraction the thumb is removed and the patient is asked to close on the anterior teeth, maintaining the jaw in a slightly protrusive position. **F,** When the patient has rested a moment, he or she is instructed to open maximally. If the disc has been reduced, a normal range of movement (48 mm) will be possible.

health to exist. Therefore when the disc could not be restored to proper position, a surgical repair of the joint appeared to be necessary. Over years of studying this condition we have learned that surgery may not be necessary for most patients. Studies[102-113] have revealed that over time many patients achieve relatively normal joint function even with the disc permanently dislocated. With these studies in mind it would seem appropriate to follow a more conservative approach that would encourage adaptation of the retrodiscal tissues. Patients with permanent disc dislocation should be given a stabilization appliance that will reduce forces to the retrodiscal tissues (i.e., decrease bruxism).[101] Only when this and the supportive therapies fail to reduce pain should surgical procedures be considered. (The indications for surgical intervention are discussed later in this chapter.)

Supportive Therapy

Supportive therapy for a permanent disc dislocation should begin with educating the patient about the condition. Because of the restricted range of mouth opening, many patients try to force their mouth to open wider. If this is attempted too strongly, it will only aggravate the intracapsular tissues, producing more pain. Patients should be encouraged not to open too wide, especially immediately following the dislocation. With time and tissue adaptation they will be able to return to a more normal range of movement (usually greater than 40 mm).[103,104,106-109,111] Gentle, controlled jaw exercise may be helpful in regaining mouth opening,[114,115] but care should be taken against being too aggressive to avoid more tissue injury. The patient must be told that this will take time, as much as 1 year or more for full range of motion.

The patient should also be told to decrease hard biting, not chew gum, and generally avoid anything that aggravates the condition. If pain is present, heat or ice may be used. NSAIDs are indicated for pain and inflammation. Joint distraction and phonophoresis over the joint area may be helpful.

Surgical Considerations for Condyle-Disc Derangement Disorders. Disc displacements and dislocations develop from alterations in the structural integrity of the condyle-disc complex. A definitive treatment that may be considered for such derangements is surgical correction. The goal of surgery should be to return the disc to a normal functional relationship with the condyle. Although this approach seems logical, it is also aggressive. Surgery therefore should be considered only when conservative nonsurgical therapy fails to adequately resolve the symptoms and/or progression of the disorder and it has been adequately determined that the source of pain is intracapsular structures. The patient should be instructed regarding the likely results of surgery and the medical risks and should weigh those factors against quality of life. The decision to undergo surgery should be made by the patient after acquiring all the needed information.

When indications show that the clinician needs to be more aggressive with disc derangement disorder, the first procedure that should be considered is an *arthrocentesis*. In this procedure, two needles are placed into the joint and sterile saline solution is passed through, lavaging the joint. This procedure is conservative, and studies suggest that it is helpful in reducing symptoms in a significant number of patients.[116-125] The lavage is thought to eliminate much of the algogenic substances and secondary inflammatory mediators that produce the pain.[126] The long-term effects of arthrocentesis are positive in maintaining the patient relatively pain free.[121,122,125,127] It is certainly the most conservative "surgical procedure" that can be offered and therefore has an important role in managing intracapsular disorders.

During arthrocentesis it is common to place a steroid into the joint at the completion of the procedure. Some surgeons have also suggested placing sodium hyaluronate in the joint.[128,129] Although this may have some benefit, further studies are necessary to determine the long-term benefit of including this treatment.

In cases of disc dislocation without reduction, a single needle can be introduced into the joint and fluid can be forced into the space in an attempt to free the articular surfaces. This technique is called "pumping the joint" and may improve the success of manual manipulation for a closed lock.[128,130-134]

Arthrocentesis has even proved to be helpful for short-term relief of rheumatoid arthritis symptoms.[135] Twelve rheumatoid arthritic patients receiving arthrocentesis were statistically improved 6 weeks postprocedure for both pain and dysfunction.

Another relatively conservative surgical approach for treating these intracapsular disorders is *arthroscopy*. With this technique an arthroscope is placed into the superior joint space and the intracapsular structures are visualized on a monitor. Joint adhesions can be identified and eliminated, and the joint can be significantly mobilized. This procedure appears to be quite successful in reducing symptoms and improving range of movement.[119,123,125,127,136-150] Interestingly, arthroscopy does not correct the disc position, but instead success is more likely achieved by improving disc mobility.[151-154]

When indicated, the joint may need to be opened for reparative procedures. Open-joint surgery is generally called *arthrotomy*. A variety of arthrotomy procedures can be performed. When a disc is displaced or dislocated, the most conservative surgical procedure is a discal repair or *plication*.[155-160] During a plication procedure a portion of the retrodiscal tissue and inferior lamina is removed, and the disc is retracted posteriorly and secured with sutures.

Difficulty arises if the disc has been damaged and can no longer be maintained for use in the joint. Then the choice becomes removal or replacement of the disc. Removal of the disc is called a *discectomy* (sometimes meniscectomy).[161-165] It leaves a bone-to-bone articulation, which is likely to produce some osteoarthritic changes. However, these changes may not produce pain.[165-167] Another choice is to remove the disc and replace it with a substitute. Early discal implants that were suggested[168] included medical Silastic, which had limited success.[169] In the 1980s Proplast-Teflon discal implants were used, but considerable problems arose with the material disintegrating and producing inflammatory reaction.[170-173] Dermal,[174-180] temporal fascial flaps,[181] fat tissue,[182,183] and auricular cartilage grafts[184-186] have also been used. Unfortunately the dental profession has not found a suitable permanent replacement for the articular disc, so when removal is necessary, significant compromise in function often occurs. A predominant thought at this time is to simply remove the disc (discectomy) and allow the natural adaptation process to restore function of the joint. This appears to be a better alternative than to attempt to replace it with something that may actually compromise the natural adaptive process.

Surgery on the TMJ should never be performed without serious consideration of the consequences. No joint that is surgically entered can be expected to function again as normal. A certain amount of scarring that restricts mandibular movement almost always occurs. There is also a high degree of postsurgical adhesion, probably secondary to hemarthrosis.[187,188] In addition, the risks of damage to the facial nerve must not be ignored. Because all these risks are great, surgery should be reserved only for patients who do not respond adequately to the more conservative therapies. This is probably less than 5% of patients seeking treatment for intracapsular disorders.

STRUCTURAL INCOMPATIBILITY OF THE ARTICULAR SURFACES

Structural incompatibility of the articular surfaces can originate from any problem that disrupts normal joint functioning. It may be trauma, a pathologic process, or merely related to excessive mouth opening. In some cases it is excessive static interarticular pressure. In others it is alterations in the bony surfaces (e.g., a spicule) or in the articular disc (a perforation) that impede normal function (Fig. 13-12). These disorders are characterized by deviating movement patterns that are repeatable and difficult to avoid.

Four categories of structural incompatibility exist: (1) deviation in form, (2) adhesions, (3) subluxation, and (4) spontaneous dislocation.

DEVIATION IN FORM

Deviation in form includes a group of disorders that are created by changes in the smooth articular surface of the joint and disc. These changes produce an alteration in the normal pathway of condylar movement.

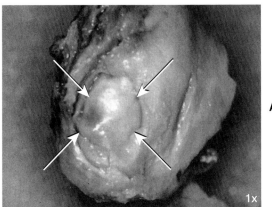

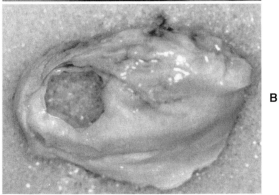

Fig. 13-12 A, This specimen shows the condyle and disc together. The perforation in the disc exposes the lateral pole of the condyle *(arrows).* **B,** The disc has been removed from the condyle so that the perforation can be more easily visualized. *(Courtesy Dr. L.R. Bean, University of Kentucky, Lexington.)*

Cause

The cause of most deviations in form is trauma. The trauma may have been a sudden blow or the slow trauma associated with microtrauma. Certainly loading of bony structures causes alterations in form.

History

Patients often report a long history related to these disorders. Many of these disorders are not painful and therefore may go unnoticed by the patient.

Clinical Characteristics

A patient with a deviation in the form of the condyle, fossa, or disc will commonly show a repeated alteration in the pathway of the opening and closing movements. When a click or deviation in opening is noted, it will always occur at the same position of opening and closing. Deviations in form may or may not be painful.

Definitive Treatment

Because the cause of deviation in form of an articular surface is actual change in structure, the definitive approach is to return the altered structure to normal form. This may be accomplished by a surgical procedure. In the case of bony incompatibility, the structures are smoothed and rounded. If the disc is perforated or misshapen, attempts are made to repair it (discoplasty). Because surgery is a relatively aggressive procedure, it should be considered only when pain and dysfunction are unmanageable. Most deviations in form can be managed by supportive therapies.

Supportive Therapy

In most cases the symptoms associated with deviations in form can be adequately managed by patient education. The patient should be encouraged, when possible, to learn a manner of opening and chewing that avoids or minimizes the dysfunction. Deliberate new opening and chewing strokes can become habits if the patient works toward this goal. In some cases the increased interarticular pressure associated with bruxism can accentuate the dysfunction associated with deviations in form. If this is the case, a stabilization appliance may be useful to decrease the muscle hyperactivity. However, the appliance is used only if muscle hyperactivity is suspected. If pain is associated, analgesics may be necessary to prevent the development of secondary central excitatory effects.

ADHERENCES AND ADHESIONS

Adherences represent a temporary sticking of the articular surfaces during normal joint movements. Adhesions are more permanent and are caused by a fibrosis attachment of the articular surfaces. Adherences and adhesions may occur between the disc and condyle or the disc and fossa.

Cause

Adherences commonly result from prolonged static loading of the joint structures. If the adherence is maintained, the more permanent condition of adhesion may develop.[189] Adhesions may also develop secondary to hemarthrosis caused by macrotrauma or surgery.[187]

History

Adherences that develop occasionally but are broken or released during function can be diagnosed only through the history. Usually the patient will report a long period when the jaw was statically loaded (such as clenching during sleep). This period is followed by a sensation of limited mouth opening. As the patient tries to open, a single click is felt and normal range of movement is immediately returned. The click or catching sensation does not return during opening and closing unless the joint is again statically loaded for a prolonged time. These patients typically report that in the morning the jaw appears "stiff" until they pop it once and normal movement is restored.

Patients with adhesions will often report a restriction in the opening range of movement. The degree of restriction is related to the location of the adhesion. Adhesions present clinically similar to adherences, but movement does not typically free the restriction.

Clinical Characteristics

Adherences present with temporary restriction in mouth opening until the click occurs, whereas adhesions present with a more permanent limitation in mouth opening. The degree of restriction is dependent on the location of the adhesion. If the adhesion affects only one joint, the opening movement will deflect to the ipsilateral side. When adhesions are permanent, the dysfunction can be great. Adhesions in the inferior joint cavity cause a sudden, jerky movement during opening. Those in the superior joint cavity restrict movement to rotation and thus limit the patient to 25 or 30 mm of opening. During mouth opening, adhesions between disc and fossa will tend to force the condyle across the anterior border of the disc. As the disc is thinned and the anterior capsular and collateral ligaments elongated, the condyle moves over the disc and onto the attachment of the superior lateral pterygoid muscle. In these cases the disc becomes dislocated posteriorly (Fig. 13-13). The possibility of a posterior disc dislocation has been debated for some time. Evidence does exist supporting this possibility.[190,191] However, it is far less common than an anterior dislocation and is more likely to be closely related to adhesions between the disc and the fossa. As mentioned in Chapter 10, a posterior dislocation will present entirely different clinical symptoms from an anterior dislocation. Often with a posterior disc dislocation, the patient opens normally but has difficulty getting the teeth back into occlusion.

The symptoms associated with adhesions are constant and repeatable. Pain may or may not be present. If pain is a symptom, it is normally associated with attempts to open the mouth, which elongates ligaments.

Definitive Treatment

Because adherences are associated with prolonged static loading of the articular surfaces, definitive therapy is directed toward decreasing

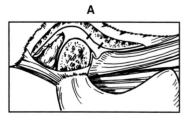
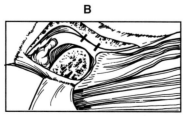
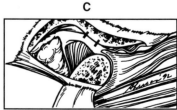

Fig. 13-13 A to **C,** Posterior dislocation of the disc secondary to an adhesion between the superior surface of the disc and the fossa.

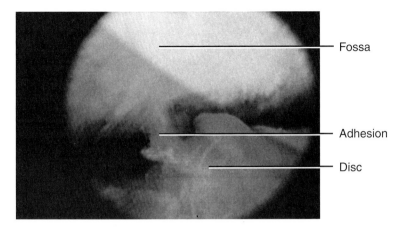

Fossa

Adhesion

Disc

Fig. 13-14 Arthroscopic view of an adhesion between the disc and the fossa. *(Courtesy Dr. Terry Tanaka, Chula Vista, Calif.)*

loading to these structures. Loading may be related to either diurnal or nocturnal clenching. Diurnal clenching is best managed by patient awareness and physical self-regulation techniques (see Chapter 11). When nocturnal clenching or bruxism is suspected, a stabilization appliance is indicated for decreasing the muscle hyperactivity. In some instances the articular surfaces may be roughened or abraded, leading to a condition that may promote the development of adherences. The stabilization appliance will often change the relationship of these areas, lessening the likelihood of adherences.

When adhesions are present, breaking the fibrous attachment is the only definitive treatment. This can often be achieved with arthroscopic surgery (Fig. 13-14).[150,192-198] Not only does the surgery break up adhesions, but as previously discussed, the lavage used to irrigate the joint during the procedure assists in decreasing symptoms.

Importantly, because surgery is relatively aggressive, definitive treatment for adhesions should be performed only when necessary. Adhesion disorders that are painless and produce only minor dysfunction are more appropriately treated by supportive therapy.

Supportive Therapy
The restriction of some adhesion problems can be improved with passive stretching, ultrasound, and distraction of the joint (Fig. 13-15). These types of treatment tend to loosen the fibrous attachments,

allowing more freedom for movement. Caution should be taken not to be too aggressive with the stretching technique, however, because this can tear tissues and produce inflammation and pain. In many instances, when pain and dysfunction are minimal, patient education is the most appropriate treatment. Having the patient limit opening and learn appropriate patterns of movement that do not aggravate the adhesions can lead to normal functioning (Fig. 13-16).

SUBLUXATION

Subluxation or, as it is sometimes called, *hypermobility*, is a clinical description of the condyle as it

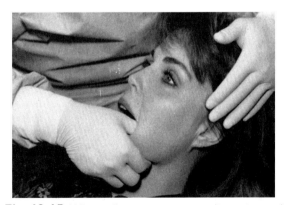

Fig. 13-15 When adhesions are recent, distraction and mobilization of the joint can sometimes be helpful in breaking them.

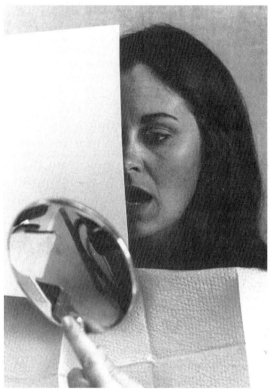

Fig. 13-16 Sometimes the patient can be trained to open in a manner that will minimize or even eliminate the dysfunction associated with a disc derangement disorder. Using a mirror helps guide the straight-downward direction with minimum translation. In some cases a straight edge is helpful in observing the midline during opening.

moves anterior to the crest of the articular eminence. It is not a pathologic condition but reflects a variation in anatomic form of the fossa.

Cause

As just stated, subluxation is usually a result of the anatomic form of the fossa. Patients who have a steep short posterior slope of the articular eminence followed by a longer flat anterior slope seem to display a greater tendency toward subluxation.[199] Subluxation results when the disc is maximally rotated on the condyle before full translation of condyle-disc complex occurs. The last movement of the condyle becomes a sudden quick jump forward, leaving a clinically noticeable preauricular depression.

History

The patient reports a locking sensation whenever the mouth is opened too wide. The patient can return the mouth to the closed position but often reports a little difficulty.

Clinical Characteristics

During the final stage of maximal mouth opening, the condyle can be seen to suddenly jump forward with a "thud" sensation. This is not reported as a subtle clicking sensation.

Definitive Treatment

The only definitive treatment for subluxation is surgical alteration of the joint itself. This can be accomplished by an eminectomy,[200-203] which reduces the steepness of the articular eminence and thus decreases the amount of posterior rotation of the disc on the condyle during full translation. In most cases, however, a surgical procedure is far too aggressive for the symptoms experienced by the patient. Therefore much effort should be directed at supportive therapy in an attempt to eliminate the disorder or at least reduce the symptoms to tolerable levels.

Supportive Therapy

Supportive therapy begins by educating the patient regarding the cause and which movements create the interference. The patient must learn to restrict opening so as not to reach the point of translation that initiates the interference. On occasion, when the interference cannot be voluntarily resolved, an intraoral device (Fig. 13-17) to restrict movement is employed.[204] Wearing the device attempts to develop a myostatic contracture of the elevator muscles, thus limiting opening to the point of subluxation. The device is worn continuously for 2 months and then removed, allowing the contracture to limit opening.

SPONTANEOUS DISLOCATION

This condition is commonly referred to as an *open lock*. It can occur following wide-open mouth procedures such as having a dental appointment. With a spontaneous dislocation both the condyles and the discs are often dislocated out of their normal positions.

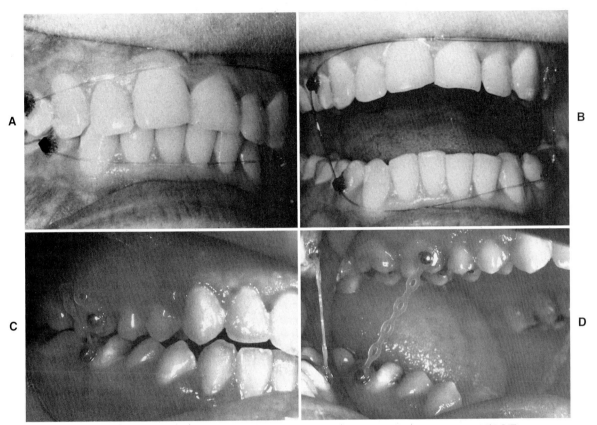

Fig. 13-17 SEVERAL INTRAORAL DEVICES USED TO RESTRICT MOUTH OPENING. A, Orthodontic tubes are bonded to the canines, and a plastic fishing line is threaded and tied. **B,** The line limits the mandibular opening just short of subluxation. If the patient opens wider, the line will become tight, restricting opening to the desired distance. This device is worn for 2 months to achieve a myostatic contracture of the elevator muscles. When it is removed, maximum opening will not reach the point of subluxation. **C,** Another method of restricting mouth opening uses intraarch orthodontic elastics attached to buttons bonded to the teeth. **D,** As the patient attempts to open the mouth, the elastics resist the movement, restricting the opening.

Cause

When the mouth opens to its fullest extent, the condyle is translated to its anterior limit. In this position the disc is rotated to its most posterior extent on the condyle. If the condyle moves beyond this limit, the disc can be forced through the disc space and trapped in this anterior position as the disc space collapses as a result of the condyle moving superiorly against the articular eminence (Fig. 13-18, *A* to *C*). This same spontaneous dislocation can also occur if the superior

lateral pterygoid contracts during the full limit of translation, pulling the disc through the anterior disc space. When a spontaneous dislocation occurs, the superior retrodiscal lamina cannot retract the disc because of the collapsed anterior disc space. Spontaneous reduction is further aggravated when the elevator muscles contract because this activity increases the interarticular pressure and further decreases the disc space. The reduction becomes even more unlikely when the superior or inferior lateral pterygoid

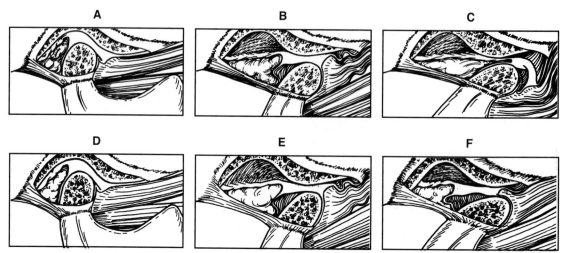

Fig. 13-18 A to **C,** Spontaneous dislocation of the temporomandibular joint results in an "open lock" with the disc dislocated anterior to the condyle. **D** to **F,** Spontaneous dislocation with the disc dislocated posterior to the condyle.

experiences myospasms, which pull the disc and condyle forward.

Spontaneous dislocation of the TMJ can occur in any joint if the condyle is brought anterior to the crest of the eminence. Although the disc has been described as being forced anterior to the condyle, it has also been demonstrated that the disc may be trapped posterior to the condyle[205] (Fig. 13-18, *D* to *F*). In either condition the condyle becomes trapped in front of the eminence, resulting in the patient's inability to close the mouth.

Although a spontaneous dislocation commonly occurs secondary to a wide-opening experience, it may also be caused by sudden contraction of the inferior lateral pterygoid or infrahyoid muscles. This activity may be the result of a spasm or cramp. Earlier chapters discuss this experience. This condition is relatively rare and should not be confused with the anatomic considerations previously mentioned. In some individuals the spontaneous dislocation becomes unprovoked and repeated secondary to uncontrolled muscle contraction. This may be associated with an oromandibular dystonia that has its original in the central nervous system. Diagnosing this dystonia is important because the management is quite different than that used to manage the anatomic conditions previously discussed.

History

The patient presents with the mouth in an open position and the lack of ability to close it. The condition immediately followed a wide-opening movement such as a yawn or a dental procedure. Because the patient cannot close the mouth, he or she is often quite distressed with the condition.

Some patients may report a sudden and unprovoked open lock that repeats itself several times a week or even daily. This presentation is significant for an oromandibular dystonia.

Clinical Characteristics

The patient remains in a wide-open mouth condition. Pain is commonly present secondary to the patient's attempts to close the mouth.

Definitive Treatment

Definitive treatment is directed toward increasing the disc space, which allows the superior retrodiscal lamina to retract the disc. Other muscle functions, however, cannot be ignored. Because the mandible is locked open in this disorder, the patient can be quite distressed and will generally tend to contract the elevators in an attempt to close it in the normal manner. This activity aggravates the spontaneous dislocation. When attempts are being made to reduce the dislocation, the patient must open

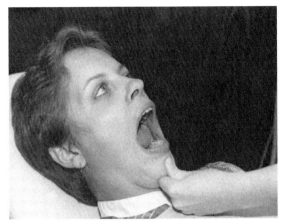

Fig. 13-19 REDUCTION OF A SPONTANEOUS DISLOCATION. Slight posterior pressure to the chin while the patient is opening wide (as in a yawn) will often reduce the dislocation.

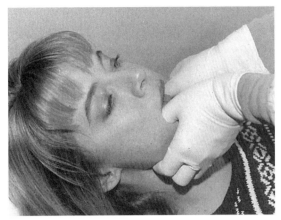

Fig. 13-20 Spontaneous dislocations can be reduced by wrapping the thumbs with gauze and placing them intraorally over the second molars. Downward force is applied on the molars while upward force is applied in the anterior region of the mouth (chin). The effect is to distract both condyles and increase the discal space. As soon as the discal space is wide enough to allow the disc to pass through it, the dislocation will reduce. The mandible should not be forced back or the mouth forced close. Because sudden reduction is common, gauze is placed to protect the thumbs from biting force.

wide as though yawning. This will activate the mandibular depressors and inhibit the elevators. At the same time, slight posterior pressure applied to the chin will sometimes reduce a spontaneous dislocation (Fig. 13-19). If this is not successful, the thumbs are placed on the mandibular molars and downward pressure is exerted as the patient is asked to yawn (Fig. 13-20). This will usually provide enough space to recapture normal disc position.

Because a certain degree of tension exists in the tissues, the reduction is usually accompanied by a sudden closure of the mouth. To protect the thumbs from this sudden closure, it is advisable to wrap each one with gauze. If the spontaneous dislocation is still not reduced, it is likely that the inferior lateral pterygoid is in myospasm, preventing posterior positioning of the condyle. When this occurs, it is appropriate to inject the lateral pterygoid with local anesthetic without a vasoconstrictor in an attempt to eliminate the myospasms and promote relaxation. If the elevators appear to be in myospasm, local anesthetic is also helpful.

When spontaneous dislocation becomes chronic or recurrent and it is determined that the anatomic relationship of the condyle and fossae are etiologic considerations, the traditional definitive treatment has been a surgical

approach to alter the anatomy. This is normally an eminectomy.[203,206-208]

When anatomic considerations are guilty of producing this condition, surgically reducing the eminence is successful. However, when the spontaneous dislocation is produced by muscle contraction, surgical intervention should be avoided because it does not address etiology. Instead, therapy needs to be directed toward reducing muscle activity. When repeated episodes of open locking are associated with an oromandibular dystonia, a more appropriate treatment is the use of botulinum toxin. Botulinum toxin injected into the dystonic muscle can reduce this condition for 3 to 4 months. Typically the best approach is to inject botulinum toxin into the inferior lateral pterygoid muscles, bilaterally using electromyographic guidance. In many cases this is a safe and effective way to reduce or even eliminate spontaneous dislocation of the condyle.[209-211] The patient should be recalled in 3 to 4 months to determine whether there is any recurrence of the problem. This seems to be the typical time it takes for the muscle to recover from the botulinum toxin and return to normal. If the symptoms return, repeated injections may be considered.

Supportive Therapy

The most effective method of treating spontaneous dislocation is prevention. Prevention begins with the same supportive therapy described for subluxation because this is often the precursor of the dislocation. When a spontaneous dislocation is recurrent, the patient is taught the reduction technique. As with subluxation, some chronic recurrent dislocations can be definitively treated by a surgical procedure. However, surgery is considered only after supportive therapy has failed to eliminate or reduce the problem to an acceptable level.

INFLAMMATORY DISORDERS OF THE TEMPOROMANDIBULAR JOINT

Inflammatory disorders of the TMJ are generally characterized by continuous joint area pain, often accentuated by function. Because the pain is constant, it can also result in secondary central excitatory effects such as cyclic muscle pain, hyperalgesia, and referred pain. These effects may confuse the examiner in establishing a primary diagnosis, which can lead to improper treatment selection. In other words, the patient who is treated for local muscle soreness that is secondary to an inflammatory disorder will not respond completely until the inflammatory condition is controlled.

Although some inflammatory conditions are easily identified by history and examination, many are not. Inflammatory conditions of the joint structures often occur simultaneously with or secondary to other inflammatory disorders. The four categories of inflammatory disorders are synovitis, capsulitis, retrodiscitis, and the arthritides. A few inflammatory conditions involve associated structures that are discussed in this section. The inflammatory disorders are discussed separately for cases in which a specific diagnosis can be established. When a general inflammatory condition is

noted but the exact structures involved are difficult to identify, a combination of these treatments is indicated.

SYNOVITIS AND CAPSULITIS

The conditions of synovitis and capsulitis are discussed together because there is no simple way to differentiate them on a clinical basis. They can only be distinguished from each other by visualizing the tissues through arthroscopy or arthrotomy. Also, because the conservative treatment is the same for both, it is appropriate to discuss them together.

Cause

The cause of capsulitis and synovitis is either trauma or a spreading of infection from an adjacent structure. If an infection is present, it needs to be addressed with proper medical support such as an antibiotic medication. This text does not discuss this type of therapy. The majority of inflammatory conditions in the joint are secondary to macrotrauma or microtrauma to the tissues within the joint.[126,212,213] This represents a sterile inflammation, and antibiotics are not indicated.

History

The most significant finding in capsulitis and synovitis is a history of macrotrauma. Trauma such as a blow to the chin received during an accident or a fall is common. Even turning into a wall or an accidental bump to the chin from an elbow can lead to traumatic capsulitis. Trauma is most likely to cause injury to the capsular ligament when the teeth are separated.

Clinical Characteristics

When capsulitis or synovitis is present, any movement that tends to elongate the capsular ligament will accentuate the pain. The pain is reported to be directly in front of the ear, and the lateral aspect of the condyle is usually tender to palpation.

Definitive Treatment

When the cause of capsulitis and synovitis is macrotrauma, the condition is self-limiting because the trauma is no longer present. Therefore no definitive treatment is indicated for the inflammatory condition. Of course, when recurrence of trauma is likely, efforts are made to protect the joint from any further injury (i.e., athletic appliance). When synovitis is present secondary to the microtrauma associated with a disc derangement, the disc derangement should be treated.

Supportive Therapy

The patient is instructed to restrict all mandibular movement within painless limits. A soft diet, slow movements, and small bites are necessary. Patients who complain of constant pain should receive mild analgesics such as an NSAID. Thermotherapy of the joint area is often helpful, and the patient is instructed to apply moist heat for 10 to 15 minutes four or five times throughout the day.[214,215] Ultrasound therapy can also be helpful for these disorders and is instituted two to four times per week. On occasion, when an acute traumatic injury has been experienced, a single injection of corticosteroid to the capsular tissues is helpful.[216,217] Repeated injections, however, are contraindicated (see Chapter 11).[218] In some instances muscle hyperactivity can coexist with the capsulitis or synovitis. As has been mentioned, muscle hyperactivity can affect the outcome of the inflammatory disorder. Therefore when this activity is suspected, appropriate therapy is initiated (see Chapter 11).

RETRODISCITIS

An inflammatory condition of the retrodiscal tissues is referred to as *retrodiscitis*. This is a relatively common intracapsular disorder.

Cause

The cause of retrodiscitis is usually trauma. Two distinct types of trauma need to be considered: extrinsic and intrinsic. Extrinsic trauma is created by a sudden movement of the condyle into the retrodiscal tissues. When a blow to the chin is received, the condyles are likely to be forced posteriorly into the retrodiscal tissues. Gross posterior displacement is resisted by both the outer oblique and the inner horizontal portions of the temporomandibular ligament. This ligament is so effective that a severe blow will often fracture the neck of

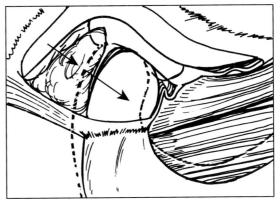

Fig. 13-21 RETRODISCITIS. Trauma to the retrodiscal tissues can lead to swelling. With swelling of these tissues, the condyle can be displaced anteriorly and inferiorly. This results in an acute malocclusion that clinically appears as a lack of posterior tooth contacts on the ipsilateral side.

the condyle instead of displacing it posteriorly. However, with both severe and mild trauma the possibility exists that the condyle will be momentarily forced into the retrodiscal tissues. These tissues often respond to this type of trauma with inflammation, which leads to swelling. Swelling of the retrodiscal tissues can force the condyle forward, resulting in an acute malocclusion[219] (Fig. 13-21). When such a condition exists, the patient complains of an inability to bite on the posterior teeth on the ipsilateral side, and if force is applied, increased pain is elicited in the offending joint. On occasion, trauma to the retrodiscal tissues will cause intracapsular hemarthrosis. This is a serious complication in retrodiscitis and may lead to adhesions and/or ankylosis of the joint.[220]

Retrodiscitis caused by intrinsic trauma is a different problem. Intrinsic trauma to the retrodiscal tissues is likely to occur when an anterior displacement or dislocation of the disc is present. As the disc becomes more anteriorly positioned, the condyle assumes a position on the posterior border of the disc, as well as on the retrodiscal tissues (Fig. 13-22). In many instances these tissues cannot withstand forces provided by the condyle, and the intrinsic trauma causes inflammation.

Retrodiscitis caused by these two different etiologies is likely to present with the same clinical characteristics. This is a problem because

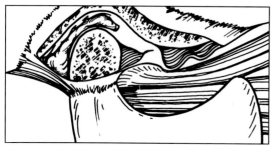

Fig. 13-22 As the disc becomes more anteriorly displaced or dislocated, the condyle rests more on the posterior border of the disc and retrodiscal tissues.

the treatment is different. Therefore the history is extremely important in determining proper therapy.

History

Patients experiencing retrodiscitis caused by extrinsic trauma will report the incidence in the history. Usually patients know exactly what produced their pain condition, which is important because the cause is no longer present.

Patients experiencing retrodiscitis caused by intrinsic trauma will report a more subtle history with a gradual onset of the pain problem. They are also likely to report the progressive onset of the condition (i.e., clicking, catching). Noting this is important because, in this case, the cause of the disorder is still present.

Clinical Characteristics

Retrodiscitis produces constant preauricular pain that is accentuated with jaw movement. Clenching the teeth usually increases the pain. If the tissues swell, a loss of posterior occlusal contact can occur on the ipsilateral side.

Because the treatment of retrodiscitis is different according to cause, the various treatments are discussed separately.

Definitive Treatment for Retrodiscitis from Extrinsic Trauma

Because the causative factor of macrotrauma is generally no longer present, there is no definitive treatment indicated. Therefore supportive therapy to establish optimum conditions for healing is generally the most effective treatment. When trauma is likely to recur, care must be taken to protect the joint.

Supportive Therapy for Retrodiscitis from Extrinsic Trauma

Supportive therapy begins with careful observation of the occlusal condition. If no evidence of acute malocclusion is found, the patient is given analgesics for pain and instructed to restrict movement to within painless limits and begin a soft diet. To decrease the likelihood of ankylosis, however, movement is encouraged. Ultrasound and thermotherapy are often helpful in reducing pain. If pain persists for several weeks, a single intracapsular injection of corticosteroids may be used in isolated cases of trauma, but repeated injections are contraindicated.[218] As symptoms resolve, the reestablishment of normal mandibular movement is encouraged.

When an acute malocclusion exists, clenching the teeth can further aggravate the inflamed retrodiscal tissues. A stabilization-type appliance should be fabricated to provide occlusal stability while the tissues repair. This appliance will lessen further loading of the retrodiscal tissues. The appliance must be regularly adjusted as the retrodiscal tissues return to normal (see the last section in this chapter).

Definitive Treatment for Retrodiscitis from Intrinsic Trauma

Unlike extrinsic trauma, intrinsic trauma often remains and continues to cause injury to the tissues. Definitive treatment therefore is directed toward eliminating the traumatic condition. When retrodiscitis is a result of an anteriorly displaced or dislocated disc with reduction, treatment is directed toward establishing a proper condyle-disc relationship. An anterior positioning appliance is used to reposition the condyle off the retrodiscal tissues and onto the disc. This often immediately relieves the pain. The appliance is usually worn only at night, allowing the mandible to assume a normal relationship in the fossa during the day. The treatment sequence for anteriorly displaced and dislocated discs with reduction is followed from this point forward.

Supportive Therapy for Retrodiscitis from Intrinsic Trauma

Supportive therapy begins with voluntarily restricting use of the mandible to within painless limits. Analgesics are prescribed when pain is not resolved with the positioning appliance. Thermotherapy and ultrasound can be helpful in controlling symptoms. Because the inflammatory condition is often chronic, intraarticular injection of corticosteroids is generally not indicated.

ARTHRITIDES

Arthritis means inflammation of the articular surfaces of the joint. Several types of arthritides can affect the TMJ. The following categories are used: osteoarthritis, osteoarthrosis, and polyarthritides.

Osteoarthritis

Osteoarthritis is one of the most common arthritides affecting the TMJ. The clinician therefore needs to understand this disorder and its natural course of progression. Osteoarthritis has also been referred to as *degenerative joint disease*.

Cause. The most common causative factor that either causes or contributes to osteoarthritis is overloading of the articular structures of the joint. This may occur when joint surfaces are compromised by disc dislocation and retrodiscitis. It would appear that this condition is not a true inflammatory response. Rather, it is a noninflammatory condition in which the articular surfaces and their underlying bone deteriorate. The precise cause is unknown, but it is generally thought[34,36,221-224] to be caused by mechanical overloading of the joint. When bony changes are active, the condition is often painful and referred to as *osteoarthritis*.

When the precise cause of the osteoarthritis can be identified, the condition is referred to as *secondary osteoarthritis*. For example, a disc dislocation without reduction can produce a secondary osteoarthritic condition. When the cause of the arthritic condition cannot be determined, it is referred to as *primary osteoarthritis*.

History. The patient with osteoarthritis usually reports unilateral joint pain that is aggravated by mandibular movement. The pain is usually constant but often worsens in the late afternoon or evening.

Secondary central excitatory effects are frequently present.

Clinical Characteristics. Limited mandibular opening is characteristic because of the joint pain. A soft end feel is common unless the osteoarthritis is associated with an anteriorly dislocated disc. Crepitation can typically be felt, especially if the condition has been present for some time. Lateral palpation of the condyle increases the pain, as does manual loading of the joint (see Chapter 10). The diagnosis is usually confirmed by TMJ radiographs, which will reveal evidence of structural changes in the subarticular bone of the condyle or fossa (flattening, osteophytes, erosions; see Chapter 9) (Figs. 13-23 and 13-24). One must appreciate that a patient may have symptoms for as long as 6 months before there is enough demineralization of bone to show up radiographically. Therefore in early cases of osteoarthritis, radiographs may appear normal and are not helpful in confirming the diagnosis.

Definitive Treatment. Because mechanical overloading of the joint structures is the major causative factor, treatment should attempt to decrease this loading. If possible, an attempt should be made to correct the condyle-disc relationship (anterior positioning appliance therapy). Unfortunately, osteoarthritis is usually associated with chronic derangements and therefore positioning appliances are not always helpful.

When muscle hyperactivity is suspected, a stabilization appliance is indicated to decrease the loading force. If this appliance accentuates the joint pain, a slight forward positioning into a pain-free condylar position needs to be developed. The patient is instructed to wear the appliance during sleep. During waking hours, however, an awareness of parafunctional activity is also necessary, along with attempts to control it voluntarily. Any oral habits that create pain in the joint must be identified and discouraged. Physical self-regulations techniques can also be helpful and should be initiated. If the patient finds relief in wearing the appliance through the day, this is encouraged.

Supportive Therapy. Before therapy begins for osteoarthritis, the clinician needs to understand the natural course of this disorder. In most instances osteoarthritis is a self-limiting disorder.[75,76,221,225-228]

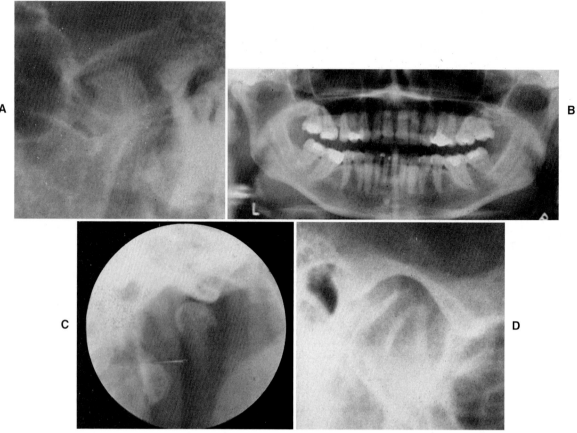

Fig. 13-23 OSTEOARTHRITIS. A, Transcranial view. Note the flattened articular surfaces and the osteophyte. **B,** Panoramic view showing the changes in the left temporomandibular joint. **C,** Transpharyngeal view of the left condyle. The alteration in form, especially the osteophyte (lipping), is shown. **D,** Transcranial view showing erosion of the lateral pole of the condyle.

As joint structures become less loaded, whether by definitive treatment or by natural remodeling processes, symptoms resolve. Long-term studies of disc derangement disorders and osteoarthritis[229] have suggested that the majority of patients seem to pass through three stages, each made up of two phases.

The first stage includes the phases of joint clicking and catching (pain may or may not be present). The second stage includes restriction of movement (locking) and pain. The third stage contains a phase in which there is a decrease in pain but joint sounds are present, followed by a second phase in which there is a return to the normal range of

painless movement with a reduction of joint sounds. Patients seem to follow this course of osteoarthritis even without treatment. It appears that approximately 80% of the patients progress through these three stages, with 60% showing the clinical manifestations of each of the six phases.

Understanding that this type of arthritide is often self-limiting affects the type of treatment indicated. Certainly no routine indication for aggressive therapy exists. Conservative, supportive therapy is all that is indicated for most patients. Some clinicians have even questioned that if the disorder is self-limiting, why even treat it? Studies[230] do show that conservative treatment is

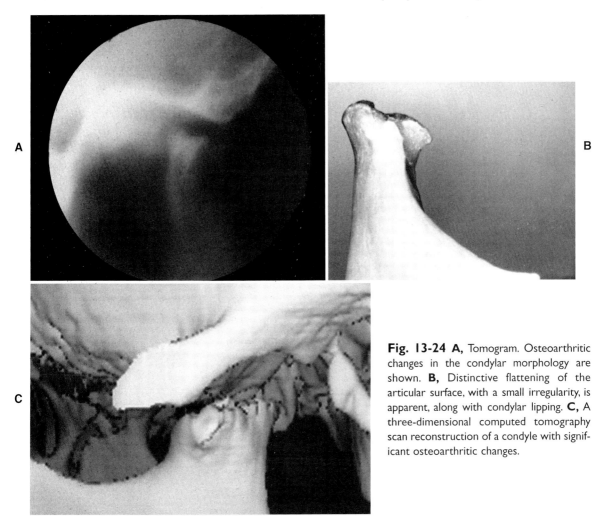

Fig. 13-24 A, Tomogram. Osteoarthritic changes in the condylar morphology are shown. **B,** Distinctive flattening of the articular surface, with a small irregularity, is apparent, along with condylar lipping. **C,** A three-dimensional computed tomography scan reconstruction of a condyle with significant osteoarthritic changes.

indicated for most patients because it is likely to reduce symptoms quicker and perhaps speed up the adaptive process.

Supportive therapy for osteoarthritis begins with an explanation of the disease process to the patient. Reassurance is given that the condition normally runs a course of degeneration and then repair. The symptoms usually follow a standard bell curve, becoming more severe for the first 4 to 7 months, then leveling off around 8 to 9 months, and finally lessening from 10 to 12 months. Along with the fabrication of an appliance in a comfortable mandibular position, pain medication and antiinflammatory agents are prescribed

to decrease the general inflammatory response. The patient is instructed to restrict movement to within painless limits. A soft diet is instituted. Thermotherapy is usually helpful in reducing symptoms. Passive muscle exercises within painless limits are encouraged to lessen the likelihood of myostatic or myofibrotic contracture of the elevator muscles, as well as to maintain function of the joint. Because the inflammatory condition is chronic, intracapsular injections of corticosteroids are contraindicated.

In most cases osteoarthritis is successfully managed with this supportive therapy and time. However, some patients have symptoms so severe that they are not successfully managed with this technique. When symptoms remain intolerable after 1 or 2 months of supportive therapy, a single injection of corticosteroids to the involved joint is indicated in an attempt to control symptoms.[231] If this is unsuccessful, it may be advisable to consider surgical intervention.

On occasion, after the symptoms associated with osteoarthritis have resolved, the sequelae of the disorder may need to be treated. If the osteoarthritis was unilateral and severe, a significant amount of subarticular bone may have been lost. This condition has been referred to as *idiopathic condylar resorption*.[232-234] With idiopathic condylar resorption the bone loss is usually rapid, resulting in a sudden loss of posterior support in the involved condyle. The mandible can then shift to the ipsilateral side. The posterior teeth on that side become fulcrums for the mandible as it shifts. The result is heavy occlusal contacts on the ipsilateral side and a posterior open bite on the contralateral side (Figs. 13-25 and 13-26).

Osteoarthrosis

Now that the natural course of osteoarthritis is understood, osteoarthrosis has meaning. When bony changes are active, the condition is

called *osteoarthritis*. As remodeling occurs the condition can become stable, yet the bony morphology remains altered. This condition is referred to as *osteoarthrosis*.

Cause. As with osteoarthritis, the cause of osteoarthrosis is joint overloading. When joint loading is mild, bony remodeling occurs without symptoms. This is nature's way of adapting to the functional demands of the system. If functional demands exceed adaptability, osteoarthritis begins. Once the adaptive process has caught up to the functional demands, osteoarthrosis remains.

History. Because osteoarthrosis represents a stable adaptive phase, symptoms are not reported by the patient. The past history may reveal a period of time when symptoms were present (osteoarthritis).

Clinical Characteristics. Osteoarthrosis is confirmed when structural changes in the subarticular bone are seen on radiographs but no clinical symptoms of pain are reported by the patient. Crepitation is common.

Definitive Treatment. Because osteoarthrosis represents an adaptive process, no therapy is indicated for the condition. In the past, some clinicians would take radiographs of the TMJs and, after seeing bone changes, would suggest treatment for these changes. In the absence of clinical symptoms

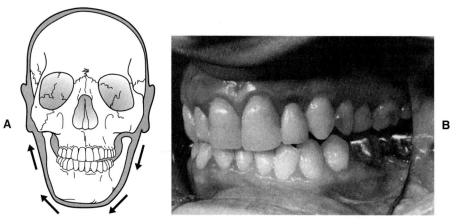

Fig. 13-25 Osteoarthritis or traumatic arthritis can lead to significant loss of subarticular bone in the condyle. **A,** Once significant bone loss has occurred in the right condyle and the right masseter and temporal muscles contract, the condyle moves more superiorly to contact the opposing articular surface. This causes heavy posterior tooth contacts on the right side. The left condyle is forced inferiorly by the fulcruming effect of the right molars, and a left posterior open bite is created. **B,** Clinical results of significant subarticular bone loss.

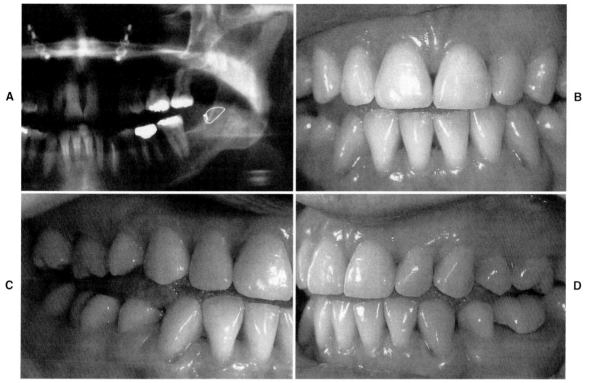

Fig. 13-26 A, This radiograph reveals idiopathic condylar resorption of the left condyle. The majority of this bone loss occurred in a 3-month period of time. **B,** As a consequence of this significant and rapid bone loss, the mandible was shifted to the left side, where only the left second molars contact. **C,** As the left masseter and temporal muscles contract, the mandible is shifted to the left, resulting in a significant posterior open bite on the patient's right side. **D,** Only the second molars contact on the affected side.

(i.e., joint pain), treatment of this arthritide is contraindicated. The only treatment that may need to be considered is if the bony changes in the condyle have been significant enough to alter the occlusal condition. If orthopedic instability has been produced, dental therapy may need to be considered. This, however, is quite rare.

Polyarthritides

The polyarthritides represent a group of arthritic conditions that are less common but certainly can occur in the TMJ. These arthritides present similar symptoms and clinical findings as osteoarthritis but have different, specific causes. Identifying the particular arthritide is important so that the cause can be properly addressed. Once the cause is

addressed, supportive therapy follows similar guidelines to the other arthritides. The following six categories are discussed briefly: traumatic arthritis, infectious arthritis, rheumatoid arthritis, hyperuricemia, psoriatic arthritis, and ankylosing spondylitis. If interested, the reader can find a more complete description in other references.

Traumatic Arthritis. When the condyle receives sudden macrotrauma, a secondary arthritic condition can develop.[235,236] This traumatic arthritic condition can lead to sudden loss of subarticular bone, which may lead to a change in the occlusal condition.[237] A similar condition called *avascular necrosis* has been reported in the hip, but at this time it has not been well documented in the TMJ.

Definitive treatment. Because gross trauma is the most common cause of traumatic arthritis, definitive treatment is not indicated. The trauma is no longer present. When future trauma is expected, the jaw should be protected (e.g., a mouth protector for sports).

Supportive therapy. Supportive therapy begins with rest. Jaw use should be decreased, with a soft diet instituted (small bites and slow chewing). Nonsteroidal antiinflammatory medications are given to reduce the inflammation. Moist heat is often helpful. If symptoms do not resolve in a reasonable time (7 to 10 days), physical therapy (ultrasound) may be indicated. A stabilization appliance is indicated if there is increased pain to occlude the teeth or if bruxism is present.

Although rare, a change in the occlusal condition can occur when significant bony support is lost. When this occurs, dental therapy may be indicated to improve the orthopedic stability. Dental therapy should not begin until symptoms have been totally resolved. The use of a bone scan can be helpful in determining the amount of bony activity in the involved joint.

Infectious Arthritis. Occasionally, a bacterial infection can invade the TMJ.[238,239] The most likely cause of such infectious arthritis is trauma such as a puncture wound. A spreading infection from adjacent structures is also possible.

Definitive treatment. Definitive treatment for an infectious arthritis is to initiate appropriate antibiotic medication to eliminate the invading organism. If the infection has spread from an adjacent structure, the original source of the infection must be treated.

Supportive therapy. Emphasis should not be placed on supportive therapy because it plays only a minor role in managing the disorder. After the infection has been controlled, supportive therapy may be considered and should be directed at maintaining or increasing the normal range of mandibular movement to avoid postinfection fibrosis or adhesions. Passive exercises and ultrasound may be helpful.

Rheumatoid Arthritis. Rheumatoid arthritis is a chronic systemic disorder of unknown cause. This condition produces a persistent inflammatory synovitis that leads to the destruction of the articular surfaces and subarticular bone.[240-245] This condition is likely related to an autoimmune disorder with a strong genetic factor.[246] About 50% of patients with rheumatoid arthritis will present with TMJ complaints.[247] About 80% of rheumatoid patients are seropositive for rheumatoid factor.[248] Although not conclusive, this test is helpful in identifying rheumatoid arthritis. In one radiographic study[249] two thirds of the patients with rheumatoid arthritis demonstrated erosive changes in the TMJs.

Definitive treatment. Because the cause of rheumatoid arthritis is unknown, there is no definite treatment.

Supportive therapy. Supportive therapy for rheumatoid arthritis is directed toward pain reduction. Sometimes a stabilization appliance can decrease forces on the articular surfaces and thereby decrease pain. This is especially helpful when clenching or bruxism is suspected. Arthrocentesis and arthroscopic procedures may be helpful with the acute symptoms associated with rheumatoid arthritis.[135,147]

The occlusion of rheumatoid patients should be closely monitored because gross loss of condylar support can cause major occlusal changes. A common finding in advanced rheumatoid arthritis is heavy posterior occlusal contacts with the development of an anterior open bite,[250] which can greatly compromise the patient's function (Fig. 13-27).[251] Because rheumatoid arthritis usually affects both joints, the open bite is most often symmetric. Improvement of the occlusion is always a possibility, but the clinician must be aware that rheumatoid arthritis has no known cause and often goes through periods of remission only to be active again later. During a remission period the clinician may suggest restoring the occlusal condition to a more orthopedically stable relationship. However, at some time in the future there is a great possibility that the condition will become active again and more bone may be lost. This makes permanently treating the malocclusion risky and unpredictable.

Hyperuricemia (Gout). Hyperuricemia or gout is an arthritic condition in which an increase in serum urate concentration precipitates urate crystals (monosodium urate monohydrate) in certain joints. The distal extremities are most commonly

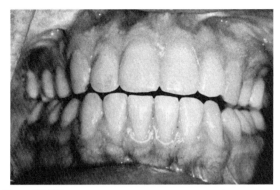

Fig. 13-27 Rheumatoid arthritis commonly causes a significant and relatively rapid loss of the articular bone of both condyles. With this loss of posterior support to the mandible, the posterior teeth begin to contact heavily. These teeth act as fulcrums by which the mandible rotates, collapsing posteriorly and opening anteriorly. The result is an anterior open bite.

affected with the great toe being involved 90% of the time.[252] Gout is primarily a condition of adult males, with women accounting for only 5% of the reported cases.[253,254] A genetic factor appears to be involved in this disorder. A serum laboratory test can be used to diagnosis hyperuricemia.

Definitive treatment. Because an increase in the serum uric acid level is responsible for the symptoms of gout, definitive treatment is directed toward lowering this level. The most effective method may be merely the elimination of certain foods from the diet. However, because this is a systemic problem, gout is usually best managed on a medical basis by the patient's physician.

Supportive therapy. No supportive therapy for gout exists. The patient's physician will be treating the patient on a medical basis.[255]

Psoriatic Arthritis. Psoriatic arthritis is an inflammatory condition that affects approximately 6% of patients with psoriasis.[253,256-259] Because psoriasis occurs in only 1.2% of the general population, this is not a common TMJ arthritide. Patients usually report a history of chronic psoriatic skin lesions, which helps establish the diagnosis. Although this disorder can clinically appear as rheumatoid arthritis, serologic tests for RH factors are negative. Radiographic changes associated with osteoarthrosis are common.[260]

Definitive treatment. Because the cause of psoriasis and psoriatic arthritis is unknown, there is no definitive treatment available.

Supportive therapy. Because this condition is a systemic disorder, the major treatment should be directed by a rheumatologist. When the TMJ is involved, certain supportive therapies can be applied. Often NSAIDs are helpful. Gentle physical therapy to maintain joint mobility is important because hypomobility is often a consequence of this disorder. On occasion moist heat and ultrasound therapy may reduce symptoms and increase joint mobility.

Ankylosing Spondylitis. A chronic inflammatory disease of unknown cause, ankylosing spondylitis primarily affects the vertebral column. The TMJ is only involved in 4% of the cases, and this condition affects only 1% of the general population. Therefore it is quite rare. This condition is more common in males than females and produces a generalized stiffness in the involved joints. The clinician should be suspicious of ankylosing spondylitis when a patient reports with a painful, hypomobile joint, no history of trauma, and neck or back complaints.[261-265]

Definitive treatment. Because the cause of ankylosing spondylitis is unknown, no definitive treatment is available at this time.

Supportive therapy. Because this condition is a systemic disorder, the major treatment should be directed by a rheumatologist. As with psoriatic arthritis, if the TMJ is involved, certain supportive therapies can be applied. Often NSAIDs are helpful. Gentle physical therapy to improve joint mobility is indicated, but care should be taken not to be too aggressive and increase symptoms. On occasion moist heat and ultrasound therapy may also be helpful.

INFLAMMATORY DISORDERS OF ASSOCIATED STRUCTURES

Associated structures of the masticatory system can become inflamed, producing painful symptoms. Two such structures are tendons and ligaments. Inflammation of these is commonly associated with chronic elongation or distractive forces. Hyperactive muscles are a frequent cause of tendon and ligament inflammation. Two conditions produce this: temporalis tendonitis and stylomandibular ligament inflammation.

Temporalis Tendonitis

The large fan-shaped temporalis muscle inserts inferiorly on the coronoid process. Chronic hyperactivity of this muscle can create a tendonitis (similar to tennis elbow).[266-269] The condition is characterized by pain during function (e.g., chewing or yawning). Another common complaint is retroorbital pain. Intraoral palpation of the attachment of the ligament to the coronoid process elicits significant pain; local anesthetic blocking of this area eliminates the pain.

Definitive Treatment. Definitive treatment is directed toward resting the muscle. A stabilization appliance may be used if clenching or bruxism is suspected. Instituting physical self-regulation techniques can be helpful in resting the muscle.

Supportive Therapy. Painful symptoms from a temporalis tendonitis should be managed with analgesics so that any central excitatory effects are minimized. Antiinflammatory medications are also advised. Physical therapy (e.g., ultrasound) may be helpful, and on occasion an injection of corticosteroid into the tendon followed by rest will be effective.

Stylomandibular Ligament Inflammation

Inflammation of the stylomandibular ligament has been described by Ernest et al.[267] The main symptom is pain at the angle of the mandible radiating up to the joint and ear. Protrusion of the mandible seems to aggravate the pain because this movement elongates the ligament. An injection of local anesthetic to this region will significantly reduce the patient's complaint.

Definitive Treatment. As with temporalis tendonitis, rest is an appropriate treatment. Instituting physical self-regulation techniques can be helpful in resting the muscle. A stabilization appliance is not likely to have a positive effect, however, unless the patient reports an association between the pain and parafunctional activity.

Supportive Therapy. Supportive therapy consists of analgesics and antiinflammatory medications. Ultrasound may also be of some help.

When symptoms are persistent, an injection of local anesthetic or corticosteroid into the attachment of the ligament at the angle of the mandible may help resolve the condition.[270]

GENERAL CONSIDERATIONS WHEN TREATING ACUTE TRAUMA TO THE TEMPOROMANDIBULAR JOINT

Patients who experience acute trauma to the TMJ are managed differently than those with chronic conditions. At the initial examination the clinician should evaluate for any soft and hard tissue damage. Hard tissue damage such as a maxillary or mandibular fracture including a condylar fracture will often produce a significant acute malocclusion, as well as an altered opening pathway (deflections). Radiographs should be taken following significant trauma to determine damage to bony structures and the teeth. Fractures to the bones or teeth need to be identified immediately so that proper treatment can begin.

Once the hard tissues have been examined and initially managed, the soft tissues of the joint need to be evaluated. Treatment for soft tissue damage is escalated according to the severity of the symptoms. If there is no significant change in range of movement and little pain, the patient is merely told to decrease use, begin a soft diet, and generally rest the jaw for 2 weeks. Patients should be reminded to not chew gum and to decrease parafunctional activities when possible. The patient is instructed to return to the office if there is any increase in pain, and an appointment is set for reevaluation in 2 weeks.

Patients with significant pain and a marked decrease in the range of movement should be closely evaluated for any acute malocclusion. If no acute malocclusion is noted, treatment should be escalated to include mild analgesics for pain and physical therapy to the pain site. For the first 24 to 36 hours following the trauma, ice can be repeatedly placed over the joint for 5 minutes at 15-minute intervals. After 1 to 2 days, ice is discontinued and moist heat is applied repeatedly throughout the day. Function should be restricted to painless limits so as not to initiate central excitatory effects.

Patients who have significant pain and demonstrate an acute malocclusion may need to receive additional treatment. As already discussed, acute trauma to retrodiscal tissues can produce swelling, temporarily displacing the condyle slightly forward away from the musculoskeletally stable position. This produces a disengagement of the ipsilateral posterior teeth. When the patient attempts to occlude the posterior teeth, pain is elicited as force is placed on the painful retrodiscal tissues. A stabilization appliance would be appropriate for this patient in order to keep the condyle from loading the retrodiscal tissues during healing. This is especially true if bruxism is present. The stabilization appliance is fabricated in a comfortable closing position for the patient and not necessarily in the normal musculoskeletally stable position of the condyle. As the acute symptoms resolve, the retrodiscal tissues will return to normal, allowing the condyle to resume the musculoskeletally stable position. As this occurs the clinician will need to adjust the appliance to obtain the proper fit.

As the pain resolves, the patient needs to be reevaluated for any residual symptoms. Joint movement should be reinitiated as soon as possible so as to avoid fibrous adhesions. Residual changes in the condyle-disc complex should be evaluated. If a disc derangement disorder is present, it should be managed as previously described.

Case Reports

Case 1

A 27-year-old insurance salesman came to the dental office complaining of a single click in the right TMJ on opening. He reported that the joint sound had begun 2 days after his third molars were removed (under general anesthesia) 3 weeks earlier. Some relatively slight pain (3/10) was associated with the clicking, but the patient was able to function normally. The pain was not aggravated with jaw function.

The single click occurred in the right TMJ at an interincisal distance of 4 mm of opening immediately after clenching. The muscle and joint examinations did not reveal any pain or tenderness except when the mouth was opened to the point of the click. At this moment slight pain was felt. Biting on a single tongue depressor between the posterior teeth eliminated the click. The occlusal examination

revealed a healthy dentition with no missing or carious teeth. A centric relation (CR)–to–intercuspal position (ICP) slide of 0.5 mm with anterior eccentric guidance existed. A panoramic radiograph revealed normally healing third molar extraction sites and no other abnormalities. Transcranial radiographs of the TMJ revealed no bony or functional abnormalities. No other significant findings were disclosed by the clinical examination.

DIAGNOSIS. The patient was diagnosed with disc displacement secondary to acute trauma received during either intubations or third molar extractions.

TREATMENT. An anterior positioning appliance that increased the vertical dimension 1 mm and repositioned the mandible approximately 1 mm anteriorly was fabricated. At this position the click was eliminated. The patient was instructed to wear the appliance at night while sleeping and during the day if necessary to reduce pain. After 8 weeks of this therapy the patient reported that the clicking was almost gone and was present only during heavy chewing. The patient was informed that this residual clicking might always be present. He did not seem to be concerned. The use of the appliance was gradually reduced. At the next regular 6-month recall appointment, the patient reported no pain and was experiencing a click only occasionally. ■

Case 2

A 32-year-old female secretary complained of right TMJ tenderness and sounds. She also reported generalized facial muscle tightness with occasional tenderness. The joint complaints had been present for 4 days and had been recurring about every 2 months. The history revealed no trauma or previous treatment for the prior episodes. It appeared that there was a relationship between the recurrence of joint symptoms and a heavy workload associated with alternate monthly deadlines.

The clinical examination revealed a single click in the right TMJ at 3 mm of opening. The joint was tender to palpation (score, 1). The left joint was asymptomatic. The examination also revealed that the right masseter muscle and left and right temporalis muscles were tender (score, 1). The left masseter, left sternocleidomastoid, and posterior neck muscles were painful (score, 2). The right lateral pterygoid muscle was also painful to functional manipulation (score, 3). The occlusal examination disclosed a generally healthy dentition with moderate wear on the canines and posterior teeth. The woman had no missing teeth, caries, or significant periodontal disease. A panoramic radiograph was found to be within normal limits. No other significant findings occurred on the clinical examination.

DIAGNOSIS. The primary diagnosis was disc displacement. The secondary diagnosis was local muscle soreness.

Both these diagnoses were related to parafunctional activity associated with increases in emotional stress.

TREATMENT. The relationship of the patient's heavy workload, emotional stress, and parafunctional activity to the condition, as well as the symptoms produced, were discussed with the patient. Alternate work patterns were suggested to lighten peak workloads. Physical self-regulation techniques were initiated, and the patient was instructed to spend at least 20 minutes per day developing these skills. A stabilization appliance was fabricated. It eliminated the joint sound. The patient was instructed to wear the appliance while sleeping and during the day only if needed to reduce pain. After 1 week she reported about 50% reduction of symptoms. After 2 weeks the symptoms were nearly completely reduced, and in 1 additional week all symptoms were eliminated. The patient then discontinued the use of the appliance but continued to develop her physical self-regulation skills. If at some time in the future the symptoms returned, she was to use these skills to reduce the symptoms. If the symptoms were not immediately reduced, appliance therapy would be reinstituted. During a regular 6-month recall appointment the patient reported two episodes, which were managed successfully with physical self-regulation skills. ∎

Case 3

A 42-year-old female homemaker came to the dental office with left TMJ pain and sounds. Associated with the symptoms was occasional muscle pain. The symptoms had begun approximately 10 months earlier and had gradually gotten worse. She commented that she could no longer open without "popping" of the left joint. She was unable to associate any specific event relating to the onset of the symptoms. However, if she yawned, the pain and clicking were increased for several hours.

The clinical examination revealed reciprocal clicking in the left TMJ. The initial click occurred at 10 mm of opening, and the closing click at 5 mm. A minimum thickness of two tongue blades between the posterior teeth eliminated the joint sounds. The left TMJ was tender to palpation (score, 1), especially during movements that accentuated the sounds. The right joint was asymptomatic. No unusual findings occurred in the panoramic radiograph regarding the general shape and contour of the TMJs. The clinical examination revealed muscle tenderness in the left and right masseters, the left temporalis, and the left sternocleidomastoid (all scores, 1). The left lateral pterygoid muscle was painful to functional manipulation (score, 2). The occlusal examination revealed a healthy dentition, without any sign of dental disease. No other significant findings were identified on the clinical examination.

DIAGNOSIS. The diagnosis was disc displacement with reduction.

TREATMENT. An anterior positioning appliance was fabricated that positioned the mandible forward enough to eliminate the reciprocal clicking in the left TMJ. The patient was instructed to wear this appliance while sleeping and during the day if needed for pain. She was also told to restrict mandibular movements to within painless limits. A mild analgesic was prescribed to be taken on a regular basis for 10 days. In 1 week she returned, reporting that the joint had not "popped" but she needed to wear the appliance a considerable period of time during the day. Since she began wearing the appliance, her pain had almost completely resolved.

After 9 weeks of this therapy she reported no joint pain but a residual clicking. At that time she reported that she was able to reduce wearing the appliance to only nighttime use. After 3 months the clicking had lessened but was still present. She was told that this joint sound would likely be permanent but hopefully there would not be a return of pain. She was instructed to wear the appliance at night only and to call if any pain returned. ∎

Case 4

A 48-year-old male mill worker reported to the dental office complaining of right TMJ sounds. The popping had been present for 15 years and had never caused any pain or discomfort. He had decided to call the office after reading an article in the paper describing treatment for this problem.

The clinical examination revealed a single click in the right TMJ at 31 mm of opening with no associated pain or tenderness. The click could not be eliminated with two tongue depressors placed bilaterally between the posterior teeth. Transcranial radiographs revealed no unusual functional findings or bony changes. The clinical examination for muscle pain was negative. The occlusal examination disclosed a full complement of natural teeth in the maxillary arch, all of which were in good repair. Three missing molars in the mandibular arch had been adequately replaced by a tooth-supported removable partial denture. A 1.5-mm, straight-forward slide existed from the CR to the ICP. Slight-to-moderate tooth wear was evident on the anterior and posterior teeth. No other significant findings were uncovered in the history or clinical examination.

DIAGNOSIS. The diagnosis was chronic adapted disc displacement with reduction.

TREATMENT. The history and examination revealed that this disc displacement was chronic and asymptomatic. No evidence indicated that it was a progressive disorder. In fact, more evidence suggested that the joint tissues had physiologically adapted to the condition. Therefore no definitive treatment was prescribed for this patient. The patient was provided education regarding the cause of the clicking, and he was dismissed with the advice that if the joint sounds changed or became painful, he should return for evaluation. ∎

Case 5

A 27-year-old female telephone operator reported that she was experiencing some jaw locking. She reported that during the past 2.5 months her right TMJ had been making sounds and on occasion had felt as if it were going to get "stuck." She stated that since yesterday, after an episode of clenching, she has not been able to open her mouth completely. Now her jaw feels locked, and the sounds are no longer present. This is the first time that her jaw had actually become locked. She reports little pain unless she tries to open her mouth wide. At that time there is pain in front of her right ear.

The clinical examination revealed tenderness of the right TMJ (score, 1) and no symptoms associated with the left joint. No joint sounds were heard. The patient's maximum interincisal opening was 26 mm with a hard end feel. She had a normal range of lateral movement to the right side (10 mm), but left lateral movement was limited to 4 mm and elicited pain on the right side. The clinical examination for the muscle was negative except for tenderness in the right masseter (score, 1). A complete natural dentition was present, in a good state of repair. Although the occlusal condition looked clinically normal, the patient complained that "the back teeth didn't seem to bite right." A panoramic radiograph was within normal limits with normal TMJ anatomy. No other significant findings were uncovered on clinical examination.

DIAGNOSIS. The diagnosis was disc dislocation without reduction secondary to parafunctional activity.

TREATMENT. An explanation of the disorder was given, and the appropriate treatment was explained to the patient. Because the disc dislocation occurred only 2 days ago, an attempt was made to manually reposition the disc back into its normal position. The manual manipulation was successful, but shortly after closing the disc dislocation recurred. An anterior positioning appliance was fabricated to position the mandible approximately 3 mm anterior to the ICP. The mandible was once again manipulated, and the disc was again successfully reduced. The appliance was immediately placed, and the patient closed in the forward position as determined by the appliance. Repeated opening and closing in this position failed to dislocate the disc. The patient was then instructed to wear the appliance continuously, removing it only for oral hygiene for the next 2 to 3 days. At that time the patient was asked to begin removing the appliance 1 to 2 hours a day, adding 1 to 2 hours each day until it was

only used at nighttime. She was rescheduled to return to the office in 1 week for a follow-up appointment.

She returned in 1 week and reported that the jaw had not relocked but that she was experiencing some muscle pain. The temporalis and masseters were tender bilaterally (score, 1). Analgesics were prescribed along with simple self-regulation techniques. The patient was instructed to continue reducing the use of the appliance to only during the nighttime, allowing the mandible to assume its predislocation position. After 2 weeks she reported feeling comfortable with no recurrence of dislocation. For the next 4 weeks the joint did not lock, but she stated that the right TMJ was feeling "tight" and she was aware of clenching on the teeth again. She related this to job stresses. The appliance was converted to a stabilization type for nocturnal bruxism. She was to wear the appliance during sleep, but she could also wear it during the day at times of high stress and diurnal parafunctional activity. Physical self-regulation strategies were provided and encouraged.

At the 1-year recall appointment, she related that occasionally she would wear the appliance when her muscles or joint began feeling tight. There was no recurrence of joint locking. The patient reported a general reduction in the problem since changing jobs 3 months earlier. ∎

Case 6

A 31-year-old male executive reported to the dental office complaining of tightness and occasional clicking of the left TMJ. The symptoms began shortly after he received a six-unit maxillary anterior fixed partial denture 6 days earlier. He stated that his occlusion had never felt comfortable, and now the joint symptoms were making it more difficult to function. No previous history of this type of problem or any joint discomfort was reported.

The clinical examination revealed tenderness in the right and left temporalis and the left masseter (score, 1). The left lateral pterygoid area was also painful to functional manipulation (score, 2). The examination also revealed tenderness of the left TMJ (score, 1) and a single click in this joint at 4 mm of opening. The occlusal examination revealed relatively sound posterior occlusal contacts and good anterior guidance when the patient was examined in the reclined position in the dental chair. However, when the patient was placed in an upright (alert feeding) position, heavy occlusal contacts existed on the new anterior fixed partial denture, which disallowed stable posterior tooth contacts. These contacts were on the inclines of the lingual fossae of the maxillary crowns, which forced the mandible to be positioned more posteriorly. No symptoms existed in the right joint. Radiographs revealed no unusual functional or articular surface findings. No other significant findings were uncovered in the history or clinical examination.

DIAGNOSIS. The diagnosis was disc displacement with reduction secondary to heavy anterior tooth contact that displaced the mandible posteriorly.

TREATMENT. The heavy occlusal contacts on the new six-unit fixed partial denture were reduced until stable posterior tooth contacts were reestablished. The occlusion was adjusted to contact primarily on the posterior teeth and only lightly on the anterior teeth in the upright position. The eccentric guidance was reevaluated and slightly adjusted to ensure disocclude of the posterior teeth during eccentric movements. The patient was asked to return to the office in 1 week for an evaluation. At that visit he related that by the next day the clicking, along with most of the muscle soreness, had resolved. There was no recurrence of the disorder at the 6-month recall appointment. ■

Case 7

A 42-year-old salesman reported to a dental office for the restoration of several posterior teeth. Immediately following the removal of the rubber dam, the patient could not close his mouth. The patient repeatedly attempted to close and with each failure became increasingly uncomfortable and frustrated. He had earlier related that when opening wide, the joint would commonly hesitate and jump forward, but there was no pain associated with this movement or any history of previous locking.

The clinical examination revealed that the mandible appeared to be positioned anteriorly and opened with the anterior teeth approximately 35 mm apart. The occlusal examination revealed that the posterior teeth were relatively close to their occluding teeth, but the anterior teeth were not. Eccentric movements were nearly impossible for the patient to achieve.

DIAGNOSIS. The diagnosis was spontaneous dislocation secondary to opening wide for a long dental appointment.

TREATMENT. The patient was first asked to open wider while gentle pressure was applied to the chin in a posterior direction. This manipulation failed to resolve the dislocation. The dentist's thumbs were wrapped with gauze, and the rest of the fingers were used to grasp the mandible. Firm but controlled force was placed on the second molars, distracting the condyle away from the fossa. As soon as this inferior distraction force was applied, the mandible immediately reduced itself and the occlusion was reestablished. The patient was reassured with an explanation of the problem. Because he had reported a history of subluxation, he was instructed to maintain normal function within the range that did not provoke this condition. Whenever possible any wide-open mouth procedures were discouraged. It was suggested that food be cut into small pieces, requiring minimal opening. The patient was asked to return to the dental office if recurrence was a problem.

No recurrence was reported at the 6-month and 1-year recall appointments. ■

Case 8

A 17-year-old male high school student reported to the dental office with severe pain in the left TMJ. He had been in a car accident 4 days earlier, and his head had hit the dashboard. He received several cuts around the cheek, eye, and chin. He was treated in a hospital emergency department for these injuries and released. On the day after the accident, his left TMJ was tender and became progressively more painful each day. At the time of his visit the pain was constant and accentuated with mandibular movement. He had no symptoms in this joint before the accident.

The clinical examination revealed an extremely painful left joint (score, 3). The right joint was asymptomatic. No joint sound or noticeable swelling occurred in the joint area. The patient could open only 22 mm interincisally without pain. His maximum opening was 45 mm. The muscle examination disclosed tenderness in the left masseter and right and left temporales (score, 1). The intraoral examination revealed a complete and healthy complement of teeth with no obvious dental disease. No evidence of trauma to any teeth existed. The occlusal condition was within normal limits, and the patient reported that he could bite on his posterior teeth without eliciting pain. Transcranial radiographs revealed no obvious bony changes but restricted functional movement in the left TMJ. Panoramic and anteroposterior (AP) radiographs failed to identify any evidence of condylar fracture. No other significant findings were noted in either the history or clinical examination.

DIAGNOSIS. The diagnosis was capsulitis secondary to extrinsic trauma.

TREATMENT. The patient was instructed to restrict all mandibular movement to within painless limits and to eat only a soft diet. Clock-regulated analgesics were prescribed to control pain. He was encouraged to apply moist heat to the painful joint area for 10 to 15 minutes four to six times a day. Because there was no evidence of parafunctional activity, appliance therapy was not instituted. The patient was asked to return in 3 days, at which time he reported that the pain had decreased but was still present at a significant level. He commented that heat helped considerably. The patient was referred to a physical therapist, who provided ultrasound therapy three times a week for the next 2 weeks. In 1 week he reported that most of the pain had resolved. After 1 additional week of this therapy, he was no longer experiencing pain and was able to resume normal function. Recall visits revealed no recurrence of symptoms. ■

Case 9

A 23-year-old female college student reported that she had been feeling severe pain in the right TMJ beginning 2 days earlier after she had fallen off her bike and hit her chin on the sidewalk. The patient reported that the pain is increased when she moves her jaw and that "her bite had changed." Any attempt to force her teeth back into her old bite was painful. She had no previous history of any type of pain in this joint. However, on occasion she had been aware of left joint sounds.

The clinical examination revealed pain in the right TMJ (score, 2) and no tenderness in the left (score, 1). No noticeable sounds occurred in either joint. The maximum comfortable interincisal opening was 17 mm with a maximum opening of 41 mm. The muscle examination revealed some tenderness of the right temporalis (score, 1). The occlusal examination revealed a relatively normal healthy dentition in a good state of repair. No teeth were missing, and posterior support appeared to be sound. Pain was increased in the right TMJ with manual manipulation into the musculoskeletally stable position. Asking the patient to clench on her posterior teeth significantly increased her pain. When a tongue depressor was placed between the posterior teeth on the right side, clenching did not elicit pain. However, when the tongue depressor was placed on the left side and the patient was asked to clench, significant pain was felt in the right TMJ area. Panoramic and AP radiographs did not disclose any evidence of fracture of the condyle. Transcranial radiographs revealed normal function and subarticular surfaces. No other significant findings were uncovered in the history or clinical examination.

DIAGNOSIS. The diagnosis was retrodiscitis secondary to extrinsic trauma.

TREATMENT. The patient was instructed to restrict all mandibular movement to within painless limits and to begin a soft diet. Analgesics were suggested to control the pain. Thermotherapy was instituted four to six times a day. The patient returned in 5 days and reported that pain was still present and most severe on awakening in the morning. The muscle and joint examination now revealed that other muscles had become tender to palpation: the left and right masseters, the right temporalis, the occipitalis, and the right sternocleidomastoideus (all scores, 1). At this time the clinician considered that parafunctional activity was a coexistent factor and was influencing the outcome of the retrodiscitis.

An occlusal appliance was fabricated in a comfortable mandibular position, and the patient was instructed to wear this during sleep or any time that clenching or bruxing was noticed. Physical self-regulation techniques were provided to the patient. Clock-regulated NSAID therapy (600 mg ibuprofen three times a day) was also initiated. The patient returned in 1 week, reporting 50% reduction of the symptoms.

The same therapy was continued, and in 1 more week she had no symptoms. She was encouraged to continue wearing the appliance at night for 4 more weeks to promote complete healing of the retrodiscal tissues. At that time appliance therapy was discontinued. She reported no recurrence of the symptoms during a 1-year recall appointment. ▪

Case 10

A 34-year-old female homemaker came to the dental office with pain in the right TMJ joint. She reported that this joint had been clicking for several years but approximately 2 months ago became "locked." At that time she could not open her mouth completely. She reported that initially there was no pain unless she tried to force her mouth open. During the past month she has noticed more pain.

The clinical examination revealed a maximum comfortable interincisal opening of 25 mm and a maximum opening of 27 mm. She was able to move the mandible normally in a right lateral direction but was severely restricted in the left lateral movement. The muscle examination disclosed tenderness in the right and left temporal and right and left masseter muscles (all scores, 1). The occlusal examination revealed several missing posterior teeth with considerable drifting of the remaining molars and premolars. The anterior teeth exhibited signs of heavy occlusal contact. When she was asked to clench on her posterior teeth, pain was elicited in the right joint. Biting on a separator did not accentuate the pain but in fact relieved it. Transcranial radiographs revealed limited movement in the right joint. The subarticular surfaces of both joints appeared normal. No other significant findings were reported in the history or clinical examination.

DIAGNOSIS. The diagnosis was an anteriorly dislocated disc of the right TMJ with associated retrodiscitis.

TREATMENT. Initially a stabilization appliance was fabricated, but it was immediately determined that this was not able to reduce the right TMJ pain associated with clenching. The appliance was converted to a slight anterior positioning appliance that was able to bring the condyle slightly forward off the retrodiscal tissues (only 1 to 2 mm forward). This almost immediately eliminated the patient's pain. After 8 weeks of wearing the appliance at night and occasionally during the day, the symptoms resolved. At this time the patient was asked to reduce wearing the appliance, but when she did the pain returned. The appliance was converted to a stabilization type, and she was instructed to wear it at night and during the day as needed for the pain. Over the next 4 weeks, she reported having no pain but needed to wear the appliance most of the time. The musculoskeletally stable position was located with a bilateral manual manipulation technique. This revealed no significant orthopedic instability. After 4 more weeks of appliance therapy the patient still reported the need to wear the appliance each night. Treatment considerations and options were presented to the patient, and an arthrocentesis was selected. The arthrocentesis was performed, and over the next 3 weeks the patient reported significant pain reduction. Over the next year the patient reported two episodes of joint tenderness, which resolved with a soft diet, physical self-regulation techniques, and the nighttime use of the appliance. ■

Case 11

A 47-year-old female college professor came to the dental office complaining of chronic right TMJ pain. She was able to locate it by placing her finger over the distal aspect of the right condyle. The pain had been present for 6 weeks and seemed to be getting worse. It was always present, although less in the morning, and it became worse as the day progressed. She was aware of a grinding sound in her right TMJ. Movement accentuated the pain. On questioning the patient, it was discovered that the right TMJ had "locked" 9 to 10 months previously and she had only recently begun to regain a more normal opening range. She commented that her wide opening was still limited compared with what it had been 1 year ago.

The clinical examination revealed pain in the right TMJ (score, 2) that was accentuated with movement (score, 3). The left joint was only slightly tender to palpation during function (score, 1). The patient experienced pain at 20 mm of interincisal opening but could open to 36 mm maximally. During opening there was a deflection of the midline to the right side. Definite crepitation in the right TMJ was noted. The muscle examination revealed tenderness of the left and right masseters, the left and right temporalis, and the left sternocleidomastoid (score, 1). The occlusal examination disclosed one missing molar in each posterior quadrant that had been replaced by fixed partial dentures. The crown and bridge had originally been constructed to develop a coincident CR and ICP. However, it was noted that in the upright (alert feeding) position the anterior teeth contacted more heavily than the posterior teeth. Adequate guidance was provided by the anterior teeth during eccentric movement. The fixed partial dentures had been present for a little more than a year. A panoramic radiograph revealed a definite alteration in the subarticular surfaces in the right condyle consistent with osteoarthritis. Tomographic radiographs were ordered, and they confirmed the presences of osteoarthritic changes in the right condyle. No history of any systemic arthritic conditions was reported, and no other significant findings were evident in the history or occlusal examination.

DIAGNOSIS. The primary diagnosis was osteoarthritis secondary to functional anterior disc dislocation without reduction. The secondary diagnosis was protective co-contraction and local muscle soreness secondary to chronic joint pain.

TREATMENT. The patient was informed of the cause and prognosis of osteoarthritis. She was told that the disease is often self-limiting but that the course of the symptoms might last 8 to 12 months. It was emphasized that conservative therapy is usually successful in controlling pain and helps to limit the inflammatory process.

A stabilization appliance was fabricated and tested for comfort. In the alert feeding position it relieved forces on the anterior teeth. The patient could clench while wearing the appliance without eliciting pain. She was to wear it at night while sleeping and during certain times of the day if it relieved the pain. She was also to restrict jaw movement to within painless limits and begin a soft diet. Physical self-regulation techniques were provided to the patient, and she was encouraged to use these daily. Analgesic and antiinflammatory medications were prescribed on a regular basis for 4 weeks. Thermotherapy was suggested several times each day.

Because the heavy anterior tooth contacts in the upright alert feeding position were suspected as a causative factor leading to the dislocation of the disc, these were reduced, which allowed the posterior teeth to occlude more heavily. The patient returned in 1 week, reporting a considerable decrease in pain. The same therapy was continued, and she began passive exercises within painless limits to maintain a normal range of movement. She complained that she had a limited range of painless movement but was reassured that with time this would change. The therapy continued for 1 month, and she returned to the office. At that time there was only occasional pain, generally associated with movements extending into the border ranges. She was encouraged, and treatment continued. After 6 months she was no longer experiencing pain and had regained a comfortable opening range of 39 mm.

One year after the initial visit, a second panoramic radiograph revealed the form of the condyle to be the same as in the pretreatment radiograph. Because the symptoms had subsided 6 months earlier, it was assumed that the condyle had progressively remodeled to a phase of osteoarthrosis. ■

Case 12

A 55-year-old salesman reported to the dental office complaining of bilateral TMJ pain that had been relatively constant for 2 weeks and was accentuated by movement. He could open only 11 mm without pain, but his maximum opening was 42 mm. In questioning, it was identified that this type of pain had been experienced 1 year earlier and had seemed to resolve without treatment. Although there was no history of trauma, when questioned regarding other arthritic conditions he commented that his great right toe and left fingers also had become painful. This corresponded to the previous episodes of pain.

The clinical examination revealed bilateral TMJ pain during movements (score, 2). The muscle examination did not disclose any significant tenderness. The occlusal examination revealed a complete natural dentition in relatively good repair, with a 1.5-mm slide from CR to ICP. A cross-bite relationship existed in the left premolar area. A panoramic radiograph showed normal subarticular surfaces and range of movement.

Blood studies for serum uric acid levels were ordered, and the results confirmed hyperuricemia.

DIAGNOSIS. The diagnosis was hyperuricemia (gout).

TREATMENT. The patient was referred to his physician for systemic management of the condition. ■

References

1. Rieder CE, Martinoff JT, Wilcox SA: The prevalence of mandibular dysfunction. Part I: sex and age distribution of related signs and symptoms, *J Prosthet Dent* 50:81-88, 1983.

2. De Laat A, Steenberghe DV: Occlusal relationships and temporomandibular joint dysfunction. I. Epidemiologic findings, *J Prosthet Dent* 54:835-842, 1985.

3. Gazit E, Lieberman M, Eini R, Hirsch N, Serfaty V et al: Prevalence of mandibular dysfunction in 10-18 year old Israeli schoolchildren, *J Oral Rehabil* 11:307-317, 1984.

4. Swanljung O, Rantanen T: Functional disorders of the masticatory system in southwest Finland, *Community Dent Oral Epidemiol* 7:177-182, 1979.

5. Osterberg T, Carlsson GE: Symptoms and signs of mandibular dysfunction in 70-year-old men and women in Gothenburg, Sweden, *Community Dent Oral Epidemiol* 7:315-321, 1979.

6. Solberg WK, Woo MW, Houston JB: Prevalence of mandibular dysfunction in young adults, *J Am Dent Assoc* 98:25-34, 1979.

7. Keeling SD, McGorray S, Wheeler TT, King GJ: Risk factors associated with temporomandibular joint sounds in children 6 to 12 years of age, *Am J Orthod Dentofacial Orthop* 105:279-287, 1994.

8. De Kanter RJ, Truin GJ, Burgersdijk RC, Van 't Hof MA, Battistuzzi PH et al: Prevalence in the Dutch adult population and a meta-analysis of signs and symptoms of temporomandibular disorder, *J Dent Res* 72:1509-1518, 1993.

9. Salonen L, Hellden L, Carlsson GE: Prevalence of signs and symptoms of dysfunction in the masticatory system: an epidemiologic study in an adult Swedish population, *J Craniomandib Disord* 4:241-250, 1990.

10. Spruijt RJ, Wabeke KB: An extended replication study of dental factors associated with temporomandibular joint sounds, *J Prosthet Dent* 75:388-392, 1996.

11. Kononen M, Waltimo A, Nystrom M: Does clicking in adolescence lead to painful temporomandibular joint locking? *Lancet* 347:1080-1081, 1996.

12. Milam SB, Zardeneta G, Schmitz JP: Oxidative stress and degenerative temporomandibular joint disease: a proposed hypothesis, *J Oral Maxillofac Surg* 56:214-223, 1998.

13. Nitzan DW: The process of lubrication impairment and its involvement in temporomandibular joint disc displacement: a theoretical concept, *J Oral Maxillofac Surg* 59:36-45, 2001.

14. Nitzan DW, Nitzan U, Dan P, Yedgar S: The role of hyaluronic acid in protecting surface-active phospholipids from lysis by exogenous phospholipase A(2), *Rheumatol (Oxford)* 40:336-340, 2001.

15. Nitzan DW, Marmary Y: The "anchored disc phenomenon": a proposed etiology for sudden-onset, severe, and persistent closed lock of the temporomandibular joint, *J Oral Maxillofac Surg* 55:797-802; discussion 802-803, 1997.

16. Yamaguchi A, Tojyo I, Yoshida H, Fujita S: Role of hypoxia and interleukin-1beta in gene expressions of matrix metalloproteinases in temporomandibular joint disc cells, *Arch Oral Biol* 50:81-87, 2005.

17. Israel HA, Diamond B, Saed Nejad F, Ratcliffe A: The relationship between parafunctional masticatory activity and arthroscopically diagnosed temporomandibular joint pathology, *J Oral Maxillofac Surg* 57:1034-1039, 1999.

18. Wright WJ Jr: Temporomandibular disorders: occurrence of specific diagnoses and response to conservative management. Clinical observations, *Cranio* 4:150-155, 1986.

19. Seligman DA, Pullinger AG: Association of occlusal variables among refined TM patient diagnostic groups, *J Craniomandib Disord* 3:227-236, 1989.

20. Solberg WK, Bibb CA, Nordstrom BB, Hansson TL: Malocclusion associated with temporomandibular joint changes in young adults at autopsy, *Am J Orthod* 89:326-330, 1986.

21. Tsolka P, Walter JD, Wilson RF, Preiskel HW: Occlusal variables, bruxism and temporomandibular disorders: a clinical and kinesiographic assessment, *J Oral Rehabil* 22:849-856, 1995.

22. Williamson EH, Simmons MD: Mandibular asymmetry and its relation to pain dysfunction, *Am J Orthod* 76:612-617, 1979.

23. De Boever JA, Adriaens PA: Occlusal relationship in patients with pain-dysfunction symptoms in the temporomandibular joint, *J Oral Rehabil* 10:1-7, 1983.

24. Brandt D: Temporomandibular disorders and their association with morphologic malocclusion in children. In Carlson DS, McNamara JA, Ribbens KA, editors: *Developmental aspects of temporomandibular joint disorders*, Ann Arbor, 1985, University of Michigan Press, pp 279-288.

25. Thilander B: Temporomandibular joint problems in children. In Carlson DS, McNamara JA, Ribbens KA, editors: *Developmental aspects of temporomandibular joint disorders*, Ann Arbor, 1985, University of Michigan Press, pp 89-98.

26. Bernal M, Tsamtsouris A: Signs and symptoms of temporomandibular joint dysfunction in 3 to 5 year old children, *J Pedod* 10:127-140, 1986.

27. Nilner M: Functional disturbances and diseases of the stomatognathic system. A cross-sectional study, *J Pedod* 10:211-238, 1986.

28. Stringert HG, Worms FW: Variations in skeletal and dental patterns in patients with structural and functional alterations of the temporomandibular joint: a preliminary report, *Am J Orthod* 89:285-297, 1986.

29. Gunn SM, Woolfolk MW, Faja BW: Malocclusion and TMJ symptoms in migrant children, *J Craniomandib Disord* 2:196-200, 1988.

30. Dworkin SF, Huggins KH, LeResche L, Von Korff M, Howard J et al: Epidemiology of signs and symptoms in temporomandibular disorders: clinical signs in cases and controls, *J Am Dent Assoc* 120:273-281, 1990.

31. Glaros AG, Brockman DL, Acherman RJ: Impact of overbite on indicators of temporomandibular joint dysfunction, *J Craniomandib Pract* 10:277-281, 1992.

32. McNamara JA Jr, Seligman DA, Okeson JP: Occlusion, orthodontic treatment, and temporomandibular disorders: a review, *J Orofac Pain* 9:73-90, 1995.

33. Hirsch C, John MT, Drangsholt MT, Mancl LA: Relationship between overbite/overjet and clicking or crepitus of the temporomandibular joint, *J Orofac Pain* 19:218-225, 2005.

34. Stegenga B, de Bont LG, Boering G, van Willigen JD: Tissue responses to degenerative changes in the temporomandibular joint: a review, *J Oral Maxillofac Surg* 49:1079-1088, 1991.

35. Dijkgraaf LC, de Bont LG, Boering G, Liem RS: The structure, biochemistry, and metabolism of osteoarthritic cartilage: a review of the literature, *J Oral Maxillofac Surg* 53:1182-1192, 1995.

36. Stegenga B: *Temporomandibular joint osteoarthrosis and internal derangement: diagnostic and therapeutic outcome assessment*, Groningen, The Netherlands, 1991, Drukkerij Van Denderen BV.

37. Harkins SJ, Marteney JL: Extrinsic trauma: a significant precipitating factor in temporomandibular dysfunction, *J Prosthet Dent* 54:271-272, 1985.

38. Moloney F, Howard JA: Internal derangements of the temporomandibular joint. III. Anterior repositioning splint therapy, *Aust Dent J* 31:30-39, 1986.

39. Weinberg S, Lapointe H: Cervical extension-flexion injury (whiplash) and internal derangement of the temporomandibular joint, *J Oral Maxillofac Surg* 45:653-656, 1987.

40. Pullinger AG, Seligman DA: Trauma history in diagnostic groups of temporomandibular disorders, *Oral Surg Oral Med Oral Pathol* 71:529-534, 1991.

41. Westling L, Carlsson GE, Helkimo M: Background factors in craniomandibular disorders with special reference to general joint hypermobility, parafunction, and trauma, *J Craniomandib Disord* 4:89-98, 1990.

42. Pullinger AG, Seligman DA: Association of TMJ subgroups with general trauma and MVA, *J Dent Res* 67:403-409, 1988.

43. Pullinger AG, Monteriro AA: History factors associated with symptoms of temporomandibular disorders, *J Oral Rehabil* 15:117-123, 1988.

44. Bakland LK, Christiansen EL, Strutz JM: Frequency of dental and traumatic events in the etiology of temporomandibular disorders, *Endod Dent Traumatol* 4:182-185, 1988.

45. Steed PA: Etiological factors and temporomandibular treatment outcomes: the effects of trauma and psychological dysfunction, *Funct Orthod* 14:17-20, 1997.

46. Kolbinson DA, Epstein JB, Senthilselvan A, Burgess JA: A comparison of TMD patients with or without prior motor vehicle accident involvement: initial signs, symptoms, and diagnostic characteristics, *J Orofac Pain* 11:206-214, 1997.

47. Farrar WB: Differentiation of temporomandibular joint dysfunction to simplify treatment, *J Prosthet Dent* 28:629-636, 1972.

48. Tallents RH, Katzberg RW, Miller TL, Manzione J, Macher DJ et al: Arthrographically assisted splint therapy: painful clicking with a nonreducing meniscus, *Oral Surg Oral Med Oral Pathol* 61:2-4, 1986.

49. Raustia AM, Pyhtinen J: Direct sagittal computed tomography as a diagnostic aid in the treatment of an anteriorly displaced temporomandibular joint disk by splint therapy, *Cranio* 5:240-245, 1987.

50. Simmons HC III, Gibbs SJ: Recapture of temporomandibular joint disks using anterior repositioning appliances: an MRI study, *Cranio* 13:227-237, 1995.

51. Summer JD, Westesson PL: Mandibular repositioning can be effective in treatment of reducing TMJ disk displacement. A long-term clinical and MR imaging follow-up, *Cranio* 15:107-120, 1997.

52. Simmons HC III, Gibbs SJ: Anterior repositioning appliance therapy for TMJ disorders: specific symptoms relieved and relationship to disk status on MRI, *Cranio* 23:89-99, 2005.

53. Joondeph DR: Long-term stability of mandibular orthopedic repositioning, *Angle Orthod* 69:201-209, 1999.

54. Anderson GC, Schulte JK, Goodkind RJ: Comparative study of two treatment methods for internal derangement of the temporomandibular joint, *J Prosthet Dent* 53:392-397, 1985.

55. Lundh H, Westesson PL, Kopp S, Tillstrom B: Anterior repositioning splint in the treatment of temporomandibular joints with reciprocal clicking: comparison with a flat occlusal splint and an untreated control group, *Oral Surg Oral Med Oral Pathol* 60:131-136, 1985.

56. Okeson JP: Long-term treatment of disk-interference disorders of the temporomandibular joint with anterior repositioning occlusal splints, *J Prosthet Dent* 60:611-616, 1988.

57. Lundh H, Westesson PL, Jisander S, Eriksson L: Disk-repositioning onlays in the treatment of temporomandibular joint disk displacement: comparison with a flat occlusal splint and with no treatment, *Oral Surg Oral Med Oral Pathol* 66:155-162, 1988.

58. Davies SJ, Gray RJ: The pattern of splint usage in the management of two common temporomandibular disorders.

Part I: the anterior repositioning splint in the treatment of disc displacement with reduction, *Br Dent J* 183: 199-203, 1997.

59. Williamson EH, Rosenzweig BJ: The treatment of temporomandibular disorders through repositioning splint therapy: a follow-up study, *Cranio* 16:222-225, 1998.

60. Tecco S, Festa F, Salini V, Epifania E, D'Attilio M: Treatment of joint pain and joint noises associated with a recent TMJ internal derangement: a comparison of an anterior repositioning splint, a full-arch maxillary stabilization splint, and an untreated control group, *Cranio* 22:209-219, 2004.

61. Lundh H, Westesson PL, Kopp S: A three-year follow-up of patients with reciprocal temporomandibular joint clicking [see comments], *Oral Surg Oral Med Oral Pathol* 63:530-533, 1987.

62. Vincent SD, Lilly GE: Incidence and characterization of temporomandibular joint sounds in adults, *J Am Dent Assoc* 116:203-206, 1988.

63. Heikinheimo K, Salmi K, Myllarniemi S, Kirveskari P: Symptoms of craniomandibular disorder in a sample of Finnish adolescents at the ages of 12 and 15 years, *Eur J Orthod* 11:325-331, 1989.

64. Tallents RH, Katzberg RW, Murphy W, Proskin H: Magnetic resonance imaging findings in asymptomatic volunteers and symptomatic patients with temporomandibular disorders, *J Prosthet Dent* 75:529-533, 1996.

65. Dibbets JM, van der Weele LT: Signs and symptoms of temporomandibular disorder (TMD) and craniofacial form, *Am J Orthod Dentofacial Orthop* 110:73-78, 1996.

66. Sato S, Goto S, Nasu F, Motegi K: Natural course of disc displacement with reduction of the temporomandibular joint: changes in clinical signs and symptoms, *J Oral Maxillofac Surg* 61:32-34, 2003.

67. Magnusson T, Egermark I, Carlsson GE: A longitudinal epidemiologic study of signs and symptoms of temporomandibular disorders from 15 to 35 years of age, *J Orofac Pain* 14:310-319, 2000.

68. Magnusson T, Egermarki I, Carlsson GE: A prospective investigation over two decades on signs and symptoms of temporomandibular disorders and associated variables. A final summary, *Acta Odontol Scand* 63:99-109, 2005.

69. Greene CS: Long-term outcome of TMJ clicking in 100 MPD patients, *J Dent Res* 61:218, 1982 (abstract).

70. Okeson JP, Hayes DK: Long-term results of treatment for temporomandibular disorders: an evaluation by patients, *J Am Dent Assoc* 112:473-478, 1986.

71. Bush FM, Carter WH: TMJ clicking and facial pain, *J Dent Res* 62:1217, 1983 (abstract).

72. Magnusson T: Five-year longitudinal study of signs and symptoms of mandibular dysfunction in adolescents, *Cranio* 4:338-344, 1986.

73. Magnusson T, Carlsson GE, Egermark I: Changes in clinical signs of craniomandibular disorders from the age of 15 to 25 years, *J Orofac Pain* 8:207-215, 1994.

74. De Leeuw R, Boering G, Stegenga B, de Bont LG: Clinical signs of TMJ osteoarthrosis and internal derangement 30 years after nonsurgical treatment, *J Orofac Pain* 8:18-24, 1994.

75. De Leeuw R, Boering G, Stegenga B, de Bont LG: Symptoms of temporomandibular joint osteoarthrosis and internal derangement 30 years after non-surgical treatment, *Cranio* 13:81-88, 1995.

76. De Leeuw R, Boering G, Stegenga B, de Bont LG: Radiographic signs of temporomandibular joint osteoarthrosis and internal derangement 30 years after nonsurgical treatment, *Oral Surg Oral Med Oral Pathol Oral Radiol Endod* 79:382-392, 1995.

77. Randolph CS, Greene CS, Moretti R, Forbes D, Perry HT: Conservative management of temporomandibular disorders: a posttreatment comparison between patients from a university clinic and from private practice, *Am J Orthod Dentofacial Orthop* 98:77-82, 1990.

78. Greene CS, Laskin DM: Long-term evaluation of treatment for myofascial pain-dysfunction syndrome: a comparative analysis, *J Am Dent Assoc* 107:235-238, 1983.

79. Greene CS, Laskin DM: Long-term status of TMJ clicking in patients with myofascial pain and dysfunction [published erratum appears in *J Am Dent Assoc* 117:558, 1988] [see comments], *J Am Dent Assoc* 117:461-465, 1988.

80. Brooke RI, Grainger RM: Long-term prognosis for the clicking jaw [published erratum appears in *Oral Surg Oral Med Oral Pathol* 67:131, 1989], *Oral Surg Oral Med Oral Pathol* 65:668-670, 1988.

81. Adler RC: A comparison of long-term post-management results of condylar-repositioned patients, *J Dent Res* 65:339, 1986 (abstract).

82. Tallents RH, Katzberg R, Macher DJ, Roberts CA, Sanchez-Woodworth R: Use of protrusive splint therapy in anterior disk displacement of the temporomandibular joint: a 1- to 3-year follow-up, *J Prosthet Dent* 63:336-341, 1990.

83. Butterworth JC, Deardorff WW: Passive eruption in the treatment of craniomandibular dysfunction: a posttreatment study of 151 patients, *J Prosthet Dent* 67: 525-534, 1992.

84. Dolwick MF: Symptomatology in TMJ surgical patients: a long-term follow-up, *J Dent Res* 66:1185, 1987 (abstract).

85. Montgomery MT, Gordon SM, Van Sickels JE, Harms SE: Changes in signs and symptoms following temporomandibular joint disc repositioning surgery, *J Oral Maxillofac Surg* 50:320-327, 1992.

86. Solberg WK, Hansson TL, Nordstrom B: The temporomandibular joint in young adults at autopsy: a morphologic classification and evaluation, *J Oral Rehabil* 12:303-305, 1985.

87. Akerman S, Kopp S, Rohlin M: Histological changes in temporomandibular joints from elderly individuals. An autopsy study, *Acta Odontol Scand* 44:231-239, 1986.

88. Isberg A, Isacsson G, Johansson AS, Larson O: Hyperplastic soft-tissue formation in the temporomandibular joint associated with internal derangement. A radiographic and histologic study, *Oral Surg Oral Med Oral Pathol* 61:32-38, 1986.

89. Hall MB, Brown RW, Baughman RA: Histologic appearance of the bilaminar zone in internal derangement of the temporomandibular joint, *Oral Surg Oral Med Oral Pathol* 58:375-381, 1984.

90. Scapino RP: Histopathology associated with malposition of the human temporomandibular joint disc, *Oral Surg Oral Med Oral Pathol* 55:382-397, 1983.

91. Salo L, Raustia A, Pernu H, Virtanen K: Internal derangement of the temporomandibular joint: a histochemical study, *J Oral Maxillofac Surg* 49:171-176, 1991.

92. Blaustein DI, Scapino RP: Remodeling of the temporomandibular joint disk and posterior attachment in disk displacement specimens in relation to glycosaminoglycan content, *Plast Reconstr Surg* 78:756-764, 1986.

93. Pereira FJ Jr, Lundh H, Westesson PL, Carlsson LE: Clinical findings related to morphologic changes in TMJ autopsy specimens, *Oral Surg Oral Med Oral Pathol* 78:288-295, 1994.

94. Pereira FJ Jr, Lundh H, Westesson PL: Morphologic changes in the temporomandibular joint in different age groups. An autopsy investigation, *Oral Surg Oral Med Oral Pathol* 78:279-287, 1994.

95. Pereira FJ, Lundh H, Eriksson L, Westesson PL: Microscopic changes in the retrodiscal tissues of painful temporomandibular joints, *J Oral Maxillofac Surg* 54:461-468, 1996.

96. Pereira FJ Jr, Lundh H, Westesson PL: Age-related changes of the retrodiscal tissues in the temporomandibular joint, *J Oral Maxillofac Surg* 54:55-61, 1996.

97. Kirk WS Jr: Magnetic resonance imaging and tomographic evaluation of occlusal appliance treatment for advanced internal derangement of the temporomandibular joint, *J Oral Maxillofac Surg* 49:9-12, 1991.

98. Choi BH, Yoo JH, Lee WY: Comparison of magnetic resonance imaging before and after nonsurgical treatment of closed lock, *Oral Surg Oral Med Oral Pathol* 78:301-305, 1994.

99. Chen CW, Boulton JL, Gage JP: Effects of splint therapy in TMJ dysfunction: a study using magnetic resonance imaging, *Aust Dent J* 40:71-78, 1995.

100. Lundh H, Westesson PL: Long-term follow-up after occlusal treatment to correct abnormal temporomandibular joint disk position, *Oral Surg Oral Med Oral Pathol* 67:2-10, 1989.

101. Schmitter M, Zahran M, Duc JM, Henschel V, Rammelsberg P: Conservative therapy in patients with anterior disc displacement without reduction using 2 common splints: a randomized clinical trial, *J Oral Maxillofac Surg* 63:1295-1303, 2005.

102. Lundh H, Westesson PL, Eriksson L, Brooks SL: Temporomandibular joint disk displacement without reduction. Treatment with flat occlusal splint versus no treatment, *Oral Surg Oral Med Oral Pathol* 73:655-658, 1992.

103. Vichaichalermvong S, Nilner M, Panmekiate S, Petersson A: Clinical follow-up of patients with different disc positions, *J Orofac Pain* 7:61-67, 1993.

104. Chung SC, Kim HS: The effect of the stabilization split on the TMJ closed lock, *J Craniomandib Pract* 11:95-101, 1993.

105. Tasaki MM, Westesson PL, Isberg AM, Ren YF, Tallents RH: Classification and prevalence of temporomandibular joint disk displacement in patients and symptom-free volunteers, *Am J Orthod Dentofacial Orthop* 109:249-262, 1996.

106. Kai S, Kai H, Tabata O, Shiratsuchi Y, Ohishi M: Long-term outcomes of nonsurgical treatment in nonreducing anteriorly displaced disk of the temporomandibular joint, *Oral Surg Oral Med Oral Pathol Oral Radiol Endod* 85:258-267, 1998.

107. Kurita K, Westesson PL, Yuasa H, Toyama M, Machida J et al: Natural course of untreated symptomatic temporomandibular joint disc displacement without reduction, *J Dent Res* 77:361-365, 1998.

108. Sato S, Takahashi K, Kawamura H, Motegi K: The natural course of nonreducing disk displacement of the temporomandibular joint: changes in condylar mobility and radiographic alterations at one-year follow up, *Int J Oral Maxillofac Surg* 27:173-177, 1998.

109. Sato S, Goto S, Kawamura H, Motegi K: The natural course of nonreducing disc displacement of the TMJ: relationship of clinical findings at initial visit to outcome after 12 months without treatment, *J Orofac Pain* 11: 315-320, 1997.

110. Sato S, Kawamura H, Nagasaka H, Motegi K: The natural course of anterior disc displacement without reduction in the temporomandibular joint: follow-up at 6, 12, and 18 months, *J Oral Maxillofac Surg* 55:234-238; discussion 238-239, 1997.

111. Sato S, Kawamura H: Natural course of non-reducing disc displacement of the temporomandibular joint: changes in electromyographic activity during chewing movement, *J Oral Rehabil* 32:159-165, 2005.

112. Minakuchi H, Kuboki T, Maekawa K, Matsuka Y, Yatani H: Self-reported remission, difficulty, and satisfaction with nonsurgical therapy used to treat anterior disc displacement without reduction, *Oral Surg Oral Med Oral Pathol Oral Radiol Endod* 98:435-440, 2004.

113. Imirzalioglu P, Biler N, Agildere AM: Clinical and radiological follow-up results of patients with untreated TMJ closed lock, *J Oral Rehabil* 32:326-331, 2005.

114. Nicolakis P, Erdogmus B, Kopf A, Ebenbichler G, Kollmitzer J et al: Effectiveness of exercise therapy in patients with internal derangement of the temporomandibular joint, *J Oral Rehabil* 28:1158-1164, 2001.

115. Cleland J, Palmer J: Effectiveness of manual physical therapy, therapeutic exercise, and patient education on bilateral disc displacement without reduction of the temporomandibular joint: a single-case design, *J Orthop Sports Phys Ther* 34:535-548, 2004.

116. Nitzan DW, Dolwick MF, Martinez GA: Temporomandibular joint arthrocentesis: a simplified treatment for severe, limited mouth opening, *J Oral Maxillofac Surg* 49: 1163-1167, 1991.

117. Dembo J, Okeson JP, Kirkwood C, Falace DA: Long-term effects of temporomandibular joint lavage, *J Dent Res* 252, 1993.

118. Murakami K, Hosaka H, Moriya Y, Segami N, Iizuka T: Short-term treatment outcome study for the management of temporomandibular joint closed lock. A comparison of arthrocentesis to nonsurgical therapy and arthroscopic lysis and lavage, *Oral Surg Oral Med Oral Pathol Oral Radiol Endod* 80:253-257, 1995.

119. Fridrich KL, Wise JM, Zeitler DL: Prospective comparison of arthroscopy and arthrocentesis for temporomandibular joint disorders, *J Oral Maxillofac Surg* 54:816-820, 1996.

120. Cascone P, Spallaccia F, Rivaroli A: Arthrocentesis of the temporomandibular joint. Long-term results, *Minerva Stomatol* 47:149-157, 1998.

121. Nitzan DW, Samson B, Better H: Long-term outcome of arthrocentesis for sudden-onset, persistent, severe closed lock of the temporomandibular joint, *J Oral Maxillofac Surg* 55:151-157; discussion 157-158, 1997.

122. Carvajal WA, Laskin DM: Long-term evaluation of arthrocentesis for the treatment of internal derangements of the temporomandibular joint, *J Oral Maxillofac Surg* 58:852-855; discussion 856-857, 2000.

123. Goudot P, Jaquinet AR, Hugonnet S, Haefliger W, Richter M: Improvement of pain and function after arthroscopy and arthrocentesis of the temporomandibular joint: a comparative study, *J Craniomaxillofac Surg* 28:39-43, 2000.

124. Sakamoto I, Yoda T, Tsukahara H, Imai H, Enomoto S: Comparison of the effectiveness of arthrocentesis in acute and chronic closed lock: analysis of clinical and arthroscopic findings, *Cranio* 18:264-271, 2000.

125. Sanroman JF: Closed lock (MRI fixed disc): a comparison of arthrocentesis and arthroscopy, *Int J Oral Maxillofac Surg* 33:344-348, 2004.

126. Chang H, Israel H: Analysis of inflammatory mediators in temporomandibular joint synovial fluid lavage samples of symptomatic patients and asymptomatic controls, *J Oral Maxillofac Surg* 63:761-765, 2005.

127. Reston JT, Turkelson CM: Meta-analysis of surgical treatments for temporomandibular articular disorders, *J Oral Maxillofac Surg* 61:3-10, 2003.

128. Sato S, Oguri S, Yamaguchi K, Kawamura H, Motegi K: Pumping injection of sodium hyaluronate for patients with non-reducing disc displacement of the temporomandibular joint: two year follow-up, *J Craniomaxillofac Surg* 29:89-93, 2001.

129. Alpaslan GH, Alpaslan C: Efficacy of temporomandibular joint arthrocentesis with and without injection of sodium hyaluronate in treatment of internal derangements, *J Oral Maxillofac Surg* 59:613-618; discussion 618-619, 2001.

130. Murakami KI, Iizuka T, Matsuki M, Ono T: Recapturing the persistent anteriorly displaced disk by mandibular manipulation after pumping and hydraulic pressure to the upper joint cavity of the temporomandibular joint, *Cranio* 5:17-24, 1987.

131. Totsuka Y, Nakamura T, Fukuda H, Sawada A, Uchiyama Y et al: Treatment of closed lock by mandibular manipulation assisted by hydraulic pressure in the upper cavity of the temporomandibular joint, *Oral Maxillofac Surg Clin North Am* 1:111-119, 1989.

132. Emshoff R, Rudisch A, Bosch R, Gassner R: Effect of arthrocentesis and hydraulic distension on the temporomandibular joint disk position, *Oral Surg Oral Med Oral Pathol Oral Radiol Endod* 89:271-277, 2000.

133. Emshoff R: Clinical factors affecting the outcome of arthrocentesis and hydraulic distension of the temporomandibular joint, *Oral Surg Oral Med Oral Pathol Oral Radiol Endod* 100:409-414, 2005.

134. Emshoff R, Rudisch A: Determining predictor variables for treatment outcomes of arthrocentesis and hydraulic distention of the temporomandibular joint, *J Oral Maxillofac Surg* 62:816-823, 2004.

135. Trieger N, Hoffman CH, Rodriguez E: The effect of arthrocentesis of the temporomandibular joint in patients with rheumatoid arthritis, *J Oral Maxillofac Surg* 57:537-540, 1999.

136. Carls FR, Engelke W, Locher MC, Sailer HF: Complications following arthroscopy of the temporomandibular joint: analysis covering a 10-year period (451 arthroscopies), *J Craniomaxillofac Surg* 24:12-15, 1996.

137. Nitzan DW, Dolwick MF, Heft MW: Arthroscopic lavage and lysis of the temporomandibular joint: a change in perspective, *J Oral Maxillofac Surg* 48:798-801, 1990.

138. Montgomery MT, Van Sickels JE, Harms SE, Thrash WJ: Arthroscopic TMJ surgery: effects on signs, symptoms, and disc position, *J Oral Maxillofac Surg* 47:1263-1271, 1989.

139. Montgomery MT, Van Sickels JE, Harms SE: Success of temporomandibular joint arthroscopy in disk displacement with and without reduction, *Oral Surg Oral Med Oral Pathol* 71:651-659, 1991.

140. Davis CL, Kaminishi RM, Marshall MW: Arthroscopic surgery for treatment of closed lock, *J Oral Maxillofac Surg* 49:704-707, 1991.

141. Clark GT, Moody DG, Sanders B: Arthroscopic treatment of temporomandibular joint locking resulting from disc derangement: two-year results, *J Oral Maxillofac Surg* 49:157-164, 1991.

142. White RD: Retrospective analysis of 100 consecutive surgical arthroscopies of the temporomandibular joint, *J Oral Maxillofac Surg* 47:1014-1021, 1989.

143. McCain JP, Sanders B, Koslin MG, Quinn JH, Peters PB et al: Temporomandibular joint arthroscopy: a 6-year multicenter retrospective study of 4,831 joints [published erratum appears in *J Oral Maxillofac Surg* 50:1349, 1992], *J Oral Maxillofac Surg* 50:926-930, 1992.

144. Stegenga B, de Bont LG, Dijkstra PU, Boering G: Short-term outcome of arthroscopic surgery of temporomandibular joint osteoarthrosis and internal derangement: a randomized controlled clinical trial, *Br J Maxillofac Surg* 31:3-14, 1993.

145. Murakami K, Moriya Y, Goto K, Segami N: Four-year follow-up study of temporomandibular joint arthroscopic surgery for advanced stage internal derangements, *J Oral Maxillofac Surg* 54:285-290, 1996.

146. Murakami KI, Tsuboi Y, Bessho K, Yokoe Y, Nishida M et al: Outcome of arthroscopic surgery to the temporomandibular joint correlates with stage of internal derangement: five-year follow-up study, *Br J Oral Maxillofac Surg* 36:30-34, 1998.

147. Gynther GW, Holmlund AB: Efficacy of arthroscopic lysis and lavage in patients with temporomandibular joint symptoms associated with generalized osteoarthritis or rheumatoid arthritis, *J Oral Maxillofac Surg* 56:147-151; discussion 152, 1998.

148. Kurita K, Goss AN, Ogi N, Toyama M: Correlation between preoperative mouth opening and surgical outcome after arthroscopic lysis and lavage in patients with disc displacement without reduction, *J Oral Maxillofac Surg* 56:1394-1397; discussion 1397-1398, 1998.

149. Sorel B, Piecuch JF: Long-term evaluation following temporomandibular joint arthroscopy with lysis and lavage, *Int J Oral Maxillofac Surg* 29:259-263, 2000.

150. Smolka W, Iizuka T: Arthroscopic lysis and lavage in different stages of internal derangement of the temporomandibular joint: correlation of preoperative staging to arthroscopic findings and treatment outcome, *J Oral Maxillofac Surg* 63:471-478, 2005.

151. Moses JJ, Sartoris D, Glass R, Tanaka T, Poker I: The effect of arthroscopic surgical lysis and lavage of the superior joint space on TMJ disc position and mobility, *J Oral Maxillofac Surg* 47:674-678, 1989.

152. Perrott DH, Alborzi A, Kaban LB, Helms CA: A prospective evaluation of the effectiveness of temporomandibular joint arthroscopy, *J Oral Maxillofac Surg* 48:1029-1032, 1990.

153. Gabler MJ, Greene CS, Palacios E, Perry HT: Effect of arthroscopic temporomandibular joint surgery on articular disk position, *J Craniomandib Disord* 3:191-202, 1989.

154. Moses JJ, Topper DC: A functional approach to the treatment of temporomandibular joint internal derangement, *J Craniomandib Disord* 5:19-27, 1991.

155. Dolwick MF, Sanders B: *TMJ internal derangement and arthrosis: surgical atlas*, St Louis, 1986, Mosby.

156. Benson BJ, Keith DA: Patient response to surgical and nonsurgical treatment for internal derangement of the temporomandibular joint, *J Oral Maxillofac Surg* 43:770-777, 1985.

157. McCarty WL, Farrar WB: Surgery for internal derangements of the temporomandibular joint, *J Prosthet Dent* 42:191-196, 1979.

158. Anderson DM, Sinclair PM, McBride KM: A clinical evaluation of temporomandibular joint disk plication surgery, *Am J Orthod Dentofacial Orthop* 100:156-162, 1991.

159. Dolwick MF: Disc preservation surgery for the treatment of internal derangements of the temporomandibular joint, *J Oral Maxillofac Surg* 59:1047-1050, 2001.

160. Vasconcelos BC, Porto GG, Bessa-Nogueira RV: Condylar disk plication for temporomandibular joint internal derangement treatment: surgical technique and results, *Med Oral Patol Oral Cir Bucal* 10(suppl 2): E133-138, 2005.

161. Eriksson L, Westesson PL: Long-term evaluation of meniscectomy of the temporomandibular joint, *J Oral Maxillofac Surg* 43:263-269, 1985.

162. Brown WA: Internal derangement of the temporomandibular joint: review of 214 patients following meniscectomy, *Can J Surg* 23:30-32, 1980.

163. Silver CM: Long-term results of meniscectomy of the temporomandibular joint, *Cranio* 3:46-57, 1984.

164. Tolvanen M, Oikarinen VJ, Wolf J: A 30-year follow-up study of temporomandibular joint meniscectomies: a report on five patients, *Br J Maxillofac Surg* 26:311-316, 1988.

165. Nyberg J, Adell R, Svensson B: Temporomandibular joint discectomy for treatment of unilateral internal derangements—a 5 year follow-up evaluation, *Int J Oral Maxillofac Surg* 33:8-12, 2004.

166. Holmlund AB, Gynther G, Axelsson S: Diskectomy in treatment of internal derangement of the temporomandibular joint. Follow-up at 1, 3, and 5 years, *Oral Surg Oral Med Oral Pathol* 76:266-271, 1993.

167. Takaku S, Toyoda T: Long-term evaluation of discectomy of the temporomandibular joint. *J Oral Maxillofac Surg* 52:722-726, 1994.

168. Kalamchi S, Walker RV: Silastic implant as a part of temporomandibular joint arthroplasty. Evaluation of its efficacy, *Br J Maxillofac Surg* 25:227-236, 1987.

169. Westesson PL, Eriksson L, Lindstrom C: Destructive lesions of the mandibular condyle following diskectomy with temporary silicone implant, *Oral Surg Oral Med Oral Pathol* 63:143-150, 1987.

170. Heffez L, Mafee MF, Rosenberg H, Langer B: CT evaluation of TMJ disc replacement with a Proplast-Teflon laminate, *J Oral Maxillofac Surg* 45:657-665, 1987.

171. Wagner JD, Mosby EL: Assessment of Proplast-Teflon disc replacements [published erratum appears in *J Oral Maxillofac Surg* 49:220, 1991] [see comments], *J Oral Maxillofac Surg* 48:1140-1144, 1990.

172. Kaplan PA, Ruskin JD, Tu HK, Knibbe MA: Erosive arthritis of the temporomandibular joint caused by Teflon-Proplast implants: plain film features, *AJR Am J Roentgenol* 151:337-339, 1988.

173. Valentine JD Jr, Reiman BE, Beuttenmuller EA, Donovan MG: Light and electron microscopic evaluation of Proplast II TMJ disc implants [see comments], *J Oral Maxillofac Surg* 47:689-696, 1989.

174. Tucker MR, Jacoway JR, White RP Jr: Autogenous dermal grafts for repair of temporomandibular joint disc perforations, *J Oral Maxillofac Surg* 44:781-789, 1986.

175. Zetz MR, Irby WB: Repair of the adult temporomandibular joint meniscus with an autogenous dermal graft, *J Oral Maxillofac Surg* 42:167-171, 1984.

176. Meyer RA: The autogenous dermal graft in temporomandibular joint disc surgery, *J Oral Maxillofac Surg* 46:948-954, 1988.

177. Spagnoli D, Kent JN: Multicenter evaluation of temporomandibular joint Proplast-Teflon disk implant, *Oral Surg Oral Med Oral Pathol* 74:411-421, 1992.

178. Trumpy IG, Lyberg T: Surgical treatment of internal derangement of the temporomandibular joint: long-term evaluation of three techniques, *J Oral Maxillofac Surg* 53:740-746; discussion 746-747, 1995.

179. Henry CH, Wolford LM: Treatment outcomes for temporomandibular joint reconstruction after Proplast-Teflon implant failure, *J Oral Maxillofac Surg* 51:352-358; discussion 359-360, 1993.

180. Dimitroulis G: The use of dermis grafts after discectomy for internal derangement of the temporomandibular joint, *J Oral Maxillofac Surg* 63:173-178, 2005.

181. Umeda H, Kaban LB, Pogrel MA, Stern M: Long-term viability of the temporalis muscle/fascia flap used for

temporomandibular joint reconstruction, *J Oral Maxillofac Surg* 51:530-533; discussion 534, 1993.

182. Dimitroulis G: The interpositional dermis-fat graft in the management of temporomandibular joint ankylosis, *Int J Oral Maxillofac Surg* 33:755-760, 2004.

183. Wolford LM, Karras SC: Autologous fat transplantation around temporomandibular joint total joint prostheses: preliminary treatment outcomes, *J Oral Maxillofac Surg* 55:245-251; discussion 251-252, 1997.

184. Ioannides C, Freihofer HP: Replacement of the damaged interarticular disc of the TMJs, *J Craniomaxillofac Surg* 16:273-278, 1988.

185. Tucker MR, Kennady MC, Jacoway JR: Autogenous auricular cartilage implantation following discectomy in the primate temporomandibular joint, *J Oral Maxillofac Surg* 48:38-44, 1990.

186. Armstrong JW, Heit JM, Edwards RC: Autogenous conchal cartilage as a replacement after a diskectomy, *Oral Surg Oral Med Oral Pathol* 73:269-275, 1992.

187. Hall MB, Baughman R, Ruskin J, Thompson DA: Healing following meniscopathy, eminectomy, and high condylectomy in the monkey temporomandibular joint, *J Oral Maxillofac Surg* 44:177-182, 1986.

188. Bernasconi G, Marchetti C, Reguzzoni M, Baciliero U: Synovia hyperplasia and calcification in the human TMJ disk: a clinical, surgical, and histologic study, *Oral Surg Oral Med Oral Pathol Oral Radiol Endod* 84:245-252, 1997.

189. Murakami K, Segami N, Moriya Y, Iizuka T: Correlation between pain and dysfunction and intra-articular adhesions in patients with internal derangement of the temporomandibular joint, *J Oral Maxillofac Surg* 50:705-708, 1992.

190. Gallagher DM: Posterior dislocation of the temporomandibular joint meniscus: report of three cases, *J Am Dent Assoc* 113:411-415, 1986.

191. Blankestijn J, Boering G: Posterior dislocation of the temporomandibular disc, *Int J Oral Surg* 14:437-443, 1985.

192. Sanders B: Arthroscopic surgery of the temporomandibular joint: treatment of internal derangement with persistent closed lock, *Oral Surg Oral Med Oral Pathol* 62:361-372, 1986.

193. Murakami KI, Lizuka T, Matsuki M, Ono T: Diagnostic arthroscopy of the TMJ: differential diagnoses in patients with limited jaw opening, *Cranio* 4:117-126, 1986.

194. Hellsing G, Holmlund A, Nordenram A, Wredmark T: Arthroscopy of the temporomandibular joint. Examination of 2 patients with suspected disk derangement, *Int J Oral Surg* 13:69-74, 1984.

195. Nuelle DG, Alpern MC, Ufema JW: Arthroscopic surgery of the temporomandibular joint, *Angle Orthod* 56:118-142, 1986.

196. Hori M, Okaue M, Harada D, Ono M, Goto T et al: Releasing severe adhesions around the eminence and the synovial portion of the TMJ: a clinical study of combined treatment using hydraulic lavage, arthroscopic surgery and rehabilitative therapy, *J Oral Sci* 41:61-66, 1999.

197. Miyamoto H, Sakashita H, Miyata M, Goss AN, Okabe K et al: Arthroscopic management of temporomandibular closed lock, *Aust Dent J* 43:301-304, 1998.

198. Hall HD, Indresano AT, Kirk WS, Dietrich MS: Prospective multicenter comparison of 4 temporomandibular joint operations, *J Oral Maxillofac Surg* 63:1174-1179, 2005.

199. Bell WE: *Temporomandibular disorders: classification, diagnosis, management*, ed 3, Chicago, 1990, Year Book Medical, p 77.

200. Oatis GW Jr, Baker DA: The bilateral eminectomy as definitive treatment. A review of 44 patients, *Int J Oral Surg* 13:294-298, 1984.

201. Undt G, Kermer C, Rasse M: Treatment of recurrent mandibular dislocation, Part II: eminectomy, *Int J Oral Maxillofac Surg* 26:98-102, 1997.

202. Holmlund AB, Gynther GW, Kardel R, Axelsson SE: Surgical treatment of temporomandibular joint luxation, *Swed Dent J* 23:127-132, 1999.

203. Williamson RA, McNamara D, McAuliffe W: True eminectomy for internal derangement of the temporomandibular joint, *Br J Oral Maxillofac Surg* 38:554-560, 2000.

204. Bell WE: *Temporomandibular disorders: classification, diagnosis, management*, ed 3, Chicago, 1990, Year Book Medical, pp 328-342.

205. Kai S, Kai H, Nakayama E, Tabata O, Tashiro H et al: Clinical symptoms of open lock position of the condyle. Relation to anterior dislocation of the temporomandibular joint, *Oral Surg Oral Med Oral Pathol* 74:143-148, 1992.

206. Pogrel MA: Articular eminectomy for recurrent dislocation, *Br J Maxillofac Surg* 25:237-243, 1987.

207. Helman J, Laufer D, Minkov B, Gutman D: Eminectomy as surgical treatment for chronic mandibular dislocations, *Int J Oral Surg* 13:486-489, 1984.

208. Puelacher WC, Waldhart E: Miniplate eminoplasty: a new surgical treatment for TMJ-dislocation, *J Craniomaxillofac Surg* 21:176-178, 1993.

209. Daelen B, Koch A, Thorwirth V: Botulinum toxin treatment of neurogenic dislocation of the temporomandibular joint, *Mund Kiefer Gesichtschir* 2(suppl 1): S125-129, 1998.

210. Daelen B, Thorwirth V, Koch A: Treatment of recurrent dislocation of the temporomandibular joint with type A botulinum toxin, *Int J Oral Maxillofac Surg* 26:458-460, 1997.

211. Moore AP, Wood GD: Medical treatment of recurrent temporomandibular joint dislocation using botulinum toxin A, *Br Dent J* 183:415-417, 1997.

212. Murakami K, Segami N, Fujimura K, Iizuka T: Correlation between pain and synovitis in patients with internal derangement of the temporomandibular joint, *J Oral Maxillofac Surg* 49:1159-1161, 1991.

213. Dimitroulis G: The prevalence of osteoarthrosis in cases of advanced internal derangement of the temporomandibular joint: a clinical, surgical and histological study, *Int J Oral Maxillofac Surg* 34:345-349, 2005.

214. Zarb GA, Speck JE: The treatment of mandibular dysfunction. In Zarb GA, Carlsson GE, editors: *Temporomandibular joint: function and dysfunction*, St Louis, 1979, Mosby, pp 382-389.

215. Gray RJ, Quayle AA, Hall CA, Schofield MA: Physiotherapy in the treatment of temporomandibular

joint disorders: a comparative study of four treatment methods, *Br Dent J* 176:257-261, 1994.

216. Toller P: Non-surgical treatment of dysfunctions of the temporo-mandibular joint, *Oral Sci Rev* 7:70-85, 1976.

217. Alstergren P, Appelgren A, Appelgren B, Kopp S, Lundeberg T et al: The effect on joint fluid concentration of neuropeptide Y by intra-articular injection of glucocorticoid in temporomandibular joint arthritis, *Acta Odontol Scand* 54:1-7, 1996.

218. Schindler C, Paessler L, Eckelt U, Kirch W: Severe temporomandibular dysfunction and joint destruction after intra-articular injection of triamcinolone, *J Oral Pathol Med* 34:184-186, 2005.

219. Marinho LH, McLoughlin PM: Lateral open bite resulting from acute temporomandibular joint effusion, *Br J Maxillofac Surg* 32:127-128, 1994.

220. Schobel G, Millesi W, Walzke IM, Hollmann K: Ankylosis of the temporomandibular joint. Follow-up of thirteen patients, *Oral Surg Oral Med Oral Pathol* 74:7-14, 1992.

221. Stegenga B, de Bont LG, Boering G: Osteoarthrosis as the cause of craniomandibular pain and dysfunction: a unifying concept, *J Oral Maxillofac Surg* 47:249-256, 1989.

222. De Bont LG, Stegenga B: Pathology of temporomandibular joint internal derangement and osteoarthrosis, *Int J Oral Maxillofac Surg* 22:71-74, 1993.

223. Bollet AJ: An essay on the biology of osteoarthritis, *Arthritis Rheum* 12:152-163, 1969.

224. Radin EL, Paul IL, Rose RM: Role of mechanical factors in pathogenesis of primary osteoarthritis, *Lancet* 1:519-522, 1972.

225. Rasmussen OC: Temporomandibular arthropathy. Clinical, radiologic, and therapeutic aspects, with emphasis on diagnosis, *Int J Oral Surg* 12:365-397, 1983.

226. Nickerson JW, Boering G: Natural course of osteoarthrosis as it relates to internal derangement of the temporomandibular joint. In Merrill RG, editor: *Oral maxillofacial surgical clinics of North America*, Philadelphia, 1989, Saunders, pp 27-45.

227. Boering G, Stegenga B, de Bont LG: Temporomandibular joint osteoarthrosis and internal derangement. Part I: Clinical course and initial treatment, *Int Dent J* 40: 339-346, 1990.

228. De Leeuw JR, Steenks MH, Ros WJ, Lobbezoo Scholte AM, Bosman F et al: Assessment of treatment outcome in patients with craniomandibular dysfunction, *J Oral Rehabil* 21:655-666, 1994.

229. Rasmussen OC: Clinical findings during the course of temporomandibular arthropathy, *Scand J Dent Res* 89:283-288, 1981.

230. Mejersjo C: Therapeutic and prognostic considerations in TMJ osteoarthrosis: a literature review and a long-term study in 11 subjects, *Cranio* 5:69-78, 1987.

231. Kopp S, Wenneberg B, Haraldson T, Carlsson GE: The short-term effect of intra-articular injections of sodium hyaluronate and corticosteroid on temporomandibular joint pain and dysfunction, *J Oral Maxillofac Surg* 43:429-435, 1985.

232. Wolford LM, Cardenas L: Idiopathic condylar resorption: diagnosis, treatment protocol, and outcomes, *Am J Orthod Dentofacial Orthop* 116:667-677, 1999.

233. Arnett GW, Milam SB, Gottesman L: Progressive mandibular retrusion-idiopathic condylar resorption. Part II, *Am J Orthod Dentofacial Orthop* 110:117-127, 1996.

234. Arnett GW, Milam SB, Gottesman L: Progressive mandibular retrusion—idiopathic condylar resorption. Part I, *Am J Orthod Dentofacial Orthop* 110:8-15, 1996.

235. Mayne JG, Hatch GS: Arthritis of the temporomandibular joint, *J Am Dent Assoc* 79:125-130, 1969.

236. Pinals RS: Traumatic arthritis and allied conditions. In McCarty DJ, editor: *Arthritis and allied conditions: a textbook of rheumatology*, ed 10, Philadelphia, 1985, Lea & Febiger.

237. Schellhas KP, Piper MA, Omlie MR: Facial skeleton remodeling due to temporomandibular joint degeneration: an imaging study of 100 patients, *AJNR Am J Neuroradiol* 11:541-551, 1990.

238. Leighty SM, Spach DH, Myall RW, Burns JL: Septic arthritis of the temporomandibular joint: review of the literature and report of two cases in children, *Int J Oral Maxillofac Surg* 22:292-297, 1993.

239. Jeon HS, Hong SP, Cho BO, Mulyukin A, Choi JY et al: Hematogenous infection of the human temporomandibular joint, *Oral Surg Oral Med Oral Pathol Oral Radiol Endod* 99:E11-17, 2005.

240. Appelgren A, Appelgren B, Kopp S, Lundeberg T, Theodorsson E: Neuropeptide in arthritic TMJ and symptoms and signs from the stomatognathic system with special consideration to rheumatoid arthritis, *J Orofac Pain* 9:215-225, 1995.

241. Zide MF, Carlton DM, Kent JN: Rheumatoid disease and related arthropathies. I. Systemic findings, medical therapy, and peripheral joint surgery, *Oral Surg Oral Med Oral Pathol* 61:119-125, 1986.

242. Seymour R, Crouse V, Irby W: Temporomandibular ankylosis secondary to rheumatoid arthritis, *Oral Surg Oral Med Oral Pathol* 40:584-589, 1975.

243. Koh ET, Yap AU, Koh CK, Chee TS, Chan SP et al: Temporomandibular disorders in rheumatoid arthritis, *J Rheumatol* 26:1918-1922, 1999.

244. Helenius LM, Hallikainen D, Helenius I, Meurman JH, Kononen M et al: Clinical and radiographic findings of the temporomandibular joint in patients with various rheumatic diseases. A case-control study, *Oral Surg Oral Med Oral Pathol Oral Radiol Endod* 99:455-463, 2005.

245. Atsu SS, Ayhan-Ardic F: Temporomandibular disorders seen in rheumatology practices: a review. *Rheumatol Int* 26:781-787, 2006.

246. Germain BF, Vasey FB, Espinoza LR: Early recognition of rheumatoid arthritis, *Compr Ther* 5:16-22, 1979.

247. Tabeling HJ, Dolwick MF: Rheumatoid arthritis: diagnosis and treatment, *Fla Dent J* 56:16-18, 1985.

248. Braunwald E, Isselbacher KJ: *Harrison's principles of internal medicine*, ed 11, New York, 1987, McGraw-Hill.

249. Akerman S, Jonsson K, Kopp S, Petersson A, Rohlin M: Radiologic changes in temporomandibular, hand, and

foot joints of patients with rheumatoid arthritis, *Oral Surg Oral Med Oral Pathol* 72:245-250, 1991.

250. Marini I, Vecchiet F, Spiazzi L, Capurso U: Stomatognathic function in juvenile rheumatoid arthritis and in developmental open-bite subjects, *ASDC J Dent Child* 66:30-35, 1999.

251. Harper RP, Brown CM, Triplett MM, Villasenor A, Gatchel RJ: Masticatory function in patients with juvenile rheumatoid arthritis, *Pediatr Dent* 22:200-206, 2000.

252. Holmes EW: Clinical gout and the pathogenesis of hyperuricemia. In McCarty DJ, editor: *Arthritis and allied conditions: a textbook of rheumatology*, ed 10, Philadelphia, 1985, Lea & Febiger, pp 134-139.

253. Koorbusch GF, Zeitler DL, Fotos PG, Doss JB: Psoriatic arthritis of the temporomandibular joints with ankylosis. Literature review and case reports, *Oral Surg Oral Med Oral Pathol* 71:267-274, 1991.

254. Kurihara K, Mizuseki K, Saiki T, Wakisaka H, Maruyama S et al: Tophaceous pseudogout of the temporomandibular joint: report of a case, *Pathol Int* 47:578-580, 1997.

255. Barthelemy I, Karanas Y, Sannajust JP, Emering C, Mondie JM: Gout of the temporomandibular joint: pitfalls in diagnosis, *J Craniomaxillofac Surg* 29:307-310, 2001.

256. Wilson AW, Brown JS, Ord RA: Psoriatic arthropathy of the temporomandibular joint, *Oral Surg Oral Med Oral Pathol* 70:555-558, 1990.

257. Ulmansky M, Michelle R, Azaz B: Oral psoriasis: report of six new cases, *J Oral Pathol Med* 24:42-45, 1995.

258. Zhu JF, Kaminski MJ, Pulitzer DR, Hu J, Thomas HF: Psoriasis: pathophysiology and oral manifestations, *Oral Dis* 2:135-144, 1996.

259. Dervis E, Dervis E: The prevalence of temporomandibular disorders in patients with psoriasis with or without psoriatic arthritis, *J Oral Rehabil* 32:786-793, 2005.

260. Kononen M, Wolf J, Kilpinen E, Melartin E: Radiographic signs in the temporomandibular and hand joints in patients with psoriatic arthritis, *Acta Odontol Scand* 49:191-196, 1991.

261. Ramos-Remus C, Perez-Rocha O, Ludwig RN, Kolotyluk DR, Gomez-Vargas A et al: Magnetic resonance changes in the temporomandibular joint in ankylosing spondylitis, *J Rheumatol* 24:123-127, 1997.

262. Ramos-Remus C, Major P, Gomez-Vargas A, Petrikowski G, Hernandez-Chavez A et al: Temporomandibular joint osseous morphology in a consecutive sample of ankylosing spondylitis patients, *Ann Rheum Dis* 56:103-107, 1997.

263. Major P, Ramos-Remus C, Suarez Almazor ME, Hatcher D, Parfitt M et al: Magnetic resonance imaging and clinical assessment of temporomandibular joint pathology in ankylosing spondylitis, *J Rheumatol* 26:616-621, 1999.

264. Ramos-Remus C, Perez Rocha O, Ludwig RN, Kolotyluk DR, Gomez-Vargas A et al: Magnetic resonance changes in the temporomandibular joint in ankylosing spondylitis, *J Rheumatol* 24:123-127, 1997.

265. Chow TK, Ng WL, Tam CK, Kung N: Bilateral ankylosis of temporomandibular joint secondary to ankylosing spondylitis in a male Chinese, *Scand J Rheumatol* 26:133-134, 1997.

266. Ernest EA: Temporal tendonitis: a painful disorder that mimics migraine headache, *J Neurol Orthoped Surg* 8:160-165, 1987.

267. Ernest EA: Three disorders that frequently cause temporomandibular joint pain: internal derangement, temporal tendonitis, and Ernest syndrome, *J Neurol Orthoped Surg* 7:189-193, 1987.

268. Ernest EA III, Martinez ME, Rydzewski DB, Salter EG: Photomicrographic evidence of insertion tendonosis: the etiologic factor in pain for temporal tendonitis, *J Prosthet Dent* 65:127-131, 1991.

269. Shankland WE II: Common causes of nondental facial pain, *Gen Dent* 45:246-253; quiz 263-264, 1997.

270. Shankland WE II: Ernest syndrome as a consequence of stylomandibular ligament injury: a report of 68 patients, *J Prosthet Dent* 57:501-506, 1987.

Classification System Used for Diagnosing Temporomandibular Disorders

Bolded type indicates the disorders discussed in this chapter.

I. Masticatory muscle disorders *(Chapter 12)*
  A. Protective co-contraction
  B. Local muscle soreness
  C. Myospasm
  D. Myofascial pain
  E. Centrally mediated myalgia
  F. Fibromyalgia
  G. Centrally mediated motor disorders

II. Temporomandibular joint (TMJ) disorders *(Chapter 13)*
  A. Derangements of the condyle-disc complex
    1. Disc displacements
    2. Disc dislocations with reduction
    3. Disc dislocation without reduction
  B. Structural incompatibility of the articular surfaces
    1. Deviation in form
      a. Disc
      b. Condyle
      c. Fossa
    2. Adherences and adhesions
      a. Disc to condyle
      b. Disc to fossa
    3. Subluxation
    4. Spontaneous dislocation
  C. Inflammatory disorders of the TMJ
    1. Synovitis and capsulitis
    2. Retrodiscitis
    3. Arthritides
      a. Osteoarthritis
      b. Osteoarthrosis
      c. Polyarthritides
        i. Traumatic arthritis
        ii. Infectious arthritis
        iii. Rheumatoid arthritis
        iv. Hyperuricemia
        v. Psoriatic arthritis
        vi. Ankylosing spondylitis
    4. Inflammatory disorders of associated structures
      a. Temporal tendonitis
      b. Stylomandibular ligament inflammation
  D. General considerations when treating acute trauma to the TMJ

III. **Chronic mandibular hypomobility *(Chapter 14)***
  A. Ankylosis
    1. Capsular fibrosis
    2. Bony
  B. Muscle contracture
    1. Myositis
      a. Passive stretching
      b. Resistant-opening exercises
    2. Myofibrotic
  C. Coronoid process impedance

IV. **Growth disorders *(Chapter 14)***
  A. Congenital and developmental bone disorders
    1. Agenesis
    2. Hypoplasia
    3. Hyperplasia
    4. Neoplasia
  B. Congenital and developmental muscle disorders
    1. Hypotrophy
    2. Hypertrophy
    3. Neoplasia

Treatment of Chronic Mandibular Hypomobility and Growth Disorders

14

CHAPTER

"Although rare, never forget the other possibilities."

— JPO

The preceding two chapters addressed the most common categories of temporomandibular disorders observed in the general practice of dentistry. This chapter deals with the remaining two categories: chronic mandibular hypomobility and growth disorders. Even though these disorders occur less frequently than the others, it is equally important that they be appropriately managed with proper definitive and supportive therapy.

CHRONIC MANDIBULAR HYPOMOBILITY

The predominant feature of this disorder is the inability of the patient to open the mouth to a normal range. Chronic mandibular hypomobility is rarely accompanied by painful symptoms or progressive destructive changes. Therefore the rationale to instigate treatment should be carefully considered. When mandibular movement is so restricted that function is significantly impaired, treatment is indicated. When pain is associated with chronic hypomobility, it usually originates from an inflammatory reaction secondary to movement beyond the patient's restriction. This may occur as a result of either the patient's attempt to open beyond the restriction or extrinsic trauma that forces the mandible beyond the restriction. When inflammatory symptoms are present, treatment is indicated to resolve the inflammation.

However, when a patient presents with chronic mandibular hypomobility and is still able to function normally without pain, the best therapy is often no treatment. Supportive therapy may sometimes be helpful, but definitive therapy is often contraindicated.

Chronic mandibular hypomobility is subdivided into three categories according to cause: ankylosis, muscle contracture, and coronoid impedance.

ANKYLOSIS

By definition, *ankylosis* means abnormal immobility of a joint. The two basic types of ankylosis are differentiated by the tissues that limit the mobility: (1) fibrous and (2) bony. A fibrous ankylosis is most common and can occur between the condyle and the disc or between the disc and the fossa. A bony ankylosis of the temporomandibular joint (TMJ) would occur between the condyle and fossa, and therefore the disc would have to have been absent from the discal space before the ankylosis. Bony ankyloses are rare and represent a more chronic and extensive disorder. Because the cause and treatment of fibrous and bony ankyloses are similar, they are discussed together.

Cause

The most common cause of ankylosis is hemarthrosis secondary to macrotrauma.[1-4] Fibrous ankylosis represents a continued progression of joint adhesions (see Chapter 13) that gradually create a significant limitation in joint movement. Chronic inflammation aggravates the disorder, leading to

455

the development of more fibrous tissue. When bony structures become involved, bony ankylosis is more likely.

History

Patients report limited mouth opening without any pain. The patient is aware that this condition has been present for a long time and may not even feel that it poses a significant problem.

Clinical Characteristics

In many cases of ankylosis the condyle can still rotate, suggesting adhesions in the superior joint space. When this occurs, movement may still be possible in the inferior joint space between the condyle and the inferior surface of the disc.

Therefore the patient may be able to open approximately 25 mm interincisally; lateral movements are restricted. The clinical examination discloses a relatively normal range of lateral movement to the affected side but restricted movement to the unaffected side (Fig. 14-1). During mouth opening the opening pathway deflects to the ipsilateral side. No condylar movement is felt or visualized on a radiograph. When the ankylosis is bony, it can often be visualized on a radiograph or computed tomographic (CT) scan.

Definitive Treatment

Because the patient generally has some movement (although restricted), definitive treatment may not be indicated. If function is inadequate or the

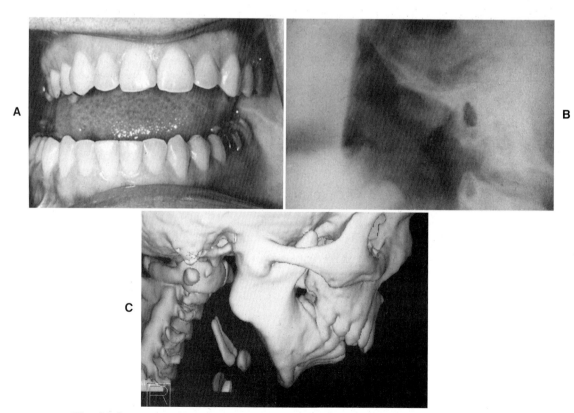

Fig. 14-1 A, Maximum opening with a fibrous ankylosis of the right temporomandibular joint. The limitation is accompanied by marked deflection of the midline to the affected side. **B,** Osseous ankylosis. Dense bone surrounds the entire joint structure. **C,** Three-dimensional computed tomographic reconstruction of the condyle of a 3-year-old patient reveals a complete osseous ankylosis. *(Courtesy Dr. J. Van Sickles, University of Kentucky, Lexington.)*

restriction is intolerable, surgery is the only definitive treatment available.[5] Arthroscopic surgery is the least aggressive surgical procedure, so it should be considered. Unfortunately many ankylosed joints are too attached to be freed with arthroscopy, and other surgical procedures need to be considered.[2,4,6-11] When surgical therapy is called for, remember that the elevator muscles are likely to be in a state of myostatic contracture and must be appropriately treated after the ankylosis is resolved.

Supportive Therapy
Because ankylosis is normally asymptomatic, generally no supportive therapy is indicated. However, if the mandible is forced beyond its restriction (i.e., by trauma), injury to the tissues can occur. If pain and inflammation result, supportive therapy is called for and consists of voluntarily restricting movement to within painless limits. Analgesics, along with deep heat therapy, can also be used.

Capsular Fibrosis
Another cause of mandibular hypomobility related to fibrotic changes is capsular fibrosis. The capsular ligament that surrounds the TMJ is partly responsible for limiting the normal range of joint movement. If it becomes fibrotic, its tissues can tighten or be restricted. As these tissues become fibrotic, the movement of the condyle within the joint is also restricted, creating a condition of chronic mandibular hypomobility. Capsular fibrosis is usually a result of inflammation, which can be secondary to inflammation of the adjacent tissues but is more commonly caused by trauma. The trauma may be an extrinsic force (e.g., a blow to the face), a surgical procedure, or an intrinsic force associated with abuse of the jaw.

Definitive Treatment. Because of two considerations, definitive treatment for capsular fibrosis is almost always contraindicated. First, capsular fibrosis usually restricts only the outer range of mandibular movement and is not a major functional problem for the patient.

Second, because the changes are fibrotic, therapy falls within the surgical range. However, surgery is one of the etiologic factors that can create this disorder. Therefore a surgical procedure to free

the fibrous restrictions must be carefully weighed, in view of the fact that it could lead to further fibrosis on healing.

Supportive Therapy. Because capsular fibrosis is normally asymptomatic, no supportive therapy is indicated. On occasion, when the mandible is forced beyond the capsular restriction (i.e., trauma), symptoms can begin. These are often related to the inflammatory reaction of the traumatized tissues. When this condition exists, the patient is treated with the same supportive therapy as for capsulitis.

MUSCLE CONTRACTURE

Contracture means a painless shortening of a muscle. The two types of contracture are myostatic and myofibrotic. Contracture of the elevator muscles can produce chronic mandibular hypomobility.

Myostatic Contracture
Cause. Myostatic contracture results when a muscle is kept from fully lengthening (stretching) for a prolonged time. The restriction may be caused by full lengthening, which causes pain in an associated structure. Therefore myostatic contracture is often secondary to another disorder. As an example, if a patient wore an anterior positioning appliance continuously, the inferior lateral pterygoid muscle would not be allowed to fully lengthen. A myostatic contracture can develop that disallows the condyle to immediately return to the musculoskeletally stable position. If this occurs and the patient removes the appliance, the posterior teeth will not occlude (a posterior open bite). This was a common adverse effect when anterior positioning appliances were used 24 hours per day. However, when these appliances are used only part time, as suggested in this text, this effect is rarely observed.

History. The patient reports a long history of restricted jaw movement. It may have begun secondary to a pain condition that has now resolved.

Clinical Characteristics. Myostatic contracture is characterized by painless limitation of mouth opening.

Definitive Treatment. Importantly, the original etiologic factor that created the myostatic contracture must be identified. If this condition still exists, it must be eliminated before effective treatment of the contracture can result. Once the original cause has been eliminated, definitive treatment is directed toward the gradual lengthening of the involved muscles. This lengthening is an attempt to reestablish the original resting length of the muscles and must be done slowly over many weeks. If pain is elicited, protective co-contraction can result and this treatment will fail. The resting length of the muscles can be reestablished by two types of exercise: passive stretching and resistant opening.

Passive stretching. Passive stretching of the elevator muscles is accomplished when the patient opens to the full limit of movement and then gently stretches beyond the restriction. The stretching should be gentle and momentary so as not to traumatize the muscle tissues and initiate pain or an inflammatory reaction.[12,13] Sometimes it is possible to assist the stretching by placing the fingers between the teeth and initiating the stretch as the patient relaxes (Fig. 14-2). Extreme care must be taken with this technique. These passive stretching exercises are performed gently over a reasonable

amount of time; the best results are achieved with weeks of therapy (not days). Too much force applied too soon can create an inflammatory reaction in the tissues being stretched.

Resistant-opening exercises. Resistant-opening exercises take advantage of the neurologic reflex system to aid in relaxation of the elevator muscles. Remember that the mandibular elevators and depressors function according to reciprocal inhibition. In other words, to elevate the mandible, the elevator muscles must be contracted at the same time and to the same length as the depressor muscles are relaxed. The neurologic stretch reflex helps control this activity. When local muscle soreness is present in one of the muscle groups, full lengthening of the muscle becomes difficult. A neurologic feedback can be used to help achieve relaxation. This is accomplished by initiating mild contraction of the antagonistic muscle groups. When the elevator muscles will not properly relax, contraction of the depressors provided by resistance to opening feeds neurologic input to the elevator muscles to relax. This has been referred to as *reflex relaxation.*[14]

Resistant-opening exercises are accomplished by instructing the patient to place the fingers under the chin. Opening is then attempted against the resistance (Fig. 14-3). Resistant-opening exercises consist

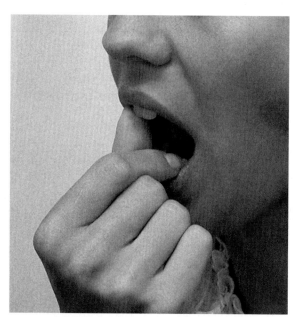

Fig. 14-2 PASSIVE STRETCHING EXERCISE. With the mandible opened to the point of restriction, the fingers are placed between the teeth. Momentary gentle force is applied to stretch the elevator muscles. This exercise should not produce pain.

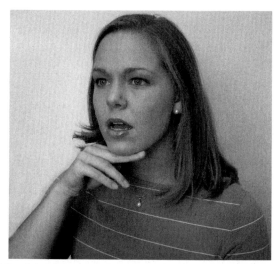

Fig. 14-3 RESISTANT-OPENING EXERCISE. The mouth is opened against finger resistance.

of 10 repetitions repeated two or three times per day. The resistant force provided by the fingers is gentle and should not induce painful symptoms. Passive stretching of the elevator muscles is done both before and after each set of resistance exercises. When lateral restrictions are present, lateral resistant exercises can also be used in a similar manner but are less often indicated (Fig. 14-4).

When passive and resistant exercises are properly employed for a patient with mandibular hypomobility, no painful symptoms result. Any pain that does develop is normally associated with an inflammatory reaction in the tissues. Pain therefore implies too much, too soon, and should clue the patient and therapist to decrease the force and sometimes the number of repetitions being used. Remember, effective treatment may take weeks and should not be rushed.

Supportive Therapy. Because definitive treatment should not create symptoms, supportive therapy is of little use in the treatment of myostatic contracture or, for that matter, in any chronic mandibular hypomobility. When symptoms do occur, analgesics can be helpful and should accompany a decrease in the intensity of the exercise program. Thermotherapy and ultrasound are also helpful.

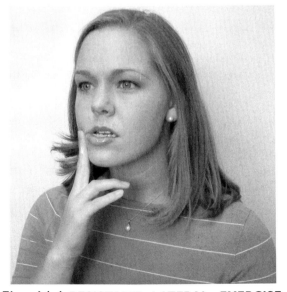

Fig. 14-4 RESISTANT LATERAL EXERCISE. The mouth is moved laterally against finger resistance.

Myofibrotic Contracture

Cause. Myofibrotic contracture occurs as a result of excessive tissue adhesions within the muscle or its sheaths. These fibrosis tissue adhesions prevent the muscle fibers from sliding over themselves, disallowing full lengthening of the muscle. Common causes of myofibrotic contracture are myositis and trauma to the muscle.

History. The history for myofibrotic contracture reveals a previous muscle injury or a long-term restriction in the range of movement. The patient has no complaints of pain. Sometimes the patient will not even be aware of the limited range of opening because it has been present for so long.

Clinical Characteristics. Myofibrotic contracture is characterized by painless limitation of mouth opening. Lateral condylar movement is usually unaffected. Thus if the diagnosis is difficult, radiographs showing limited condylar movement during opening but normal movement during lateral excursions may help. No acute malocclusion exists.

Definitive Treatment. In myofibrotic contracture, the muscle tissues can relax but the muscle length does not increase. Myofibrotic contracture is therefore permanent. Some elongation of the muscle can be accomplished by continuous elastic traction. This is done by linear growth of the muscle and is slow and limited by the muscle tissue health and adaptability.[12] Generally, definitive treatment is the surgical detachment of the muscles involved. If surgical intervention is indicated, it must be noted that the function of the uninvolved muscles has also been chronically restricted and the muscles are likely to be in a state of myostatic contracture. Once a myofibrotic contracture is surgically resolved, therapy for it and the remaining elevator muscles is instituted. It should be noted that muscles that have been surgically detached often reattach with time. If the range of movement can be maintained by passive exercises, hopefully the restriction will not return.

Supportive Therapy. Because myofibrotic contracture is rarely associated with painful symptoms, supportive therapy is not indicated. When symptoms do arise, the same type of therapy suggested for myostatic contracture is instituted.

The clinician should note that it is often difficult to determine by the history and examination whether muscle contracture is myostatic or myofibrotic. In many cases the key to diagnosis lies in treatment. When treatment regains muscle length, myostatic contracture is confirmed. If treatment creates repeated symptoms without achieving increased muscle length, myofibrotic contracture is likely.

CORONOID IMPEDANCE

During mandibular opening the coronoid process passes anteroinferiorly between the zygomatic arch and the lateral surface of the maxilla. If its pathway is impeded, it will not slide smoothly and the mouth will not open fully.

Cause

Coronoid impedance is generally caused by either elongation of the process (Fig. 14-5) or the encroachment of fibrous tissue.[15-19] Because these conditions are chronic, pain is not usually present, and it is for this reason that coronoid impedance is considered to be a hypomobility disorder. The first condition, elongation of the coronoid process,[20,21] may be the result of chronic temporalis hyperactivity. (Remember, the temporales attach to the coronoid.) The suggestion has even been made[22] that elongation of the coronoid process may be associated with disc dislocations.

The second condition, tissue fibrosis, can be the result of a traumatic incident or a prior infection.[18]

When the tissues anterior and inferior to the coronoid process become fibrotic, the coronoid may not be able to move freely between the maxilla and the zygomatic arch. The trauma may be the result of a surgical procedure in the area that led to scar formation or a mandibular or maxillary fracture that was treated with zygomatic arch wiring that led to the development of fibrotic tissue in the area.

History

Patients often experience painless restriction of opening that, in many cases, followed trauma to the area or an infection. A long-standing anterior disc dislocation may also be present.

Clinical Characteristics

Limitation is evident in all movements but especially during mandibular protrusion. A straight midline opening path is commonly observed unless one coronoid process is more free than the other. If the problem is unilateral, opening will deflect the mandible to the same side as the restriction. A CT scan can be helpful in making the differential diagnosis (see Fig. 14-5, *B*).[23,24]

Definitive Treatment

Definitive treatment for coronoid impedance is alteration of the responsible tissue. Sometimes ultrasound followed by gentle passive stretching will help mobilize the structures. A true definitive

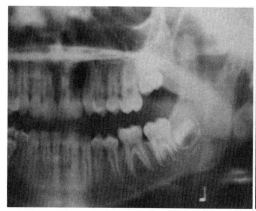

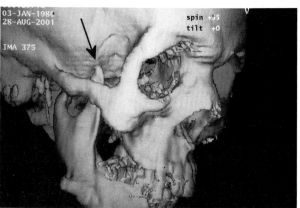

A   **B**

Fig. 14-5 A, An extremely long coronoid process. The length of the coronoid limits mandibular opening, resulting in a chronic hypomobility condition. **B,** This three-dimensional computed tomographic reconstruction reveals a long coronoid process *(arrow)* that limited mouth opening for this patient.

treatment is surgery that either shortens the coronoid process or eliminates the tissue obstruction (whichever is the cause).[25-28] Because the condition is generally painless, surgical intervention is usually contraindicated due to its aggressiveness. A surgical procedure can also create the very process that it is trying to eliminate (fibrosis). Therefore it should be considered only if function is severely impaired.

Supportive Therapy

Because coronoid impedance is normally asymptomatic, no supportive therapy is indicated. If the mandible is forced to open beyond the restriction, symptoms can result and are usually related to the inflammatory reaction of the traumatized tissues. If inflammation exists, the patient is treated with the same supportive therapy indicated for tendonitis.

GROWTH DISORDERS

Growth disorder of the masticatory system can be divided into two broad categories according to the tissues involved: (1) bone disorders and (2) muscle disorders.

CONGENITAL AND DEVELOPMENTAL BONE DISORDERS

Common growth disturbances of the bones are agenesis (no growth), hypoplasia (insufficient growth), hyperplasia (too much growth), or neoplasia (uncontrolled, destructive growth).

Cause

The cause of bone growth disorders is not completely understood. Trauma in many instances is a contributing factor and, especially in a young joint, can lead to hypoplasia of that condyle, resulting in an asymmetric shift or growth pattern.[29-34] This ultimately causes an asymmetric shift of the mandible with an associated malocclusion[35] (Figs. 14-6 and 14-7). An asymmetric growth pattern may also result from early development of rheumatoid arthritis.[36,37] In other instances trauma[38] can cause a hyperplastic reaction, resulting in an overgrowth of bone (Fig. 14-8).[39,40] This is commonly seen at the

site of an old fracture. Some hypoplastic and hyperplastic activities relate to inherent growth activities and hormonal body imbalances (e.g., acromegaly) (Fig. 14-9). It is unfortunate that many causative factors of neoplasia, especially metastases, are yet to be determined (Fig. 14-10).

History

A common characteristic of bone growth disorders is that the clinical symptoms reported by the patient are directly related to the structural changes present. Because these disorders usually produce slow changes, pain is not present and patients commonly alter function to accommodate the changes.

Clinical Characteristics

Any alteration of function or the presence of pain is secondary to structural changes. Clinical asymmetry may be noticed that is associated with and indicative of a growth or developmental interruption. Radiographs of the TMJ, as well as CT scans, are extremely important in identifying structural (bony) changes that have taken place.

Definitive Treatment

Definitive treatment for bone growth disorders must be tailored specifically to the patient's condition. Because definitive treatment for these disorders does not fall within the context of this book, other, more detailed sources should be consulted.[41,42] Generally, treatment is provided to restore function while minimizing any trauma to the associated structures. The health and welfare of the patient over his or her lifetime should always be considered. Neoplastic activity needs to be aggressively investigated and treated.[43-46]

Supportive Therapy

Because most bone growth disorders are not associated with pain or dysfunction, supportive therapy is not indicated. If pain or dysfunction arises, then treatment is rendered according to the problem identified (i.e., local muscle soreness, disc derangement, inflammation). The clinician should note that the later stages of neoplasia can result in symptoms. When neoplasia is identified, supportive therapy should not be used to mask

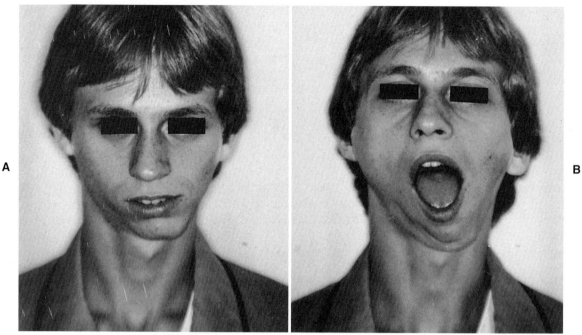

Fig. 14-6 UNILATERAL HYPOPLASIA OF THE CONDYLE. A, At an early age the left temporomandibular joint received a traumatic injury. Its condyle failed to develop normally, resulting in a shift of the midline by the normally growing right condyle. **B,** During opening there is a restricted movement pattern of the left condyle, resulting in a marked shift of the midline to that side.

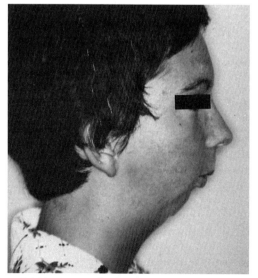

Fig. 14-7 BILATERAL HYPOPLASIA OF THE CONDYLES. The significant lack of growth in the mandible is demonstrated.

the symptoms. More definitive treatment is indicated, and the patient must be referred to appropriate dental or medical specialists.

CONGENITAL AND DEVELOPMENTAL MUSCLE DISORDERS

Common congenital or developmental muscle disorders can be divided into three categories: hypotrophy (lack of development), hypertrophy (overdevelopment), and neoplasms (uncontrolled, destructive growth).

Cause

The cause of congenital and developmental muscle disorders is largely unknown. Certainly congenital factors can play an important role, as well as certain systemic disorders (i.e., multiple sclerosis). Hypertrophic changes may be secondary to increased use such as bruxism. The cause of neoplastic muscle disorders needs further investigation.

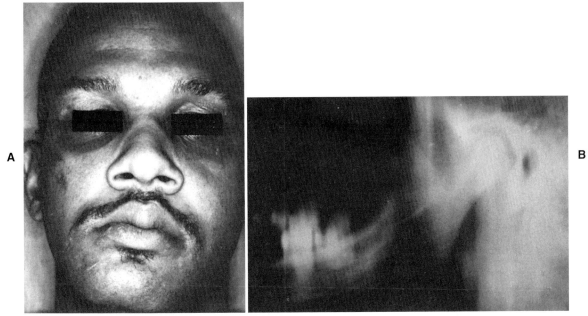

Fig. 14-8 UNILATERAL HYPERPLASIA OF THE CONDYLES. A, The midline shift to the right is a result of hyperplastic growth of the left condyle. **B,** Hyperplasia of the left condyle.

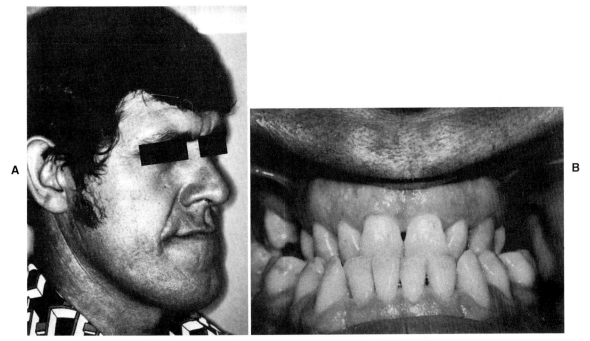

Fig. 14-9 ACROMEGALY. A, The prominence of the mandible resulting from continued growth is demonstrated. **B,** Significant malocclusion.

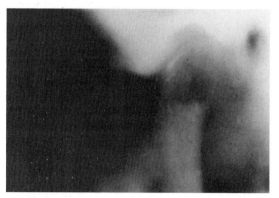

Fig. 14-10 Neoplasia of the left condyle, metastatic adenocarcinoma. *(Courtesy Dr. D. Damm, University of Kentucky, Lexington.)*

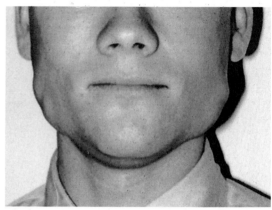

Fig. 14-11 Masseter muscle hyperplasia secondary to chronic bruxism.

History

A common characteristic of muscle hypotrophy is a feeling of muscle weakness. Patients with hypertrophic muscle changes rarely report any symptoms and may only be concerned with aesthetics (large masseters). Because these disorders usually produce slow changes, patients commonly accommodate and are unaware of the disorder.

Clinical Characteristics

The clinical characteristics of muscle growth disorders relate to the specific problem that is present. Hypotrophy is often difficult to recognize. Hypertrophy can be observed as large masseter muscles (Fig. 14-11), but appreciating normalcy for the patient may be difficult. A normal range of mandibular movement is likely to be present in any of these muscle conditions.

Definitive Treatment

Definitive treatment for muscle growth disorders must be tailored specifically to the patient's condition. Because definitive treatment for these disorders does not fall within the context of this book, other, more detailed sources should be consulted.[47] Generally, treatment is provided to restore function while minimizing any trauma to the associated structures. The health and welfare of the patient over his or her lifetime should always be considered. When hypertrophy is present secondary to bruxism, a muscle relaxation appliance should be offered. Enlarged masseter and temporalis muscles can be reduced with botulinum toxin injections (see Chapter 12); however, if the bruxing activity continues, the enlargement may return. Neoplastic activity needs to be aggressively investigated and treated.

Supportive Therapy

Because most muscle growth disorders are not associated with pain or dysfunction, supportive therapy is not indicated. If pain or dysfunction arises, then treatment is rendered according to the problem identified (e.g., local muscle soreness, disc derangement, inflammation). Be aware that the later stages of neoplasia can result in symptoms. When neoplasia is identified, supportive therapy should not be used to mask the symptoms. More definitive treatment is indicated, and the patient must be referred to appropriate dental or medical specialists.

Case Reports

Case 1

A 32-year-old salesman reported to the dental office with a chief complaint of being unable to open his mouth completely. These symptoms had begun 5 weeks ago, 1 day after a dental appointment in which he received an injection of local anesthetic. He reported that the injection site had become so tender that it was difficult to open wide without eliciting pain. The pain had subsided after 1 week without treatment, but the restriction in mandibular opening remained. When the patient came to this office, he was without any pain symptoms yet had limited opening.

The clinical examination revealed no pain, tenderness, or sounds from either joint. The maximum interincisal opening was 34 mm, and no pain was felt at this limit. Both lateral movements appeared to be only slightly restricted. The muscle examination was negative. The occlusal examination disclosed a complete natural dentition with several teeth in need of repair. There was a 2-mm straightforward and superior shift from the centric relation (CR) position to intercuspal position (ICP). Moderate tooth wear was apparent on the anterior teeth. All other occlusal findings were within normal limits. A thorough examination of the injection site failed to identify any signs or symptoms of inflammation. A panoramic radiograph taken in the open position revealed normal subarticular surfaces with bilateral functional restrictions. No other significant findings were reported in the history or clinical examination.

DIAGNOSIS. The patient was diagnosed with myostatic contracture of the elevator muscles secondary to postinjection trauma and/or infection.

TREATMENT. The history suggested that a postinjection inflammation was responsible for the myostatic contracture. Thorough examination of the injection site failed to reveal any signs of inflammation. It was suspected that this causative factor had resolved independently of treatment. Passive muscle exercises and stretching were instituted to gradually increase muscle length. The patient was instructed to perform these exercises two or three times per day and, if pain was elicited, to lessen the frequency and force used. After 1 week the patient had a maximum interincisal opening of 36 mm. He was pleased with this progress. Resistant-opening exercises were added to the passive exercises to be done at the same time each day. By the next week he could open 38 mm but was complaining of some mild soreness in the muscles. He was then instructed to reduce the force employed in the resistant and stretching exercises until no pain was felt. By the next week the symptoms had resolved, and opening was measured at 38 mm.

Over the next 4 weeks the interincisal opening reached 44 mm without pain. Exercises were discontinued on the fifth week. At the next 6-month recall the maximum interincisal opening was 46 mm. ■

Case 2

A 27-year-old policeman reported that he was troubled by restricted mandibular movement. He related that the restriction seemed to originate from the left TMJ. His symptoms

had begun 6 months ago when he was struck on the right side of the chin. At the time a mandibular fracture had been suspected but was not radiographically confirmed. The patient was treated with interarch fixation for 4 weeks. After the fixation was removed, he reported soreness in the left TMJ that was accentuated by movement. Two weeks later the limitation continued, but it remained asymptomatic for the next 5 months. The patient originally was told that the limitation would slowly improve; because it did not, he decided to seek treatment. When questioned, he revealed no major problems in functioning.

The clinical examination revealed no pain or tenderness in either joint. On opening there was a definite deflection of the mandibular midline to the left. Observation and palpation revealed movement of the right condyle during opening, but no movement could be observed in the left joint. The patient could move in a left lateral excursion 7 mm, but only 2 mm right. Maximum opening was 26 mm. The clinical examination was negative for any muscle tenderness or pain. The occlusal examination disclosed an anteriorly fixed partial denture, which had been fabricated to replace two teeth that were lost during the same incident. No CR-to-ICP slide was present. Group function guidance existed bilaterally. Panoramic and open and closed transcranial radiographs depicted the subarticular surfaces as normal. The right TMJ showed slight limitation of functional movement, whereas the left showed no movement at all. No other significant findings were reported in either the history or the clinical examination.

DIAGNOSIS. The patient was diagnosed with fibrotic ankylosis of the left joint secondary to hemarthrosis related to trauma.

TREATMENT. The nature of the disorder was explained to the patient, and it was related that the only definitive treatment would be surgery. After an evaluation and discussion of the patient's minimal dysfunctional condition, it was advised that no treatment be provided at this time. ■

Case 3

A 66-year-old retired mailman came to the dental office with pain in the left TMJ that had been constant for 3 weeks. He reported an inability to eat well because of the pain and related that this was contributing to his overall failing health. The history revealed chronic asymptomatic joint sounds with pain beginning only recently.

The clinical examination revealed pain in the left joint (score, 2), with the right joint being asymptomatic. A normal range of mandibular movement was observed (44 mm of opening and lateral excursions of 8 mm), but pain was accentuated with the movement. The muscle examination revealed pain in the right masseter and temporalis (score, 2). The left temporalis was also tender (score, 1).

The occlusal examination revealed an edentulous mouth with a 4-year-old denture that appeared to have adequately replaced the vertical dimension and provided a stable occlusal relationship. The transcranial and panoramic radiographs both disclosed a large eroded area in the posterior aspect of the left condyle. Tomograms were immediately ordered and more clearly verified the presence of a cystlike mass that had eroded the posterior aspect of the condyle. The patient was immediately referred to a surgeon for an appropriate evaluation of the radiographic findings. A surgical biopsy of the bone tissue was taken for analysis.

DIAGNOSIS. The patient was diagnosed with metastatic adenocarcinoma.

TREATMENT. Further physical examination revealed a large lesion in the left lung. This was suspected of being the primary site from which the left TMJ lesion had metastasized. The patient underwent radical surgery to remove both lesions and was started on a course of chemotherapy. ■

References

1. Guthua SW, Maina DM, Kahugu M: Management of posttraumatic temporomandibular joint ankylosis in children: case report, *East Afr Med J* 72:471-475, 1995.
2. Guven O: A clinical study on temporomandibular joint ankylosis, *Auris Nasus Larynx* 27:27-33, 2000.
3. Ferretti C, Bryant R, Becker P, Lawrence C: Temporomandibular joint morphology following post-traumatic ankylosis in 26 patients, *Int J Oral Maxillofac Surg* 34:376-381, 2005.
4. Vasconcelos BC, Bessa-Nogueira RV, Cypriano RV: Treatment of temporomandibular joint ankylosis by gap arthroplasty, *Med Oral Patol Oral Cir Bucal* 11:E66-69, 2006.
5. Kirk WS Jr, Farrar JH: Early surgical correction of unilateral TMJ ankylosis and improvement in mandibular symmetry with use of an orthodontic functional appliance—a case report, *Cranio* 11:308-311, 1993.
6. Nitzan DW, Bar-Ziv J, Shteyer A: Surgical management of temporomandibular joint ankylosis type III by retaining the displaced condyle and disc, *J Oral Maxillofac Surg* 56:1133-1138; discussion 1139, 1998.
7. Ko EW, Huang CS, Chen YR: Temporomandibular joint reconstruction in children using costochondral grafts, *J Oral Maxillofac Surg* 57:789-798, 1999.
8. Mercuri LG: Considering total temporomandibular joint replacement, *Cranio* 17:44-48, 1999.
9. Sawhney CP: Bony ankylosis of the temporomandibular joint: follow-up of 70 patients treated with arthroplasty and acrylic spacer interposition, *Plast Reconstr Surg* 77: 29-40, 1986.
10. Long X, Li X, Cheng Y, Yang X, Qin L et al: Preservation of disc for treatment of traumatic temporomandibular joint ankylosis, *J Oral Maxillofac Surg* 63:897-902, 2005.
11. Tanrikulu R, Erol B, Gorgun B, Soker M: The contribution to success of various methods of treatment of temporomandibular joint ankylosis (a statistical study containing 24 cases), *Turk J Pediatr* 47:261-265, 2005.
12. Bell WE: *Temporomandibular disorders: classification, diagnosis, management,* ed 3, Chicago, 1990, Year Book Medical, p 363.
13. Ylinen JJ, Takala EP, Nykanen MJ, Kautiainen HJ, Hakkinen AH et al: Effects of twelve-month strength training subsequent to twelve-month stretching exercise in treatment of chronic neck pain, *J Strength Cond Res* 20:304-308, 2006.
14. Schwartz L: *Disorders of the temporomandibular joint,* Philadelphia. 1959, Saunders, pp 223-225.
15. Hicks JL, Iverson PH: Bilateral coronoid hyperplasia: an important cause of restricted mandibular motion, *Northwest Dent* 72:21-24, 1993.
16. Smyth AG, Wake MJ: Recurrent bilateral coronoid hyperplasia: an unusual case, *Br J Oral Maxillofac Surg* 32:100-104, 1994.
17. Freihofer HP: Restricted opening of the mouth with an extra-articular cause in children, *J Craniomaxillofac Surg* 19:289-298, 1991.
18. Lucaya J, Herrera M, Vera J: Unilateral hyperplasia of the coronoid process in a child: a cause of restricted opening of the mouth, *Radiology* 144:528-529, 1982.
19. Kai S, Hijiya T, Yamane K, Higuchi Y: Open-mouth locking caused by unilateral elongated coronoid process: report of case, *J Oral Maxillofac Surg* 55:1305-1308, 1997.
20. Hall RE, Orbach S, Landesberg R: Bilateral hyperplasia of the mandibular coronoid processes: a report of two cases, *Oral Surg Oral Med Oral Pathol* 67:141-145, 1989.
21. Isberg AM, McNamara JA Jr, Carlson DS, Isacsson G: Coronoid process elongation in rhesus monkeys (*Macaca mulatta*) after experimentally induced mandibular hypomobility. A cephalometric and histologic study, *Oral Surg Oral Med Oral Pathol* 70:704-710, 1990.
22. Isberg A, Isacsson G, Nah KS: Mandibular coronoid process locking: a prospective study of frequency and association with internal derangement of the temporomandibular joint, *Oral Surg Oral Med Oral Pathol* 63: 275-279, 1987.
23. Munk PL, Helms CA: Coronoid process hyperplasia: CT studies, *Radiology* 171:783-784, 1989.
24. Tucker MR, Guilford WB, Thomas PM: Versatility of CT scanning for evaluation of mandibular hypomobilities, *J Maxillofac Surg* 14:89-92, 1986.
25. Gerbino G, Bianchi SD, Bernardi M, Berrone S: Hyperplasia of the mandibular coronoid process: long-term follow-up after coronoidotomy, *J Craniomaxillofac Surg* 25:169-173, 1997.
26. Loh HS, Ling SY, Lian CB, Shanmuhasuntharam P: Bilateral coronoid hyperplasia—a report with a view on its management, *J Oral Rehabil* 24:782-787, 1997.
27. Capote A, Rodriguez FJ, Blasco A, Munoz MF: Jacob's disease associated with temporomandibular joint dysfunction: a case report, *Med Oral Patol Oral Cir Bucal* 10:210-214, 2005.

28. Talmi YP, Horowitz Z, Yahalom R, Bedrin L: Coronoidectomy in maxillary swing for reducing the incidence and severity of trismus—a reminder, *J Craniomaxillofac Surg* 32:19-20, 2004.

29. Jerrell RG, Fuselier B, Mahan P: Acquired condylar hypoplasia: report of case, *ASDC J Dent Child* 58:147-153, 1991.

30. Germane N, Rubenstein L: The effects of forceps delivery on facial growth, *Pediatr Dent* 11:193-197, 1989.

31. Berger SS, Stewart RE: Mandibular hypoplasia secondary to perinatal trauma: report of case, *J Oral Surg* 35:578-582, 1977.

32. Obiechina AE, Arotiba JT, Fasola AO: Ankylosis of the temporomandibular joint as a complication of forceps delivery: report of a case, *West Afr J Med* 18:144-146, 1999.

33. Oztan HY, Ulusal BG, Aytemiz C: The role of trauma on temporomandibular joint ankylosis and mandibular growth retardation: an experimental study, *J Craniofac Surg* 15:274-282; discussion 282, 2004.

34. Defabianis P: The importance of early recognition of condylar fractures in children: a study of 2 cases, *J Orofac Pain* 18:253-260, 2004.

35. Guyuron B: Facial deformity of juvenile rheumatoid arthritis, *Plast Reconstr Surg* 81:948-951, 1988.

36. Kjellberg H, Fasth A, Kiliaridis S, Wenneberg B, Thilander B: Craniofacial structure in children with juvenile chronic arthritis (JCA) compared with healthy children with ideal or postnormal occlusion, *Am J Orthod Dentofacial Orthop* 107:67-78, 1995.

37. Stabrun AE: Impaired mandibular growth and micrognathic development in children with juvenile rheumatoid arthritis. A longitudinal study of lateral cephalographs, *Eur J Orthod* 13:423-434, 1991.

38. McGuirt WF, Salisbury PL III: Mandibular fractures. Their effect on growth and dentition, *Arch Otolaryngol Head Neck Surg* 113:257-261, 1987.

39. Jacobsen PU, Lund K: Unilateral overgrowth and remodeling processes after fracture of the mandibular condyle. A longitudinal radiographic study, *Scand J Dent Res* 80:68-74, 1972.

40. Ferguson MW, Whitlock RI: An unusual case of acquired unilateral condylar hypoplasia, *Br J Maxillofac Surg* 16:156-162, 1978.

41. Miloro M: *Principles of oral and maxillofacial surgery*, ed 2, Hamilton, Ontario, Canada, 2004, BB Decker.

42. Fonseca R, Walker R, Betts N, Barber H, Powers M: *Oral and maxillofacial trauma*, ed 3, Philadelphia, 2005, Saunders.

43. Butler JH: Myofascial pain dysfunction syndrome involving tumor metastasis. Case report, *J Periodontol* 46:309-311, 1975.

44. Weinberg S, Katsikeris N, Pharoah M: Osteoblastoma of the mandibular condyle: review of the literature and report of a case, *J Oral Maxillofac Surg* 45:350-355, 1987.

45. White DK, Chen S, Mohnac AM, Miller AS: Odontogenic myxoma. A clinical and ultrastructural study, *Oral Surg Oral Med Oral Pathol* 39:901-917, 1975.

46. Trumpy IG, Lyberg T: In vivo deterioration of Proplast Teflon temporomandibular joint interpositional implants: a scanning electron microscopic and energy-dispersive X-ray analysis, *J Oral Maxillofac Surg* 51:624-629, 1993.

47. Braunwald E, Isselbacher KJ: *Harrison's principles of internal medicine*, New York, 1987, McGraw-Hill.

Occlusal Appliance Therapy

15

CHAPTER

"The occlusal appliance: an adjunction to managing TMD."

—JPO

*A*n occlusal appliance (often called a *splint*) is a removal device, usually made of hard acrylic, that fits over the occlusal and incisal surfaces of the teeth in one arch, creating precise occlusal contact with the teeth of the opposing arch (Fig. 15-1). It is commonly referred to as a *bite guard, night guard, interocclusal appliance*, or even an *orthopedic device* (i.e., orthotic).

Occlusal appliances have several uses, one of which is to temporarily provide an occlusal condition that allows the temporomandibular joints (TMJs) to assume the most orthopedically stable joint position. They can also be used to introduce an optimum occlusal condition that reorganizes the neuromuscular reflex activity, which in turn reduces abnormal muscle activity while encouraging more normal muscle function. Occlusal appliances are also used to protect the teeth and supportive structures from abnormal forces that may create breakdown and/or tooth wear.

GENERAL CONSIDERATIONS

Appliance therapy has several favorable qualities that render it helpful for the management of many temporomandibular disorders (TMDs). Because the etiology and interrelationships of many TMDs are often complex, the initial therapy should generally be reversible and noninvasive. Occlusal appliances can offer such therapy while temporarily improving the functional relationships of the masticatory system. When an occlusal appliance is specifically designed to alter a causative factor of TMDs, even temporarily, the symptoms are also altered. In this sense the appliance becomes diagnostic. Care must be taken, however, not to oversimplify this relationship. As discussed later in this chapter, an appliance can affect a patient's symptoms in several ways. It is extremely important that, when it reduces symptoms, the precise cause-and-effect relationship be identified before irreversible therapy is begun. These considerations are necessary to ensure that more extensive treatment will produce long-term success. Occlusal appliances are equally helpful in ruling out certain causative factors. When a malocclusion is suspected of contributing to a TMD, occlusal appliance therapy can quickly and reversibly introduce a more desirable occlusal condition. If it does not affect the symptoms, the malocclusion is probably not a causative factor and certainly the need for irreversible occlusal therapy should be questioned.

Another favorable quality of occlusal appliance therapy in managing TMDs is that it is useful in reducing symptoms.[1-5] An extensive critical review of the literature[6] revealed that its effectiveness is between 70% and 90%. However, a more recent article using the Cochrane Database Systematic

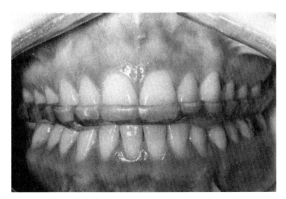

Fig. 15-1 Maxillary occlusal appliance.

FABRICATION AND ADJUSTMENT OF THE APPLIANCE

Once the proper appliance has been selected, it must be fabricated and adjusted such that the treatment goals will be successfully accomplished. Care must be taken to construct an appliance that will be both compatible with the soft tissues and provide the exact alteration in function needed to eliminate the cause. An improperly adjusted appliance will not only diminish treatment effects but may also introduce doubt on the part of both patient and dentist in the diagnosis and future treatment.

PATIENT COOPERATION

Because appliance therapy is reversible, it is effective only when the patient is wearing the appliance. Patients must be instructed regarding its appropriate use. Some appliances require extensive use, whereas others require only part-time use. Patients who do not respond favorably to this therapy should be questioned regarding their compliance with the prescribed use of the appliance. A properly selected appliance that is accurately adjusted will fail to reduce symptoms in a patient who does not wear it appropriately.

Review reported that occlusal appliances do not have a strong or reliable effect on TMD symptoms.[7] This is likely a reflection of the poor research design commonly used in earlier studies. The precise mechanism by which appliances may reduce TMD symptoms has been debated and is inconclusive at present.[8-10] The profession must provide better evidence-based data to better understand the role of appliances in TMDs. What is evident is that they are generally a reversible noninvasive modality that can help manage the symptoms of many TMDs. Therefore they are often indicated in the initial and in some long-term treatments of many TMDs.[11,12]

The success or failure of occlusal appliance therapy depends on the selection, fabrication, and adjustment of the appliance and on patient cooperation.

PROPER APPLIANCE SELECTION

Several types of appliances are used in dentistry. Each is aimed at affecting a specific causative factor. To select the proper appliance for a patient, one must first identify the major contributing factor causing the disorder. An appliance that will best affect that factor can then be selected. No single appliance is useful with all TMDs. In fact, some TMDs do not respond to appliance therapy at all. Once again, the importance of a thorough history, examination, and diagnosis is emphasized.

TYPES OF OCCLUSAL APPLIANCES

Many types of occlusal appliances have been suggested for the treatment of TMDs. The two used most frequently are (1) the stabilization appliance and (2) the anterior positioning appliance. The stabilization appliance is sometimes called a *muscle relaxation appliance* because it is primarily used to reduce muscle pain.[1,2,12,13] The anterior positioning appliance is sometimes called an *orthopedic repositioning appliance* because its goal is to change the position of the mandible in relationship to the cranium. Other types of occlusal devices are the anterior bite plane, the posterior bite plane, the pivoting appliance, and the soft or resilient appliance. The descriptions, treatment goals, and indications for these devices are reviewed in the following sections.

Because the stabilization and anterior positioning appliances are important in the treatment of TMDs, a fabrication technique for each of these is presented.

STABILIZATION APPLIANCE

Description and Treatment Goals

The stabilization appliance is generally fabricated for the maxillary arch and provides an occlusal relationship considered optimal for the patient (see Chapter 5). When it is in place, the condyles are in their most musculoskeletally stable (MS) position at the time the teeth are contacting evenly and simultaneously. Canine disocclusion of the posterior teeth during eccentric movement is also provided. The treatment goal of the stabilization appliance is to eliminate any orthopedic instability between the occlusal position and the joint position, thus removing this instability as a causative factor in the TMD (see Chapter 7).

Indications

The stabilization appliance is generally used to treat muscle pain disorders.[1,2,12] Studies[14-19] have shown that wearing it can decrease the parafunctional activity that often accompanies periods of stress. Thus when a patient reports with a TMD that relates to muscle hyperactivity such as bruxism, a stabilization appliance should be considered.[20] More recent studies are less convincing regarding the precise mechanism by which occlusal appliances help reduce TMD symptoms, but most authors still support their use.[1,2,10,12,21] The patient with local muscle soreness or chronic centrally mediated myalgia, likewise, may be a good candidate for this type of appliance. Stabilization appliances are also helpful for patients experiencing retrodiscitis secondary to trauma. This appliance can help minimize forces[22] to damaged tissues, thus permitting more efficient healing.

Simplified Fabrication Technique

The full-arch hard acrylic stabilization appliance can be used in either arch, but maxillary placement provides some advantages. The maxillary device is usually more stable and covers more tissue, which makes it more retentive and less likely to break. It is also more versatile, allowing opposing contacts to be achieved in all skeletal and molar relationships. In Class II and Class III patients, for example, achievement of proper anterior contact and guidance is often difficult with a mandibular appliance. The maxillary appliance provides increased stability because all mandibular contacts are on flat surfaces. This may not be possible with a mandibular device, especially in the anterior region. Another advantage of the maxillary appliance is the ability of certain features of the appliance to help locate the MS relationship of the condyles in the fossae. As discussed, a mandibular appliance does not afford some of these advantages. A major advantage of the mandibular appliance is that it is easier for the patient to speak with it in place. In addition, for some patients a mandibular appliance is less visible than other occlusal appliances; thus it may be more aesthetic. However, this advantage is only present if the patient needs to wear the appliance during the day (see later discussion).

Many methods have been suggested for the fabrication of occlusal appliances. One frequently used method begins with casts mounted on an articulator. Undercuts in the maxillary arch are blocked out, and the appliance is developed in wax. The waxed appliance is invested and processed with heat-cured acrylic resin and is then adjusted for final fit intraorally.[23-26] Another common technique uses mounted casts and self-curing acrylic.[27] Undercuts in the maxillary teeth are blocked out, a separating solution is applied to the casts, and the desired outline of the appliance is bordered with rope wax. Acrylic monomer and polymer are sprinkled on the maxillary cast, and the occlusion is developed by closing the mandibular cast into the setting acrylic. Eccentric guidance and the thickness of the occlusal device are developed by using an anterior guide pin and a previously developed guide table (see Chapter 20).

The following section describes a more simplified occlusal appliance fabrication technique. As with other techniques,[28-32] it does not require mounted casts. The precise position of the mandible is located with direct assistance of the muscles, minimizing cast-mounting inaccuracies.

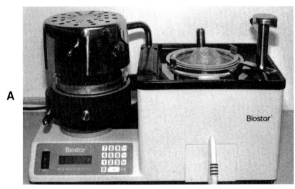
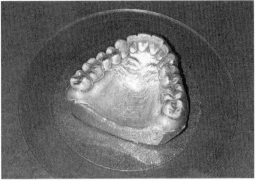

Fig. 15-2 A, A 2-mm-thick, clear resin sheet adapted to the cast with a pressure adapter (example shown is the Biostar, Great Lakes Orthodontics Products, Tonawanda, NY). **B,** Adapted resin sheet on the cast.

The finished appliance can also be inserted at the same appointment during which the impression was made. It should always be remembered, however, that the manner in which an appliance is fabricated is not important in resolving symptoms. The technique is only important to the dentist. Resolving symptoms is dependent on how well the appliance meets the treatment goals. Regardless of the technique used, it is the responsibility of the dentist to ensure that before the patient leaves the office, the appliance is correctly adjusted to meet the optimum criteria for orthopedic stability reviewed in Chapter 5. This technique is offered as a simple method of achieving these treatment goals.

Fabricating the Appliance. The fabrication of a maxillary occlusal appliance involves several steps.

An alginate impression is made of the maxillary arch. This should be free of bubbles and voids on the teeth and palate. It is poured immediately with a suitable gypsum product (preferably die stone). The impression is not inverted because a large base is not necessary. When the stone is adequately set, the cast is withdrawn from the impression. It should be free of bubbles and voids.

The excess stone labial to the teeth is trimmed on a model trimmer to the depth of the vestibule. With a pressure or vacuum adapter (Fig. 15-2, *A*), a 2-mm-thick, hard, clear sheet of resin is adapted to the cast (Fig. 15-2, *B*). Some companies offer a dual-sided resin sheet with a soft side for the teeth

and a hard side on which to develop the occlusion. This product should be considered because it offers good retention and comfort for the patient while still allowing the development of a precise occlusal contact scheme.

The outline of the appliance is then cut off the cast with a separating disk. The cut is made at the level of the interdental papilla on the buccal and labial surfaces of the teeth. The posterior palatal area is cut with a separating disk along a straight line connecting the distal aspects of each second molar (Fig. 15-3).

The adapted occlusal resin appliance is removed from the stone cast. A lathe with a hard rubber wheel can be used to eliminate excess resin in the palatal area (Fig. 15-4).

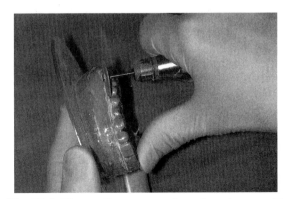

Fig. 15-3 The maxillary structure is cut from the cast with a separating disk.

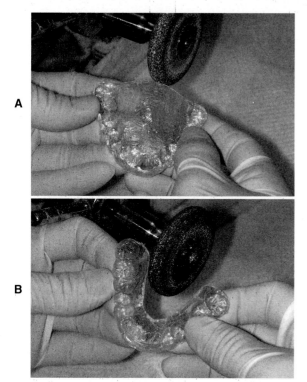

Fig. 15-4 The excess acrylic covering the palatal tissue is removed with a hard rubber wheel on a lathe. **A,** Before. **B,** After.

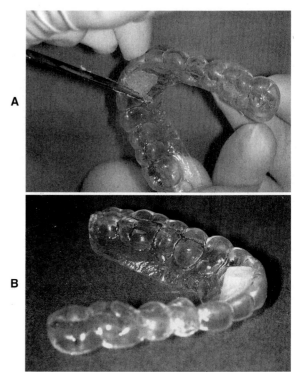

Fig. 15-5 A, Small amount of self-curing acrylic added to the anterior portion of the appliance as a stop for the lower incisor. The area of this stop is approximately 4 to 6 mm. **B,** Lateroocclusal view of the anterior stop placed on the appliance.

The lingual border of the appliance extends 10 to 12 mm from the gingival border of the teeth throughout the lingual portion of the arch. A large acrylic bur is used to smooth any rough edges. The labial border of the appliance terminates between the incisal and middle thirds of the anterior teeth. (The border around the posterior teeth may be slightly longer.) It is safer to leave the border a little longer at this time. If the occlusal appliance does not completely seat intraorally, the borders are carefully shortened until an adequate fit is obtained.

A small amount of clear, self-curing, acrylic resin is mixed in a dappen dish. As it thickens, it is added to the occlusal surface of the anterior portion of the appliance (Fig. 15-5). This acrylic will act as the anterior stop. It is approximately 4 mm wide and should extend to the region where a mandibular anterior central incisor will contact (Fig. 15-6).

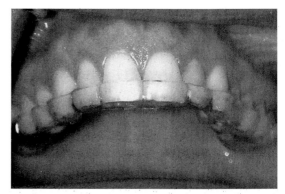

Fig. 15-6 The appliance is placed over the maxillary teeth and evaluated for proper fit. It should fit comfortably, providing adequate retention with no rocking.

Fitting the Appliance to the Maxillary Teeth. The occlusal appliance is then evaluated intraorally (see Fig. 15-6). It should fit the maxillary teeth well, offering adequate retention and stability. Lip and tongue movement should not dislodge it. Pressure applied to any portion should not cause tipping or loosening. If the borders of the appliance have been maintained near the junction of the middle and incisal thirds on the facial surfaces of the teeth, adequate retention will exist.

If it does not seat completely, it can be carefully heated extraorally with a hair dryer and reseated on the teeth. This will help achieve a well-fitting appliance. Care must be taken not to overheat the plastic or all shape may be lost.

On occasion, when the resin does not adapt well to the teeth or retention is poor, the occlusal appliance can be lined intraorally with clear self-curing acrylic resin. This can only be accomplished when using the solid acrylic sheets. When a dual surface sheet is used (soft/hard side), relining is not possible. Before a relining procedure begins, the patient is examined for any acrylic restorations (e.g., temporary crowns). The clinician should proceed with the following steps:

1. Any acrylic restorations are lubricated well with petrolatum to prevent bonding with the new acrylic.
2. A relining procedure is accomplished by mixing a small amount of self-curing acrylic resin in a dappen dish. Monomer is added to the inside of the occlusal appliance to aid in bonding of the resin. One to two millimeters of the setting acrylic resin is placed on the appliance. The setting acrylic should be dried with an air syringe, and, when it becomes tacky, the patient moistens the maxillary teeth. Then the appliance is seated on the teeth. The patient must not bite on it.
3. Any excessive setting resin is removed from the labial interproximal areas.
4. As the resin cures, the appliance is removed and replaced a number of times to avoid locking the setting acrylic resin into undercuts.
5. When the resin becomes warm, the appliance is removed for curing outside the mouth. The patient's teeth are immediately inspected and cleaned of any setting acrylic that may be left behind. After the acrylic has cured, the appliance

is inspected and any sharp edges or excess around the borders is removed. When the appliance is replaced on the teeth, adequate retention and stability should now exist.

When the occlusal device has been adequately adapted to the maxillary teeth, the occlusion is developed and refined.

Locating the Musculoskeletally Stable Position. For the stabilization appliance to be optimally effective, the condyles must be located in their most MS position, which is centric relation (CR). Two techniques have become widely used for finding CR.

The first uses the bilateral manual manipulation technique described in Chapter 9. In the normal TMJ, when the condyles are seated to the MS position the discs are properly interposed between the condyles and the articular fossae. If a disc is either functionally displaced or dislocated, the manual mandibular guiding technique will seat that condyle on retrodiscal tissues. When manual mandibular guidance produces pain in the joint, an intracapsular disorder should be suspected and the stability of this position should be questioned. Treatment should be directed toward the source of this intracapsular pain. An anterior positioning appliance might be more appropriate therapy.

A second technique uses a stop placed on the anterior region of the appliance, and the muscles are used to locate the MS position of the condyles. (This technique uses the same principles employed with the leaf gauge; see Chapter 9.) In a reclined position the patient is asked to close on the posterior teeth, which causes only one mandibular incisor to contact on the anterior stop of the appliance. The stop should provide a thickness that maintains the anterior teeth 3 to 5 mm apart. This will result in the posterior teeth being separated only 1 to 3 mm. The mandibular posterior teeth should not contact on any portion of the appliance. If the posterior teeth contact the appliance, it should be thinned to eliminated these contacts.

The contact on the anterior stop is marked with articulating paper and adjusted so that it provides a stop perpendicular to the long axis of the mandibular tooth being contacted. Importantly, no angulation to the contact should occur because

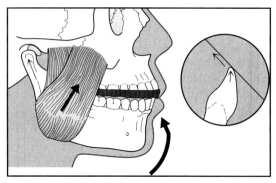

Fig. 15-7 If the anterior stop provides a distal incline, closure of the jaw will tend to deflect the mandible posteriorly, away from the most musculoskeletally stable position.

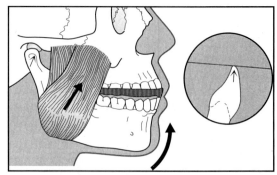

Fig. 15-9 When the anterior stop is flat and perpendicular to the long axis of the contacting mandibular incisor, the functional pull of the major elevator muscles will seat the condyles in their most superoanterior position in the fossae, resting against the posterior slopes of the articular eminences.

angulation will tend to deflect the mandibular position. If a distal inclination exists on the stop, clenching will force the mandible posteriorly (retrusively) away from the MS position (Fig. 15-7). This anterior stop should not create a retrusive force to the mandible. Likewise, the anterior stop should not be mesially inclined and create a forward shift or slide of the mandible because the clenching will tend to reposition the condyle forward, away from the most MS position (Fig. 15-8). When the anterior stop is flat and the patient closes on the posterior teeth, the functional pull of the major elevator muscles will seat the condyles in their most superoanterior position at the base of the posterior slopes of the articular eminences (Fig. 15-9).[33]

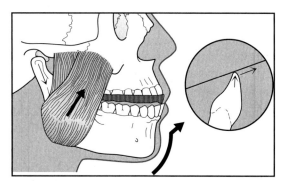

Fig. 15-8 If the anterior stop provides a mesial incline, closure of the jaw will tend to deflect the mandible anteriorly, away from the most musculoskeletally stable position.

In both techniques it is important to communicate well with the patient regarding the precise mandibular position. Because the anterior stop is flat, the patient can protrude, closing in a position anterior to MS position. This is avoided by asking the patient to close on the posterior teeth. Also, when the patient is reclining in the dental chair, gravity tends to position the mandible posteriorly. In some cases it is helpful to have the patient place the tip of the tongue on the posterior aspect of the soft palate while slowly closing.

Probably the most reliable and repeatable method of finding the MS position of the condyles is to use both techniques simultaneously. With the appliance in place and the patient reclined, the clinician should first locate the MS position with a bilateral manipulation technique. The clinician should bring the teeth close together and then ask the patient to repeatedly close on the posterior teeth. After a few closures, the contact marked on the anterior stop should become reproducible, reflecting a location of the stable mandibular position (Fig. 15-10).

Developing the Occlusion. Once the CR position has been located, the patient should become familiar with it by wearing the appliance for a few minutes. Instructions are given to tap on the anterior stop. This is helpful in influencing the neuromuscular control system that has coordinated muscle activities as related to the existing

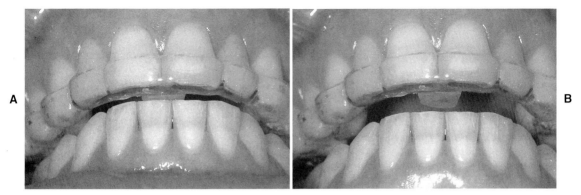

Fig. 15-10 A, Contact of the lower incisors on the anterior stop. No other contacts are present. **B,** The anterior contact is marked with articulating paper and observed to be flat and perpendicular to the long axis of the mandibular incisor.

occlusal conditions. Because the anterior stop eliminates the existing occlusal conditions, any muscle engrams associated with neuromuscular protection will be eliminated, thus promoting stabilization and allowing more complete seating of the condyles in their MS positions. When a masticatory muscle disorder exists or locating a repeatable CR position is difficult, it may be helpful to have the patient wear the appliance with only the anterior stop for 24 hours before the appliance is completed. However, although this is sometimes helpful in decreasing symptoms, there are some disadvantages, which are discussed in a later section.

When the MS position has been carefully located by the patient (with or without manual guidance), the appliance is removed from the mouth and self-curing acrylic is added to the remaining anterior and posterior regions of the occlusal surface (Fig. 15-11). Sufficient resin must be added to show the indentations of each mandibular tooth, and additional resin is added to the anterior region labial to the mandibular canines for the future guidance ramp.

Before the appliance is returned to the mouth, it is important that all free monomer is eliminated with an air syringe. Once the setting acrylic is dried of free monomer, the appliance is thoroughly rinsed with warm water. The appliance is then returned to the mouth, and a bilateral manual manipulation procedure is performed. Once the clinician believes that the condyles are properly

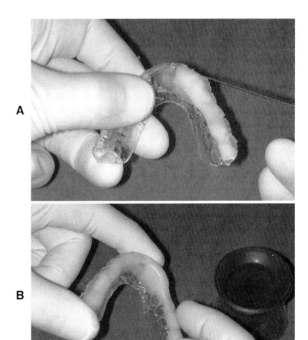

Fig. 15-11 A, Self-curing acrylic is added to the occluding surface of the appliance. **B,** All occluding areas, except the contact on the anterior stop, have been covered. The setting acrylic is dried with an air syringe and rinsed in warm water before it is placed in the patient's mouth.

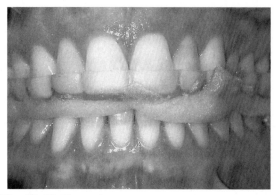

Fig. 15-12 The appliance with the setting acrylic is placed in the mouth, and the mandible is closed into centric relation on the anterior stop. Adequate resin labial to the mandibular canines provides for the future canine guidance.

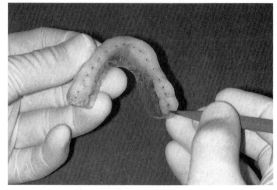

Fig. 15-13 Once the acrylic has set, the impressions of each mandibular buccal cusp tip and incisal edge are marked with a pencil. These represent the finished centric relation contacts that will be present on the finished appliance.

located, the patient is asked to close the posterior teeth into the setting acrylic (Fig. 15-12). The mandibular teeth should sink into the setting acrylic until the incisors contact the anterior stop. After 5 to 6 seconds the patient is instructed to open the mouth, and the appliance is removed. The occlusal surface of the appliance is visualized to make sure all mandibular teeth have made indentations in the setting acrylic and there is sufficient acrylic labial to the canines for the future development of eccentric guidance. The appliance can be returned to the mouth several times, each time relocating the MS position until the setting acrylic becomes firm and holds its shape. Then the appliance is removed for the final set.

Note: The appliance must be removed well before the resin produces heat. It is then allowed to bench-cure until completely hard. Placing the setting acrylic in a cup of warm water can reduce the amount of bubbles that develop in an appliance.

Adjusting the Centric Relation Contacts. The occlusal surface of the appliance is best adjusted by first marking the deepest area of each mandibular buccal cusp tip and incisal edge with a pencil (Fig. 15-13). These represent the final CR occlusal contacts that will be present when the appliance is completed. The acrylic surrounding the pencil marks is removed so that the relatively flat occlusal surface will allow eccentric freedom. The only areas preserved should be those that are anterior and labial to each mandibular canine.

These areas will create the desired contacts during mandibular movement.

Any excess acrylic is most quickly removed with a hard rubber wheel on a lathe (Fig. 15-14). The resin is flattened to the pencil marks in all areas except anterior and labial to the canines. A large acrylic bur in a slow-speed handpiece is helpful in refining and smoothing the appliance after the lathe. When the appliance has been adequately smoothed, it is returned to the mouth and the CR

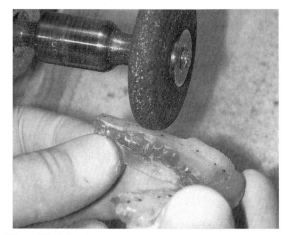

Fig. 15-14 Excess acrylic surrounding the centric contacts is removed with a hard rubber wheel on a lathe. All areas, except labial to the mandibular canines, are flattened to the contact (pencil) marks. This area will create the eccentric guidance.

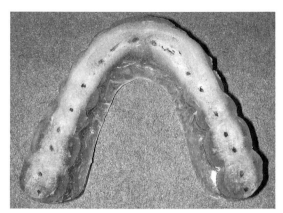

Fig. 15-15 OCCLUSAL VIEW OF WELL-ADJUSTED STABILIZATION APPLIANCE WHEN PATIENT CLOSES IN MUSCULOSKELETALLY STABLE POSITION (CENTRIC RELATION [CR]). All CR contacts are even and on flat surfaces.

contacts are marked by red articulating paper as the patient closes. All contacts, both anterior and posterior, should be carefully refined so that they will occur on flat surfaces with equal occlusal force. In many cases, normal setting shrinkage of the resin will distort the occlusal surface so that the cusp tips cannot reach the depths of the imprints and "doughnutlike" marks will result. When this occurs, the resin around each imprint must be reduced, allowing the cusps to contact completely in the fossae. The patient should be able to close and feel all the teeth contacting evenly and simultaneously on flat surfaces (Fig. 15-15).

Adjusting the Eccentric Guidance. Once the desired CR contacts have been achieved, the anterior guidance is refined. The acrylic prominences labial to the mandibular canines are smoothed. They should exhibit about a 30- to 45-degree angulation to the occlusal plane and allow the mandibular canines to pass over in a smooth and continuous manner during protrusive and laterotrusive excursions (Fig. 15-16).

The mandibular canines must be able to move freely and smoothly over the occlusal surface of the appliance. If the angulation of the prominences is too steep, the canines will restrict mandibular movement and may aggravate an existing muscle disorder. Confusion can be avoided by using a different-colored articulating paper to record the eccentric contacts. The appliance is returned to the patient's mouth. With blue articulating paper, the patient closes in CR and moves in left laterotrusive, right laterotrusive, and straight protrusive excursions. The blue articulating paper is removed and replaced with red articulating paper. Again the mandible closes in CR and the contacts are marked. The appliance is then removed and examined. Blue lines on the anterior portion depict laterotrusive and protrusive contacts of the mandibular canines and should be smooth and continuous. If a canine follows an irregular pathway or displays a catching movement, the pathway needs adjustment (Fig. 15-17).

Canine guidance must provide a smooth and gentle disocclusion of the posterior teeth. Any

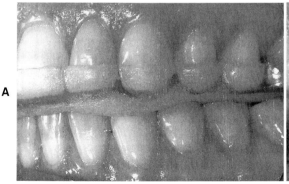
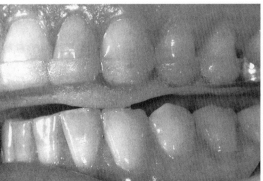

Fig. 15-16 A, The acrylic prominence labial to the canine (lateral view) is demonstrated. **B,** During a laterotrusive movement the mandibular canine disoccludes the remaining posterior teeth (canine guidance).

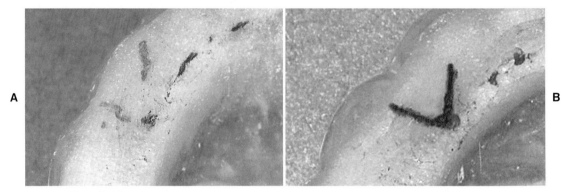

Fig. 15-17 A, The laterotrusive and protrusive guidances are not continuous, smooth-flowing contacts. These should be adjusted to produce smooth, continuous pathways as shown in **B.**

contacts marked in blue on the posterior surface of the appliance will have been made by posterior eccentric interferences and must be eliminated, leaving only the red marks of CR. Eccentric contacts of the mandibular central and lateral incisors also must be eliminated so that the predominant marks are those of the mandibular canines (Fig. 15-18).

During a protrusive movement, guidance by the mandibular canines, not the mandibular central and lateral incisors, is the goal. The mandibular incisors can be used to assist in protrusive movements; but when they are, care must be taken not to deliver the entire force of a protrusion to a single incisor. When the mandibular incisors are used for guidance during a protrusion, all latero-protrusive excursions must be examined because they will be the indicators of whether a single incisor is likely to be traumatized by a particular movement. These adjustments can take time. Often a simpler (and equally acceptable) solution is to place protrusive guidance only on the mandibular canines, thereby allowing for quick elimination of any eccentric contacts of the mandibular incisors. After these adjustments have been made, the appliance is returned to the patient's mouth to repeat the markings. Adjustments should continue until the posterior tooth contacts are only on flat surfaces in CR.

Once the stabilization appliance has been adjusted in the reclined position, the patient is raised to the upright or slightly forward head position (Fig. 15-19) and is instructed to tap lightly

on the posterior teeth. If the anterior contacts are heavier than the posterior contacts, the mandible has assumed a slightly anterior position during this postural change (see Chapter 5) and the anterior contacts need to be reduced until they are lighter than the posterior. As soon as the patient

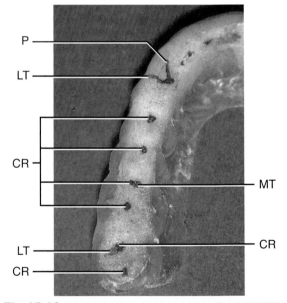

Fig. 15-18 RIGHT SIDE OF AN APPLIANCE WITH OCCLUSAL CONTACTS MARKED. The mandibular canine provides the laterotrusive *(LT)* and protrusive *(P)* guidance. The posterior portion of the appliance should reveal only centric relation *(CR)* contacts. This appliance, however, also reveals undesirable laterotrusive *(LT)* and mediotrusive *(MT)* posterior contacts. These must be eliminated.

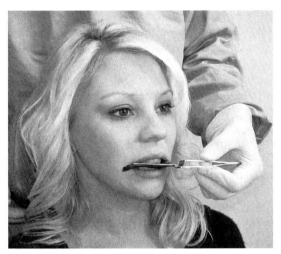

Fig. 15-19 With the patient reclined, the occlusal appliance is adjusted. Then the patient is raised to the upright head position (alert feeding position), and the occlusion is evaluated. The anterior teeth should not contact more heavily than the posterior teeth. If they do, they are marked with articulating paper and adjusted to contact more lightly.

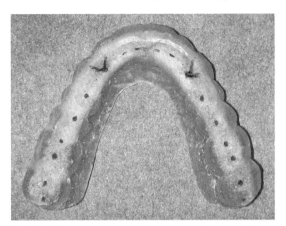

Fig. 15-20 The final occlusal contacts for a stabilization appliance.

can close lightly and feel predominantly posterior contacts, the adjustment is complete.

Note: The patient can easily protrude the mandible and contact heavily on the anterior guidance. Careful instruction may be necessary to ensure that the patient does not protrude the mandible when asked to close on the appliance. The patient should be specifically asked to close and tap on the *posterior teeth*.

Once the stabilization appliance has been properly adjusted, it is smoothed and polished. The patient should be asked to check with his or her tongue and lips for any sharp or uncomfortable areas. In some cases the acrylic extending over the labial surface of the maxillary teeth will not be important for retention and will not be needed for eccentric guidance. It can be removed from the maxillary anterior teeth to improve the aesthetics of the appliance.

Final Criteria for the Stabilization Appliance. The following eight criteria must be achieved before the patient is given the stabilization appliance (Fig. 15-20):

1. It must accurately fit the maxillary teeth, with total stability and retention when contacting the mandibular teeth and when checked by digital palpation.
2. In CR all mandibular buccal cusps and incisal edges must contact on flat surfaces with even force.
3. During protrusive movement the mandibular canines must contact the appliance with even force. The mandibular incisors may also contact it but not with more force than the canines.
4. In any lateral movement, only the mandibular canine should exhibit laterotrusive contact on the appliance.
5. The mandibular posterior teeth must contact the appliance slightly more heavily than the anterior teeth during closure.
6. In the alert feeding position the posterior teeth must contact the appliance more prominently than the anterior teeth.
7. The occlusal surface of the appliance should be as flat as possible with no imprints for mandibular cusps.
8. The occlusal appliance is polished so that it will not irritate any adjacent soft tissues.

Instructions and Adjustments. The patient is instructed in proper insertion and removal of the appliance. Finger pressure is used to align and seat it initially. Once it has been pushed onto the teeth, it may be stabilized with biting force. Removal is most easily accomplished by catching it near the first molar area with the fingernails of the index fingers and pulling the distal ends downward.

The patient is instructed to wear the appliance according to the disorder that is being treated. When a patient reports muscle pain on awaking, bruxism is suspected and nighttime use is essential. When a patient reports late-afternoon pain, diurnal muscle activity associated with emotional stress, ergonomics, and fatigue may be more important. For these patients the appliance may not be necessary during the day, and the techniques of physical self-regulation discussed in Chapter 11 should be employed. The appliance may be initially helpful during the day as a reminder of what they are doing with their teeth (cognitive awareness). As the patient masters these techniques, the appliance is no longer necessary during the day. When the disorder is retrodiscitis, the appliance may need to be worn more frequently. It has been demonstrated that myogenous pain disorders respond best to part-time use (especially nighttime use), whereas intracapsular disorders are better managed with more continuous use.[34] If wearing causes increased pain, the patient should discontinue wearing and report the problem immediately for evaluation and correction.

Initially, an increase in salivation may occur. This will resolve in a few hours. The appliance should be brushed immediately after being taken out of the mouth (with water, a dentifrice, or perhaps baking soda) to prevent the buildup of plaque and calculus and at the same time avoid any unpleasant aftertaste.

The patient is asked to return in 2 to 7 days for evaluation. At that time the occlusal marks on the appliance are reexamined. As muscles relax and symptoms resolve, a more superoanterior position of the condyle may be assumed. This change must be accompanied by adjustments of the appliance to optimum occlusal conditions. The muscle and TMJ examinations are repeated at each subsequent visit, so it can be determined whether the signs and symptoms are being eliminated.

When the symptoms are relieved by the appliance, it is likely that the proper diagnosis has been made and treatment is apparently successful. If symptoms are not relieved or improved, the appliance should be reevaluated for proper fit and occlusal contacts. If these factors are correct and the patient is wearing the appliance as instructed, the source of the disorder has probably not been affected. Either the initial diagnosis was incorrect or the muscle disorder is secondary to another condition. As discussed earlier, effective treatment of a secondary muscle disorder can occur only after elimination of the primary pain disorder.

On certain occasions, fabrication of a mandibular stabilization appliance may be desirable. Evidence suggests that maxillary and mandibular appliances reduce symptoms equally.[35] The primary advantages of the mandibular type are that it affects speech less and aesthetics may be better. The occlusal requirements of the mandibular appliance are exactly the same as those of the maxillary device (Fig. 15-21); however, because the maxillary incisors are angled labially it is impossible to develop an anterior stop on the mandibular appliance that is perpendicular to the long axis of the maxillary incisors. Therefore the muscles cannot be reliably used to help locate the MS position of the condyles. When fabricating a mandibular stabilization appliance, the clinician must rely solely on the bilateral manual manipulation technique to locate the stable joint position.

ANTERIOR POSITIONING APPLIANCE

Description and Treatment Goals
The anterior positioning appliance is an interocclusal device that encourages the mandible to assume a position more anterior than the intercuspal position (ICP). It may be useful for the management of certain disc derangement disorders because anterior positioning of the condyle may help provide a better condyle-disc relationship, thus allowing better opportunity for tissue adaptation or repair. The goal of treatment is not to alter the mandibular position permanently but only to change the position temporarily so as to enhance adaptation of the retrodiscal tissues. Once tissue adaptation has occurred, the appliance is eliminated, allowing the condyle to assume the MS position and painlessly function on the adaptive fibrous tissues (see Chapter 13).

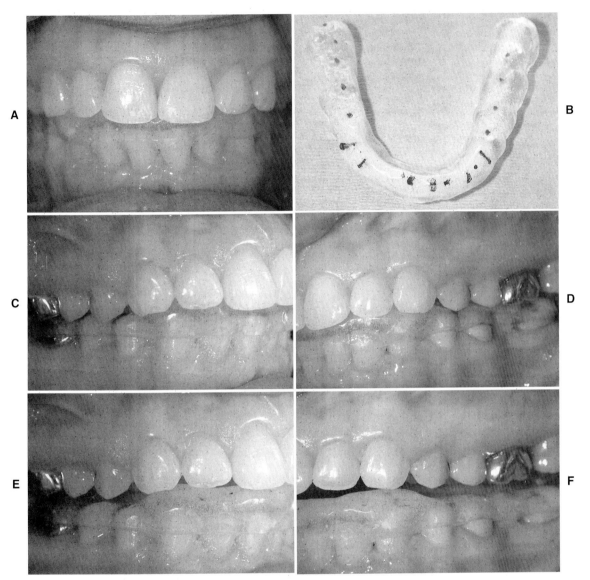

Fig. 15-21 A, Mandibular stabilization appliance. **B,** Occlusal view of a mandibular stabilization appliance with contacts and eccentric guidance marked with articulating paper. Right **(C)** and left **(D)** lateral view in the musculoskeletally stable position. Right **(E)** and left **(F)** lateral view during eccentric movement of the mandible. The presence of canine guidance is demonstrated.

Indications

The anterior positioning appliance is used primarily to treat disc displacements and disc dislocations with reduction. Patients with joint sounds (e.g., a single or reciprocal click) can sometimes be helped by it. Intermittent or chronic locking of the joint can also be treated with it. Some inflammatory disorders are managed with this appliance, especially when a slight anterior positioning of the condyles is more comfortable for the patient (e.g., retrodiscitis).

Simplified Fabrication Technique

Like the stabilization appliance, the anterior positioning appliance is a full-arch hard acrylic device that can be used in either arch. However, the maxillary arch is preferred because a guiding ramp can be more easily fabricated to direct the mandible into the desired forward position. With a mandibular appliance the guiding ramp does not achieve this forward position as easily, and thus the mandible is not controlled as well. In other words, the patient can more easily position the mandible posteriorly with the mandibular appliance.

Fabricating and Fitting the Appliance. The initial steps in fabricating a maxillary anterior positioning appliance are identical to that in fabricating a stabilization appliance. The anterior stop is constructed, and the appliance is fitted to the maxillary teeth. Because the acrylic extending over the labial surfaces of the maxillary teeth is not necessary for occlusal purposes, it can be removed to improve aesthetics. This may be important if the patient needs to wear the appliance during the day, although daytime use is rare (see Chapter 13).

Locating the Correct Anterior Position. The key to successful anterior positioning appliance fabrication is finding the most suitable position for eliminating the patient's symptoms. The anterior stop is used to locate it. The surface of the stop is adjusted so that it will be flat and perpendicular to the long axes of the mandibular incisors. The stop should not significantly increase the vertical dimension (the appliance should be as thin as possible). As with the stabilization appliance, the patient repeatedly opens and closes on the stop. When the incisors occlude with it, the posterior teeth should be close to but not actually contacting the posterior portion of the appliance. If contact occurs, the posterior portion needs to be thinned. Once this has been done, the patient closes on the stop again and the joint symptoms are evaluated. If the clicking and pain symptoms have been eliminated with only the increase in vertical dimension and improved joint stability provided by the stop, a stabilization appliance should be fabricated as previously described.

If the joint pain and clicking has not been eliminated, the patient is instructed to protrude the mandible slightly and to open and close the mouth in this position (Fig. 15-22). The joint is reevaluated for symptoms, and the anterior position that stops the clicking is located and marked with red

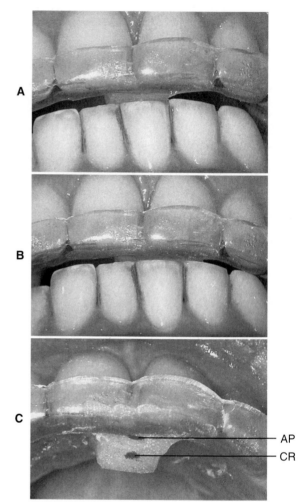

Fig. 15-22 LOCATING THE DESIRABLE ANTE-RIOR POSITION. A, Relationship of the anterior teeth to the anterior stop in centric relation. **B,** The patient protrudes slightly until an opening and closing movement occurs that eliminates the disc derangement disorder. The contact area on the anterior stop is marked with articulating paper in this position. **C,** Two contact marks are demonstrated: the centric relation *(CR)* contact and the desired anterior position that eliminates the disc derangement symptoms *(AP).*

marking paper as the patient taps on the stop. The position used should be the shortest anterior distance from MS position (CR) that eliminates the symptoms. Once this has been marked, the appliance is removed and the area of the contact is grooved approximately 1 mm deep with a small

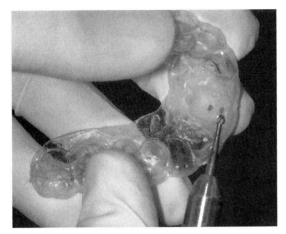

Fig. 15-23 The contact on the anterior stop, marking the desired anterior position, is grooved with a small round bur. This will assist the patient in returning to the desired mandibular position.

round bur (Fig. 15-23). This will provide a positive contact location for the mandibular incisor. The appliance is then returned to the mouth and the patient locates the groove and taps into it. Once the proper location for the incisor has been found, the patient opens and closes, returning to this position, while the joint symptoms are evaluated. There should be no joint sounds during opening and closing. Joint pain during clenching should also be reduced or eliminated. Myogenous pain originating from the superior lateral pterygoid, however, will not be eliminated because this muscle is active during clenching. Functional manipulation techniques may be helpful in differentiating this pain (see Chapter 9).

If no signs or symptoms are noted, this position is verified as the correct anterior position for the appliance. If the joint symptoms are still present, the position is unsatisfactory and a new one must be ascertained.

The treatment goals of the anterior positioning appliance are to eliminate joint sounds and pain. However, although eliminating joint sounds may help determine the proper mandibular position, the absence of sounds does not necessarily indicate that the condyle is resting on the intermediate zone of the disc. Both arthrography[36] and computed tomographic scanning[37] have disclosed that even

when joint sounds are eliminated by the anterior positioning appliance, some discs remain displaced or dislocated. It has been suggested that more sophisticated techniques such as arthroscopy[38] or magnetic resonance imaging[39,40] be used to assist in locating the optimum mandibular position for the appliance. This would undoubtedly be helpful, but most practitioners are likely to find these techniques both impractical and too costly. Thus it is more feasible to establish the position initially by using clinical joint sounds and, if the appliance fails to reduce symptoms, then call on the more sophisticated techniques for assistance.

When the joint symptoms have been eliminated and verified by the anterior stop, the appliance is taken out of the patient's mouth and self-curing acrylic is added to the remaining occlusal surface so that all occlusal contacts can be established (Fig. 15-24).

The clinician should note that the anterior stop should not be covered by the acrylic. An excess of acrylic is placed in the anterior palatal area, which will be located lingual to the mandibular anterior teeth when occluded. The setting acrylic is dried with an air syringe and rinsed in warm water, and the appliance is then returned to the mouth. The patient is asked to close slowly into the grooved area on the anterior stop. Initial closure may be

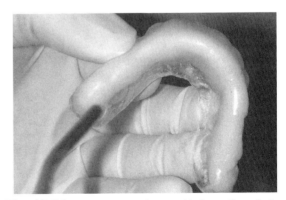

Fig. 15-24 Self-curing acrylic is added to all occluding areas of the appliance except the anterior stop. A prominence of resin is formed lingual to the future contacts of the mandibular anterior teeth. This will form the retrusive guiding ramp. The setting acrylic is dried with an air syringe and then rinsed in warm water before it is placed in the patient's mouth.

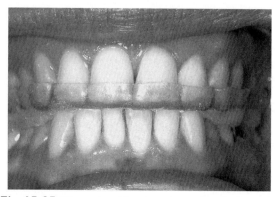

Fig. 15-25 The patient bites into the setting acrylic at the desired anterior position as determined by the groove.

assisted by instructing the patient into the proper position (Fig. 15-25). Because the patient may not be able to close directly into the groove, a slightly more anterior position is encouraged, and, once the anterior stop is contacted, the patient can slowly bring the mandible posteriorly until the groove is felt. In this manner the setting acrylic that will be the anterior guiding ramp will not be disturbed. When the anterior teeth are felt to contact in the groove on the anterior stop, the position is verified by opening and closing a few times (Fig. 15-26). When the resin becomes firm and before heat is produced, the appliance is removed and allowed to bench-cure.

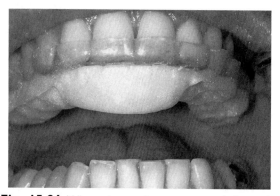

Fig. 15-26 When the teeth are separated from the setting acrylic, the imprints formed by the mandibular teeth can be seen. The resin lingual to the anterior teeth is demonstrated. This will provide the retrusive guidance.

Adjusting the Occlusion. Like the stabilization appliance, the anterior positioning appliance requires flat occlusal contacts for all occluding teeth. The difference with this appliance is the anterior guiding ramp, which requires the mandible to assume a more forward position to the ICP (Fig. 15-27).

The appliance is evaluated, and gross excesses are removed with a hard rubber wheel on the lathe. An acrylic bur in a slow-speed handpiece smoothes the acrylic resin. Flat occlusal contacts are developed for the posterior teeth, and the large lingual ramp in the anterior region is only smoothed. The appliance is returned to the mouth, and the patient closes in the forward position. After a few taps on red articulating paper the appliance is removed and evaluated. Sound contact should be visible on all cusp tips. In many cases the setting resin will shrink slightly, not allowing the cusp tips to reach the depths of the imprints, and doughnutlike marks result. When this occurs, the resin around each imprint must be reduced, allowing the cusps to contact completely in the fossae. A well-adjusted appliance allows contact on all teeth evenly and simultaneously in the established forward position (Fig. 15-28). If the patient wishes to retrude the mandible, the prominent anterior guidance ramp will contact the mandibular incisors and during the closing movement return the mandible to the desired forward position (Fig. 15-29). The ramp is developed into a smooth sliding surface so as not to promote catching or locking of the teeth in any position.

Final Criteria for the Anterior Positioning Appliance. The following five criteria should be met by the anterior positioning appliance before it is given to the patient:

1. It should accurately fit the maxillary teeth with total stability and retention when in contact with the mandibular teeth and when checked by digital palpation.
2. In the established forward position, all the mandibular teeth should contact it with even force.
3. The forward position established by the appliance should eliminate the joint symptoms during opening and closing to and from that position.

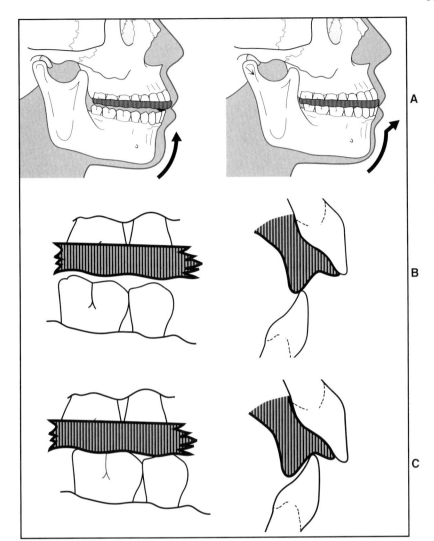

Fig. 15-27 A, The anterior positioning appliance causes the mandible to assume a forward position, creating a more favorable condyle-disc relationship. **B,** During normal closure the mandibular anterior teeth contact in the anterior guiding ramp provided by the maxillary appliance. **C,** As the mandible rises into occlusion, the ramp causes it to shift forward into the desired position that will eliminate the disc derangement disorder. At the desired forward position, all teeth contact to maintain arch stability.

4. In the retruded range of movement, the lingual retrusive guidance ramp should contact and, on closure, direct the mandible into the established therapeutic forward position.
5. The appliance should be smoothly polished and compatible with adjacent soft tissue structures.

Instruction and Adjustments. As with the stabilization appliance, instructions regarding insertion and removal of the anterior positioning appliance are given, as well as advice on its proper care. The patient is instructed to wear the appliance only at night. During the day the appliance should not be worn so that normal function of the condyle will promote the development of fibrotic connective tissue in the retrodiscal tissue. If the patient reports pain during the day, the appliance may be worn for short periods of time through the day to reduce the pain. As soon as the pain is resolved, the use of the appliance is limited to nighttime only (see Chapters 13 and 16).

Some clinicians prefer to use a mandibular anterior positioning appliance because this may be more acceptable from a functional and aesthetic standpoint. Functional and aesthetic concerns are only important if the appliance is to

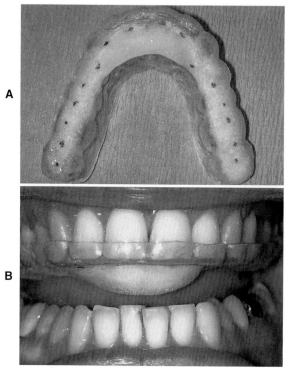

Fig. 15-28 A, The contact of all the teeth and the prominent anterior guidance ramp are demonstrated in this occlusal view of the maxillary anterior positioning appliance. **B,** Frontal view of the maxillary anterior positioning appliance.

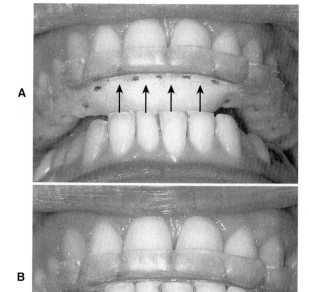

Fig. 15-29 A, Anterior guidance ramp as the patient attempts to close into maximum intercuspation. The mandibular anterior teeth contact the ramp. **B,** The ramp guides the mandible forward into the position that will eliminate the disc derangement disorder.

be worn during the day. As just mentioned, this is rarely necessary for most patients with disc displacement and dislocations with reduction. If a mandibular appliance is used, the patient must be instructed to maintain the forward position dictated by the mandibular appliance. The maxillary appliance is best for nighttime use because the patient cannot consciously maintain the forward position. It is likely that during sleep the mandible will retrude and the maxillary appliance (with the prominent retrusive ramp) will better restrict this movement (Fig. 15-30).

The length of time that the appliance is worn will be determined by the type, extent, and chronicity of the disorder. The health and age of the patient are also factors in treatment (see Chapter 13).

ANTERIOR BITE PLANE

Description and Treatment Goals

The anterior bite plane is a hard acrylic appliance worn over the maxillary teeth, providing contact with only the mandibular anterior teeth (Fig. 15-31). It is primarily intended to disengage the posterior teeth and thus eliminate their influence on the function of the masticatory system.

Indications

The anterior bite plane has been suggested[41-44] for the treatment of muscle disorders related to orthopedic instability or an acute change in the occlusal condition (Fig. 15-32). Parafunctional activity may also be treated with it for short periods. Some major complications can arise when an

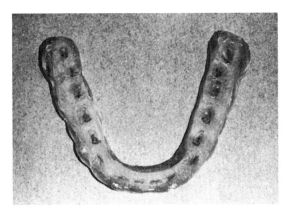

Fig. 15-30 MANDIBULAR ANTERIOR POSITION-ING APPLIANCE. Unlike the stabilization appliance, each centric cusp on this appliance fits into a small depression or fossa, which dictates the desired forward position. This appliance is only used when a daytime mandibular position-ing is necessary to reduce symptoms. As soon as symptoms are controlled during the day, the appliance is eliminated. The nighttime use of the maxillary positioning appliance is continued until adequate tissue adaptation has occurred.

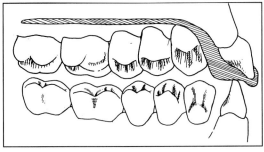

Fig. 15-31 ANTERIOR BITE PLANE. This appliance provides occlusal contacts only on the anterior teeth.

anterior bite plane or any appliance that covers only a portion of one arch is used. The unopposed posterior teeth have the potential to supraerupt. If the appliance is worn continuously for several weeks or months, there is a great likelihood that the unopposed mandibular posterior teeth will supraerupt. When this occurs and the appliance is removed, the anterior teeth will no longer contact and the result will be an anterior open bite.

Anterior bite plane therapy must be closely moni-tored and used only for short periods. The same treatment effect can be accomplished with the stabilization appliance, and therefore this is usually a better choice. When a full-arch device is fabricated and adjusted, supraeruption cannot occur regardless of the length of time the appli-ance is worn.

Recently a device has been marketed as new and helpful for the management of headache. This appliance has been named by its inventor[45] the Nociceptive Trigeminal Inhibition Tension Suppression System (NTI TSS) or NTI. The concept is not new, only a resurrected idea from the litera-ture on anterior bite planes. In fact, it is an anterior bite plane that only allows the anterior central incisors to occlude. The initial paper suggested that the NTI was only slightly more effective than standard appliance therapy for the reduction of headache pain.[46] However, the authors of this study did not compare the NTI with a stabilization appliance that would have represented the gold standard for appliance therapy. Instead, they compared it with a bleaching tray that has never been evaluated for headache pain. Comparing two unknowns is a fatal flaw in research design and therefore its results are invalid. In a more scientif-ically designed double-blind randomized parallel trial,[47] the NTI was not more effective than a stabi-lization appliance for TMD and headache symp-toms. Al Quran[48] also found that the NTI was not more effective than a stabilization appliance for TMDs. In still another well-designed, randomly controlled study,[49] the NTI was not as effective as a stabilization appliance in almost all measured parameters. In fact, an interesting and likely important finding was that 1 of 15 patients devel-oped an anterior open bite with the NTI, whereas none of the patients wearing a stabilization appli-ance had any occlusal changes. This suggests that the NTI poses a greater risk factor for permanently changing the occlusion than the stabilization appliance.

There is little doubt that occlusal appliances can reduce some headaches in some individuals.[50-53] What needs further investigation is what type of headaches respond to what type of appliances. The data are strongly lacking at this time. The ideal appliance should have maximum effectiveness with minimal adverse side effects and be cost effective.

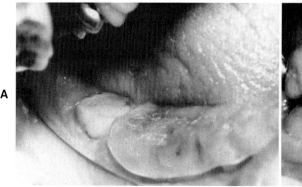
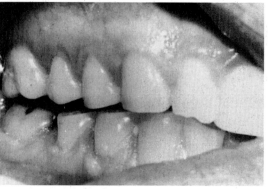

A

B

Fig. 15-32 A, This patient has been wearing a mandibular appliance for 4 months. The second mandibular molar was not included in it. While the appliance was being worn, the second molar supraerupted. **B,** When the appliance was removed and the patient was asked to occlude, only the erupted second molar contacted the maxillary molar. Wearing this appliance has created an anterior open bite.

The profession needs to scientifically determine this appliance and not quickly jump to unfounded claims of those with business interests.

POSTERIOR BITE PLANE

Description and Treatment Goals
The posterior bite plane is usually fabricated for the mandibular teeth and consists of areas of hard acrylic located over the posterior teeth and connected by a cast metal lingual bar (Fig. 15-33). The treatment goals of the posterior bite plane are

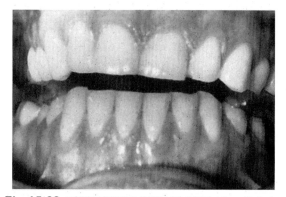

Fig. 15-33 POSTERIOR BITE PLANE. Note that this appliance provides occlusal contact only on the posterior teeth.

to achieve major alterations in vertical dimension and mandibular positioning.

Indications
Posterior bite planes have been advocated in cases of severe loss of vertical dimension or when there is a need to make major changes in anterior positioning of the mandible.[54] Some therapists[55,56] have suggested that this appliance be used by athletes to improve athletic performance. At present, however, scientific evidence does not support this theory.[57,58]

The use of this device may be helpful for certain disc derangement disorders, although this appliance has not been studied well for this condition. As with the anterior bite plane, the major concern surrounding this appliance is that it occludes with only part of the dental arch and therefore allows potential supraeruption of the unopposed teeth and/or intrusion of the occluded teeth (Fig. 15-34). Constant and long-term use should be discouraged. In most cases, when disc derangement disorders are treated, the entire arch should be included, as with the anterior positioning appliances.

PIVOTING APPLIANCE

Description and Treatment Goals
The pivoting appliance is a hard acrylic device that covers one arch and usually provides a single

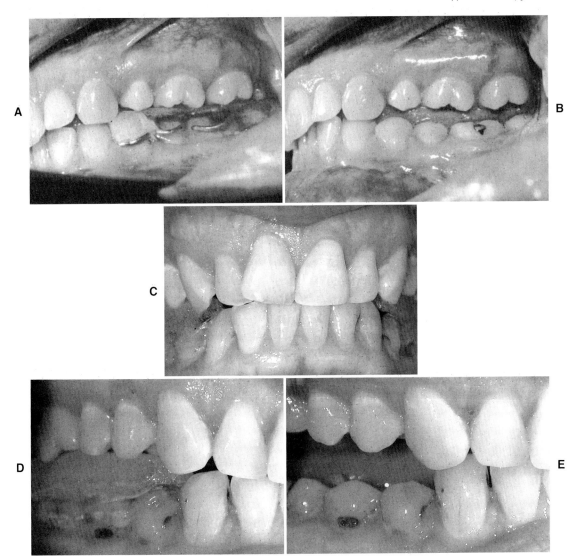

Fig. 15-34 This patient had been wearing this posterior bite appliance continuously for approximately 1 year. **A,** With the appliance in place, all teeth contact. **B,** When the appliance is removed, it can be easily seen that the posterior teeth no longer contact in the intercuspal position. This appliance has either intruded the posterior teeth or allowed supraeruption of the anterior teeth (or both). **C,** Anterior view of another patient who had been wearing a posterior bite appliance for several years. The anterior teeth are occluding normally. **D,** Lateral view with the appliance in place. **E,** When the appliance is removed, a significant posterior open bite results. This undesirable occlusal change depicts the major disadvantage of this type of occlusal appliance.

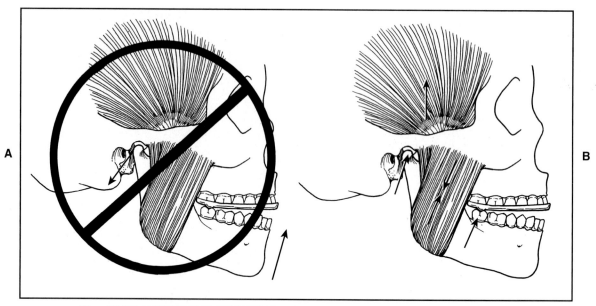

Fig. 15-35 POSTERIOR PIVOTING APPLIANCE. A, Many clinicians believe that this device will cause condylar distraction; however, this has not been documented. **B,** Because the pivot is anterior to the force of the elevator muscles (masseter and temporalis), the joint is seated to the musculoskeletally stable position while force is applied to the posterior tooth contacting the pivot. Studies suggest that such an appliance loads the joints; it does not distract the joints. Distraction occurs only if extraoral force is applied upward on the chin.

posterior contact in each quadrant (Fig. 15-35). This contact is usually established as far posteriorly as possible. When superior force is applied under the chin, the tendency is to push the anterior teeth close together and pivot the condyles downward around the posterior pivoting point.

Indications

The pivoting appliance was originally developed with the idea that it would reduce interarticular pressure and thus unload the articular surfaces of the joint. This was thought to be possible when the anterior teeth moved closer together, creating a fulcrum around the second molar, pivoting the condyle downward and backward away from the fossa. However, such an effect can occur only if the forces that close the mandible are located anterior to the pivot. Unfortunately, the forces of the elevator muscles are located primarily posterior to the pivot, which therefore disallows any pivoting

action. Whereas it was originally suggested[42] that this therapy would be helpful in treating joint sounds, it now appears that the anterior positioning appliance is more suitable for this purpose because it provides better control of positional changes. Perhaps one positive effect that a pivoting appliance may offer in a disc displacement or dislocation patient is that the pivot does not restrict the mandibular position and therefore the patient may close and position the mandible more downward and forward to avoid the pivot. If this occurs the condyle would be positioned off the retrodiscal tissues, providing a therapeutic effect on the disorder.[59] This thought is speculative, and scientific research is necessary to better understand whether this appliance has any use in dentistry.

The pivoting appliance has also been advocated for the treatment of symptoms related to osteoarthritis of the TMJs.[60] It has also been suggested that the device be inserted and elastic bandages wrapped from the chin to the top of the head to decrease forces on the joint. Manual extraoral force to the chin can also be used to decrease intraarticular pressure.

Studies[33,61,62] demonstrated that a pivoting appliance without extraoral force actually seats the condyles in an anterosuperior position in the fossae. Thus it does not unload the TMJs. In another study, however, Mocayo[63] found that when patients place their lips together and bite on a bilateral pivoting appliance, there is an average of 1.3 mm condylar lowering in the fossa as revealed by tomograms. These contradicting studies reveal the need for more investigations.

The only appliance that can routinely distract a condyle from the fossa is a unilateral pivot appliance. When a unilateral pivot is placed in the second molar region, closing the mandible on it will load the contralateral joint and slightly distract the ipsilateral one (i.e., increase the discal space).[33] The biomechanics of this appliance might appear to be indicated for the treatment of an acute unilateral disc dislocation without reduction. However, there is no scientific evidence at present that such a treatment is effective in reducing the disc. This device should not be used for longer than 1 week because it is likely to intrude the second molar used as the pivot (Fig. 15-36).

SOFT OR RESILIENT APPLIANCE

Description and Treatment Goals
The soft appliance is a device fabricated of resilient material that is usually adapted to the maxillary teeth. Treatment goals are to achieve even and simultaneous contact with the opposing teeth. In many instances this is difficult to accomplish precisely because most of the soft materials do not adjust readily to the exact requirements of the neuromuscular system.

Indications
Soft appliances have been advocated for several uses. Unfortunately, little evidence exists to support many of these. Certainly the most common and well-substantiated indication is as a protective device for persons likely to receive trauma to their dental arches (Fig. 15-37). Protective athletic splints decrease the likelihood of damage to the oral structures when trauma is received.[64-66]

Soft appliances have also been recommended for patients who exhibit high levels of clenching and bruxism.[42,60] It seems reasonable that they should help dissipate some of the heavy loading forces encountered during parafunctional activity. Soft appliances have not been shown to decrease bruxing activity. In fact, in one study Okeson[18]

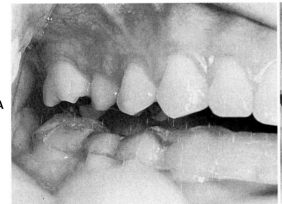
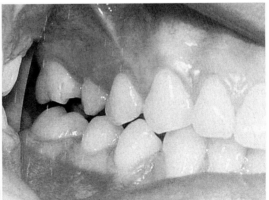

A

B

Fig. 15-36 A, Clinical photo of a mandibular pivoting appliance. Only the maxillary first molar contacts the appliance. **B,** The patient wore this appliance continuously for only 2 weeks. When it was removed, the occlusion changed. The maxillary first molar was intruded out of occlusal contact.

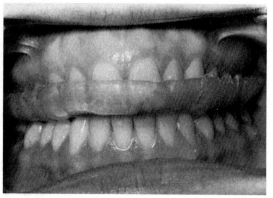

Fig. 15-37 SOFT OR RESILIENT APPLIANCE.
This is used primarily for protection during athletic activities.

demonstrated that nocturnal masseter electromyographic activity was increased in 5 of 10 subjects with a soft appliance. In the same study 8 of the 10 subjects had significant reduction of nocturnal electromyographic activity with a hard stabilization appliance. (Only one subject showed reduction of activity with the soft appliance.) Other studies[67,68] evaluating the effectiveness of hard and soft appliances on symptoms showed that although soft appliances can reduce symptoms, hard appliances seem to reduce symptoms more quickly and effectively. Hard appliances seem to reduce the electromyographic activity of the masseter and temporalis muscles more than soft appliances while controllably clenching the teeth.[69] In a more recent study[70] short-term use of soft appliances was shown to be more helpful than palliative therapy and no therapy in reducing TMD symptoms. Recently Truelove et al.[71] demonstrated that hard and soft appliances both seem to reduce TMD symptoms.

Scientific evidence[14,15,17-19,32,72-74] supports the use of hard appliances for reduction of symptoms related to clenching and bruxing activity. Soft appliances have been less documented in the scientific literature, but a few more recent studies suggest that they may be helpful in some patients for short-term use.[75]

Soft appliances have been advocated for patients who suffer from repeated or chronic sinusitis resulting in extremely sensitive posterior teeth.[76] In some maxillary sinusitis cases the posterior teeth (with roots extending into the sinus area) become extremely sensitive to occlusal forces. A soft appliance may help decrease the symptoms, although definitive treatment is directed toward the sinusitis.

COMMON TREATMENT CONSIDERATIONS OF APPLIANCE THERAPY

As previously stated, a wealth of research evidence indicates that occlusal appliance therapy is a successful treatment in reducing symptoms in 70% to 90% of TMDs. However, much controversy exists over the exact mechanism by which occlusal appliances reduce symptoms. In earlier studies many authors concluded[6,14,15,17-19,72] that occlusal appliances decrease muscle activity (particularly parafunctional activity). When muscle activity is decreased, myogenous pain decreases. The reduced muscle activity also lessens the forces placed on the TMJs and other structures within the masticatory system. When these structures are unloaded, the associated symptoms decrease. Some of the controversy that still exists is over which specific features of an appliance decrease muscle activity. Unfortunately, many clinicians fabricate an occlusal device and, as symptoms resolve, it confirms to them their predetermined diagnosis. They then immediately direct permanent treatment toward the feature of the masticatory system that they believe the appliance has affected. In some instances they may be right; however, in other cases, this treatment may be quite inappropriate.

Before any permanent therapy is begun, one needs to be aware that at least seven general features are common to all appliances, which may explain why occlusal appliances reduce symptoms associated with TMDs. Each of these possibilities must be considered before any permanent occlusal therapy is attempted:

1. *Alteration of the occlusal condition*: All occlusal appliances temporarily alter the existing occlusal condition. A change, especially toward a more stable and optimum condition, generally decreases muscle activity, which may result in the reduction of symptoms. This concept has

been accepted for years and is often considered by many to be the only manner by which occlusal appliances affect TMD symptoms. This approach reflects a narrow view and may lead the clinician to make unnecessary permanent occlusal changes. Before any permanent changes are begun, the following six additional considerations need to be considered.

2. *Alteration of the condylar position*: Most appliances alter condylar position to either a more MS or a more structurally compatible and functional position. This effect on the joint stability can be responsible for a decrease in symptoms.

3. *Increase in the vertical dimension*: All interocclusal appliances temporarily increase the patient's vertical dimension. This effect is universal regardless of treatment goals. It has been demonstrated that an increase in vertical dimension can temporarily decrease muscle activity[77-79] and symptoms.[80] Therefore this change may be responsible for the symptom reduction.

4. *Cognitive awareness*: Patients who wear occlusal appliances become more aware of their functional and parafunctional behavior. The appliance acts as a constant reminder to alter activities that may affect the disorder. As cognitive awareness is increased, factors that contribute to the disorder are decreased. The result is a decrease in the symptoms.[81-84]

5. *Placebo effect*: As with any treatment, a placebo effect can result.[85,86] Studies[87,88] suggest that approximately 40% of the patients suffering from certain TMDs respond favorably to such treatment. A positive placebo effect may result from the competent and reassuring manner in which the doctor approaches the patient and provides the therapy. This favorable doctor-patient relationship, accompanied by an explanation of the problem and reassurance that the appliance will be effective, often leads to a decrease in the emotional stress experienced by the patient, which may be the significant factor responsible for the placebo effect.

6. *Increased peripheral input to the central nervous system* (CNS): As discussed in Chapter 7, nocturnal muscle hyperactivity appears to have its source in the CNS. Any change at the peripheral sensory input seems to have an inhibitory effect on this CNS activity.[89] When an occlusal appliance is placed between the teeth, it provides a change in peripheral sensory input and thus decreases CNS-induced bruxism. The appliance does not cure bruxism; it only inhibits the bruxing tendency while it is being worn. Studies[19,90,91] show that even after long-term use of an appliance, bruxism returns if use of the device is stopped. Also, when an individual wears an appliance every night, there may still be a return of bruxism as the patient accommodates to the altered sensory input.[92]

7. *Regression to the mean*: Regression to the mean is a statistical term that addresses the common fluctuation of symptoms associated with chronic pain conditions.[93] If one follows the symptoms of a TMD patient over time, it will be noted that the intensity of the pain often varies on a daily basis. Some days will be quite painful, whereas other days are more tolerable. If the patient is asked to rate the intensity of the pain each day on a visual analog scale with 0 being no pain and 10 the worst possible pain ever, the patient may report an average day to be 3. This would represent his or her mean pain score. However, some days the pain may reach a 7 or 8 but then often with time the pain returns to its mean level of 3. Patients most commonly report to the dental office when the pain intensity is great because that is often the factor that motivates them to seek treatment. When the clinician provides therapy (such as an occlusal appliance) and the symptoms reduce to the average level of 3, one must question whether the reduction of symptoms was actually the therapeutic effect of the treatment or whether the patient's symptoms merely regressed to the mean. This factor can be confusing to the clinician and may lead to misdirection of future treatment. Uncontrolled short-term studies that report success of various therapies need to be questioned regarding their actual effect. Was the symptom reduction caused by the actual therapeutic effect of the modality, or was it regression to the mean? The importance of well-controlled, blinded studies becomes obvious when attempting to answer this question.[86]

When a patient's symptoms are reduced by occlusal appliance therapy, each of these seven factors must be considered as responsible for the success. Permanent treatment should be delayed until significant evidence exists to rule out the other factors. For example, a patient reports severe pain associated with masticatory muscle soreness. A clinical examination reveals an obvious loss of vertical dimension. A device is fabricated to reestablish that dimension. In 1 week the patient reports feeling no symptoms. Initially it appears that the increase in vertical dimension has been responsible for the relief of symptoms, but the other six factors cannot be ruled out. Before a permanent alteration of the vertical dimension is undertaken, attempts must be made to verify the effect of vertical dimension changes or rule out the other factors. The appliance should be gradually thinned while maintaining the same occlusal contact and condylar position. The significance of this decrease of the vertical dimension is confirmed if the symptoms return as the appliance is thinned. Requesting the patient to continue wearing the appliance at the correct vertical dimension for 4 to 6 weeks will often decrease the placebo effect because this effect is greatest during the initial contact with the patient. If the patient remains comfortable, the likelihood of a placebo effect is diminished. After 4 to 6 weeks of appliance therapy with no return of symptoms, the patient should be asked to remove the appliance for several days. Recurrence of the symptoms may confirm the diagnosis of decreased vertical dimension, but it does not exclude the other factors such as the occlusal condition or the condylar position. If the symptoms do not return, then other factors (e.g., cognitive awareness, placebo effect, bruxing associated with emotional stress, regression to the mean) must be considered. Emotional stress is often cyclic and self-limiting and may contribute to the escalation of local muscle soreness.

Importantly, any sudden change in vertical dimension seems to have a positive effect on reducing many TMD symptoms (especially myalgia). This effect, however, may only be temporary[94] and does not indicate that a permanent change in vertical dimension would continue to resolve the symptoms. Studies[95] do not suggest that vertical dimension is a major contributor to TMD. Therefore much care should be taken to establish the correct causative factor before any change in vertical dimension is undertaken.

In summary, although occlusal appliances may have some diagnostic value, conclusions regarding the rationale for their success must not be hastily made. Before any permanent treatment plan is begun, ample evidence must exist that the treatment will be of benefit to the patient. For example, extensive occlusal therapy is not normally proper treatment for parafunctional activity associated with high levels of emotional stress.

References

1. Wahlund K, List T, Larsson B: Treatment of temporomandibular disorders among adolescents: a comparison between occlusal appliance, relaxation training, and brief information, *Acta Odontol Scand* 61:203-211, 2003.
2. Ekberg E, Nilner M: Treatment outcome of appliance therapy in temporomandibular disorder patients with myofascial pain after 6 and 12 months, *Acta Odontol Scand* 62:343-349, 2004.
3. Kuttila M, Le Bell Y, Savolainen-Niemi E, Kuttila S, Alanen P: Efficiency of occlusal appliance therapy in secondary otalgia and temporomandibular disorders, *Acta Odontol Scand* 60:248-254, 2002.
4. Ekberg E, Nilner M: A 6- and 12-month follow-up of appliance therapy in TMD patients: a follow-up of a controlled trial, *Int J Prosthodont* 15:564-570, 2002.
5. Wassell RW, Adams N, Kelly PJ: The treatment of temporomandibular disorders with stabilizing splints in general dental practice: one-year follow-up, *J Am Dent Assoc* 137:1089-1098, 2006; quiz 1168-1089.
6. Clark GT: Occlusal therapy: occlusal appliances. *The president's conference on the examination, diagnosis and management of temporomandibular disorders*, Chicago, American Dental Association, 1983, pp 137-146.
7. Al-Ani MZ, Davies SJ, Gray RJ, Sloan P, Glenny AM: Stabilisation splint therapy for temporomandibular pain dysfunction syndrome, *Cochrane Database Syst Rev* CD002778, 2004.
8. Forssell H, Kalso E, Koskela P, Vehmanen R, Puukka P et al: Occlusal treatments in temporomandibular disorders: a qualitative systematic review of randomized controlled trials, *Pain* 83:549-560, 1999.
9. Ekberg EC, Vallon D, Nilner M: Occlusal appliance therapy in patients with temporomandibular disorders. A double-blind controlled study in a short-term perspective, *Acta Odontol Scand* 56:122-128, 1998.

10. Kreiner M, Betancor E, Clark GT: Occlusal stabilization appliances. Evidence of their efficacy, *J Am Dent Assoc* 132:770-777, 2001.

11. Yatani H, Minakuchi H, Matsuka Y, Fujisawa T, Yamashita A: The long-term effect of occlusal therapy on self-administered treatment outcomes of TMD, *J Orofac Pain* 12:75-88, 1998.

12. Ekberg E, Vallon D, Nilner M: The efficacy of appliance therapy in patients with temporomandibular disorders of mainly myogenous origin. A randomized, controlled, short-term trial, *J Orofac Pain* 17:133-139, 2003.

13. Shi CS, Wang HY: Postural and maximum activity in elevators during mandible pre- and post-occlusal splint treatment of temporomandibular joint disturbance syndrome, *J Oral Rehabil* 16:155-161, 1989.

14. Solberg WK, Clark GT, Rugh JD: Nocturnal electromyographic evaluation of bruxism patients undergoing short term splint therapy, *J Oral Rehabil* 2:215-223, 1975.

15. Clark GT, Beemsterboer PL, Solberg WK, Rugh JD: Nocturnal electromyographic evaluation of myofascial pain dysfunction in patients undergoing occlusal splint therapy, *J Am Dent Assoc* 99:607-611, 1979.

16. Clark GT, Rugh JD, Handelman SL: Nocturnal masseter muscle activity and urinary catecholamine levels in bruxers, *J Dent Res* 59:1571-1576, 1980.

17. Fuchs P: The muscular activity of the chewing apparatus during night sleep. An examination of healthy subjects and patients with functional disturbances, *J Oral Rehabil* 2: 35-48, 1975.

18. Okeson JP: The effects of hard and soft occlusal splints on nocturnal bruxism, *J Am Dent Assoc* 114:788-791, 1987.

19. Sheikholeslam A, Holmgren K, Riise C: A clinical and electromyographic study of the long-term effects of an occlusal splint on the temporal and masseter muscles in patients with functional disorders and nocturnal bruxism, *J Oral Rehabil* 13:137-145, 1986.

20. Kurita H, Kurashina K, Kotani A: Clinical effect of full coverage occlusal splint therapy for specific temporomandibular disorder conditions and symptoms, *J Prosthet Dent* 78:506-510, 1997.

21. Dao TT, Lavigne GJ: Oral splints: the crutches for temporomandibular disorders and bruxism? *Crit Rev Oral Biol Med* 9:345-361, 1998.

22. Dos Santos JD Jr, de Rijk WG: Vectorial analysis of the equilibrium of forces transmitted to TMJ and occlusal biteplane splints, *J Oral Rehabil* 22:301-310, 1995.

23. Askinas SW: Fabrication of an occlusal splint, *J Prosth Dent* 28:549-551, 1972.

24. Bohannan H, Saxe SR: Periodontics in general practice. In Morris AL, Bohannan HM, editors: *The dental specialties in general practice*, Philadelphia, 1969, Saunders, pp 294-300.

25. Shulman J: Bite modification appliances—planes, plates and pivots, *Va Dent J* 49:27-30, 1972.

26. Kornfeld M: *Mouth rehabilitation*, ed 2, St Louis, 1974, Mosby.

27. Becker CM, Kaiser DA, Lemm RB: A simplified technique for fabrication of night guards, *J Prosthet Dent* 32:582-589, 1974.

28. Shore NA: A mandibular autorepositioning appliance, *J Am Dent Assoc* 75:908-911, 1967.

29. Grupe HE, Gromeh JJ: Bruxism splint, techniques using quick cure acrylic, *J Periodontol* 30:156-157, 1959.

30. Hunter J: Vacuum formed bite raising appliances for temporomandibular joint dysfunction, *Dent Tech* 27: 39-40, 1974.

31. Okeson JP: A simplified technique for biteguard fabrication, *J Ky Dent Assoc* 29:11-16, 1977.

32. Okeson JP: Biteguard therapy and fabrication. In Lundeen HC, Gibbs CH, editors: *Advances in occlusion*, Boston, 1982, John Wright PSG, pp 220-226.

33. Ito T, Gibbs CH, Marguelles-Bonnet R, Lupkiewicz SM, Young HM et al: Loading on the temporomandibular joint with five occlusal conditions, *J Prosthet Dent* 56:478-484, 1986.

34. Wilkinson T, Hansson TL, McNeill C, Marcel T: A comparison of the success of 24-hour occlusal splint therapy versus nocturnal occlusal splint therapy in reducing craniomandibular disorders, *J Craniomandib Disord* 6:64, 1992.

35. Schumann S et al: Comparative efficacy of maxillary and mandibular splints for TMD, *J Dent Res* 70(special issue):1441, 1991 (abstract).

36. Roberts CA, Tallents RH, Katzberg RW, Sanchez-Woodworth RE, Manzione JV et al: Clinical and arthrographic evaluation of temporomandibular joint sounds, *Oral Surg Oral Med Oral Pathol* 62:373-376, 1986.

37. Manco LG, Messing SG: Splint therapy evaluation with direct sagittal computed tomography, *Oral Surg Oral Med Oral Pathol* 61:5-11, 1986.

38. Manzione JV, Tallents R, Katzberg RW, Oster C, Miller TL: Arthrographically guided splint therapy for recapturing the temporomandibular joint meniscus, *Oral Surg Oral Med Oral Pathol* 57:235-240, 1984.

39. Moritz M, Behr M, Held P, Dammer R, Niederdellmann H: Comparative study of results of electronic axiography with results of magnetic resonance imaging including MRI-assisted splint therapy, *Acta Stomatol Belg* 92:35-38, 1995.

40. Cohen SG, MacAfee KA II: The use of magnetic resonance imaging to determine splint position in the management of internal derangements of the temporomandibular joint, *Cranio* 12:167-171, 1994.

41. Ramfjord SP, Ash MM: *Occlusion*, ed 3, Philadelphia, 1983, Saunders.

42. Posselt U: *Physiology of occlusion and rehabilitation*, ed 2, Philadelphia, 1968, FA Davis.

43. Krogh-Poulsen WG, Olsson A: Management of the occlusion of the teeth. In Schwartz L, Chayes CM, editors: *Facial pain and mandibular dysfunction*, Philadelphia, 1969, Saunders, pp 236-280.

44. Bruno SA: Neuromuscular disturbances causing temporomandibular dysfunction and pain, *J Prosthet Dent* 26: 387-395, 1971.

45. Boyd J: *The NTI TSS appliance* (website): http://www.drjim-boyd.com. Accessed 2000.

46. Shankland WE II: Migraine and tension-type headache reduction through pericranial muscular suppression: a preliminary report, *Cranio* 19:269-278, 2001.

47. Jokstad A, Mo A, Krogstad BS: Clinical comparison between two different splint designs for temporomandibular disorder therapy, *Acta Odontol Scand* 63:218-226, 2005.

48. Al Quran FA, Kamal MS: Anterior midline point stop device (AMPS) in the treatment of myogenous TMDs: comparison with the stabilization splint and control group, *Oral Surg Oral Med Oral Pathol Oral Radiol Endod* 101:741-747, 2006.

49. Magnusson T, Adiels AM, Nilsson HL, Helkimo M: Treatment effect on signs and symptoms of temporomandibular disorders—comparison between stabilisation splint and a new type of splint (NTI). A pilot study, *Swed Dent J* 28:11-20, 2004.

50. Wright EF, Clark EG, Paunovich ED, Hart RG: Headache improvement through TMD stabilization appliance and self-management therapies, *Cranio* 24:104-111, 2006.

51. Bondemark L, Lindman R: Craniomandibular status and function in patients with habitual snoring and obstructive sleep apnea after nocturnal treatment with a mandibular advancement splint: a 2-year follow-up, *Eur J Orthod* 22:53-60, 2000.

52. Ekberg E, Vallon D, Nilner M: Treatment outcome of headache after occlusal appliance therapy in a randomized controlled trial among patients with temporomandibular disorders of mainly arthrogenous origin, *Swed Dent J* 26:115-124, 2002.

53. Kemper JT Jr, Okeson JP: Craniomandibular disorders and headaches, *J Prosthet Dent* 49:702-705, 1983.

54. Gelb H: *Clinical management of head, neck and TMJ pain and dysfunction,* Philadelphia, 1977, Saunders.

55. Bodenham RS: A biteguard for athletic training. A case report, *Br Dent J* 129:85-86, 1970.

56. Smith SD: Muscular strength correlated to jaw posture and the temporomandibular joint, *N Y State Dent J* 44:278-285, 1978.

57. Schubert MM, Guttu RL, Hunter LH, Hall R, Thomas R: Changes in shoulder and leg strength in athletes wearing mandibular orthopedic repositioning appliances, *J Am Dent Assoc* 108:334-337, 1984.

58. Yates JW, Koen TJ, Semenick DM, Kuftinec MM: Effect of a mandibular orthopedic repositioning appliance on muscular strength, *J Am Dent Assoc* 108:331-333, 1984.

59. Yin X, Zhang D: [Clinical observation of TMJDS treated with pivot splint], *Chung Hua Kou Chiang Hsueh Tsa Chih* 31:357-359, 1996.

60. Watts DM: *Gnathosonic diagnosis and occlusal dynamics,* New York, 1981, Praeger.

61. Sato H, Ukon S, Ishikawa M, Ohki M, Kitamori H: Tomographic evaluation of TMJ loading affected by occlusal pivots, *Int J Prosthodont* 13:399-404, 2000.

62. Christensen LV, Rassouli NM: Experimental occlusal interferences. Part V. Mandibular rotations versus hemimandibular translations, *J Oral Rehabil* 22:865-876, 1995.

63. Moncayo S: Biomechanics of pivoting appliances, *J Orofac Pain* 8:190-196, 1994.

64. Stenger JM, Lawson EA, Wright JM, Ricketts J: Mouthguards: protection against shock to head, neck and teeth, *J Am Dent Assoc* 69:273-281, 1964.

65. Seals RR Jr, Morrow RM, Kuebker WA, Farney WD: An evaluation of mouthguard programs in Texas high school football, *J Am Dent Assoc* 110:904-909, 1985.

66. Garon MW, Merkle A, Wright JT: Mouth protectors and oral trauma: a study of adolescent football players, *J Am Dent Assoc* 112:663-665, 1986.

67. Block SL, Apfel M, Laskin DM: The use of resilient latex rubber bite appliance in the treatment of MPD syndrome, *J Dent Res* 57(special issue):92, 1978 (abstract).

68. Nevarro E, Barghi N, Rey R: Clinical evaluation of maxillary hard and resilient occlusal splints, *J Dent Res* 57(special issue):1313, 1985 (abstract).

69. Al Quran FA, Lyons MF: The immediate effect of hard and soft splints on the EMG activity of the masseter and temporalis muscles, *J Oral Rehabil* 26:559-563, 1999.

70. Wright E, Anderson G, Schulte J: A randomized clinical trial of intraoral soft splints and palliative treatment for masticatory muscle pain, *J Orofac Pain* 9:192-199, 1995.

71. Truelove E, Huggins KH, Mancl L, Dworkin SF: The efficacy of traditional, low-cost and nonsplint therapies for temporomandibular disorder: a randomized controlled trial, *J Am Dent Assoc* 137:1099-1107, 2006.

72. Clark GT, Beemsterboer PL, Rugh JD: Nocturnal masseter muscle activity and the symptoms of masticatory dysfunction, *J Oral Rehabil* 8:279-286, 1981.

73. Carraro JJ, Caffesse RG: Effect of occlusal splints on TMJ symptomatology, *J Prosthet Dent* 40:563-566, 1978.

74. Franks AST: Conservative treatment of temporomandibular joint dysfunction: a comparative study, *Dent Pract Dent Rec* 15:205-210, 1965.

75. Pettengill CA, Growney MR Jr, Schoff R, Kenworthy CR: A pilot study comparing the efficacy of hard and soft stabilizing appliances in treating patients with temporomandibular disorders, *J Prosthet Dent* 79:165-168, 1998.

76. Dawson PE: *Evaluation, diagnosis and treatment of occlusal problems,* St Louis, 1974, Mosby.

77. Graf H: Bruxism, *Dent Clin North Am* 13:659-665, 1969.

78. Christensen J: Effect of occlusion-raising procedures on the chewing system, *Dent Pract Dent Rec* 10:233-238, 1970.

79. Rugh JD, Drago CJ: Vertical dimension: a study of clinical rest position and jaw muscle activity, *J Prosthet Dent* 45:670-675, 1981.

80. Christensen LV, Mohamed SE, Harrison JD: Delayed onset of masseter muscle pain in experimental tooth clenching, *J Prosthet Dent* 48:579-584, 1982.

81. Rugh JD, Robbins JW: Oral habits disorders. In Ingersoll B, editor: *Behavioral aspects in dentistry,* New York, 1982, Appleton-Century-Crofts, pp 179-202.

82. Rugh JD, Solberg WK: Psychological implications in temporomandibular pain and dysfunction, *Oral Sci Rev* 7:3-30, 1976.

83. Oakley ME, McCreary CP, Clark GT, Holston S, Glover D et al: A cognitive-behavioral approach to temporomandibular dysfunction treatment failures: a controlled comparison, *J Orofac Pain* 8:397-401, 1994.

84. Mishra KD, Gatchel RJ, Gardea MA: The relative efficacy of three cognitive-behavioral treatment approaches to

temporomandibular disorders, *J Behav Med* 23:293-309, 2000.

85. Stockstill JW: The placebo effect. The placebo effect in the management of chronic myofascial pain: a review, *J Am Coll Dent* 56:14-18, 1989.

86. Dao TT, Lavigne GJ, Charbonneau A, Feine JS, Lund JP: The efficacy of oral splints in the treatment of myofascial pain of the jaw muscles: a controlled clinical trial, *Pain* 1994;56:85-94, 1994.

87. Greene CS, Laskin DM: Meprobamate therapy for the myofascial pain-dysfunction (MPD) syndrome: a double-blind evaluation, *J Am Dent Assoc* 82:587-590, 1971.

88. Greene CS, Laskin DM: Splint therapy for the myofascial pain-dysfunction (MPD) syndrome: a comparative study, *J Am Dent Assoc* 84:624-628, 1972.

89. Cassisi JE, McGlynn FD, Mahan PE: Occlusal splint effects on nocturnal bruxing: an emerging paradigm and some early results, *Cranio* 5:64-68, 1987.

90. Holmgren K, Sheikholeslam A, Riise C: Effect of a full-arch maxillary occlusal splint on parafunctional activity during sleep in patients with nocturnal bruxism and signs and symptoms of craniomandibular disorders, *J Prosthet Dent* 69:293-297, 1993.

91. Pierce CJ, Gale EN: A comparison of different treatments for nocturnal bruxism, *J Dent Res* 67:597-601, 1988.

92. Harada T, Ichiki R, Tsukiyama Y, Koyano K: The effect of oral splint devices on sleep bruxism: a 6-week observation with an ambulatory electromyographic recording device, *J Oral Rehabil* 33:482-488, 2006.

93. Whitney CW, Von Korff M: Regression to the mean in treated versus untreated chronic pain, *Pain* 50:281-285, 1992.

94. Yaffe A, Tal M, Ehrlich J: Effect of occlusal bite-raising splint on electromyographic, motor unit histochemistry and myoneuronal dimension in rats, *J Oral Rehabil* 18:343-351, 1991.

95. Rivera-Morales WC, Mohl ND: Relationship of occlusal vertical dimension to the health of the masticatory system, *J Prosthet Dent* 65:547-553, 1991.

Treatment Sequencing

16

CHAPTER

"The complexity of TMD makes developing a 'cook book' impossible, even though that is precisely what everyone would like. Here is an attempt."

—JPO

he preceding five chapters have described the specific treatment for each major temporomandibular disorder (TMD). Treatment sequencing is also an important part of managing these problems. Knowing when to institute specific treatment in the overall management of a disorder can be critical. Sometimes the success or failure of a treatment can be determined by the relative sequence in which it is introduced. In an attempt to enhance treatment effects and assist in managing these patients, this chapter describes the proper sequence of treatment for the major TMDs.

Each of the treatment sequences described is designed as an algorithm* to assist the therapist in managing the disorder. Treatment options are described for both success and failure of the previous treatment. The treatments identified are only briefly described. The appropriate chapter for each disorder should be reviewed for more specific details regarding a given treatment.

Importantly, the therapist should recognize that these sequencing diagrams are designed for the general management of a disorder and, although appropriate for most patients, may not be suitable in all instances. The sequencing diagrams are designed to accommodate a single diagnosis. When more than one diagnosis is established, the therapist must follow more than one sequencing diagram. This can become quite complicated and difficult. Therefore a good rule to follow is that if two diagnoses have been established and a conflict in treatment results, the primary diagnosis should take precedence over the secondary one.

For example, a common finding is a masticatory muscle disorder and a disc derangement disorder present concomitantly. As described in Chapter 11, these frequently appear simultaneously because one can lead to the other. When this occurs, it is helpful to determine the primary disorder so that effective treatment directed to it may also eliminate the secondary disorder. This is sometimes a difficult task. A good history and clinical examination are essential. In many patients the primary disorder becomes the one that most closely relates to the chief complaint. This is not always an accurate assumption, but when the primary diagnosis is difficult to determine, it is a good beginning point.

When a person has a disc derangement disorder and a masticatory muscle disorder concomitantly and a primary diagnosis cannot be established, it is generally advisable to treat the masticatory muscle disorder as the primary diagnosis. Therefore treatment is initially directed toward the

---

*The flow charts are presented in this discussion and again in the Appendix (for easy reference).

498

muscle symptoms. If the symptoms are not decreased in a reasonable time, therapy is then directed to the disc derangement disorder.

Another general rule in treating patients is that reversible and noninvasive forms are used to manage the disorder initially. The results of this treatment can be helpful in determining the need, if any, for more aggressive or irreversible treatment. This general rule is always applied in treating TMDs; in this manner, unnecessary irreversible treatment will be avoided.

Occasionally treatment will fail to eliminate the symptoms. When this occurs, the diagnosis must be reexamined for accuracy. Some instances may arise in which the diagnosis is accurate but the treatment is unable to alter the causative factors. A typical example is a permanent anterior dislocation of the disc. An occlusal appliance and supportive therapy may fail to reduce the symptoms. When severe pain persists, a surgical procedure may be the only alternative. The decision to undergo surgical correction of an intracapsular disorder must be made by the patient and not by the therapist. The patient must therefore be well informed in order to make the proper decision for himself or herself. The patient should decide whether to undergo surgery on the basis of two considerations: First, the patient needs to understand the success versus failure, advantages versus disadvantages, and risks of and expected results from the surgical procedure. The second consideration should be regarding the level of pain caused by the condition. Because pain is a personal, individual experience, only the patient can know the degree of suffering involved. When suffering is only occasional and mild, a surgical procedure may not be indicated. However, when it alters the quality of life, surgery becomes a viable consideration.

Only the patient can decide whether to proceed with a surgical procedure.

This chapter provides 11 flowcharts to assist the therapist in selecting and sequencing the appropriate treatment: four for masticatory muscle disorders, four for disc derangement disorders, and three for inflammatory disorders. Once the proper diagnosis has been established, these charts can be used. The list of diagnoses with the appropriate chart follows:

I. Masticatory muscle disorders
   A. Protective co-contraction (Fig. 16-1)
   B. Local muscle soreness (see Fig. 16-1)
   C. Myofascial pain (Fig. 16-2)
   D. Myospasm (Fig. 16-3)
   E. Chronic centrally mediated myalgia.(Fig. 16-4)
II. Temporomandibular joint disorders
   A. Derangement of the condyle-disc complex
      1. Disc displacement (Fig. 16-5)
      2. Disc dislocation with reduction (see Fig. 16-5)
      3. Disc dislocation without reduction (Fig. 16-6)
   B. Structural incompatibility
      1. Deviation in form (Fig. 16-7)
      2. Adhesions (see Fig. 16-7)
      3. Subluxation (Fig. 16-8)
      4. Spontaneous dislocation (see Fig. 16-8)
   C. Inflammatory disorders of the temporomandibular joint
      1. Capsulitis and synovitis (Fig. 16-9)
      2. Retrodiscitis (see Fig. 16-9)
      3. Arthritides
         a. Osteoarthritis (Fig. 16-10)
         b. Polyarthritides
            i. Infectious arthritis (Fig. 16-11)
            ii. Traumatic arthritis (see Fig. 16-9)

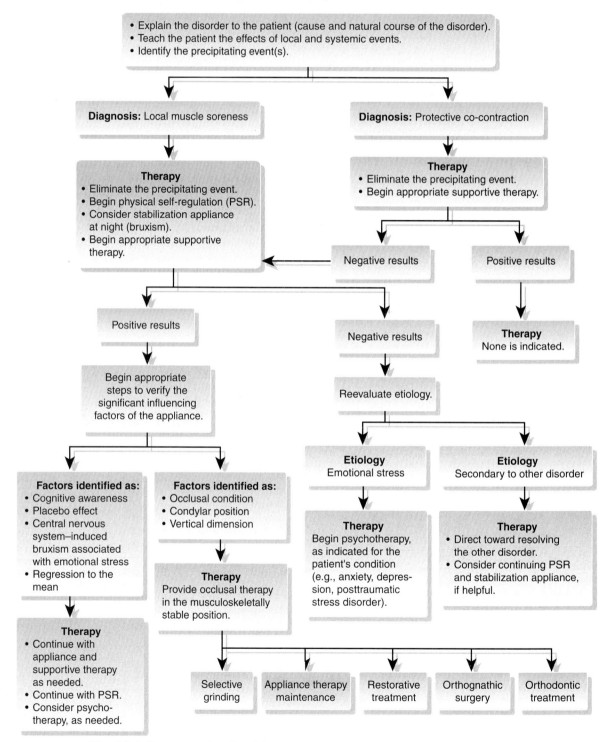

Fig. 16-1 Diagnostic algorithm for masticatory muscle disorders (subclass: protective co-contraction and local muscle soreness).

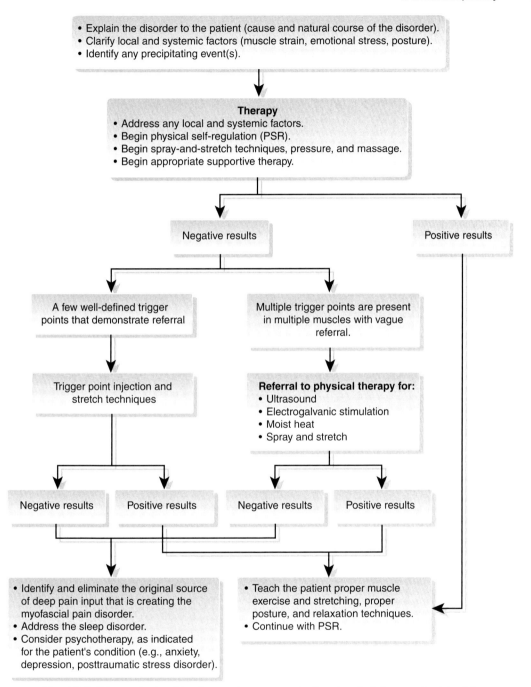

- Explain the disorder to the patient (cause and natural course of the disorder).
- Clarify local and systemic factors (muscle strain, emotional stress, posture).
- Identify any precipitating event(s).

Therapy
- Address any local and systemic factors.
- Begin physical self-regulation (PSR).
- Begin spray-and-stretch techniques, pressure, and massage.
- Begin appropriate supportive therapy.

Negative results

Positive results

A few well-defined trigger points that demonstrate referral

Multiple trigger points are present in multiple muscles with vague referral.

Trigger point injection and stretch techniques

Referral to physical therapy for:
- Ultrasound
- Electrogalvanic stimulation
- Moist heat
- Spray and stretch

Negative results

Positive results

Negative results

Positive results

- Identify and eliminate the original source of deep pain input that is creating the myofascial pain disorder.
- Address the sleep disorder.
- Consider psychotherapy, as indicated for the patient's condition (e.g., anxiety, depression, posttraumatic stress disorder).

- Teach the patient proper muscle exercise and stretching, proper posture, and relaxation techniques.
- Continue with PSR.

Fig. 16-2 Diagnostic algorithm for masticatory muscle disorders (subclass: myofascial pain).

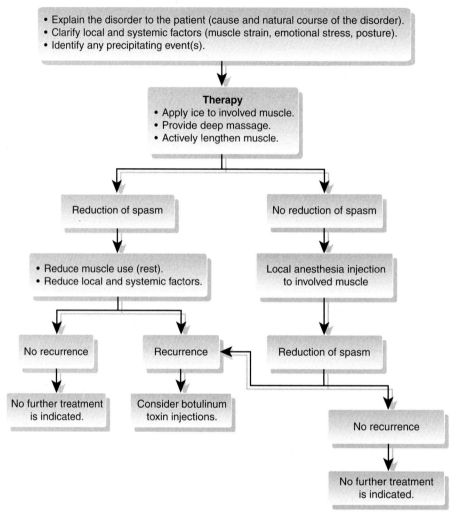

Fig. 16-3 Diagnostic algorithm for masticatory muscle disorders (subclass: myospasm).

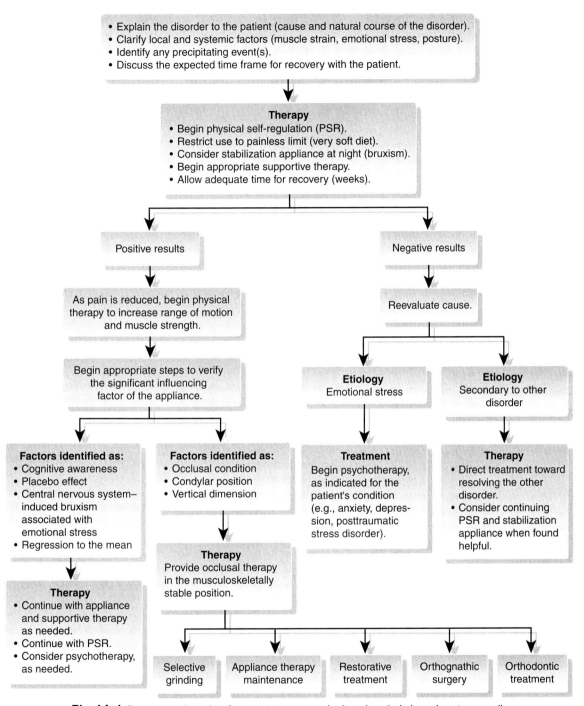

Fig. 16-4 Diagnostic algorithm for masticatory muscle disorders (subclass: chronic centrally mediated myalgia).

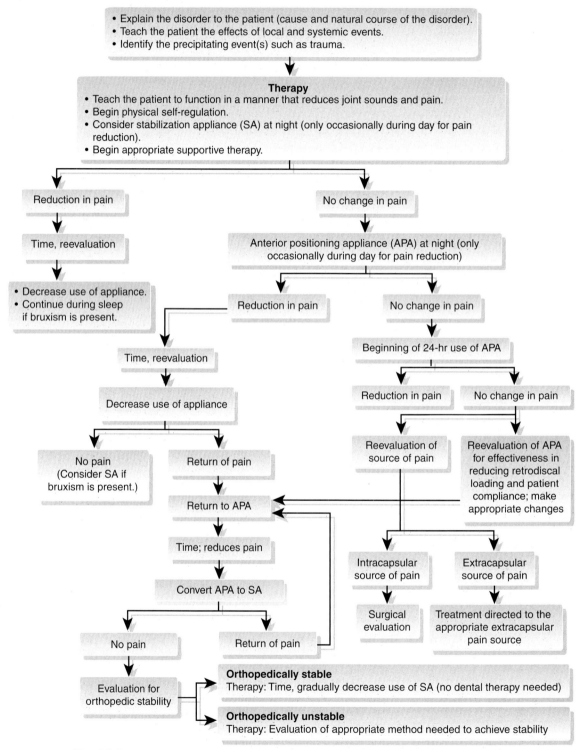

Fig. 16-5 Diagnostic algorithm for temporomandibular joint disorders (subclass: derangement of the condyle-disc complex—disc displacement and disc dislocation with reduction).

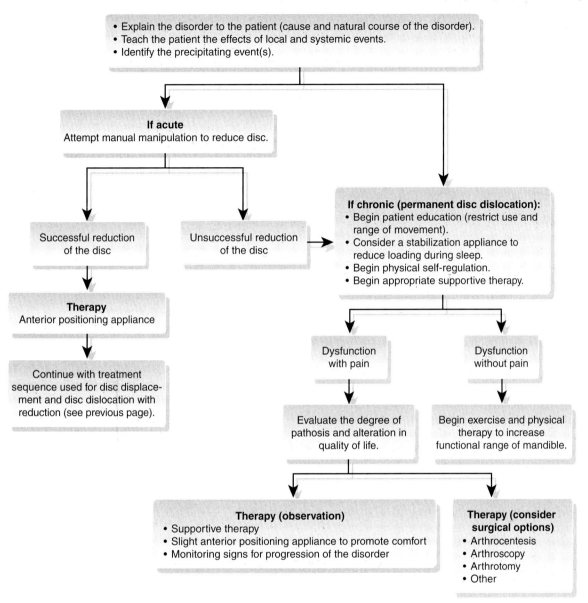

Fig. 16-6 Diagnostic algorithm of temporomandibular joint disorders (subclass: derangement of the condyle-disc complex—disc dislocation without reduction).

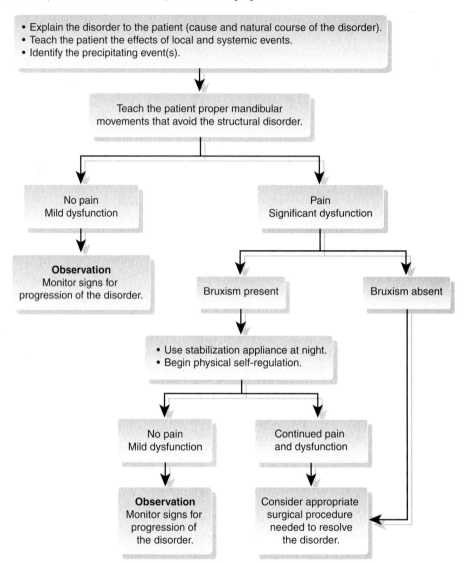

Fig. 16-7 Diagnostic algorithm of temporomandibular joint disorders (subclass: structural incompatibility—deviation in form and adhesions).

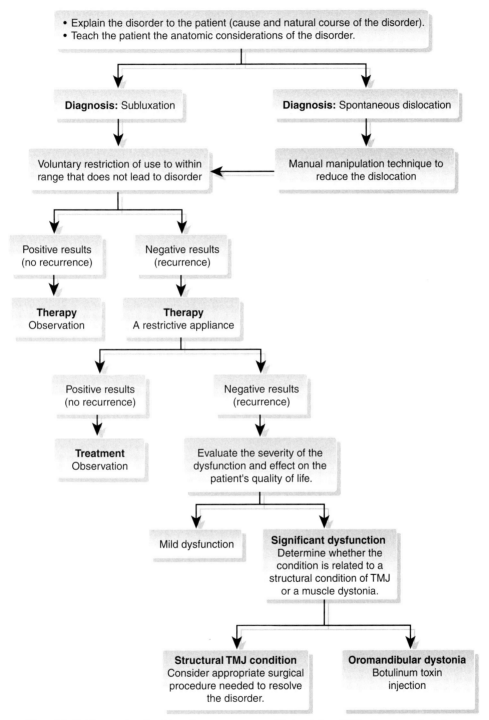

Fig. 16-8 Diagnostic algorithm for temporomandibular joint *(TMJ)* disorders (subclass: structural incompatibility—subluxation and spontaneous dislocation).

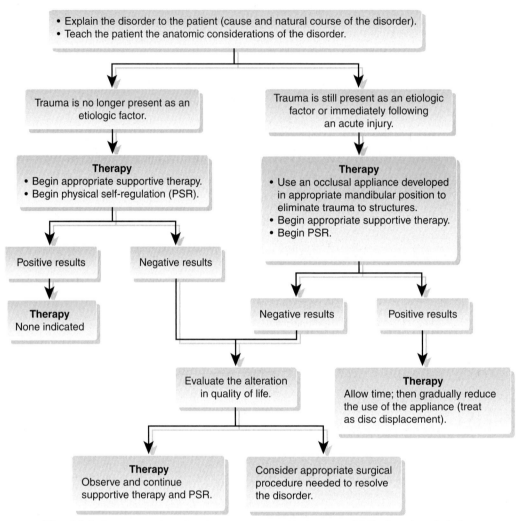

Fig. 16-9 Diagnostic algorithm for temporomandibular joint (TMJ) disorders (subclass: inflammatory disorders of the TMJ—capsulitis and synovitis, retrodiscitis, traumatic arthritis).

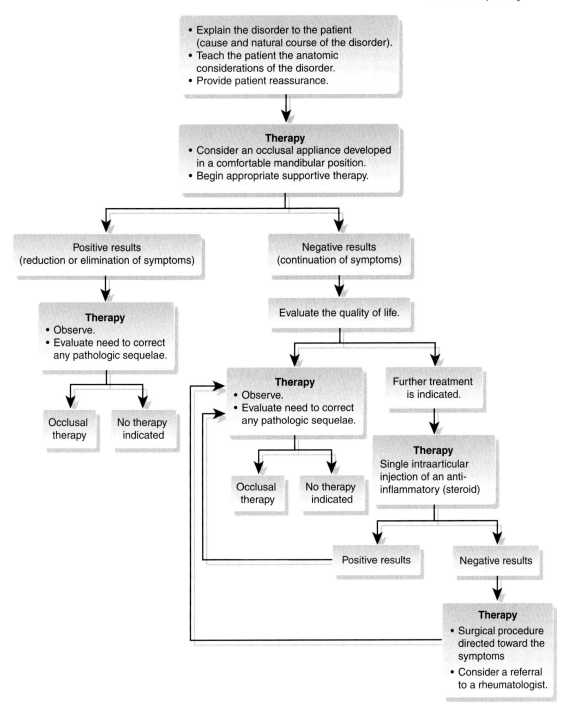

Fig. 16-10 Diagnostic algorithm for temporomandibular joint (TMJ) disorders (subclass: inflammatory disorders of the TMJ—osteoarthritis).

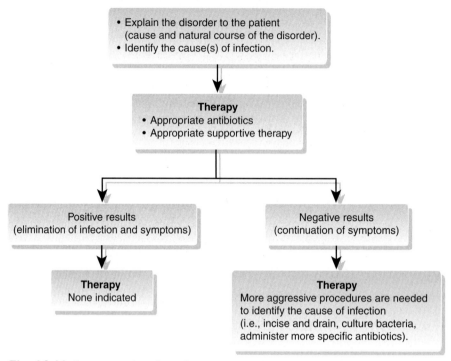

Fig. 16-11 Diagnostic algorithm of temporomandibular joint (TMJ) disorders (subclass: inflammatory disorders of the TMJ—infectious arthritis).

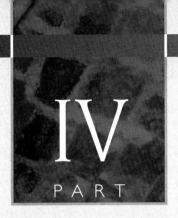

PART

IV

Occlusal Therapy

Permanent alteration of the occlusal condition is indicated for two reasons. The first and most common reason is to improve the functional relationship between the maxillary and mandibular teeth. Included in the consideration is aesthetics. Most dental procedures, in one way or another, are directed toward this goal. This may be accomplished by prosthetic procedures that replace functional tooth surfaces. It may also be accomplished by orthodontic or surgical movement of the teeth into a better functional occlusal relationship or aesthetics, or both. These procedures have nothing to do with temporomandibular disorders (TMDs).

The second reason for permanently altering the occlusal condition is as a treatment goal to eliminate a TMD. In this instance the patient may have no missing or damaged teeth, but changes are indicated because of orthopedic instability. Permanent occlusal therapy is only indicated when significant evidence exists to support a suspicion that the occlusal condition is a causative factor related to the TMD symptoms. One should not routinely alter the occlusion without such evidence.

This is not to say that occlusion is unimportant. In fact, it is the basic foundation of dentistry. Occlusal concepts need to be closely adhered to every time dental procedures are performed.

Part IV consists of four chapters that discuss various considerations of permanent occlusal therapy. The indications and need for occlusal therapy must be established with certainty before treatment begins.

General Considerations in Occlusal Therapy

17

CHAPTER

"If occlusion is found to significantly contribute to a TMD, dentistry is the only health profession that can provide lasting effect. If occlusion is not related to the TMD, it should not be altered other than for restorative or aesthetic reasons."

—JPO

Occlusal therapy is any treatment that alters a patient's occlusal condition. It can be used to improve function of the masticatory system through the influence of the occlusal contact patterns and by altering the functional jaw position. Occlusal therapy can be reversible or irreversible.

Reversible occlusal therapy temporarily alters the occlusal condition, the joint position, or both; however, when this therapy is removed, the patient's preexisting condition returns. An example would be an occlusal appliance (Fig. 17-1). When the occlusal appliance is used, it creates a favorable alteration in the occlusal contacts and joint position. When it is removed, the patient's original occlusal condition returns.

Irreversible occlusal therapy permanently alters the occlusal condition, so the original condition cannot be recovered. An example would be selective grinding of the teeth whereby the occlusal surfaces are reshaped with the goal of improving the occlusal condition and orthopedic stability. Because this procedure involves the removal of enamel, it becomes irreversible and therefore permanent. Other forms of irreversible occlusal therapy are fixed prosthetic procedures and orthodontic therapy (Fig. 17-2).

In the previous chapters, reversible occlusal therapies (occlusal appliances) were discussed as treatment for many TMDs. In the following chapters the emphasis of occlusal therapy is on the irreversible types. Because irreversible occlusal therapy is permanent, it must be provided only when it is determined to be beneficial to the patient. Two general indications suggest the need for irreversible occlusal therapy: (1) treatment of TMDs and (2) treatment in conjunction with other necessary measures that will significantly alter the existing occlusal condition.

TREATMENT OF TEMPOROMANDIBULAR DISORDERS

Irreversible occlusal therapy is indicated when sufficient evidence exists that the primary causative factor creating a TMD is the prevalent occlusal condition and/or orthopedic instability. In other words, permanent improvement of the occlusal condition is likely to eliminate the functional disturbance of the masticatory system.

At one time the dental profession believed that most TMDs were caused by malocclusion. With that belief, permanent occlusal changes became a routine part of the management of TMDs. Now that clinicians have a better understanding of the complexity of TMD, they appreciate that the occlusal condition is only one of five major causative factors that may lead to TMD (see Chapter 7). Therefore permanent occlusal therapy

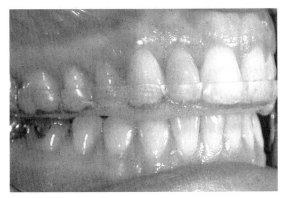

Fig. 17-1 Stabilization appliances are a form of reversible occlusal therapy.

is only indicated when significant evidence exists to support the belief that the occlusal condition is a causative factor. One should not routinely alter the occlusion without such evidence. The occlusal condition can become a causative factor in TMD in two ways: (1) via an acute change in the occlusal condition (altered sensory input) and (2) via orthopedic instability (plus loading) (see Chapter 7). Importantly, the clinician must recognize that the occlusal management of these two considerations is quite different.

Sufficient evidence to change a patient's occlusion is commonly derived through successful occlusal appliance therapy. However, the mere fact that the occlusal appliance relieves symptoms is not alone sufficient evidence to start irreversible occlusal therapy. As discussed in Chapter 15, the occlusal appliance can affect symptoms in several different manners. Effort must be made to determine which feature of the appliance is responsible for the elimination of the symptoms. When the multiple effects of occlusal appliance therapy are overlooked, an irreversible procedure such as selective grinding is likely to fail to eliminate the symptoms of the disorder. Because irreversible occlusal therapy is permanent, care is always taken to confirm the need for these procedures before they are instituted.

TREATMENT IN CONJUNCTION WITH OTHER DENTAL THERAPIES

Irreversible occlusal therapy is often indicated in the absence of any functional disturbance of the masticatory system. When patients have a dentition that is severely compromised by broken, decayed, or missing teeth, there is a need to

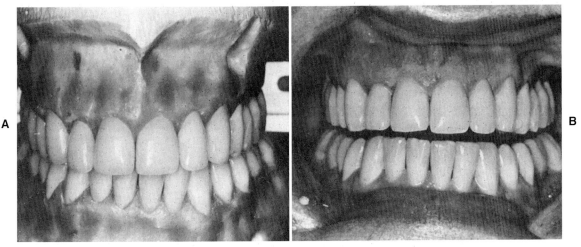

Fig. 17-2 This extensive restorative procedure is a form of irreversible occlusal therapy. **A,** Twenty-eight units of full ceramic restoration on the articulator ready for delivery to the patient. **B,** Ceramic restorations permanently cemented in the patient's mouth. *(Courtesy The Foschi Office, Bologna, Italy.)*

restore masticatory function. Restoring the dentition with operative procedures or with fixed or removable prostheses, or both, is a form of irreversible occlusal therapy. Even in the absence of any obvious TMD, the occlusal condition needs to be carefully restored to a condition that will promote and maintain health for the patient (Fig. 17-3).

Providing occlusal therapy for patients with debilitated dentitions is undoubtedly an important service provided by dentists. This type of therapy, however, can lead to interesting and important questions regarding treatment. Imagine a 24-year-old woman who comes to the dental office for a routine checkup. She has no signs of functional disturbances of the masticatory system. Examination reveals, however, that she has a significant malocclusion. The question now posed is one of prevention. Should occlusal therapy be provided to improve the occlusal condition in an attempt to prevent any future TMD? Many prominent dentists would suggest just that. Yet at this time there is no scientific evidence that this patient will at any time in the future have problems if left untreated. She is functioning within her physiologic tolerance, even though the malocclusion appears to be significant. One might think that at some time in the future perhaps her level of physiologic tolerance may be exceeded by other causes such as trauma, increased emotional stress, or deep pain input. However, no evidence in any given patient indicates that this will happen (if it did, management would likely be quite different than occlusal therapy).

The clinician should also remember that the patient's dental malocclusion may not pose a significant risk factor for TMD. The malocclusion needs to be evaluated for its relationship to the

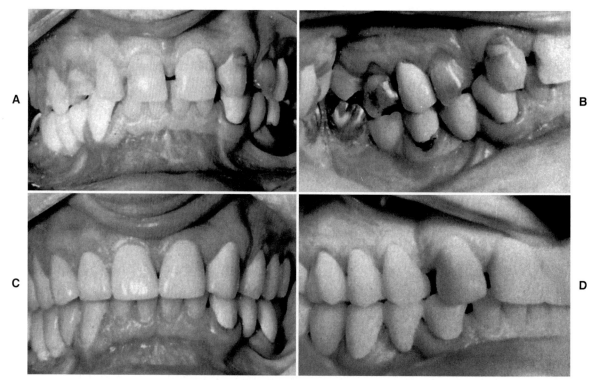

Fig. 17-3 Frontal **(A)** and lateral **(B)** views of a patient with multiple dental problems best treated by restorative procedures. Frontal **(C)** and lateral **(D)** views of the same patient after irreversible occlusal therapy has been accomplished by restorative procedures. The correction of the plane of occlusion is demonstrated.

joint positions. If the intercuspal position is in harmony with the musculoskeletally stable (MS) position of the condyles (see Chapter 5), it does not pose a significant risk factor for TMD (a stable malocclusion). This concept was presented in Chapter 7 and needs to be considered any time the clinician is developing a treatment plan for treating TMD.

At this time, with the data on hand, it is impossible to predict whether any individual patient will develop TMD. Therefore justification of prevention therapy is difficult, especially when the appropriate treatment is expensive and time consuming. If, however, extensive treatments are indicated for other reasons (e.g., aesthetics, caries, missing teeth), occlusal therapy should be provided in conjunction with the treatment so that when it is completed, optimal occlusal and orthopedic conditions will have been established.

TREATMENT GOALS FOR OCCLUSAL THERAPY

When occlusal therapy is indicated to resolve the symptoms of a TMD permanently, the specific treatment goals are determined by the reversible occlusal therapy (the occlusal appliance) that has successfully eliminated the symptoms. If a stabilization appliance has resolved the disorder, a similar occlusal condition should be introduced by the irreversible occlusal therapy. The treatment goals are therefore the same for both reversible and irreversible therapies (orthopedic stability).

When an anterior positioning appliance has eliminated the symptoms, it does not immediately suggest that permanent occlusal therapy should be completed in the forward therapeutic position. As stated in Chapter 13, the main purpose of the anterior positioning appliance is to promote adaptation of the retrodiscal tissues. Once this adaptation has occurred, the condyle should be returned to the MS position. Therefore following successful anterior positioning therapy and stabilization appliance therapy, the condyle should be in the MS position. The treatment goals of permanent occlusal therapy are to establish orthopedic stability in this position.

TREATMENT GOALS FOR THE MUSCULOSKELETALLY STABLE POSITION

Patients suffering from a masticatory muscle disorder are generally treated with a stabilization appliance that provides the optimum occlusal conditions when the condyles are in their most MS position (see Chapter 5). Patients suffering from an inflammatory disorder, as well as a severely debilitated dentition, are also best treated using this criterion. In all these conditions the treatment goals for occlusal therapy are to permit the condyles to assume their MS positions (centric relation) at the same time that the teeth are in their maximum intercuspal position (orthopedic stability). More specifically, treatment goals are as follows:

1. The condyles are resting in their most superoanterior position against the posterior slopes of the articular eminences.
2. The articular discs are properly interposed between the condyles and the fossae. In those cases when a disc derangement disorder has been treated, the condyle may now be articulating on adaptive fibrotic tissue with the disc still displaced or even dislocated. Although this condition may not be ideal, it is adaptive and should be considered functional in the absence of pain.
3. When the mandible is brought into closure in the MS position, the posterior teeth contact evenly and simultaneously. All contacts occur between centric cusp tips and flat surfaces, directing occlusal forces through the long axes of the teeth.
4. When the mandible moves eccentrically, the anterior teeth contact and disocclude the posterior teeth.
5. In the upright head position (alert feeding position) the posterior tooth contacts are more prominent than the anterior tooth contacts.

Because these treatment goals are most effective in relieving the symptoms of many TMDs, they become the treatment goals for permanent occlusal therapy. These goals also offer a stable and reproducible mandibular position, which is absolutely necessary for restoring the dentition.

As suggested in Chapter 5, it appears that when the patient is treated to this joint position and occlusal conditions, the likelihood is great that health will prevail.

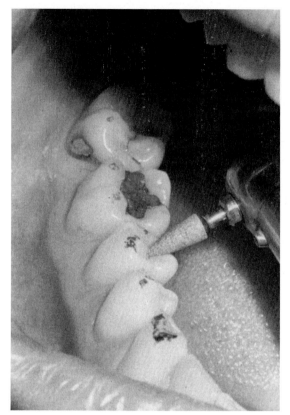

TREATMENT PLANNING FOR OCCLUSAL THERAPY

When it has been determined that occlusal therapy will benefit the patient, the proper method of treatment needs to be identified. Generally, *the best choice is to perform the fewest number of dental alterations that will fulfill the treatment goals.* Frequently only minor changes are required to alter an existing occlusion to one that is more favorable.

When only minor changes are necessary, the occlusal surfaces of the teeth can often be merely reshaped to achieve a desired occlusal contact pattern. This type of treatment is called *selective grinding* or *occlusal adjustment* (also *occlusal equilibration*) (Fig. 17-4). It involves the removal of tooth structure and is therefore limited to the thickness of the enamel. If enamel is completely removed, dentin will be exposed, posing a problem with sensitivity and dental caries.

As the interarch alignment of the teeth becomes farther from ideal, more extensive alteration of the existing occlusal conditions is necessary to meet the treatment goals. If selective grinding procedures cannot be successfully performed within the confines of the enamel, restoration of the teeth may be indicated. Crowns and fixed prosthetic procedures are used to alter an occlusal condition to the desired treatment goals (Fig. 17-5).

As the interarch alignment of the teeth becomes even poorer, crowns and fixed prosthetic procedures alone may not be able to complete the treatment goals. Posterior crowns must be fabricated such that occlusal forces are directed through the long axes of the roots. This cannot always be accomplished as the interarch malalignment becomes great. Therefore orthodontic procedures are sometimes necessary to accomplish the treatment goals. Orthodontic procedures are used to align teeth in the dental arches to a more favorable occlusal relationship (Fig. 17-6). On occasion the poor interarch tooth alignment is created by poor

Fig. 17-4 Selective grinding is a form of irreversible occlusal therapy by which the teeth are carefully reshaped to meet the occlusal treatment goals.

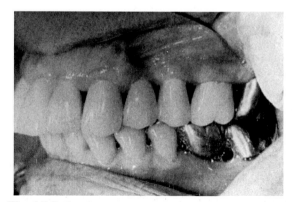

Fig. 17-5 Fixed prosthodontic procedures are a form of irreversible occlusal therapy that may be indicated when selective grinding cannot accomplish the occlusal treatment goals.

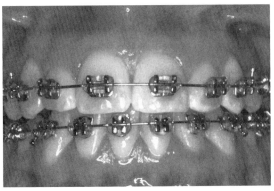

Fig. 17-6 Orthodontic therapy is a form of irreversible occlusal therapy that may be indicated when malalignment of the dental arches is so great that fixed prosthodontics cannot successfully accomplish the occlusal treatment goals.

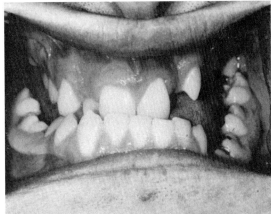

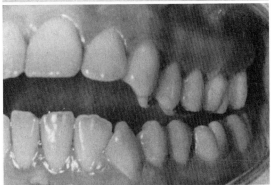

Fig. 17-7 SEVERE MALOCCLUSIONS IN TWO PATIENTS. The major factor creating these problems is the skeletal relations of the maxilla and mandible. Dental therapy alone will not be sufficient to correct the situation. A surgical procedure in conjunction with proper dental therapy (e.g., orthodontics, fixed prosthodontics) will have to be considered.

alignment of the dental arches themselves. When this condition is present, a surgical procedure to correct the skeletal malalignment (Fig. 17-7), in conjunction with orthodontics, is likely to be the most successful method of achieving the treatment goals (orthognathic surgery).

The appropriate occlusal therapy is therefore often determined by the severity of the malocclusion. The treatment choices range from selective grinding to crowns, fixed prostheses, removable prostheses, orthodontics, and even surgical correction. Combining treatments to achieve the proper treatment goals is often appropriate. For example, after orthodontic therapy is completed, a selective grinding procedure may be helpful in refining the exact contact pattern of the teeth. All these treatment options emphasize the need for developing a precise treatment plan. Two general considerations exist: (1) The simplest treatment that will accomplish the treatment goals is generally the best, and (2) treatment should never begin until the clinician can visualize the end results.

In most routine cases the final result can be easily seen, and therefore progress can be made toward that goal. However, when more complex treatments are planned, it is sometimes difficult to visualize exactly how each step or phase will contribute to the end results. With these complex cases it is advisable to seek out the information necessary to predict the final treatment results

accurately before the actual treatment begins. This is best accomplished by accurately mounting diagnostic casts on an articulator and performing the suggested treatment on the casts. For example, a selective grinding procedure performed on diagnostic casts can help determine the difficulty that will be encountered when performing this treatment in the mouth. It can also reveal the degree of tooth structure that will need to be removed (Fig. 17-8). This will help predict not only the success of the procedure but also the need for any restorative procedures after selective grinding. The patient can therefore be informed in advance of

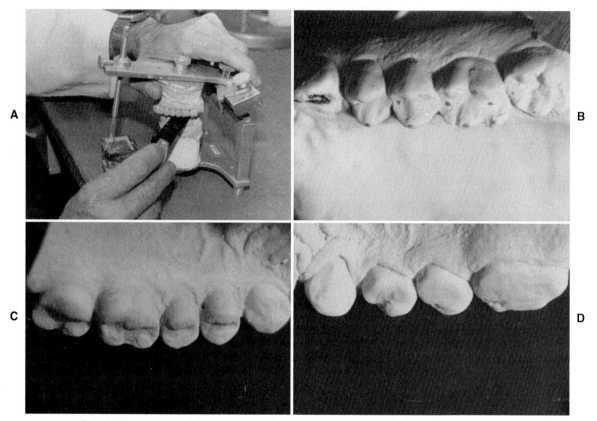

Fig. 17-8 A, For the success of selective grinding to be evaluated, the procedure must first be completed on accurately mounted diagnostic casts. **B,** Very little change in tooth form is demonstrated. Thus it appears that selective grinding is an acceptable procedure for this patient. **C** and **D,** Diagnostic casts made following selective grinding procedures are demonstrated. The amount of tooth structure removed was too extensive for selective grinding alone. Sensitive dentin has been exposed, and crowns are now indicated. These patients should have been informed of this additional treatment before the selective grinding procedure.

the number of crowns, if any, that will be necessary after the selective grinding.

When missing teeth are to be replaced by fixed prostheses, the future occlusal condition, as well as aesthetics, can be predicted by prewaxing the restoration (Fig. 17-9). This assists in determining the preparation design and also allows the patient to visualize the expected aesthetics. Orthodontic procedures can also be accomplished on the cast by sectioning teeth and moving them to the desired position (Fig. 17-10). When diagnostic casts are used in this manner, the expected final

results are easily visualized, and any problems in achieving these results are identified in advance. *Never begin occlusal treatment for a patient without being able to visualize the final result, as well as each step that will make it possible.*

RULE OF THIRDS

Selecting appropriate occlusal treatment is an important and sometimes difficult task. In most instances the choice must be made among selective grinding, crown and fixed prosthodontic

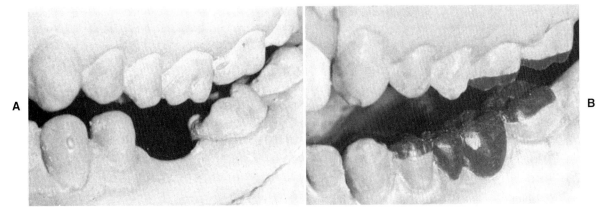

Fig. 17-9 A diagnostic prewax is used to predict the success of fixed prosthodontic procedures. **A,** Pretreatment. The missing tooth and mesial tipping of the mandibular molar are demonstrated. **B,** Posttreatment. The expected result of a fixed partial denture in conjunction with molar uprighting and third molar extraction is shown.

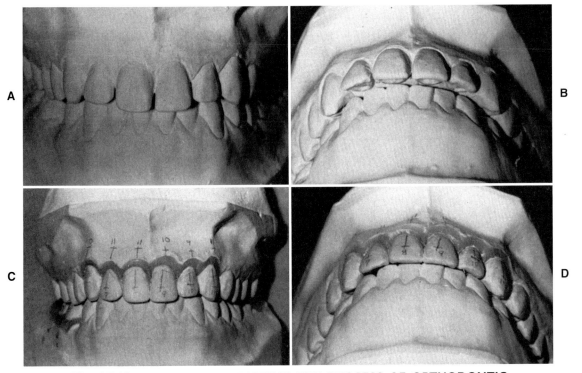

Fig. 17-10 SETUP FOR PREDICTING THE SUCCESS OF ORTHODONTIC PROCEDURES. A and **B,** Pretreatment. The generalized interdental spacing **(A)** and lack of anterior guidance **(B)** are shown. **C** and **D,** Expected results after orthodontic therapy. The teeth have been sectioned from the casts and moved to their final orthodontic positions. The resolved interdental spacing and the improved anterior guidance are demonstrated.

procedures, and orthodontics. Often the critical factor determining the appropriate treatment is the buccolingual arch discrepancy of the maxillary and mandibular posterior teeth. The extent of this discrepancy establishes which treatment will be appropriate.

This relationship is best examined by first placing the condyles in the MS position (centric relation) with a bilateral manual manipulation technique. In this position the jaws are gently closed in a hinge axis movement until the first tooth touches lightly. At this point the buccolingual relationships of the maxillary and mandibular teeth are examined. If the centric cusps are located near the opposing central fossae, only slight alterations in the occlusal condition will be necessary to achieve the treatment goals. The greater the distance that the centric cusps are positioned from the opposing fossae, the more extensive will be the treatment necessary to achieve the treatment goals.

The "rule of thirds"[1-3] has been developed to aid in determining the appropriate treatment. Each inner incline of the posterior centric cusps is divided into three equal parts. If, when the mandibular condyles are in their desired position, the centric cusp tip of one arch contacts the opposing centric cusp's inner incline in the third closest to the central fossa, selective grinding can usually be performed without damage to the teeth (Fig. 17-11, *A*).

If the opposing centric cusp tip makes contact in the middle third of the opposing inner incline (Fig. 17-11, *B*), crown and fixed prosthodontic procedures will usually be most appropriate for achieving the treatment goals. In these cases selective grinding is likely to perforate the enamel, creating the need for a restorative procedure.

If the cusp tip contacts the opposing inner incline on the third closest to the cusp tip or even on the cusp tip (Fig. 17-11, *C*), the appropriate treatment is orthodontic procedures. Crown and fixed prosthodontics in these instances will often create restorations that cannot adequately direct occlusal forces through the long axes of the roots, thus producing a potentially unstable occlusal relationship.

The "rule of thirds" is applied clinically by drying the teeth, locating the condyles in the desired position, and having the patient close lightly on marking paper in a hinge axis movement. The contact area is visualized, and its position on the incline is determined. Visualizing the buccolingual relationship of the entire arch is equally important

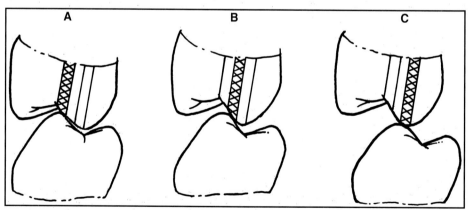

Fig. 17-11 RULE OF THIRDS. The inner inclines of the posterior centric cusps are divided into thirds. When the condyles are in the desired treatment position (centric relation) and the opposing centric cusp tip contacts on the third closest to the central fossa **(A)**, selective grinding is the most appropriate occlusal treatment. When the opposing centric cusp tip contacts on the middle third **(B)**, crowns or other fixed prosthetic procedures are generally indicated. When the opposing centric cusp tip contacts on the third closest to the opposing centric cusp tip **(C)**, orthodontics is the most appropriate occlusal treatment.

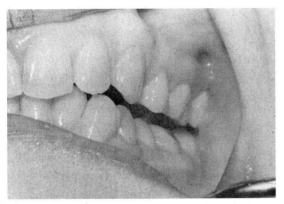

Fig. 17-12 With the condyles in centric relation position, the buccolingual discrepancy of the entire arch is easily visualized. The rule of thirds can be used to determine the most appropriate occlusal treatment.

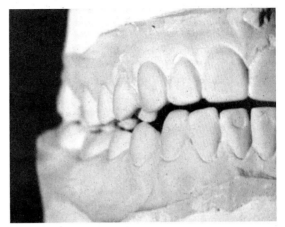

Fig. 17-13 Visualizing the occlusal relationship of the teeth is sometimes easier on the articulator than in the mouth because there is no interference from soft tissues or neuromuscular controlling mechanisms. In this instance the buccolingual discrepancy of the maxillary and mandibular first premolars becomes obvious on the diagnostic casts.

in determining appropriate treatment (Fig. 17-12). On occasion the tooth contact will not be typical of the entire arch and therefore will not be the best determinant of treatment.

In many cases the selection of treatment is obvious and can be made with confidence by merely visualizing the teeth clinically. In other instances, however, the judgment is more difficult (e.g., when the mandible is not easily guided to centric closure, when the teeth are not easily visualized). When it is difficult to determine the appropriate treatment, diagnostic casts accurately mounted on an articulator are helpful. In the absence of soft tissue, muscles, and saliva, a more accurate diagnosis can be made (Fig. 17-13). The casts are also helpful (as previously mentioned) for rehearsing the treatment to determine the degree and difficulty of success.

FACTORS THAT INFLUENCE TREATMENT PLANNING

After careful analysis of the occlusal condition, the most appropriate treatment is determined. If it has been decided that selective grinding can successfully accomplish the treatment goals without damaging the teeth, this procedure is completed. If, however, it is decided that less

conservative procedures are indicated (e.g., crowns or orthodontic therapy), other factors may need to be considered. Because these procedures involve a considerable amount of time and expense, the suggested treatment must be weighed against the potential benefits. Five factors can influence the selection of treatment: (1) symptoms, (2) condition of the dentition, (3) systemic health, (4) aesthetics, and (5) finances.

SYMPTOMS

The symptoms associated with TMDs vary greatly from patient to patient. Some patients experience short durations of mild discomfort that recurs only occasionally. When extensive restorative or orthodontic therapy is considered, it is often too extreme for the symptoms being experienced. However, when the symptoms are severe and it has been determined that occlusal therapy would be helpful (i.e., occlusal appliance therapy), these more extensive types of therapy become indicated. Therefore the severity of the symptoms can help determine the need for permanent occlusal therapy.

CONDITION OF THE DENTITION

The health of the dentition also influences the selection of treatment. When a patient has multiple missing and broken-down teeth, restorative and fixed prosthetic procedures are generally indicated—not only for the TMD but also for the general improvement in health and function of the masticatory system. On the other hand, patients with healthy and virtually unrestored dental arches that are merely poorly aligned are more likely to be best treated orthodontically rather than restoratively. In this sense the condition of the dentition influences the most appropriate occlusal therapy for the patient.

SYSTEMIC HEALTH

Although the majority of dental patients are healthy and tolerate dental procedures well, some do not. In developing an occlusal treatment plan, the systemic health of the patient always needs to be considered. The prognosis of some treatments can be greatly influenced by the general health of the patient. For example, resolving a periodontal condition may be greatly influenced by a systemic disorder such as diabetes or leukemia. Even a long dental appointment can have detrimental effects on some chronically ill patients. These considerations may greatly influence the selection of appropriate occlusal therapy.

AESTHETICS

Almost all of dentistry centers around the establishment and maintenance of function and aesthetics in the masticatory system. In treating a TMD, functional considerations are by far the most important. However, aesthetic considerations are still likely to be a major concern. When an occlusal treatment plan is being developed, aesthetic considerations should not be overlooked or underemphasized. The patient should be questioned regarding aesthetic concerns. Sometimes treatments are unacceptable because of these concerns. For example, a patient may not wear an occlusal appliance because it is aesthetically unpleasing. In other instances, aesthetics may encourage certain treatments. A patient with mild or moderate TMD symptoms may be an excellent candidate for orthodontic procedures when it is learned that this person is unhappy with his or her present appearance and wants to have improvements made. Orthodontics can then simultaneously provide improvement in both function and aesthetics, thereby more completely treating the patient's needs.

FINANCES

As with any service, the patient's ability to finance the treatment can significantly influence the treatment plan. Even though cost should not influence treatment selection, in fact it often does. Some patients who would benefit from a complete restoration of the dentition cannot afford such treatment. Alternatives must be developed. In some instances removable partial dentures, removable overlay partial dentures, or even complete dentures can provide the desirable occlusal conditions at a fraction of the cost of a full mouth reconstruction. These financial considerations can be assessed by the patient only in light of the values placed on appearance, health, and comfort, which cannot be put into any formula.

PRIORITIZING THE FACTORS

Each of these five factors needs to be considered before an appropriate occlusal treatment plan can be developed. Importantly, the clinician must realize that the priority of the factors may be different for the patient and for the therapist. When symptoms are not severe, finances and aesthetics will often be more important concerns of the patient. At the same time, however, the dentist may believe that the condition of the dentition is more important. In any case the patient's concerns must always remain foremost in the development of a successful treatment plan.

In some instances the appropriate treatment will be obvious and therapy can begin. In others, however, it may be necessary to labor over which treatment is best for the patient. When this occurs, occlusal appliance maintenance may be appropriate. Most patients who are considered for irreversible occlusal therapy have already received an occlusal appliance that has proved to be successful in relieving the TMD symptoms. In occlusal appliance maintenance the patient is encouraged to continue using the appliance as needed to relieve or eliminate symptoms. Occlusal appliance maintenance is especially appropriate when the symptoms are episodic or related to increased levels of emotional stress. Many patients can remain comfortable by using the occlusal appliance during specific times, such as while they sleep.

Others have learned that high emotional stress periods promote symptoms, and thus the occlusal appliance is worn during these times. Patients who cannot afford extensive treatment or in whom systemic health considerations prevent treatment are often good candidates for occlusal appliance maintenance. When this is suggested, it is important that the patient understand the use, care, and maintenance of the appliance. It is also extremely important that the appliance provide occlusal stops for all teeth so that prolonged use will not allow eruption of any teeth.

References

1. Burch JG: The selection of occlusal patterns in periodontal therapy, *Dent Clin North Am* 24:343-356, 1980.
2. Burch JG: Orthodontic and restorative considerations. In Clark J, editor: *Clinical dentistry; prevention, orthodontics, and occlusion*, New York, 1976, Harper & Row.
3. Fox CW, Neff P: The rule of thirds. In Fox CW, Neff P, editors: *Principles of occlusion*, Anaheim, Calif, 1982, Society for Occlusal Studies, p D1.

Use of Articulators in Occlusal Therapy

18
CHAPTER

"The articulator: a tool, not the answer."

—JPO

A dental articulator is an instrument that duplicates certain important diagnostic and border movements of the mandible. Each is designed to serve the needs that its inventor believes are the most important for a particular use. With the enormous range of opinions and uses, dozens of articulators have been developed over the years. The instrument is certainly a valuable aid in occlusal therapy; however, it should always be considered as merely an aid and not, by any means, as a form of treatment. It can help accumulate information and, when properly used, will assist in some treatment methods. It cannot, however, give back proper information without proper handling by the operator. In other words, only when the operator has a thorough understanding of the capabilities, advantages, disadvantages, and uses of the articulator can the instrument become maximally beneficial in occlusal therapy.

USES OF THE ARTICULATOR

The dental articulator can be helpful in many aspects of dentistry. In conjunction with accurate diagnostic casts that have been properly mounted, it may be used in diagnosis, treatment planning, and treatment.

IN DIAGNOSIS

Occlusal therapy involves two important phases: diagnosis and treatment. Because diagnosis always precedes and dictates the plan of treatment, it must be both thorough and accurate. Building a treatment plan on an inaccurate diagnosis will certainly lead to treatment failure.

Establishing an accurate diagnosis can be difficult because of the complex interrelationships of the various structures of the masticatory system. To arrive at an accurate diagnosis, it is essential that all the needed information be collected and analyzed (see Chapter 9). There are times during an occlusal examination when it may be necessary to evaluate the occlusal condition more closely. This is especially appropriate when a strong suspicion exists that the occlusal condition may be contributing significantly to the disorder or when the condition of the dentition strongly suggests the need for occlusal therapy. When these conditions are present, diagnostic casts are accurately mounted on an articulator to assist in evaluating the occlusal condition. The casts are mounted in the musculoskeletally stable position (centric relation [CR]) so the full range of border movements can be evaluated. If they are mounted in the intercuspation position and the patient has a CR–to–intercuspal position (ICP) slide, the more superoposterior position of the condyles cannot be located on the articulator and the occlusal conditions in this position cannot be properly evaluated.

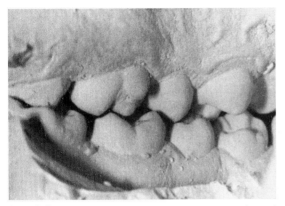

Fig. 18-1 Mounted diagnostic casts provide lingual visualization of the occlusal condition. This cannot be observed clinically.

Mounted diagnostic casts offer two major advantages in diagnosis. First, they improve the visualization of both static and functional interrelationships of the teeth. This is especially helpful in the second molar region, where the soft tissues of the cheek and tongue often prevent good visibility. They also allow lingual examination of the patient's occlusion, which cannot be viewed clinically (Fig. 18-1). Often this is essential in examining the static and dynamic functional relationships of the teeth. The second advantage of mounted diagnostic casts involves the ease of mandibular movement. On the articulator a patient's mandibular movements and resultant occlusal contacts can be observed without the influence of the neuromuscular system. Often when a patient is examined clinically, the protective reflexes of the neuromuscular system avoid damaging contacts. As a result, interferences can go unnoticed and therefore undiagnosed. When the mounted diagnostic casts are occluded, these contacts become evident (Fig. 18-2). Thus the casts can assist in a more thorough occlusal examination.

As has been emphasized in this text, however, the occlusal examination alone is not diagnostic of a disorder. The significance of the occlusal findings must be ascertained. Nevertheless, information received from properly mounted diagnostic casts can serve as an additional source of information for establishing an accurate diagnosis.

IN TREATMENT PLANNING

The most successful method of providing treatment is to develop a plan that not only eliminates the causative factors that have been identified but does so in a logical and orderly manner. Sometimes it is difficult to examine a patient clinically and determine the outcome of a particular treatment. Yet it is essential that the final results of the treatment, as well as each step needed to accomplish the treatment goals, be visualized before treatment begins. When this is not possible, properly

A 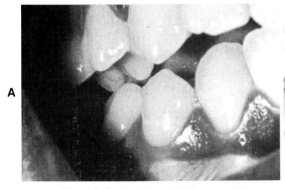 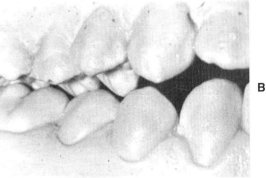 B

Fig. 18-2 A, When a left laterotrusive movement is performed, the neuromuscular system avoids the mediotrusive contact between the maxillary and mandibular first premolars. **B,** When the movement is observed on diagnostic casts mounted on the articulator, the mediotrusive contact is obvious.

mounted diagnostic casts can become an important part in treatment planning. Diagnostic casts are used to ensure that successful treatment will be achieved and can be employed in several manners depending on the treatment in question.

Selective Grinding

Frequently it is difficult to examine a patient clinically and determine whether a selective grinding procedure can be accomplished without damage to the teeth. If a quick judgment is incorrect, the dentist is likely to grind through enamel, subjecting the patient to an unplanned restorative procedure. In patients in whom the success of selective grinding is difficult to predict, the procedure is completed on properly mounted diagnostic casts and the end result visualized. When extensive tooth structure must be removed to meet the treatment goals, the patient is informed in advance that additional time will be necessary and the expense will be greater. This kind of planning encourages the patient's trust instead of doubt or disappointment (Fig. 18-3).

Functional (Diagnostic) Prewax

Often badly broken-down or missing teeth require crown or fixed prosthodontic procedures to restore normal function and occlusal stability. In some instances it is difficult to visualize exactly how the

restorations should be designed to best fulfill the treatment goals. Mounted diagnostic casts are useful in determining the feasibility of altering the functional relationship of the teeth, as well as improving the selection of a method to accomplish the treatment goals. As with selective grinding, the suggested treatment is completed on the casts. A functional prewax is developed that fulfills the treatment goals (Fig. 18-4). While the prewax is being fabricated, a proper design is developed that will be most appropriate for the specific situations encountered. The prewax will not only allow visualization of the expected final treatment but also give insight into any problems that may be encountered while reaching that goal. After it is completed, the treatment can begin with greater assurance of success.

Aesthetic (Diagnostic) Prewax

When time and money have been invested in the fabrication of anterior crowns or a fixed prosthesis and then the patient is not pleased with the aesthetic results, it is discouraging. Preexisting conditions need to be examined carefully so that the effects on the final aesthetics of a restoration can be determined. Unusual interdental spacing, tissue morphology, or occlusion will often alter the final appearance of a crown or fixed prosthesis. If the final aesthetics cannot be visualized because of

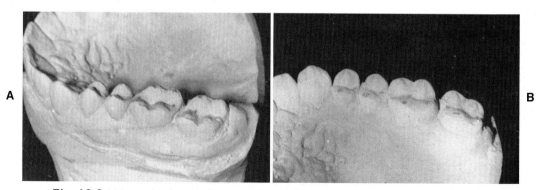

Fig. 18-3 When selective grinding is performed in advance on diagnostic casts, the final results can be easily visualized. **A,** In this instance selective grinding has not significantly altered the tooth form, and it therefore appears to be an appropriate occlusal treatment for the patient. **B,** In this instance selective grinding has significantly altered the form of the centric cusps. It will likely result in exposed dentin, requiring restorative procedures. The patient must be informed of this additional treatment before selective grinding is performed.

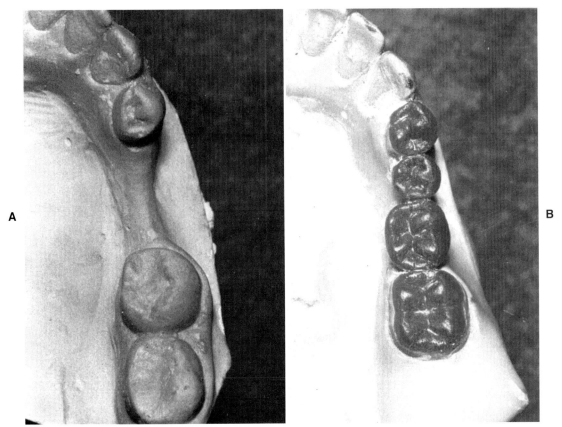

Fig. 18-4 FUNCTIONAL (DIAGNOSTIC) PREWAX. A, Pretreatment occlusal condition. **B,** The completed functional prewax helps visualize the expected result of extracting the third molar and developing a four-unit, fixed partial denture. As can now be visualized, the space will accommodate two pontics that are both smaller than the adjacent teeth.

unusual preexisting conditions, an aesthetic pre-wax is completed. This allows visualization of the most aesthetic results achievable and gives the dentist an idea as to how these results can be attained (Fig. 18-5).

If during the prewax it is apparent that the aesthetic results are undesirable, other types of treatment in conjunction with the fixed prosthesis may be necessary. This may include orthodontics, periodontics, endodontics, or a removable partial denture. After an aesthetic result is achieved, both the dentist and patient can visualize the expected appearance of the new restoration. The patient's expectations now become realistic, which minimizes any disappointment. Treatment can begin with greater assurance of success.

Orthodontic Setup

Malalignment of the dental arches is usually treated more appropriately by orthodontics. In simple routine cases, orthodontics is easily predicted. However, on occasion, a particular alignment problem or crowding of the teeth will pose a difficult problem in visualizing the final results. Then mounted diagnostic casts are helpful. With sectioning of the desired teeth from the casts and repositioning them in wax, the final results of orthodontics can be visualized (Fig. 18-6).

When extraction is being considered, the teeth to be removed are left out of the setup. The orthodontic results achieved by extraction can then be compared with the nonextraction results. The most appropriate treatment is selected by visualizing

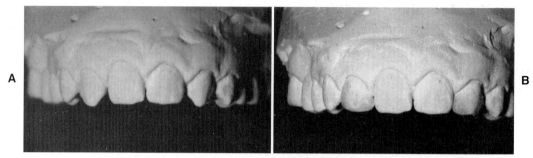

Fig. 18-5 AESTHETIC (DIAGNOSTIC) PREWAX. A, Pretreatment. The lateral incisors are missing, and the canines have moved into their position. Interdental spacing is evident. The patient was interested in improving the aesthetics of this condition. **B,** By diagnostic waxing of the canines to the more normal morphology of the lateral incisors, it is possible to achieve aesthetically satisfying results. The patient needs to be aware in advance that these teeth will be wider (mediodistally) than normal laterals. Having the patient visualize these results can help create realistic expectations.

the final results of the different treatments available. An orthodontic setup therefore provides valuable information for treatment planning. It is especially helpful in developing a treatment plan for individual tooth movements (Fig. 18-7). When complex orthodontic treatment is indicated, the orthodontic setup is helpful but cannot be the only indicator of treatment. A sound understanding of growth and development, as well as the biomechanics of tooth movement, is necessary for a successful treatment plan.

Designing Fixed Restorative Prostheses

The specific design of a fixed or removable prosthesis is generally dependent on the functional and aesthetic considerations of the mouth. Mounted diagnostic casts are helpful in designing restorations that are best able to accommodate these considerations. The occlusal requirements from a single crown to a removable partial denture can be visualized and predicted on a mounted diagnostic cast.

When a tooth is weakened by caries or a preexisting restoration, a treatment must be selected to strengthen and preserve the clinical crown. If a single-unit casting is the treatment of choice, properly mounted diagnostic casts are helpful in designing the type of restoration that will give the optimum form and function. Functional occlusal analysis of the casts can reveal areas needing additional

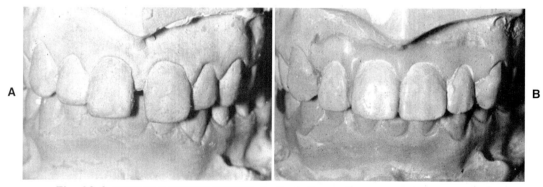

Fig. 18-6 ORTHODONTIC SETUP. A, Pretreatment (anterior view). The significant diastema between the central incisors is shown. **B,** The diastema can be successfully eliminated by orthodontically moving only the four maxillary anterior teeth.

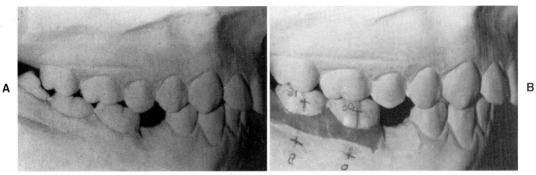

Fig. 18-7 ORTHODONTIC SETUP. A, Pretreatment (lateral view). **B,** With extraction of the third molar, the first and second molars can be successfully uprighted into a favorable occlusal relationship. A fixed partial denture is now indicated to replace the missing teeth in this mandibular quadrant.

strength for occlusal forces, as well as areas where aesthetics can be the prime consideration. In this manner a restoration is designed to meet the needs of both function and aesthetics.

The same occlusal analysis of diagnostic casts is used to design a removable partial denture for the optimum occlusal condition. Mounted diagnostic casts provide information regarding the available interarch space for a removable partial denture base, as well as which teeth are best positioned for occlusal and incisal rests. Even the prognosis of overlay dentures can be enhanced when mounted casts are used to help select the most desirable teeth to be maintained under the denture base.

Additional Uses of the Articulator and Mounted Diagnostic Casts

Mounted diagnostic casts are often helpful for patient education. Usually patients more easily understand problems that exist in the mouth if these problems are identified on diagnostic casts. In addition, they can understand a treatment plan more completely when it is demonstrated on their own diagnostic casts. This type of patient education enhances the establishment of a good working relationship with the patient. Groundwork for successful treatment begins with the patient's thorough understanding of the problems and their appropriate treatment.

IN TREATMENT

Probably the most common use of the dental articulator is in treatment. Although it cannot treat a patient, it can be an indispensable aid in developing dental appliances that will help treat the patient. It can provide the appropriate information regarding mandibular movement that is necessary to develop an appliance or restoration for occlusal harmony. Although this information could theoretically be acquired by working directly in the mouth, the articulator eliminates many factors that contribute to errors such as the tongue, cheeks, saliva, and neuromuscular control system. In some instances it is necessary to use materials that are not suitable for the oral cavity. Then the articulator becomes the only reliable method for developing an appropriate occlusal condition in the dental appliance. It is an intricate part of crown and fixed prosthodontic procedures. It is also a necessary part of the fabrication of removable partial dentures and complete dentures. Many orthodontic appliances also require the use of an articulator.

GENERAL TYPES OF ARTICULATORS

Dental articulators come in many sizes and shapes. The designs are as individual as the purposes for which they are used. To discuss and understand articulators, it is helpful to separate the various types into three general categories—nonadjustable, semiadjustable, and fully adjustable—according to their ability to adjust to and duplicate the patient's specific condylar movements. Generally the more adjustable the articulator is, the more accurate it can be in duplicating condylar movement.

In the following section each of these types of articulators is described along with the general procedures necessary for its use. The advantages and disadvantages of each are also discussed.

NONADJUSTABLE ARTICULATOR

Description
The nonadjustable articulator (Fig. 18-8) is the simplest type available. No adjustments are possible to adapt it more closely to the specific condylar movements of the patient. Many of these articulators allow for eccentric movements but only average values. Accurate duplication of an eccentric movement for a specific patient is impossible.

The only accurate and reproducible position that can be used on a nonadjustable articulator is one specific occlusal contact position (e.g., ICP). When the casts are mounted in this position on the nonadjustable articulator, they can be repeatedly separated and closed only to this position, which becomes the only repeatable and accurate position that can be used. Even the opening and closing pathways of the teeth do not accurately duplicate the pathways of the patient's teeth because the distance from the condyles to the

specific cusps is not accurately transferred to the articulator. The ICP is reproducible only when the casts are mounted on the articulator in that position. All other positions or movements (e.g., opening, protrusive, laterotrusive) do not accurately duplicate the conditions found in the patient.

Associated Procedures Required for the Nonadjustable Articulator
Because only the occlusal position in which the teeth are mounted is accurately duplicated, arbitrary mounting procedures are used to locate and fix the casts. Generally the casts are held together with the teeth in maximum intercuspation and located equidistant between the maxillary and mandibular components of the articulator. Mounting stone is then placed between the mandibular cast and the mandibular component of the articulator, firmly adhering these together. The maxillary cast is likewise attached to the maxillary component of the articulator. When the mounting stone is set, the casts can be separated and the simple hinge of the articulator will accurately return the casts to the position maintained during mounting.

The clinician should note that the casts must be mounted with the teeth contacting in the desired occlusal position. If a wax record that separates the teeth is used, an inaccurate ICP will be developed. This occurs because the actual hinge axis of the patient's mandible is not accurately duplicated on the nonadjustable articulator. (For a more complete explanation, see Taking Centric Relation Interocclusal Records at an Increased Vertical Dimension.)

Advantages and Disadvantages of the Nonadjustable Articulator
Using a nonadjustable articulator has two distinct advantages. The first is expense. This articulator is relatively inexpensive, and the dentist can thus afford to purchase as many as will support the needs of the practice. The second advantage is the usually small amount of time invested in mounting the casts on the articulator. Because the mounting procedure is arbitrary, no procedures are necessary to obtain information from the patient that will assist in mounting the casts.

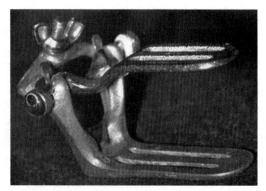

Fig. 18-8 A nonadjustable articulator.

Therefore the casts are mounted in a minimum of time.

Although these advantages can be helpful, the disadvantages of the nonadjustable articulator often far outweigh the advantages. Because this articulator accurately reproduces only one contact position, a restoration cannot be properly prepared to meet the occlusal requirements of the eccentric movements of the patient. With such a small amount of control of the occlusal condition on the articulator, the dentist must be prepared to spend necessary time adjusting the restorations intraorally in the appropriate eccentric movements. This can be costly. Also, if considerable grinding is necessary, poor anatomic form and occlusal relationships may result.

SEMIADJUSTABLE ARTICULATOR

Description

The semiadjustable articulator (Fig. 18-9) permits more variability in duplicating condylar movement than does the nonadjustable articulator. It usually has three types of adjustments that can lead to close duplication of condylar movements for any individual patient. Therefore not only can an occlusal contact position be accurately duplicated, but when the teeth are moved eccentrically from this position, the resulting contact pattern will nearly duplicate the contact pattern found in the patient's mouth. As a result, more information regarding the patient's specific movements can be stored in the articulator for use when subsequent restorations are being developed. The most common adjustments found on the semiadjustable articulator are the (1) condylar inclination, (2) lateral translation movement (or Bennett angle), and (3) intercondylar distance.

Condylar Inclination. The angle at which the condyle descends along the articular eminence in the sagittal plane can have a great effect on the fossa depth and cusp height of the posterior teeth (see Chapter 6). With a semiadjustable articulator this angulation is altered to duplicate the angle present in a specific patient. Therefore a restoration can be fabricated with appropriate fossa depth and cusp height that will harmonize with the patient's existing occlusal condition.

Bennett Angle. In a laterotrusive movement the angle at which the orbiting condyle moves inward (as measured in the horizontal plane) can have a significant effect on the width of the central fossa of the posterior teeth (see Chapter 6). The angle described by the inward movement of the condyle is referred to as the *Bennett angle*. Appropriate adjustment of it can assist in developing restorations that will more nearly fit the existing occlusal condition of the patient.

Most semiadjustable articulators allow for a Bennett angle movement of the orbiting condyle to be only a straight line from the centric position in which the casts are mounted to the maximum laterotrusive position. A few also provide adjustment for immediate and progressive Bennett angle movements. When a significant immediate lateral translation movement is present, these articulators provide a more accurate duplication of condylar movement.

Intercondylar Distance. The distance between the rotational centers of the condyles can have an effect on the mediotrusive and laterotrusive pathways of the posterior centric cusps over their opposing occlusal surfaces (in the horizontal plane) (see Chapter 6). The semiadjustable articulator allows for adjustments that permit the intercondylar distance on the articulator to duplicate very nearly the intercondylar distance of the patient. Proper adjustment will aid in the development of a restoration with an occlusal anatomy that is in close harmony with the eccentric pathways of the centric cusp in the patient's mouth.

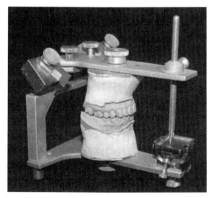

Fig. 18-9 A semiadjustable articulator (Whip-Mix).

Associated Procedures Required for the Semiadjustable Articulator

Because this articulator can be adjusted, information must be acquired from the patient so that proper adjustments can be made. Three procedures are necessary to adjust the semiadjustable articulator accurately: (1) a face-bow transfer, (2) a CR interocclusal record, and (3) eccentric interocclusal records.

Face-Bow Transfer. The primary use of the face-bow transfer is to mount the maxillary cast accurately on the articulator. It uses three distinct reference points (two posterior and one anterior) to locate the cast on the articulator. The posterior references are the hinge axis of each condyle, and the anterior is an arbitrary point.

Most semiadjustable articulators do not attempt to locate the exact hinge axis for the patient; instead they rely on a predetermined point that has been shown to be near the hinge axis in most patients. Using this arbitrary hinge axis as the posterior reference allows the maxillary cast to be mounted on the articulator at a distance from the condyles similar to that found in the patient. The anterior reference point is arbitrary and is usually established by the manufacturer so that the maxillary cast will be appropriately positioned between the maxillary and mandibular components of the articulator. In some articulators the anterior reference is the bridge of the nose; in others it is located a specific distance superior to the incisal edges of the maxillary anterior teeth.

The intercondylar distance is measured when the posterior determinants are located. This is done by measuring the width of the patient's head between the posterior determinants and subtracting a standard amount that compensates for the distance lateral to each center of rotation of the condyles. The measurement is then transferred by the face-bow to the articulator, with allowances for the appropriate intercondylar distance to be adjusted on the articulator. When the intercondylar distance has been adjusted, the face-bow is appropriately fixed to the articulator and the maxillary cast can be mounted to the maxillary component of the articulator (Fig. 18-10).

The Centric Relation Interocclusal Record. To mount the mandibular cast to the articulator, the articulator must be appropriately oriented to the maxillary cast. This is accomplished by finding the desired mandibular position and maintaining this relationship while the mandibular cast is attached to the articulator with mounting stone. The ICP is often an easy position to locate because the teeth generally fall quickly into the maximum intercuspal relationship. When hand articulating the casts in the ICP is difficult or unstable, the patient is instructed to close completely into a warm wax wafer. The wafer is then placed between the casts (Fig. 18-11). This type of interocclusal record assists in mounting the cast in the ICP.

The clinician should remember, however, that when the casts are mounted in the ICP, most

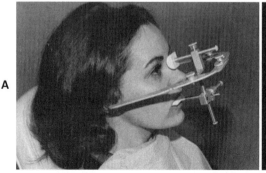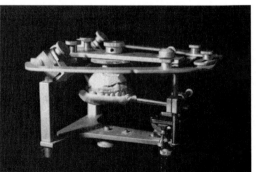

A **B**

Fig. 18-10 The face-bow is used to mount the maxillary cast on the maxillary component of the articulator at a distance from the rotating centers of the condyles that is identical to this distance on the patient. **A,** Face-bow properly positioned. **B,** The face-bow is then transferred to the articulator for mounting of the maxillary cast.

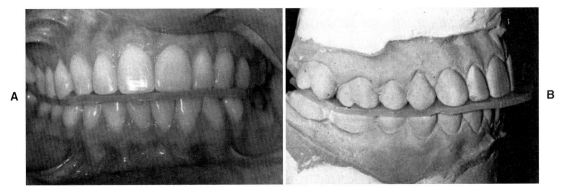

Fig. 18-11 An interocclusal record is used for mounting the mandibular cast on the mandibular component of the articulator. **A,** A wax wafer can be used to capture the desired interocclusal position. The wax is heated, and the teeth are closed in the desired position. **B,** The wax record is then air chilled, removed from the patient's mouth, and placed on the maxillary cast, and the mandibular cast is appropriately positioned in it. In this relationship the mandibular cast is mounted on the mandibular component of the articulator.

articulators do not allow for any further posterior movement of the condyles. For patients with a CR-to-ICP slide, mounting the cast in maximum intercuspation prevents any possibility of locating the CR position on the articulator. In other words, if the casts are mounted in ICP, any range of movement available posterior to ICP cannot be observed on the articulator. Because this movement can play a significant role in occlusal therapy, it is often appropriate to mount the cast in the CR position. In this condylar position an unstable occlusal relationship often exists; therefore an interocclusal record needs to be developed that stabilizes the arch relationship.

Once a stable interocclusal record has been developed with the condyles in the CR position, the record can be transferred to the articulator and the mandibular cast can be mounted to the mandibular component of the articulator. Once the cast is mounted, the interocclusal record is removed, allowing the teeth to close into the initial CR contact. The mandibular cast is then observed as it shifts into the more stable ICP, revealing the CR-to-ICP slide. When the casts are mounted in this manner, the CR-to-ICP range of movement can be observed and used to develop subsequent restorations.

The clinician should note that the CR interocclusal record is taken at a vertical dimension that is slightly greater than the initial tooth contact in CR. If a vertical dimension is used that is less, the record will be perforated by the occluding teeth and the result will be tooth contacts that can shift the mandibular position. On the other hand, if the interocclusal record is taken at an increased vertical dimension, inaccuracies can result when the record is removed and the teeth are allowed to contact. These inaccuracies occur when the exact hinge axis location has not been duplicated (see Taking Centric Relation Interocclusal Records at an Increased Vertical Dimension).

Eccentric Interocclusal Records. Eccentric interocclusal records are used to adjust the articulator so that it will follow the appropriate condylar movement of the patient. Wax is commonly used for these records.

An appropriate amount of wax is heat softened and placed over the posterior teeth. The patient separates the teeth slightly and then makes a laterotrusive border movement. With the mandible in a laterotrusive position, the teeth close into—but not through—the softened wax (Fig. 18-12). The wax is chilled with air and removed. This record captures the exact position of the teeth during a specific border movement. It also captures the accurate position of the condyles during the laterotrusive movement. When it is returned to the mounted casts and the teeth bite into it, the condylar movement in

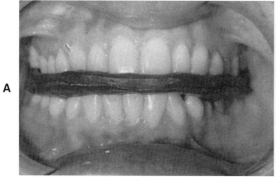

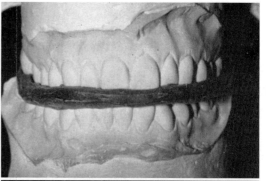

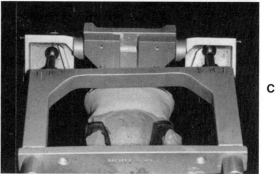

Fig. 18-12 LATEROTRUSIVE INTEROC-CLUSAL RECORD. A, Wax is placed between the teeth, and the mandible is shifted in a right laterotrusive movement. In this position the mandibular teeth are closed into the wax record. **B,** The wax record is air chilled and placed on the maxillary cast. The mandibular cast is moved to fit into the record. **C,** When the wax record is in place, the left condyle can be seen to have begun its orbiting pathway forward, downward, and inward around the right rotating condyle. This is appropriately recorded, and adjustments are made for it in the articulator.

the patient is visualized by the same movement on the articulator. The condylar inclination and Bennett angle adjustments are then appropriately altered to duplicate this specific condylar position. By means of interocclusal records in both right and left laterotrusive, as well as protrusive, border movements, the articulator is adjusted to duplicate the eccentric movements of the patient.

The clinician should note that the condylar guidance is the adjustment on the articulator that regulates the angle at which the condyle descends from the CR position during a protrusive or laterotrusive movement. The normal form of the skull is such that this pathway is generally curved (Fig. 18-13). Most semiadjustable articulators, however, are limited to providing a straight pathway. When a patient has an immediate or progressive side shift, the pathway is often not a straight line. If a laterotrusive interocclusal record is taken when the teeth are beyond the end-to-end relationship of the working canines, the orbiting condyle will move downward and forward to position *C* (see Fig. 18-13). This results in a relatively small Bennett angle *(c)*. If, however, an interocclusal record is

taken only 3 to 5 mm from the CR position, the recording will express more closely the immediate and progressive shift of the patient (position *B*). This will result in a greater Bennett angle *(b)*. Because the clinician is concerned with any movement that may result in tooth contact, it is logical that the first 3 to 5 mm of movement is most critical. If the smaller angle is used for the fabrication of posterior crowns, a relatively narrow fossa will be developed. When these crowns are placed in the mouth and the greater side shift is expressed, the crowns will contact during a mediotrusive movement and the result will be a nondesirable occlusal interference. To avoid this error, the lateral interocclusal record should be taken at no more than 5 mm of eccentric movement.

Advantages and Disadvantages of the Semiadjustable Articulator

The adaptability of the semiadjustable articulator to the patient's specific condylar movements provides a significant advantage over the nonadjustable instrument. Restorations that more closely fit the occlusal requirements of the patient can be

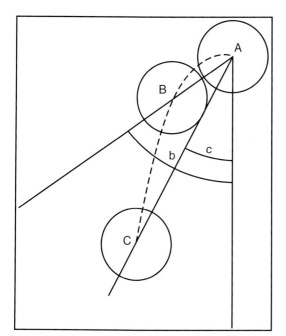

Fig. 18-13 Circle *A* represents the condyle in the centric relation (CR) position (horizontal view). The dotted line is the pathway of the orbiting condyle that exhibits a significant progressive lateral translation movement. If a laterotrusive interocclusal record is taken 3 to 5 mm from the CR position (as seen in position *B*), the resultant Bennett angle will be angle *b*. If a second laterotrusive interocclusal record is taken 7 to 10 mm from the CR position (as seen in position *C*, which is beyond the canine end-to-end relationship), a Bennett angle *(c)* will be acquired. Because the potential for tooth contacts is much greater near the CR position, the interocclusal record should be taken at position *B*.

nonadjustable type; however, again the increased benefits usually far outweigh the increased cost.

FULLY ADJUSTABLE ARTICULATOR

Description
The fully adjustable articulator (Fig. 18-14) is the most sophisticated instrument in dentistry for duplicating mandibular movement. By virtue of the numerous adjustments that are available, this articulator is capable of repeating most of the precise condylar movements depicted in any individual patient: (1) condylar inclination, (2) Bennett angle or immediate lateral shift, (3) rotating condylar movement (working condyle), and (4) intercondylar distance.

Condylar Inclination. As on the semiadjustable articulator, the angle at which the condyle descends on the fully adjustable articulator during protrusive and laterotrusive movements can be altered. Whereas the semiadjustable articulator can usually provide a condylar movement only in a straight pathway, the fully adjustable articulator is capable of adjusting the condylar pathway to duplicate the angle and curvature of the patient's condylar movement.

Bennett Angle (Lateral Translation Movement). The fully adjustable articulator has adjustments that permit duplication of both the patient's Bennett angle and the immediate lateral

fabricated, thus minimizing the need for intraoral adjustments. Generally the semiadjustable articulator is an excellent instrument for routine dental treatment.

One disadvantage of the semiadjustable articulator when compared with the nonadjustable type is that initially more time is necessary to transfer information from the patient to the articulator. However, this time is minimal and generally well worth the effort because it can save much time in the intraoral adjustment phase of the procedure. Another disadvantage of the semiadjustable articulator is that it is more expensive than the

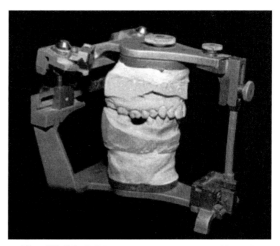

Fig. 18-14 A fully adjustable articulator (Denar).

translation movement of the patient's orbiting condyle. As already discussed, many semiadjustable articulators cannot duplicate this exact pathway because only flat surfaces are available to guide the condyle. When the exact characteristics of the orbiting condylar movement are duplicated, the correct groove placement and fossa width can be more precisely developed in a posterior restoration.

Rotating Condylar Movement. During a laterotrusive movement, the rotating (working) condyle does not purely rotate around a fixed point (see Chapter 6) but can move slightly laterally. This lateral shift can also have a superior, inferior, forward, or backward component, which can influence the fossa depth and cusp height, as well as the ridge and groove direction developed in the posterior teeth. The rotating condylar movement affects both the working and the nonworking sides but has its greatest effect on the working side. Semiadjustable articulators do not have the ability to compensate for this movement. The fully adjustable articulators can be set so that the pathway of the rotating condyle on the articulator will duplicate that of the patient.

Intercondylar Distance. As on the semiadjustable articulator, the distance between the rotating centers of the condyles on the fully adjustable articulator can be modified to match that in the patient. Often three general settings are available on the semiadjustable articulator: small, medium, and large. The setting that most closely fits the patient is used. With the fully adjustable articulator, a complete range of intercondylar distances can be selected. Therefore the intercondylar adjustment is set at the precise millimeter distance as determined from the patient. This then allows a more accurate duplication of this distance and thus minimizes errors in the eccentric pathways of the centric cusps.

Associated Procedures Required for the Fully Adjustable Articulator

Three procedures are necessary to use the fully adjustable articulator effectively: (1) an exact hinge axis location, (2) a pantographic recording, and (3) a CR interocclusal record.

Exact Hinge Axis Location. With the semiadjustable articulator, an arbitrary or average condylar hinge axis is used for the face-bow transfer. Transferring information from the patient to the fully adjustable articulator, however, begins with locating the exact hinge axis of the condyles. This procedure is accomplished by using a device known as the *hinge axis locator*, which is attached to the maxillary and mandibular teeth and extends extraorally posteriorly to the condylar regions (Fig. 18-15). A grid attached to the maxillary teeth is located in the general area of the condyle. A stylus attached

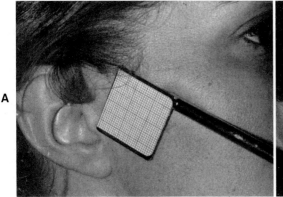
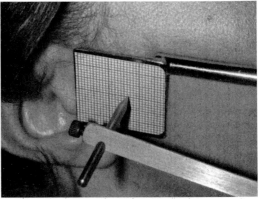

A **B**

Fig. 18-15 HINGE AXIS LOCATION. A, A grid attached to the maxillary teeth is positioned over the area of the condyle. **B,** A stylus attached to the mandibular teeth is positioned over the grid. The mandible is rotated open and closed in the hinge axis position, and the stylus is adjusted until it rotates only about a specific point. The point about which it rotates is the hinge axis, and the area is marked on the tissues adjacent to the point of the stylus.

to the mandibular teeth is positioned over the grid. The mandible is then arched in a hinge axis movement, and the stylus is adjusted until it does not move from its location but merely rotates about a point. When the adjustment is completed, the stylus is positioned directly over the exact hinge axis of the condyle. This area is marked by placing a dot on the surface of the skin.

Pantographic Recording. The fully adjustable articulator has the ability to duplicate mandibular movement precisely. For this to be accomplished, information regarding the patient's specific movements must be acquired.

The eccentric interocclusal records used for the semiadjustable articulator are not adequate for this purpose. With the fully adjustable articulator a pantograph is used to identify the precise condylar movements of the patient. This instrument reveals on several recording tables the exact pathway of the jaw during critical border movements (Fig. 18-16).

A pantograph is made up of two components: a mandibular component, which is attached to the mandibular teeth and usually supports six recording tables, and a maxillary component, which is attached to the maxillary teeth and supports six styluses. When the maxillary and mandibular components are in place, the styluses are situated directly on the recording tables. The two components are attached temporarily to the teeth. When they are in place, the maxillary and

mandibular arches contact only a central bearing point. Therefore movement that occurs, especially in the posterior region of the pantograph, is determined by the patient's condyles moving against the discs and fossae. The posterior portions of the mandibular component are placed over the exact hinge axis of each condyle.

There are two recording tables located near each condyle. One records the movement of the condyle in the horizontal plane, while at the same time the other records the movement in the vertical plane. In addition, two anterior tables record the lateral movements of the mandible in the horizontal plane. When the pantographic tracing is made, three border movements are generally recorded: protrusive, right laterotrusive, and left laterotrusive. As the mandible precisely executes these movements, the recording tables also move, causing the styluses (which are stationary) to scribe a line across the table. The typical pantographic recording for both the vertical and the horizontal tables is depicted in Fig. 18-17. The mandibular movements and resultant recordings are illustrated in Fig. 18-18.

After the tracings have been completed, the pantograph is stabilized and then removed from the patient. It serves two important functions: First, it acts as a facebow to transfer the maxillary cast to the articulator in an exact relationship to the condyles; second, it stores all the needed information for adjusting the articulator to the precise condylar movements of the patient (this is accomplished by transferring the pantograph from the patient to the articulator). The articulator is then systematically adjusted until each stylus passes directly over the corresponding tracing that represents the patient's condylar movement. When all six styluses pass over their corresponding tracings in all three movements, the articulator is adjusted to duplicate the condylar movements of the patient.

Centric Relation Interocclusal Record. The hinge axis location and pantographic tracings provide information needed to mount the maxillary cast and adjust the articulator to the patient's specific condylar movements. As with the semiadjustable articulator, an interocclusal record is necessary to mount the mandibular cast on the fully adjustable

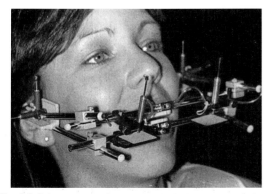

Fig. 18-16 PANTOGRAPH. Two anterior tables (horizontal) are present. In the posterior area two tables exist for each condyle (one vertical and one horizontal).

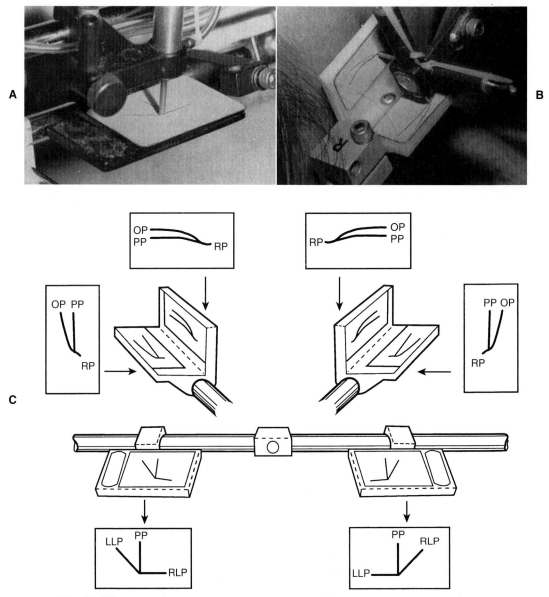

Fig. 18-17 A, Typical recording on the anterior table. **B,** Typical recording on the posterior (horizontal and vertical) tables. **C,** Typical records for all six tables. *LLP,* Left laterotrusive pathway; *OP,* pathway of orbiting condyle; *PP,* pathway of protruding condyle; *RLP,* right laterotrusive pathway; *RP,* pathway of rotating condyle.

articulator in proper relation to the maxillary teeth. In order for the full range of movement to be observed, the interocclusal record is developed in the CR position.

Taking centric relation interocclusal records at an increased vertical dimension. When the exact hinge

axis is located and transferred to the articulator, the opening and closing pathways of the teeth in the terminal hinge movement are the same in the patient's mouth as on the articulator. This is true because the distances from the centers of rotation of the condyles to any given cusp are exactly the

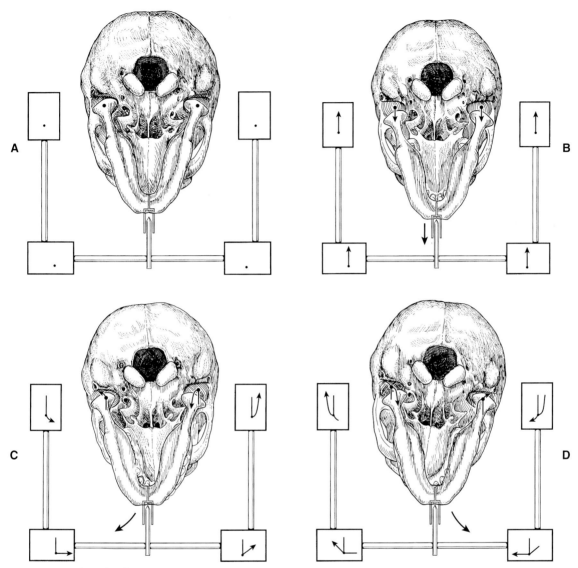

Fig. 18-18 A, Pantograph recordings. In this drawing the condyles are in the centric relation position to begin the pantographic tracing. No movements have been recorded yet. **B,** The pantograph tracings of a protrusive movement on all four recording tables are demonstrated. **C,** The pantograph tracings of a right laterotrusive movement on all four recording tables are shown. **D,** The pantograph tracings of a left laterotrusive movement on all four recording tables are demonstrated.

same in the patient's mouth as on the articulator. When this condition exists, the thickness of the interocclusal record has no effect on the accuracy of the mounting.

However, when an arbitrary or average hinge axis is used to mount the maxillary cast (as with nonadjustable and semiadjustable articulators), the likelihood is great that the distances between the centers of rotation of the condyles and any given cusp will not be the same in the mouth as on the articulator. Therefore the hinge axis opening and closing pathway of the cusps will not be exactly the same. If the mandibular cast is mounted in the ICP, this discrepancy has no clinical significance because the only difference is in the opening pathway (which has no occlusal contact considerations). Yet a significant discrepancy can exist if the arbitrary hinge axis is used to mount the maxillary cast and an interocclusal record at

an increased vertical dimension is used to mount the mandibular cast. Because the closure arcs for the patient and the articulator are not identical, when the interocclusal record is removed the cast will arc closed on a different pathway, resulting in a different occlusal contact position from that seen in the patient's mouth (Fig. 18-19).

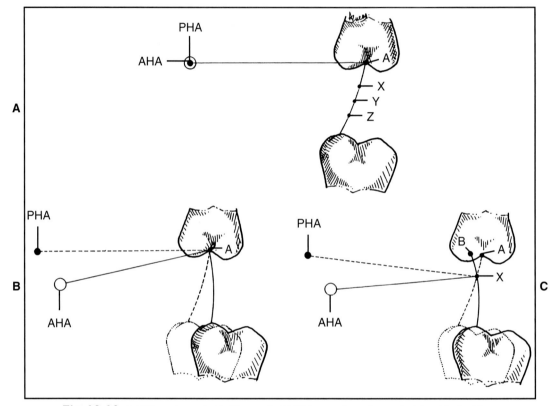

Fig. 18-19 A, When the patient's hinge axis *(PHA)* is transferred to coincide with the hinge axis of the articulator *(AHA)*, the arcs of closure for the patient and the articulator are identical. Therefore an interocclusal record at any degree of opening *(X, Y,* and *Z)* will provide an arc of closure to the desired occlusal position *(A).* **B,** When the exact hinge axis is not located, it is more likely that a difference will exist between PHA and AHA. The AHA is inferior and anterior to the PHA. When this occurs, the opening and closing pathways (arcs) are different. If an interocclusal record is taken with the teeth in the desired occlusal position *(A),* the difference in these two pathways has no clinical significance because there are no occlusal contacts during the opening and closing movements. The important feature is that both closing pathways return to the mandible to the desired occlusal position. **C,** The PHA and the AHA are not the same as shown in **B.** However, when an interocclusal record taken at an increased vertical dimension *(X)* is used in mounting the cast, the mandibular teeth are at a proper distance from the PHA but not the AHA. When the record is removed, the teeth close on an arcing pathway around the AHA and not the PHA. Because this pathway is different from the patient's, the resulting contact position will be different (not *A* but *B*). Therefore when the PHA is not transferred to the articulator, the record should be taken at the desired occlusal position where the restorations will be fabricated. Taking an interocclusal record at an increased vertical dimension will introduce error at the occlusal contact position.

Generally, the thicker the interocclusal record, the greater the chances of introducing inaccuracies when mounting.

As a rule, interocclusal records are most accurate when taken at the vertical dimension of occlusion where the restorations will be developed (with the teeth in contact). Records taken in this manner are accurate when both arbitrary and exact hinge axis locations are used. If it is necessary to take a record at an increased vertical dimension (with the teeth apart), however, the exact hinge axis should be located and transferred to the articulator. When a semiadjustable articulator is being used, it is often impossible to transfer the location of the exact hinge axis to the articulator. Then error in mounting is inevitable. It is important in these cases to minimize the thickness of the record, which in turn will minimize the degree of error. Such errors must be compensated for when the restorations are taken to the mouth.

In some instances a treatment plan is developed that requires increasing the patient's vertical dimension of occlusion on the articulator by developing appropriate restorations. Then an exact hinge axis location is indicated. Restorations developed at an increased vertical dimension on the cast will not accurately fit the patient unless the pathway of opening and closing is the same in the patient as it is on the articulator. Exact hinge axis location is necessary to achieve this.

Advantages and Disadvantages of the Fully Adjustable Articulator

The major advantage of this articulator is its ability to duplicate mandibular movement. When it is used properly, restorations that precisely fit the patient's occlusal requirements can be developed. Therefore a minimum amount of intraoral adjustment is necessary, resulting in a stable and anatomic interocclusal relationship.

The major disadvantages of the fully adjustable articulator are that it is usually expensive and a considerable amount of time must be invested initially in transferring information properly from the patient to the articulator. This time and expense must be weighed against the benefits. Simple restorative procedures do not justify the use of the fully adjustable articulator. It is generally easier to use a semiadjustable instrument and compensate for its shortcomings by adjusting the restorations in the mouth. However, when extensive restorative treatment is being planned, the initial expense and investment of time are often well worthwhile in the development of precise-fitting restorations.

SELECTION OF AN ARTICULATOR

The selection of an articulator must be based on four factors: (1) recognition of certain characteristics of the patient's occlusion, (2) the extent of the restorative procedures planned, (3) understanding of the limitation of the articulator system, and (4) the skills of the clinician.

CHARACTERISTICS OF THE PATIENT'S OCCLUSION

As described in Chapter 6, two factors determine mandibular movement: the anterior tooth guidance and the posterior condylar guidance. When a patient has adequate and immediate anterior guidance, these tooth contacts generally dominate in controlling mandibular movement. The posterior condylar guidance usually has little, if any, effect on the posterior eccentric tooth contacts. Because one of the most important functions of an articulator is to provide the influence of the posterior determinants, a less sophisticated articulator system can be used successfully for this patient. However, when a patient manifests poor anterior guidance resulting from missing or malaligned anterior teeth, the predominant factors of mandibular movement are the posterior determinants. Generally in this case a more sophisticated articulator system is indicated.

EXTENT OF THE RESTORATIVE PROCEDURES

One of the primary reasons for using an articulator is to minimize the need for intraoral adjustment of the restorations being planned. Therefore the more sophisticated the instrument, the greater the likelihood that restorations can be fabricated with minimum adjustment. However, the chair time required to use a sophisticated, fully adjustable articulator often makes it impractical for the fabrication of a single crown. Generally a more extensive treatment plan requires a more sophisticated articulator system. When minor procedures are indicated, it is often easier to compensate for the shortcomings of the simpler instruments by adjusting the restorations intraorally.

UNDERSTANDING THE LIMITATIONS OF THE ARTICULATOR SYSTEM

The advantages and disadvantages of each articulator system must be understood if the proper instrument is to be selected. The dentist must be aware that before a restoration can be permanently placed in a patient's mouth, it must meet all the criteria of optimum functional occlusion. Some of the simple articulators provide only a small portion of the information necessary to reach this goal. Therefore after a restoration has been fabricated the dentist must be prepared to make the necessary adjustments that will enable it to meet the criteria for optimum functional occlusion (see Chapter 5) before it is permanently placed in the patient's mouth.

Fig. 18-20 shows that the shortcomings of the simple articulator require more compensation than those of a more sophisticated device. The fully adjustable articulator therefore appears to be a better instrument. As previously mentioned, however, this factor must be considered along with the complexity of the treatment plan.

Actually, each articulator system has its own indications, as follows:

1. Because the *nonadjustable* articulator is simplest, the dentist may be directed toward it. For patients with adequate and immediate anterior guidance, this type may be successfully used for the fabrication of a single crown. However, remember that additional chair time is required for the necessary intraoral adjustments that will compensate for the shortcomings of this instrument.

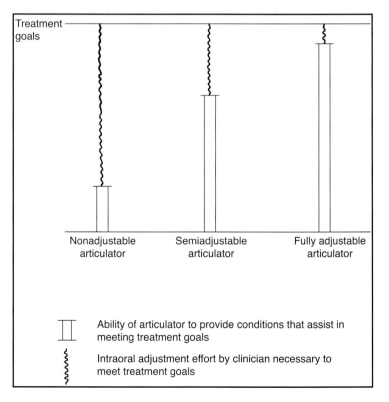

Fig. 18-20 CONTRIBUTION OF EACH TYPE OF ARTICULATOR IN REACHING THE TREATMENT GOALS. The wavy lines, representing the effort that must be provided by the clinician during the intraoral adjustment phase to meet the goals for the restoration, do not necessarily show the length of time of treatment because the complexity of treatment has not been considered in this illustration.

2. A more practical selection for a single crown is the *semiadjustable* articulator. This instrument is capable of closely reproducing mandibular movement and therefore decreasing intraoral adjustment time when compared with the nonadjustable articulator. The semiadjustable instrument is especially helpful in fabricating a crown for the patient with minimal anterior guidance. Although a little more time is necessary initially to transfer information from the patient to the articulator, this is usually offset by the decreased intraoral adjustment time.

3. Whereas the semiadjustable articulator is a good instrument for routine fixed prosthetic procedures, the increasing complexity of the treatment plan often necessitates that the *fully adjustable* articulator be considered. It is certainly indicated for complex full mouth reconstructions and when alterations in the vertical dimension of occlusion are being considered.

Fig. 18-20 illustrates that the nonadjustable articulator can provide only the minimum amount of information that is necessary to fabricate a restoration. The semiadjustable articulator gives more information, and therefore the restoration can be fabricated to meet the criteria for optimum functional occlusion more closely. Yet it has certain limitations, and the dentist must be prepared to make the necessary adjustments to meet these before permanently placing the restoration. A fully adjustable articulator can provide all the necessary information to attain optimum functional occlusion; however, because of minor clinical and operator errors, these criteria may not be perfectly met. Therefore it is necessary to examine the restoration carefully and, when called for, make the changes that will allow development of an optimum occlusion.

SKILLS OF THE CLINICIAN

Of note is that an articulator is only as accurate as the clinician who uses it. When care is not exercised in acquiring information from the patient for adjusting the articulator or when casts are inaccurately mounted, the usefulness of any articulator is greatly diminished. As depicted in Fig. 18-20, each articulator can be adequate for an operator who has mastered the skills necessary to use it to its fullest capability. However, when the skills of the clinician are considered, Fig. 18-20 may not be totally accurate. In other words, a semiadjustable articulator in the hands of a knowledgeable clinician may be of greater assistance in treatment than a fully adjustable articulator in the hands of an inexperienced operator.

Selective Grinding

"Selective grinding: one of the most difficult and demanding procedures in dentistry."

—JPO

*S*elective grinding is a procedure by which the occlusal surfaces of the teeth are precisely altered to improve the overall contact pattern. Tooth structure is selectively removed until the reshaped teeth contact in such a manner as to fulfill the treatment goals. Because this procedure is irreversible and involves the removal of tooth structure, it is of limited usefulness. Therefore proper indications must exist before it is considered.

INDICATIONS

A selective grinding procedure can be used to (1) assist in managing certain temporomandibular disorders (TMDs) and (2) complement treatment associated with major occlusal changes.

ASSIST IN MANAGING CERTAIN TEMPOROMANDIBULAR DISORDERS

Selective grinding is indicated when sufficient evidence exists that permanent alteration of an occlusal condition will reduce or eliminate the symptoms associated with a specific TMD. This evidence cannot be determined by the severity of the malocclusion. As discussed in Chapter 7, the severity of the malocclusion does not correlate

well with symptoms, partly because of the great variation in patients' physiologic tolerances and also because the malocclusion may not reflect orthopedic instability (a stable malocclusion). The evidence for the need to permanently change the occlusal condition is obtained through reversible occlusal therapy (e.g., occlusal appliance therapy). Selective grinding is indicated when (1) the occlusal appliance has eliminated the TMD symptoms *and* (2) attempts to identify the feature of the appliance that affects the symptoms have revealed that it is the occlusal contact or jaw position. When these conditions exist, it is likely that if the occlusal condition provided by the appliance was permanently introduced in the dentition, the disorder would resolve. Then there would be a basis for confidence, and selective grinding could be pursued.

COMPLEMENT TREATMENT ASSOCIATED WITH MAJOR OCCLUSAL CHANGES

The most common reason to consider selective grinding for a patient is as part of a treatment plan that will result in a major change in the existing occlusal condition. This reason for the treatment is not associated with a TMD but entails a significant restoration or reorganization of the occlusal condition. When major occlusal changes are planned, treatment goals should be established that will provide optimum occlusal conditions when the treatment is completed. If extensive crown and fixed prosthodontic procedures are necessary, selective grinding may be indicated before treatment begins so that a stable functional mandibular position is established to which the restorations can be fabricated.

In summary, selective grinding is indicated to improve an occlusal condition only when sufficient evidence exists that this alteration will assist in the management of a TMD or in conjunction with an already established need for major occlusal treatment. At this time no evidence indicates that prophylactic selective grinding benefits the patient.

PREDICTING THE OUTCOME OF SELECTIVE GRINDING

Remember that even when alteration of the occlusal condition is indicated, a selective grinding procedure may not be the treatment of choice. Selective grinding is appropriate only when alterations of the tooth surfaces are minimal so that all corrections can be made within the enamel structure. When the malalignment of teeth is great enough that achieving the treatment goals will penetrate the enamel, selective grinding must be accompanied by proper restorative procedures. Exposure of dentin poses problems (increased sensitivity, caries susceptibility, and wear) and therefore should not be left untreated. It is extremely important that the treatment outcome of selective grinding be accurately predicted before treatment begins. Both the operator and the patient must know and be prepared in advance for the results of the selective grinding procedure. Patient acceptance and rapport are not strengthened when, after the procedure is completed, additional crowns necessary to restore the dentition are added to the treatment plan.

The success in achieving the treatment goals using a selective grinding procedure alone is determined by the degree of malalignment of the teeth. Because it is necessary to work within the confines of the enamel, only minimal corrections can be made. The "rule of thirds" (see Chapter 17) is helpful in predicting the success of a selective grinding procedure. It deals with the buccolingual arch discrepancy when the condyles are in the musculoskeletally stable position (Fig. 19-1).

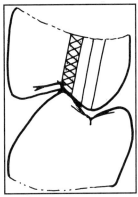

Fig. 19-1 THE RULE OF THIRDS—SELECTIVE GRINDING. In using the rule of thirds, the inner incline of the centric cusps is divided into thirds. With the condyles in the desired treatment position (centric relation), the mandible is closed to tooth contact. If the initial contact of the lower centric cusp is on the third closest to the central fossa of the opposing tooth (as shown here), selective grinding can be successfully accomplished. The nearer the location of this contact to the middle third, the more likely selective grinding will lead to exposure of dentin and the need for restorative procedures.

The anteroposterior discrepancy also needs to be considered. It is best examined by visualizing the centric relation (CR)–to–intercuspal position (ICP) slide, which is observed by locating the mandible in the musculoskeletally stable position (CR) and, with a hinge axis movement, bringing the teeth into light contact. Once the buccolingual discrepancy of the posterior teeth is examined (rule of thirds), the patient applies force to the teeth. An anterosuperior shift of the mandible from CR to ICP will be noted. The shorter the slide, the more likely it is that selective grinding can be accomplished within the confines of the enamel. Normally an anterior slide of less than 2 mm can be successfully eliminated by a selective grinding procedure.

The direction of the slide in the sagittal plane can also influence the success or failure of selective grinding. Both the horizontal and the vertical components of the slide should be examined. Generally, when the slide has a great horizontal component, it is more difficult to eliminate within the confines of the enamel (Fig. 19-2). If it is almost parallel with the arc of closure (large vertical

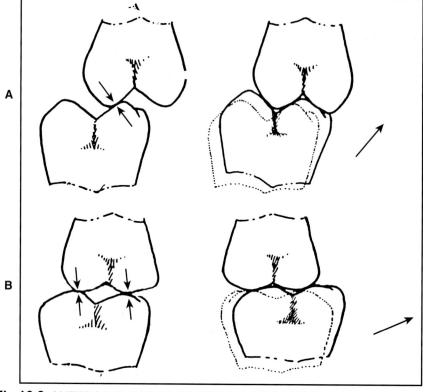

Fig. 19-2 ANTEROPOSTERIOR DIRECTION OF THE SLIDE. A, When the cusps are relatively tall (sharp), the direction of the centric relation–to–intercuspal position (CR-to-ICP) slide is predominantly vertical. **B,** When the cusps are relatively flat, the CR-to-ICP slide has a greater horizontal component. The more horizontal the component, the greater the difficulty in accomplishing selective grinding within the confines of the enamel.

component), eliminating it is usually easier. Therefore both the distance and direction of the slide are helpful in predicting the outcome of selective grinding.

After the CR slide has been examined, the position of the anterior teeth is evaluated. These teeth are important because they will be used to disocclude the posterior teeth during eccentric movements. With the condyles in their treatment position (CR), the mandible is once again closed until the first tooth contacts lightly. An attempt is made to visualize the relationship of the maxillary and mandibular anterior teeth as though the arc of closure were continuing until the patient's vertical dimension of occlusion was achieved. This represents the

position of the anterior teeth after the premature CR contacts have been eliminated. An attempt is made to predict the type and adequacy of the future anterior guidance.

Predicting the treatment outcome in a patient with well-aligned teeth and a very short CR slide is relatively easy. Equally easy is determining that a patient with a 6-mm horizontal slide and poorly aligned teeth is not a good candidate for this procedure alone. The problem with predicting the outcome of selective grinding arises with the patient who is between these two extremes. Therefore when it is difficult to determine the outcome of selective grinding, accurate diagnostic casts are carefully mounted on an articulator so that further analysis can be made. Tooth alignment and the CR slide are more easily evaluated on mounted diagnostic casts. When doubt still exists, selective grinding is carefully performed on the diagnostic casts so that the final results can be visualized. Teeth that are severely altered should be treatment planned for crowns. Once the results of the selective grinding are visualized, the potential benefits of the procedure can be weighed against any additional treatment needed to restore the dentition. These considerations must be evaluated before a selective grinding procedure is suggested to the patient.

IMPORTANT CONSIDERATIONS IN SELECTIVE GRINDING

After the determination has been made that there are proper indications for selective grinding and treatment results have been adequately predicted, the procedure can begin. It is advisable, however, not to rush into treatment without thoroughly explaining the procedure to the patient. In some cases the success or failure of the treatment will hinge on the acceptance and assistance of the patient. The clinician should explain that small areas of the teeth interfere with the normal functioning of the jaw and that the goal is to eliminate these so that normal function can be restored. The patient should be aware that although this procedure may take some time, the changes are slight and often difficult to visualize in the mirror. Any questions regarding the procedure should be discussed and explained before the procedure begins. The treatment outcome must be thoroughly explained, especially if any restorative procedures will be necessary.

From the technical point of view, selective grinding can be a difficult and tedious procedure. It should not be initiated haphazardly or without a complete understanding of the treatment goals. A well-performed selective grinding will enhance function of the masticatory system. On the other hand, a poorly performed selective grinding may actually create problems with masticatory function and even accentuate occlusal interferences that have been previously overlooked by the neuromuscular

system (creating what has been called a *positive occlusal awareness*). It may therefore initiate functional problems. A well-executed selective grinding procedure does not lead to positive occlusal awareness. Rather, the condition usually occurs in patients with high levels of emotional stress or other emotional problems. It is best avoided by (1) being sure that there are proper indications for selective grinding (emotional stress is not a major factor) and (2) carrying out the procedure carefully and precisely.

The effectiveness of selective grinding can be greatly influenced by the operator's ability to manage the patient. Because the procedure demands precision, careful control of the mandibular position and tooth contacts is essential. The patient's muscular activity must be properly restrained during the procedure so that the treatment goals can be accomplished. Therefore conditions that exist during the procedure should promote patient relaxation. Selective grinding is performed in a quiet and peaceful setting. The patient is reclined in the dental chair and approached in a soft, gentle, and understanding manner. Encouragement is given when success in relaxing and aiding the operator is achieved. When it is advantageous for the operator to guide the mandible to a desired position, the movement is performed slowly and deliberately so as not to elicit protective muscle activity. The success of a selective grinding procedure is dependent on all these considerations.

TREATMENT GOALS FOR SELECTIVE GRINDING

Although selective grinding involves the reshaping of teeth, the mandibular position to which the teeth are altered is also critical. Selective grinding should begin with locating the musculoskeletally stable (CR) position of the condyles. This is done using the bimanual manipulation technique described in Chapter 9. In the patient with a TMD, an occlusal appliance may have been used to help determine the stable joint position. If for any reason the condylar position is in question, selective grinding should not be initiated until a stable, reproducible position has been achieved.

The occlusal treatment goals for selective grinding are as follows:

1. With the condyles in the musculoskeletally stable (CR) position and the articular discs properly interposed, all possible posterior teeth contact evenly and simultaneously between centric cusp tips and opposing flat surfaces.
2. When the mandible is moved laterally, laterotrusive contacts on the anterior teeth disocclude the posterior teeth.
3. When the mandible is protruded, contacts on the anterior teeth disocclude the posterior teeth.
4. In the upright head position (alert feeding position) the posterior teeth contact more heavily than the anterior teeth.

Several methods can be used to achieve these goals. The one described in this chapter consists of developing (1) an acceptable CR contact position and (2) an acceptable laterotrusive and protrusive guidance.

DEVELOPING AN ACCEPTABLE CENTRIC RELATION CONTACT POSITION

The goal of this step is to create desirable tooth contacts when the condyles are in their musculoskeletally stable (CR) position. In many patients an unstable occlusal condition exists in CR and creates a slide to the more stable ICP. A major goal of selective grinding is to develop a stable intercuspal contact position when the condyles are in the CR position.

Another way of describing this goal is to refer to it as *elimination of the CR slide*. A slide of the mandible is created by the instability of contacts between opposing tooth inclines. When the cusp tip contacts a flat surface in CR and force is applied by the elevator muscles, no shift occurs. Thus the goal in achieving acceptable contacts in ICP is to alter or reshape all inclines into either cusp tips or flat surfaces. Cusp tip–to–flat surface contacts are also desirable because they effectively direct occlusal forces through the long axes of the teeth (see Chapter 5).

The CR slide can be classified as anterosuperior, anterosuperior and to the right, and anterosuperior and to the left. Each is created by specific opposing inclines. A basic understanding of these makes establishing an acceptable CR position much more simple.

Anterosuperior Slide

The slide from CR to maximum intercuspation may follow a pathway that is straightforward and superior in the sagittal plane. The slide is caused by contact between the mesial inclines of the maxillary cusps and the distal inclines of the mandibular cusps (Fig. 19-3).

Anterosuperior and *Right* Slide

The CR slide may be anterosuperior with a right lateral component (i.e., moving to the right). When there is a lateral component, it is caused by the inner and outer inclines of the posterior teeth.

When a right lateral slide is created by opposing tooth contacts on the right side of the arch, it is because of the inner inclines of the maxillary lingual cusps against the inner inclines of the mandibular

Fig. 19-3 ANTEROSUPERIOR SLIDE.
The mesial inclines of the maxillary teeth *(small arrows)*, which oppose the distal inclines of the mandibular teeth, cause this type of mandibular slide *(large arrow)* from centric relation to intercuspal position. *D,* Distal; *M,* mesial.

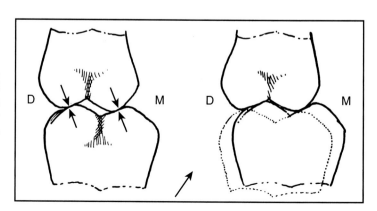

buccal cusps. Because these are also the locations for mediotrusive contacts, they are sometimes called *mediotrusive CR interferences* (Fig. 19-4, *A*).

When a right lateral slide is created by opposing tooth contacts on the left side of the arch, two contacting surfaces may be responsible: the inner inclines of the maxillary buccal cusps against the outer inclines of the mandibular buccal cusps, or the outer of the maxillary lingual cusps against the inner of the mandibular lingual cusps. Because these inclines are also the areas for laterotrusive contacts, they are sometimes called *laterotrusive CR interferences* (Fig. 19-4, *B*).

Anterosuperior and Left Slide

The CR slide may be anterosuperior with a left lateral component. When a left lateral shift is present, the opposing inclines that create it are the same as those that create the right lateral shift but are present on the opposite teeth (Fig. 19-5).

Understanding the exact location of the contacting inclines can greatly assist in the selective grinding procedure. Of course, these types of incline locations are accurate only if the normal buccolingual alignment is present. When posterior teeth are in crossbite, the location of the contacting inclines changes.

With these principles in mind, the clinician can begin the selective grinding procedure.

Achieving the Centric Contact Position

The patient reclines in the dental chair, and CR is bimanually located. The teeth are lightly brought together, and the patient identifies the tooth that is felt to contact first. The mouth is then opened, and the teeth are thoroughly dried with an air syringe or cotton roll. Thin articulating paper held with forceps is placed on the side identified as having the first contact. The mandible is again guided to CR and the teeth contact, lightly tapping on the paper.

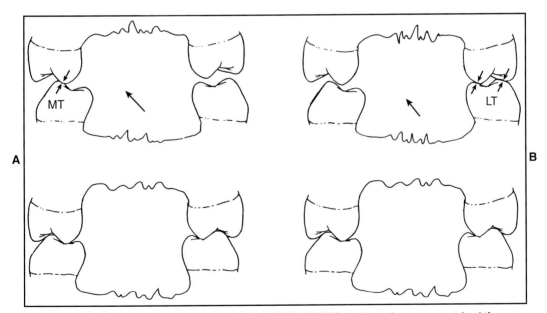

Fig. 19-4 ANTEROSUPERIOR AND RIGHT SLIDE. Inclines that create a right shift of the mandible from centric relation (CR) to intercuspal position can be located on both sides of the arches. **A,** The inclines on the right side *(small arrows)* that cause a right shift of the mandible are the inner inclines of the maxillary lingual cusps against the inner inclines of the mandibular buccal cusps (mediotrusive CR interferences). **B,** The inclines *(small arrows)* located on the left side that cause a right shift of the mandible *(large arrow)* are either the inner inclines of the maxillary buccal cusps against the outer inclines of the mandibular buccal cusps or the outer inclines of the maxillary lingual cusps against the inner inclines of the mandibular lingual cusps (laterotrusive CR interferences). *LT,* Laterotrusive; *MT,* mediotrusive.

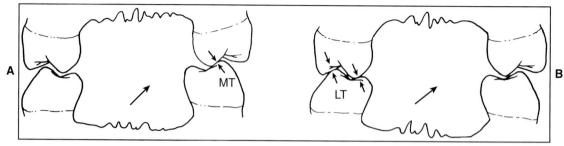

Fig. 19-5 ANTEROSUPERIOR AND LEFT SLIDE. Similar to the right slide, inclines that create a left shift of the mandible from centric relation (CR) to intercuspal position can be located on both sides of the dental arches. These areas are similar to those causing the right shift but on the opposite side of the dental arches. **A,** Mediotrusive CR interferences *(small arrows)* on the left side shift the mandible to the left. **B,** Laterotrusive CR interferences *(small arrows)* on the right side shift the mandible to the left. *LT,* Laterotrusive; *MT,* mediotrusive.

The contact areas are located for the maxillary and mandibular teeth. One or both of the contacts will be on an incline, either the mesial and distal inclines (Fig. 19-6) or the buccal and lingual inclines (Fig. 19-7). To eliminate the CR slide, these inclines must be reshaped into cusp tips or flat surfaces.

A small Dura-Green polishing stone in a high-speed handpiece is an acceptable method for reshaping tooth surfaces. It is advisable, however, that beginning students use a Green stone in a slow-speed handpiece to avoid removing too much tooth structure too quickly. When confidence and expertise are gained, the high-speed handpiece can be used. It will achieve good results in a reasonable time with less tooth-to-bone vibration and therefore generally more comfort for the patient.

When a contact is found on an incline close to a centric cusp tip, it is eliminated. With this area eliminated, the likelihood is greater that the next time the posterior teeth come together the contact area will be shifted up closer to the cusp tip (Figs. 19-6, *B;* 19-7, *B;* and 19-8). When a contact area is located on an incline near the central fossa area, the incline is reshaped into a flat surface. This is often called *hollow grinding* because the fossa area is widened slightly (Figs. 19-6, *D;* 19-7, *D;* and 19-9). The clinician should remember that the buccolingual relationship of the maxillary and mandibular teeth cannot be altered because this is

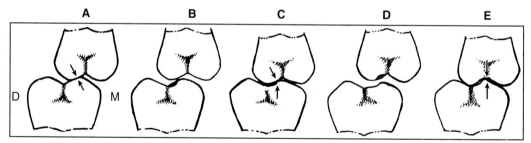

Fig. 19-6 SELECTIVE GRINDING SEQUENCE IN CENTRIC RELATION (CR).
A, In CR a mesial incline of the maxillary tooth contacts a distal incline *(arrows)* of the mandibular tooth. **B,** The contact closest to the cusp tip is located on the mandibular tooth. This incline is eliminated, allowing only the cusp tip to contact. **C,** During the next closure this mandibular cusp tip contacts the mesial incline *(arrows)* of a maxillary cusp. **D,** This incline is reshaped into a flat surface (i.e., hollow grinding). **E,** On the next closure the mandibular cusp tip can be seen to contact the maxillary flat surface *(arrows),* and the treatment goals for this pair of contacts are achieved. *D,* Distal; *M,* mesial.

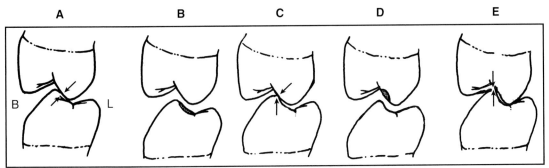

Fig. 19-7 SELECTIVE GRINDING SEQUENCE IN CENTRIC RELATION (CR) (MESIAL VIEW). A, In CR an inner incline of the maxillary tooth contacts an inner incline of the mandibular tooth. **B,** The contact area closest to the tip is located on the mandibular centric cusp. This incline is eliminated, allowing only the cusp tip to contact. **C,** During the next closure the mandibular cusp tip contacts the inner incline of the maxillary centric cusp. **D,** This incline is reshaped into a flat surface (hollow grinding). **E,** On the next closure the mandibular cusp tip contacts the maxillary flat surface, and the treatment goals for this pair of contacts are achieved. *B,* Buccal; *L,* lateral.

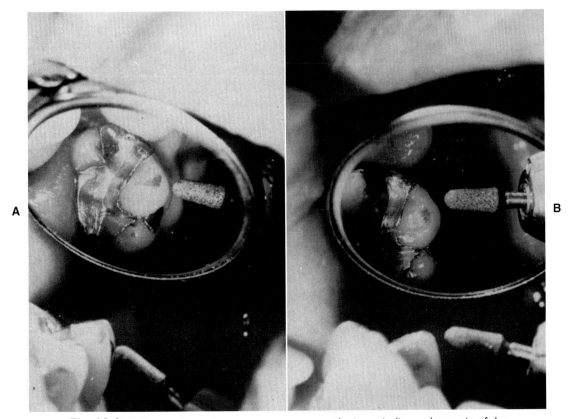

Fig. 19-8 A, In centric relation a contact occurs on the inner incline and cusp tip of the maxillary molar. **B,** The contact area is altered such that only the cusp tip contacts on the next closure.

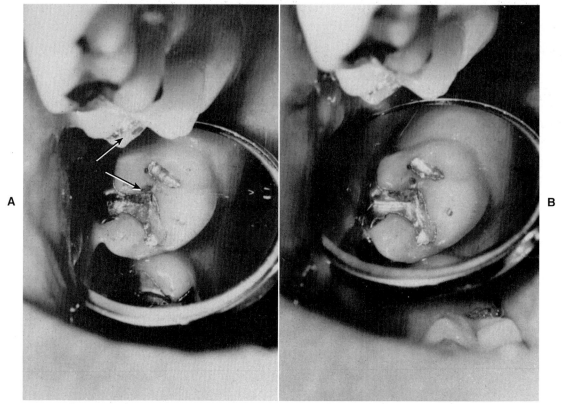

Fig. 19-9 A, In centric relation a contact occurs on the inner incline near the central fossa of this maxillary molar *(arrows)*. **B,** The contact area is reshaped into a flat surface by elimination of the incline, leaving only a flat surface (hollow grinding).

determined by the interarch widths when the condyles are in CR. Therefore the only way that a cusp tip can contact a flat surface is for the fossa area to be widened and a new flat area created.

Once these incline areas have been adjusted, the teeth are redried, remarked, and reevaluated. If inclines are still present, they are readjusted in a similar manner until only the cusp tip contacts a flat surface. Once this has been achieved, the contact relationship between the two areas is stable. However, these two contacts are not the only ones necessary to achieve a stable CR position. As adjustments are made, other teeth will also come into contact and must be adjusted by the same sequence and technique.

The opposing incline contacts in CR are at an increased vertical dimension of occlusion. As the inclines are eliminated, the contact position begins to approach the patient's original vertical dimension of occlusion, which is maintained by the ICP. As closure occurs, more teeth come into contact. Each pair of contacts is evaluated and adjusted to cusp tips and flat surfaces. All contacting incline areas must be eliminated.

As the CR contacts are developed, sound cusp tip–to–flat surface contacts are established but often at a greater vertical dimension than the ICP. Therefore it is likely that these new contacts will not allow the other posterior teeth to contact (Fig. 19-10). When this occurs, these contacts are reduced slightly so that the remaining teeth can occlude.

Even though cusp tip–to–flat surface contacts are desirable, these areas must be reduced to permit full contact of the remaining teeth. Generally it is important for function and stability to maintain

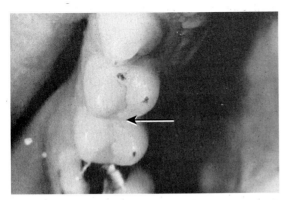

Fig. 19-10 DESIRABLE CUSP TIP AND FLAT SURFACE CONTACTS ON MAXILLARY PREMO-LARS. However, a mandibular buccal cusp does not contact the mesial marginal ridge of the maxillary second premolar *(arrow)*. The existing contacts must be adjusted to permit the remaining cusp in the opposing arch to contact this marginal ridge.

prominent cusp tips. Thus the appropriate contact area to reduce is the flat surface. However, the clinician should make one other consideration. As a fossa area is reduced, the centric cusp becomes situated more deeply in the fossa. The deeper a cusp tip is located in a fossa, the more likely it is to contact an opposing incline during eccentric movements. Because eliminating posterior tooth contacts is one of the goals of selective grinding, it is most efficient to address this condition at this time. Therefore the decision to reduce either the

cusp tip or the flat surface is made by visualizing the cusp tip as it executes the various eccentric movements.

When a cusp tip does not contact an opposing tooth surface during eccentric movements, the opposing flat surface is reduced (Fig. 19-11). When a cusp tip does contact an opposing tooth surface, the cusp tip is reduced (Fig. 19-12). This reduction not only assists in establishing CR contacts on other posterior teeth but also reduces the likelihood of undesirable eccentric posterior tooth contacts when the anterior guidance is developed. When altering either a cusp tip or a flat surface, the same shape must be maintained so that the desired contact will be reestablished as the vertical dimension approaches the original values of the patient.

The CR contacts are marked and adjusted until all available posterior centric cusps are contacting evenly and simultaneously on flat surfaces. Ideally there should be four CR contacts on each molar and two on each premolar. Because selective grinding involves only the removal of tooth structure and cannot control all tooth surfaces or positions, sometimes less than ideal circumstances result. A minimum goal that must be achieved is for every opposing tooth to have at least one CR contact. If this is not done, then drifting of unopposed teeth can occur and the result may be reestablishment of undesirable tooth contacts.

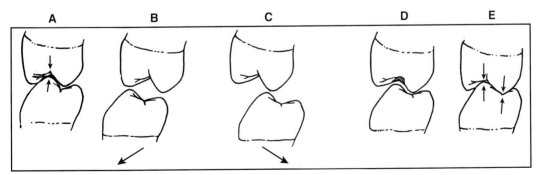

Fig. 19-11 A, The mandibular buccal cusp prematurely contacts *(small arrows),* preventing contact of the maxillary lingual cusp. **B,** No contact during a laterotrusive movement is demonstrated *(large arrow).* **C,** No contact during a mediotrusive movement is shown *(large arrow).* **D,** The fossa area opposing the mandibular buccal cusp is reduced. **E,** This reduction allows contact of the maxillary lingual cusp tip.

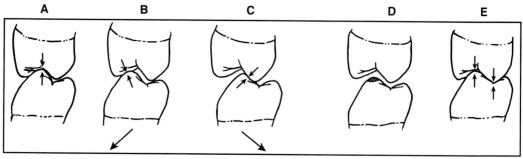

Fig. 19-12 A, The mandibular buccal cusp prematurely contacts, preventing contact of the maxillary lingual cusp. Contacts also occur **(B)** during a laterotrusive movement and **(C)** during a mediotrusive movement. **D,** The mandibular buccal cusp is shortened. **E,** This allows contact of the maxillary lingual cusp tip *(small arrows)*.

Anterior teeth that contact heavily during the development of posterior CR contacts are reduced. It is generally acceptable to reduce these contacts equally on both the maxillary and the mandibular anterior teeth until the posterior teeth are reestablished as the more prominent contacts. When the anterior teeth are being adjusted, it is vitally important to visualize the future guidance contacts that will soon be developed. If it is determined that by grinding more on either a maxillary or a mandibular tooth the guidance can be improved, this should be done.

An acceptable CR position has been developed when equal and simultaneous contacts occur between cusp tips and flat surfaces on all posterior teeth. When the mandible is guided to CR and force is applied, no shift or slide occurs. (No inclines create a slide.) When the patient closes and taps in CR position, all the posterior teeth are felt evenly. If a tooth contacts more heavily, it is carefully reduced until it contacts evenly with the other posterior teeth.

DEVELOPING AN ACCEPTABLE LATERAL AND PROTRUSIVE GUIDANCE

The goal of this step in selective grinding is to establish a sound and functional complement of tooth contacts that will serve to guide the mandible through the various eccentric movements.

As discussed in Chapter 5, posterior teeth are not usually good candidates to accept the forces of eccentric mandibular movement. The anterior teeth, especially the canines, are much better. Therefore under optimum conditions, the canines should contact during laterotrusive movements and disocclude all the posterior teeth (bilaterally). When the canines are in proper alignment, this goal is achieved. Often, however, they are not properly positioned to contact immediately during a laterotrusive movement. Because selective grinding deals only with the removal of tooth structure, this lack of contact cannot be corrected. When it occurs, the teeth that are best able to accept the lateral forces should contact and guide the mandible until the canines can contact and assist in the movement.

Laterotrusive contacts are best accepted by several posterior teeth closest to the anterior portion of the mouth (e.g., the premolars). In other words, when the canines are not positioned such that they can immediately provide laterotrusive guidance, a group function guidance is established. In this instance the mandible is laterally guided by the premolars and even the mesiobuccal cusps of the first molars. As soon as there is adequate movement to bring the canines into contact, they are used to assist in the movement.

Importantly, the clinician should remember that this laterotrusive movement is not static but dynamic. Tooth contacts must be properly controlled during the entire movement until the canines pass over each other, allowing the anterior incisors to contact (which is termed the *cross-over position*). During this dynamic movement all teeth

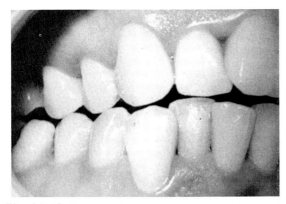

Fig. 19-13 Early in a laterotrusive movement it appears that a group function is present. However, at this particular position only the first premolars contact. This type of contact is likely to result in traumatic forces to these teeth. Such contacts must be reduced to allow the other teeth to participate in the group function guidance.

providing guidance in the group function should contact evenly and smoothly. If it is noticed that the first premolar is responsible for all guidance during a particular portion of the movement, this tooth may experience traumatic forces, usually resulting in mobility (Fig. 19-13). Selective grinding adjusts this tooth until it contacts evenly with the remaining teeth during the laterotrusive movement.

1. Acceptable laterotrusive contacts occur between the buccal cusps and not the lingual cusps. Lingual laterotrusive contacts, as well as mediotrusive contacts, are always eliminated because they produce eccentric occlusal instability.
2. As with lateral movements, protrusive movements are best guided by the anterior teeth and not the posterior teeth. During a straight protrusive movement the mandibular incisors pass down the lingual surfaces of the maxillary incisors, disoccluding the posterior teeth. During any lateroprotrusive movement the lateral incisors can also be involved in the guidance. As the movement becomes more lateral, the canines begin to contribute to the guidance.

Technique

After the CR contacts are established, they should never be altered. All adjustments for the eccentric contacts occur around the CR contacts without altering them.

The patient closes in CR, and the relationship of the anterior teeth is visualized. It is then determined whether immediate canine guidance is possible or a group function guidance is necessary (Fig. 19-14).

When a group function is indicated, the teeth that can assist in the guidance must be selected. The patient moves the mandible through the various lateral and protrusive excursions to reveal the most desirable contacts. In some instances gross mediotrusive contacts will actually disocclude the anterior teeth and make it difficult to visualize the best guidance (Fig. 19-15). When this occurs, it is

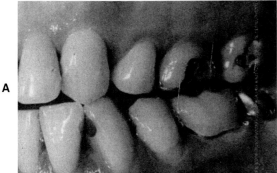
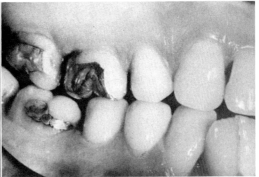

A **B**

Fig. 19-14 A, Canine guidance. The canines contact, disoccluding the posterior teeth during a laterotrusive movement. **B,** Group function guidance. Many posterior teeth participate in guiding the mandible during a laterotrusive movement.

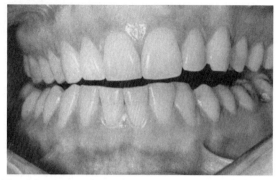

Fig. 19-15 During a right laterotrusive movement there is significant mediotrusive contact on the left third molars. This discludes the right side and must be eliminated before the type of laterotrusive guidance on the right side can be evaluated.

advisable to eliminate the mediotrusive contacts before determining the best guidance relationship.

Once the desirable guidance contacts have been determined, they are refined and the remaining eccentric contacts eliminated. To ensure that the already established CR contacts are not altered, two different marking papers are used. The teeth are dried, and blue marking paper is placed between them. The patient closes and taps on the posterior teeth. Then from the CR position a right excursion is made with return to centric, followed by a left excursion with return to centric. Finally, a straight protrusive movement is made with return to centric. The mouth is then opened, the blue paper is removed and replaced with red paper, and the patient closes and taps on the CR contacts. The red paper is removed, and the contacts are inspected. All eccentric contacts are now marked in blue, and the CR contacts are marked in red. The blue eccentric contacts are adjusted to meet the determined guidance condition without altering any red CR contacts. A red dot with a blue streak extending from it is typically seen (Fig. 19-16). This type of marking reveals that the red centric cusp tip contacts an opposing tooth incline during a particular eccentric movement.

When performing a selective grinding procedure it is extremely helpful to have a thorough understanding of the various locations of eccentric contacts. This will allow immediate identification

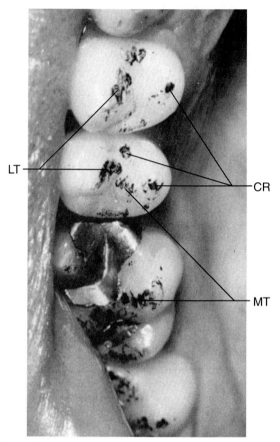

Fig. 19-16 Blue marking paper is used for the eccentric contacts, and red paper for the centric relation *(CR)* contacts. In this instance laterotrusive *(LT)* and mediotrusive *(MT)* contacts are present around the CR contacts.

of contacts that are desirable and those that must be eliminated.

During a lateral movement, laterotrusive contacts can occur between the inner inclines of the maxillary buccal cusps and the outer inclines of the mandibular buccal cusps. They can also occur between the outer inclines of the maxillary lingual cusps and the inner inclines of the mandibular lingual cusps. Mediotrusive contacts can occur between the inner inclines of the maxillary lingual cusps and the inner inclines of the mandibular buccal cusps. When the occlusal surfaces of the posterior teeth are visualized, there are certain areas of the teeth on which each of the contact areas can be found (Fig. 19-17). A comprehensive

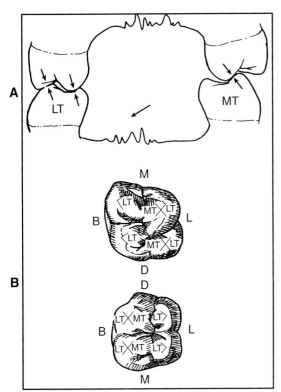

Fig. 19-17 When teeth occlude in a normal buccolingual relation, eccentric contacts occur on predictable areas of the teeth. **A,** Right lateral movement. **B,** Potential areas of contact on the maxillary and mandibular first molars. *B,* Buccal; *D,* distal; *L,* lingual; *LT,* laterotrusive; *M,* mesial; *MT,* mediotrusive.

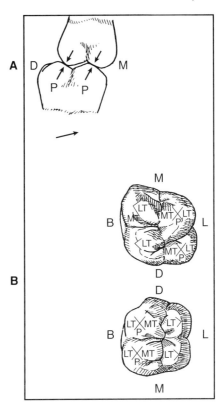

Fig. 19-18 A, Potential areas of posterior tooth contact *(small arrows)* during a protrusive movement *(large arrow).* **B,** All the potential areas of eccentric contacts on maxillary and mandibular first molars. *B,* Buccal; *D,* distal; *L,* lateral; *LT,* laterotrusive; *M,* mesial; *MT,* mediotrusive; *P,* protrusive.

understanding of these areas can simplify the selective grinding procedure.

During a protrusive movement, posterior protrusive contacts can occur between the distal inclines of the maxillary lingual cusps and the mesial inclines of the mandibular buccal cusps. When these potential contact sites are added to the occlusal surface of the posterior teeth, it is possible to visualize all the potential areas of eccentric contacts on the posterior teeth (Fig. 19-18).

Procedure for Canine Guidance. When the anterior tooth relationship provides for canine guidance, all blue marks on the posterior teeth are eliminated without alteration of the established CR contacts (red). Once this is accomplished, the teeth are redried and the blue eccentric and red centric marking procedure is repeated. Often several adjustments are necessary to achieve the

desired results. At the completion of this procedure the posterior teeth reveal only red CR contacts on the cusp tips and flat surfaces. The canines reveal the blue laterotrusive contacts, and the incisors (with possibly the canines) reveal the blue protrusive contacts (Fig. 19-19).

Procedure for Group Function Guidance. When the anterior tooth relationship is such that a group function is necessary for the guidance, all the blue contacts on the posterior teeth are not eliminated. Because selected posterior teeth are necessary to assist in the guidance, care must be taken not to eliminate these contacts. The desirable contacts are the laterotrusive on the buccal cusps of the premolars and the mesiobuccal cusp of the first molar. When the selective grinding procedure is completed, the occlusal condition

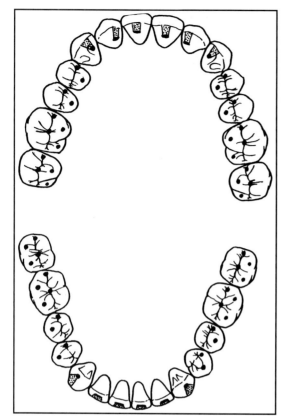

Fig. 19-19 DESIRED RESULTS OF A SELECTIVE GRINDING PROCEDURE. In this instance a canine guidance was achieved.

reveals only the red CR contacts on the posterior teeth (except for the blue laterotrusive contacts on the buccal cusps that are necessary to assist in the guidance). The canines reveal the blue laterotrusive contacts as the movement becomes great enough to disocclude these teeth. The incisors reveal the blue protrusive contacts (Fig. 19-20).

As discussed in an earlier chapter, the neuromuscular system that controls mandibular movement is protective. Tooth contacts that create interferences with normal function are avoided by protective reflex mechanisms. This protection exists during normal function but not usually during subconscious parafunctional activity. In other words, contacts likely to be present during parafunctional activities are avoided during examination of the teeth. These need to be identified and eliminated during a selective grinding procedure so that

they will not be present during parafunctional times. They are best identified by assisting the patient through the laterotrusive movements.[1]

As depicted in Fig. 19-21, force is applied to the inferior border and angle of the mandible in a superomedial direction as the patient moves in the mediotrusive direction. It assists the condyle in making a border movement that may not occur during normal function but can occur during parafunctional activity. Any tooth contacts that occur during this assisted movement are identified and eliminated during the selective grinding procedure.

EVALUATION IN THE UPRIGHT HEAD POSITION (ALERT FEEDING POSITION)

The selective grinding procedure is not complete until the upright head position has been evaluated. Because most such procedures are performed in a reclined position, there has been no consideration of postural changes of the jaw position in the preceding discussion. Evaluation for postural changes of the mandible must be accomplished before the patient is dismissed.

In the upright position with the head tilted forward approximately 30 degrees (placing the Frankfort plane 30 degrees off horizontal), the patient closes on the posterior teeth. Determining whether a postural change in the mandibular position has occurred that will cause anterior tooth contacts to be heavier than posterior tooth contacts is important. If this has occurred, the anterior tooth contacts are reduced slightly until the posterior teeth contact more heavily. Care must be taken in questioning the patient that the information received is valid. When the question is asked merely whether the anterior teeth contact more heavily, the patient may protrude slightly onto the guidance and check for contact; in this position the anterior tooth contacts will feel heavier and the patient will therefore answer affirmatively, with the result that a portion of the established guidance will be unnecessarily removed.

The most successful way to question a patient in the alert feeding position is to ask him or her to close the mouth and then tap the posterior teeth together. While this is being done, the patient is asked whether

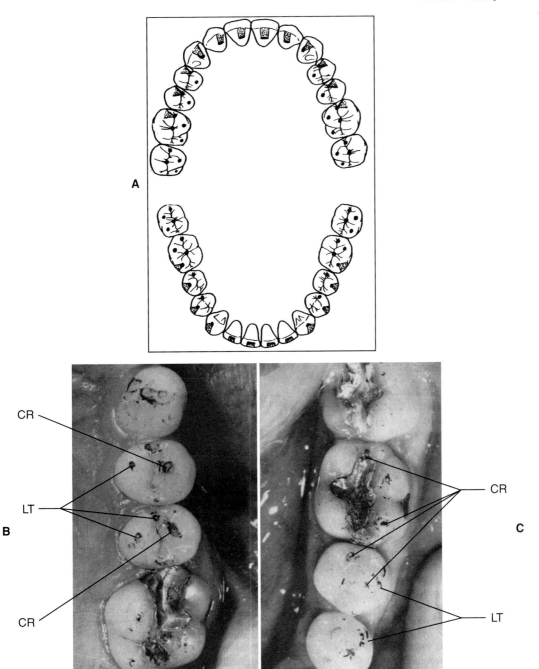

Fig. 19-20 A, Desired results of a selective grinding procedure. In this instance a group function guidance was achieved. **B** and **C,** Maxillary and mandibular teeth after a selective grinding procedure is completed. Note that group function guidance has been developed. The centric relation *(CR)* contacts have been developed on cusp tips and flat surfaces. Laterotrusive *(LT)* contacts are seen on canines and premolars. No mediotrusive contacts exist.

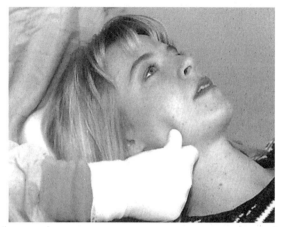

Fig. 19-21 ASSISTED MANDIBULAR MOVEMENT. Force is applied to the angle of the mandible in a mediosuperior direction to assist in identifying mediotrusive contacts.

the posterior teeth contact predominantly, the anterior teeth contact predominantly, or both anterior and posterior teeth contact equally. If the posterior teeth are contacting predominantly, minimal postural change has occurred and the selective grinding procedure is complete. If, however, the anterior teeth are contacting heavily or both anterior and posterior teeth are contacting evenly, a final adjustment in the alert feeding position is necessary. In this upright position the anterior teeth are dried, and red marking paper is placed between them. The patient again taps on the posterior teeth. Any red CR contacts on the anterior teeth are slightly reduced until the patient reports feeling predominantly the posterior teeth contacting. Normally one or two adjustments will accommodate for this postural change of the mandible. As soon as the posterior teeth are felt more predominantly, the selective grinding procedure is complete.

Patient Instructions

After the selective grinding procedure, the patient's muscles may feel tired. This is a normal finding, especially when the procedure has been accomplished during a long appointment. The patient can be informed that some teeth may feel gritty when rubbed together, but these will become smooth and polished within a few days.

Patients need not concentrate on any mandibular positions or tooth contacts to assist in the effectiveness of this procedure. Those who make a conscious effort to explore the occlusal conditions may likely find contacts not identified during the procedure and become concerned. The overall effect of such activity is generally muscle hyperactivity. Asking the patient to relax the muscles and keep the teeth from contacting is often the best advice.

PARTIAL SELECTIVE GRINDING

In some instances the patient may need only a partial selective grinding. For example, a prominent mediotrusive contact restricts mandibular movement during function. The initial reaction might be to eliminate it without altering any other feature of the occlusion. Although this could provide more freedom of mandibular movement, some precautions need to be considered before such partial selective grinding is undertaken.

If a mediotrusive contact is eliminated without regard to the stability of the tooth in the ICP, the tooth may be removed from occlusion and may then drift in such a way that the contact is reestablished or perhaps a new intercuspal relationship is introduced that precludes any permanent benefit from the grinding even though sufficient enamel has been removed (Fig. 19-22). On occasion, teeth that have been taken out of occlusion will not re-erupt and this introduces the problem of loss of ICP. As occlusal contacts are lost, the acute perception of mandibular position by the periodontal ligaments is also lost. This often leads to the patient constantly seeking a stable occlusal position, resulting in muscle hyperactivity (protective co-contraction). The condition is most effectively treated by returning the teeth to occlusal contact through restorative procedures. The development of a precise and stable ICP is essential for this patient.

Partial selective grinding is not indicated when orthopedic instability has been identified as the major causative factor creating a TMD. In this instance partial selective grinding relies only on the operator's guesswork in determining which interferences need to be eliminated. Complete selective grinding is the only method of improving orthopedic instability.

In a few instances, however, partial selective grinding may be helpful. When a patient complains of

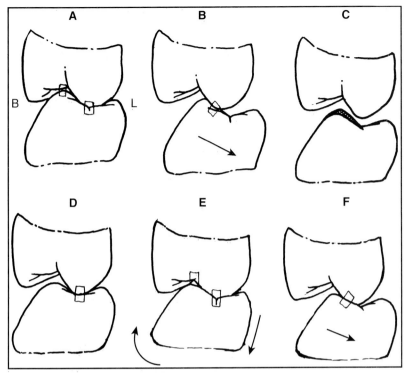

Fig. 19-22 Partial selective grinding can create undesirable tooth relationships. **A,** Stable intercuspal relation. **B,** A mediotrusive contact is present *(arrow).* **C,** The mediotrusive contact is removed without regard for the intercuspal position (ICP) or the mandibular buccal cusp. **D,** The centric contact on the mandibular buccal cusp has now been lost in the ICP. **E,** Drifting of the tooth can occur, which reestablishes cusp contact *(arrow).* **F,** Concomitant with this repositioning is the reestablishment of the undesirable mediotrusive contact *(arrow).* B, Buccal; L, lateral.

symptoms associated with a new restoration (acute changes in the occlusal condition), the restoration should be carefully examined. If undesirable contacts are present, they are eliminated to conform with the existing occlusal condition. When a single tooth is experiencing mobility or pulpitis, sometimes its occlusion should be adjusted to lessen the applied forces. One must understand that complete removal of the tooth from occlusal contact is only a temporary treatment. As the tooth re-erupts into occlusion, eccentric contact on it may reestablish the preexisting condition. It is generally better to lighten the tooth in the ICP while eliminating all eccentric contacts. This will maintain the tooth in a stable functional relationship while decreasing the likelihood of recurrent symptoms.

When mobility and pulpitis are present, partial selective grinding is considered to be only supportive therapy. It rarely affects the causative factors that create the problems. When a tooth becomes hypersensitive or mobile with no evidence of periodontal disease, parafunctional activity should be suspected. Partial selective grinding can assist in decreasing the symptoms associated with that tooth but will rarely affect the parafunctional activity. In these instances treatment that will decrease the parafunctional activity should be considered.

Reference

1. Okeson JP, Dickson JL, Kemper JT: The influence of assisted mandibular movement on the incidence of nonworking tooth contact, *J Prosthet Dent* 48:174-177, 1982.

Restorative Considerations in Occlusal Therapy

20

CHAPTER

"Restoring the teeth is basic to the practice of dentistry."

—JPO

*I*n the general practice of dentistry, the greatest number of procedures is in some form restorative. The rationale for providing this treatment is the replacement or rebuilding of missing tooth structure. Unfortunately, the influence that these procedures have on the occlusal condition of the teeth is often underemphasized. Most restorative procedures cannot be performed without influencing to some degree the existing occlusal condition. The potential effect of restorative procedures on the occlusion is obvious when a complete reconstruction of the dentition is being considered. However, one should be aware that even an occlusal amalgam can have a significant effect on the occlusion when the restoration is undercarved or overcarved.

On occasion, a series of small and seemingly insignificant changes will occur slowly over a period, resulting in a gradual loss of occlusal stability. These often go unnoticed by the patient until significant occlusal interferences have resulted. By contrast, abrupt changes in the occlusion are usually quickly noticed by the patient and therefore are often resolved before difficult consequences arise.

It is important to consider that all restorative procedures are, in some degree, a form of occlusal therapy. This statement is not always true, however, because some restorations do not replace occluding surfaces (e.g., a buccal pit restoration on a mandibular first molar or an anterior crown for a patient with an anterior open bite). Nevertheless, the vast majority of restorations do involve occluding surfaces. Because restorative procedures can affect the occlusal condition, when it is determined that occlusal therapy is indicated to resolve a temporomandibular disorder (TMD), restorative procedures can often provide the necessary occlusal changes to meet the treatment goals. Because restorative procedures use both addition and subtraction of tooth surfaces, a greater degree of occlusal change can be accomplished with these than with only selective grinding.

Restorative procedures and occlusal therapy should generally be considered inseparable. When restorative procedures are indicated primarily to eliminate dental caries and rebuild teeth, care must be taken to redevelop a sound functional occlusion. When they are indicated primarily as occlusal therapy, the same care must be taken to rebuild the teeth to sound aesthetics and a form compatible with the adjacent tissues.

In this chapter, restorative procedures are divided into two types: (1) operative and (2) fixed prosthodontic. Operative procedures are those in which the final restorations are fabricated intraorally (e.g., an amalgam, a composite resin). Fixed prosthodontic procedures are those that involve extraoral fabrication with final adjustment and cementation in the mouth (e.g., inlays, onlays, full crowns, fixed partial dentures). Although in this chapter little emphasis is placed on the removable partial denture, the same occlusal considerations are appropriate.

OPERATIVE CONSIDERATIONS IN OCCLUSAL THERAPY

Unfortunately, when operative techniques are discussed in the literature, little emphasis is usually placed on occlusal considerations. The success or failure of the procedure, however, relies not only on the margins and contours of the restorations but also on the occlusal relationship.

TREATMENT GOALS

To stabilize a tooth and provide optimum functional conditions, one must accomplish certain treatment goals. These can be divided into (1) tooth contacts and (2) mandibular position.

Treatment Goals for Tooth Contacts

Posterior Contacts. After an operative procedure, the new restoration must provide stability of both the opposing and the adjacent tooth so that drifting or eruption will not occur. When the mandible closes, the new restoration must provide for even, simultaneous, and harmonious occlusion with the existing posterior tooth contacts. It should direct forces through the long axes of the teeth. In many cases, before the restoration this stability and axial loading have been provided by reciprocating inclines as a cusp fit into an opposing fossa. Carving an amalgam back into a reciprocating incline contact relationship is often a difficult task. If it is attempted and full reciprocation is not achieved (missing an incline), instability can result. Therefore it is frequently best to develop the necessary stability and axial loading by carving the restoration to a cusp tip opposing a flat surface type of contact relationship. This will fulfill the treatment goals.

Anterior Contacts. The majority of operative procedures completed on the anterior teeth are composite resin restorations and should restore the teeth to normal form and function. One occlusal requirement of the anterior teeth (as indicated in Chapter 5) is to provide guidance for the

mandible during eccentric movement. Therefore in the closing position the anterior teeth should contact with less force than the posterior teeth. During an eccentric movement, available anterior teeth should guide the mandible and disocclude the posterior teeth. In the upright head position (alert feeding position), the anterior teeth should not contact as heavily as the posterior teeth.

Treatment Goals for the Mandibular Position

When operative procedures are performed, the mandibular position at which the restorations are developed depends largely on the presence of any functional disturbance of the masticatory system. When operative procedures are performed on a patient with no functional disturbances, the restorations are generally developed in the maximum intercuspal position (ICP). If a patient has a functional disturbance of the masticatory system, it is generally best to resolve it before the operative procedure begins. If in resolving the disorder it is determined that the occlusal condition is a major causative factor, then a selective grinding procedure (when determined to be feasible) should be completed before any operative procedures. Thus the restorations can be developed into the sound occlusal relationship achieved by the selective grinding procedure.

ACCOMPLISHING THE TREATMENT GOALS

Accomplishing the treatment goals for both anterior and posterior teeth is greatly enhanced by closely examining the occlusal conditions before the operative procedure. This is done by visualizing diagnostic casts or by having the patient close on articulating paper and marking the occlusal contacts (Fig. 20-1). Knowing the location of the existing contacts can greatly assist in reestablishing these contacts on the restoration.

Posterior Contacts

Reestablishing stable posterior tooth contacts on a new amalgam restoration can be a trying task. One quickly learns that leaving a new amalgam restoration too high often results in fracture of the restoration and the need for replacement.

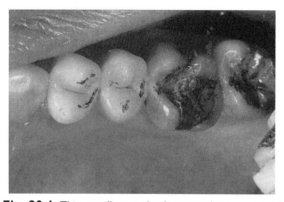

Fig. 20-1 This maxillary molar has mesial interproximal caries and will be restored. The occlusal contacts before the tooth is prepared have been marked with articulating paper. This will assist the operator in knowing which areas of the new restoration will support an occlusal contact. Of note is that the mesial marginal ridge has an occlusal contact.

Therefore a great tendency exists to overcarve the amalgam slightly and thus protect the setting amalgam from fracture. Although the immediate results are satisfying because the patient cannot detect any alteration in the occlusion, the condition that has been developed is usually unstable, allowing for drifting or eruption of the teeth until new occlusal contacts can be established. This drifting can result in undesirable tooth relationships or eccentric contacts, or both (Fig. 20-2).

Therefore amalgam restorations should be carved into and not out of occlusion. Initially the patient is asked to close gently on articulating paper, and the excess amalgam is carved away. Observing the occlusal contact before the operative procedure can provide valuable insight regarding the location and extent of carving that needs to be completed. The area of setting amalgam that opposes a centric cusp tip is carved to a flat surface. Depending on its location, the flat area will be either a marginal ridge or a central fossa. It is helpful to look for contacts on natural tooth structure. When these occur, the carving of the restoration is nearly complete. After it has been determined that the restoration is contacting evenly and simultaneously (on cusp tips and flat surfaces) with the opposing teeth, eccentric contacts are evaluated. A different-colored marking paper is helpful in identifying the eccentric contacts from the closing contacts (as in the selective grinding procedure; see Chapter 19). In most instances amalgam restorations do not serve as guidance surfaces for mandibular movement, and eccentric contact is therefore completely eliminated.

If the desired mandibular closure position is the ICP, movement posterior to this position is often possible. This movement must be evaluated so that the new restoration does not contribute any occlusal interferences in the posterior or retruded range of movement. If the initial tooth contact when the mandible is closed in centric relation (CR) is found to be on the new restoration, this surface is reduced so that the original CR contact pattern is not disturbed. In the absence of any functional disturbances, this contact pattern is considered to be physiologically acceptable and therefore no attempt is made to disrupt it.

Anterior Contacts

The initial guide used to develop anterior composite restorations is tooth morphology. When the composite is shaped and finished to the tooth's original contour, the occlusal condition is evaluated. Heavy contacts in the desired mandibular closure position are reduced. Frequently these can be detected by placing the fingers on the labial surfaces of the teeth while the patient closes and taps on the posterior teeth (Fig. 20-3). Heavy contacts tend to displace the teeth labially or cause heavy vibration (known as *fremitus*). These contacts are marked and adjusted until the fingers cannot detect any unusual displacement of the restored teeth.

When the contacts in mandibular closure have been adjusted, eccentric mandibular movements are observed. If a restoration is involved with an eccentric pathway, it should provide a smooth and unrestricted movement. Any irregularity of its surface must be smoothed to enhance this movement. A restoration that has been overcarved or overpolished, leaving a distinct catch or defect on its margin, is replaced. It is evaluated not only in straight protrusive and laterotrusive movements but also through various lateroprotrusive excursions.

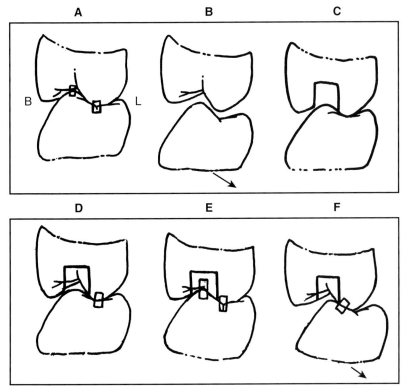

Fig. 20-2 A, In the intercuspal position (ICP), a stable occlusal relation exists. **B,** No contact during a mediotrusive movement. **C,** A preparation for an amalgam restoration has been completed on the maxillary molar. **D,** The new amalgam has been overcarved, resulting in a lack of contact with the mandibular buccal cusp. **E,** After a time the mandibular tooth shifts to a more stable occlusal position, which reestablishes contact between the mandibular buccal cusp and the restoration. **F,** Although the ICP is now stable, a mediotrusive contact has resulted.

When the restoration is adequately adjusted to the eccentric movements, the patient is brought upright in the dental chair and the alert feeding position is evaluated. Heavy contacts on the anterior teeth are reduced until the posterior teeth become more prominent.

FIXED PROSTHODONTIC CONSIDERATIONS IN OCCLUSAL THERAPY

Fixed prosthodontics affords many advantages in occlusal therapy over operative procedures. Although operative procedures involve replacing tooth surfaces, the occlusal condition is usually developed by careful removal of restorative material. In this sense, they are subject to the same limitations

as selective grinding. Fixed prosthodontics, however, uses the benefit of adding and subtracting tooth surfaces until the precise desired restoration is achieved. Because this is accomplished most often extraorally, errors stemming from poor intraoral working conditions (i.e., visibility, access, saliva) are avoided. With the appropriate use of articulators (see Chapter 18), restorations can be fabricated precisely to meet treatment goals. Once they are completed, final adjustments are made in the mouth.

TREATMENT GOALS

As with operative procedures, the treatment goals for fixed prosthodontics can be divided into tooth contacts and mandibular position.

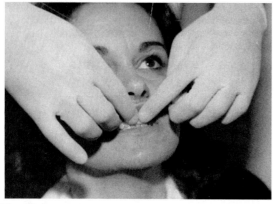

Fig. 20-3 Heavy anterior tooth contacts can be detected by placing the finger on the labial surface of the anterior teeth while the patient repeatedly closes and taps the posterior teeth together.

Treatment Goals for Tooth Contacts

Posterior Contacts. The posterior teeth should contact in a manner that provides stability while directing forces through the long axes of the teeth. Because precise tooth form can be developed, this axial loading may be accomplished by using reciprocating incline contacts around the centric cusps (known as *tripodization*) or by developing a cusp tip–to–opposing flat surface contact (Fig. 20-4). Both methods will achieve the treatment goals.

Anterior Contacts. The anterior teeth should lightly contact during closure while providing prominent contacts during eccentric movements. Because fixed prosthodontic procedures allow for greater control of the entire tooth form, the precise guidance pattern can be more carefully controlled. As with other procedures, the alert feeding position must not create heavy anterior tooth contacts.

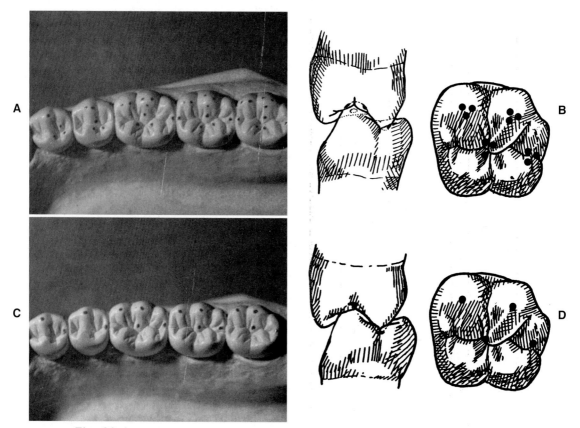

Fig. 20-4 A, Typical pattern of occlusal contacts when tripodization is used. **B,** Each centric cusp contacting an opposing fossa has three reciprocating contact areas. **C,** Typical pattern of occlusal contacts when the cusp tip–to–flat surface areas are used. **D,** Each centric cusp tip has a contact that opposes a flat surface.

Treatment Goals for the Mandibular Position

The mandibular position to which the fixed prosthodontic restorations are fabricated is determined by two factors: (1) the presence of any functional disturbance in the masticatory system and (2) the extent of the procedures indicated.

Functional Disturbances. A thorough examination of the patient must be performed before any fixed prosthetic procedures. If any functional disturbance is noted, it is treated and resolved before the procedures begin. If it is determined by reversible occlusal therapy and the other considerations discussed in Chapter 15 that the existing occlusal condition is a contributing causative factor to the disorder, a selective grinding procedure is completed so that a stable occlusal condition is developed in the desired mandibular position (CR). Once this occlusal relationship is established, the fixed restorations are developed to stabilize the occlusal condition and mandibular position.

Extent of Treatment. In patients with no signs of functional disturbance of the masticatory system, the extent of fixed prosthodontics indicated determines the mandibular position to be used in restoring the occlusion. Patients with no functional disturbance basically demonstrate that their occlusal condition falls within their physiologic tolerance.

When minor fixed restorative procedures are indicated (e.g., a single crown), it is appropriate for the restoration to be developed in harmony with the existing occlusal condition (Fig. 20-5). Therefore the crown is fabricated in the ICP and placed in harmony with the existing eccentric guidance. It is difficult to justify altering the complete occlusal condition to one considered more favorable when the patient is functioning without difficulties.

However, when a patient requires extensive fixed prosthetic procedures, the optimum mandibular position (CR) should be used regardless of the patient's apparent tolerance of the ICP (Fig. 20-6). Two considerations make this appropriate: First, the ICP is completely determined by tooth contacts. During the preparation phase of the procedure, these contacts are eliminated, causing the original ICP to be lost. A new ICP can be developed; however, there is no evidence that this position will be equally tolerated by the patient. When the ICP is lost, the most acceptable treatment is to use the most musculoskeletally stable position of the condyle as a reference in developing a stable occlusal condition. Second, this position also has the advantage of repeatability, which can assist in developing a very precise occlusal condition.

Preventing TMDs has not been documented to date (see Chapter 17). Because many factors can contribute to functional disturbances of the masticatory system, it is extremely difficult, if not impossible, to predict the future development of a TMD. Yet when an extensive amount of occlusal alteration is planned and the original occlusal contact position will be lost, it seems only logical that the most stable mandibular position should be used in rebuilding the occlusal condition. If prevention is

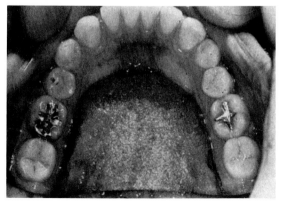

Fig. 20-5 Examination reveals little need for restorative treatment. The gold inlay fabricated for the mandibular first molar has been developed in the intercuspal position.

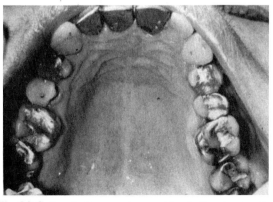

Fig. 20-6 Examination reveals a need for significant restorative treatment. It should be developed in an optimum joint position (centric relation).

possible, this position would seem to be most advantageous.

Even when a single restoration is all that is indicated, the overall health of the mouth must be considered in determining the mandibular position to which the crown will be developed. When it can be predicted that over time the patient will need more extensive fixed restorative procedures, it is wise to begin the first restoration in the CR position. This will provide a stable joint position and offer reproducibility, which allows each consecutive restoration to be fabricated in the same mandibular position. When CR is not used as a reference, it is difficult to coordinate the treatment goals for each procedure over several years. The results frequently reflect an extensively restored mouth with uncontrolled occlusal conditions.

This section can be summarized by categorizing all patients with fixed prosthetic needs into one of four groups (Table 20-1). The general treatment plan and sequence for each are presented. Because a simple illustration cannot accurately classify all patients, only extreme examples are depicted. Much thought

and analysis must go into treatment planning for patients who do not have such clear-cut needs (e.g., the patient who requires a three-unit fixed partial denture and has a 6-year history of asymptomatic clicking of the right temporomandibular joint).

ACCOMPLISHING THE TREATMENT GOALS

In planning and sequencing fixed prosthodontic treatment procedures, it is generally appropriate to develop the anterior tooth contacts first. When the anterior teeth have been developed to provide the acceptable guidance for eccentric mandibular movement, the posterior teeth can be developed in harmony with that guidance.

Anterior Contacts

Careful examination of the functional relations of the anterior teeth should be completed before beginning any anterior fixed prosthodontic procedures. The adequacy of the anterior guidance during eccentric mandibular movements should be

---

TABLE **20-1**

General Summary of Treatment Planning and Sequencing

Condition of Masticatory System	CONDITION OF DENTITION	
	Need for Minor Occlusal Alterations (e.g., One Crown)	Need for Major Occlusal Alterations (e.g., Full-Mouth Reconstruction)
Functional disturbance	**Patient Type A** Resolution of disturbance Stabilization of occlusal condition with selective grinding (when possible) Fabrication of crown to stabilize occlusal condition Fabrication of crown to existing occlusal condition (care taken not to introduce any centric or eccentric premature contacts)	**Patient Type B** Resolution of disturbance Stabilization of occlusal condition with selective grinding (when possible) Fabrication of crowns to stabilize occlusal condition
No functional disturbance	**Patient Type C** Fabrication of crown to existing occlusal condition (care taken not to introduce any centric or eccentric premature contacts)	**Patient Type D** Stabilization of occlusal condition with selective grinding Fabrication of crowns to stabilize occlusal condition

determined (i.e., the ability of the anterior teeth to disocclude the posterior teeth). The sequence in which the anterior teeth are restored depends on whether the existing anterior guidance is adequate or inadequate.

Adequate Guidance. In many instances the morphology and function of the anterior teeth provide adequate anterior guidance, yet there are indications to restore these teeth. During the preparation stage, the teeth are reduced and the characteristics of the existing guidance are obliterated. Once these characteristics are lost, the new restorations can be fabricated only arbitrarily. However, arbitrary development of the guidance often produces conditions that are less well tolerated by the patient. If the restored angle of the anterior guidance is less steep, the posterior teeth may not be disoccluded during the entire eccentric movement. If the restored angle is too steep, a restricted mandibular pattern that compromises muscle function may be developed. To avoid these complications, the precise characteristics of the anterior guidance should be preserved and the new restorations fabricated to it. The characteristics of the anterior guidance can be recorded and preserved on an articulator by a custom guidance table.

Custom anterior guidance table. A custom anterior guidance table is easily developed on most semi-adjustable articulators. The characteristics of a patient's prerestored anterior guidance are transferred to this table and maintained while the teeth are prepared. When new restorations are fabricated, the characteristics of the original guidance can be duplicated in the new restorations. Thus anterior resolutions that provide the identical guidance of the original anterior teeth are developed.

The fabrication of a custom anterior guidance table begins with accurately mounted diagnostic casts on a semiadjustable articulator. The incisal pin is pulled away from the table approximately I mm, and a small amount of self-curing acrylic resin is placed on the anterior table. The mandibular cast is occluded with the maxillary cast, which causes the incisal pin to penetrate into the setting acrylic resin (Fig. 20-7). From its occluded position the mandibular cast is slowly moved through various eccentric motions. The incisal pin is also moved

through these motions, and the resin is molded to the specific characteristics of the excursions as the pin travels along the pathway dictated by the contact pattern of the anterior teeth.

Once all of the movements have been performed, the resin is allowed to set. If the set is accurate, the incisal pin will contact the resin in all movements at the time that the maxillary and mandibular anterior teeth are contacting. If the pin or teeth do not contact in all excursions, it is likely that the resin has been slightly distorted. When this occurs, corrections must be made. If the inaccuracy is caused by the fact that the teeth do not contact, the resin can often be adjusted to allow proper movement. If the inaccuracy is a result of the pin not contacting the resin, relining the incisal guide table with new resin may be necessary.

After it has been determined that the custom anterior guidance table with the diagnostic casts is accurate, the anterior teeth are prepared for the restorations. The working casts with the dies of the prepared teeth are accurately mounted on the articulator. As the mandibular member is moved through the various eccentric excursions, the incisal pin contacts the custom-designed resin and the original guidance is demonstrated. The new restorations are developed to contact the opposing teeth during the eccentric movements guided by the incisal pin. The original anterior guidance has then been duplicated.

Inadequate Anterior Guidance. Sometimes, because of missing, malaligned, or broken-down anterior teeth, the existing anterior guidance is inadequate. For these patients the anterior teeth must be altered to furnish more acceptable guidance. Fabrication of a custom anterior guidance table from the original casts is not helpful because this only duplicates the existing inadequate guidance. The anterior teeth must be prepared for the new restorations, and provisional or temporary restorations must be fabricated.

The provisional restorations are developed to provide adequate anterior guidance and aesthetics. In some instances it may also be desirable to reposition the teeth orthodontically (Fig. 20-8). Because these provisional restorations alter the anterior guidance, patients should be observed for

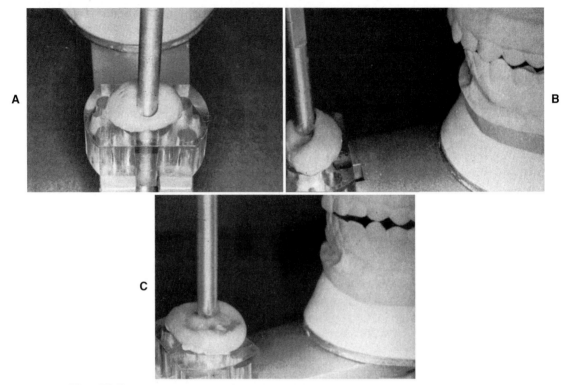

Fig. 20-7 FABRICATION OF A CUSTOM ANTERIOR GUIDANCE TABLE.
A, A small amount of setting acrylic resin is placed on the incisal table of a semiadjustable articulator. When the casts are closed, the incisal pin penetrates the acrylic resin. **B,** The mandibular cast is moved through the entire range of protrusive and lateral excursions while the resin is setting. **C,** Once the resin is set, the incisal pin should contact the incisal table at the same time that the maxillary and mandibular teeth are contacting each other during each eccentric movement.

several weeks (or even months) to determine their acceptance of this change. This trial period will determine not only the acceptability of the new guidance but also the new aesthetics. If the changes prove to be unsuccessful, the provisionals are altered until acceptable guidance and aesthetics are achieved. When guidance is proved to be acceptable, a diagnostic cast of the teeth is made. This is accurately mounted on the articulator, and the custom anterior guidance table is fabricated to the contours of the provisional restorations. Once it is decided that the table is accurate, the working cast with sectioned dies is mounted and the appropriate tooth form is developed in the final restorations, duplicating the information stored in the custom anterior guidance table.

Another method whereby adequate anterior guidance can be established is with a diagnostic prewax. With this method, diagnostic casts are mounted on an articulator and the anterior teeth are waxed to provide desirable anterior guidance and aesthetics. A diagnostic cast of the prewax is then used to fabricate the provisional anterior restorations. If these prove to be adequate for the patient, the custom anterior guidance table is fabricated on the basis of the altered diagnostic cast. If they prove to be inadequate, they are altered intraorally until adequate. Once it is determined that the restorations are adequate, a diagnostic cast of the provisionals is mounted on the articulator and the custom anterior guidance table is fabricated on the basis of this cast.

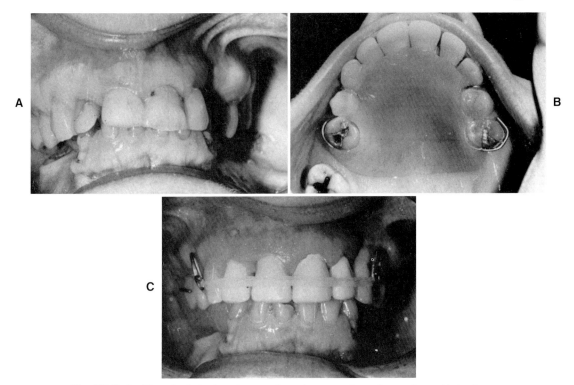

Fig. 20-8 A, These badly broken-down and poorly restored anterior teeth provide inadequate anterior guidance. **B,** The teeth have been prepared, and provisional acrylic crowns fabricated. A removable orthodontic appliance has also been inserted. **C,** The appliance provides an elastic that orthodontically retracts the anterior teeth, returning them to a more ideal position. During this treatment the provisional crowns are reshaped to provide desirable anterior guidance and aesthetics. Once this has been achieved, a diagnostic cast is made and a custom anterior guidance table is developed to be used in fabricating the permanent crowns.

Not all inadequate guidance can be corrected by fixed prosthetic procedures. As tooth malalignment and interarch discrepancy become greater, other methods such as orthodontics or orthognathic surgery may be considered. This is especially true when there are no other indications to restore the teeth (Fig. 20-9). Complete analysis of the casts before treatment is helpful in determining an appropriate treatment plan.

Posterior Contacts

When adequate anterior guidance has been achieved, the posterior teeth can be restored to provide stable occlusal steps in the CR position. When adequate guidance is present, the posterior teeth should contact only in the closed position and not during any eccentric movement. The posterior contacts must provide stability while also directing occlusal forces through the long axes of the teeth.

As mentioned earlier, this can be accomplished by developing a tripodization contact pattern for the centric cusps or by a centric cusp tip–to–flat surface contact. Each technique has advantages and disadvantages, as follows:

1. *Tripodization:* Tripodization uses opposing tooth inclines to establish a stable intercuspal relationship. Each centric cusp is developed to have three equally distributed contacts around its tip. These share the force of occlusion

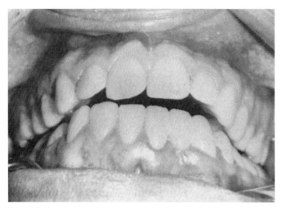

Fig. 20-9 This anterior open bite provides poor anterior guidance, which is best improved with orthodontic treatment. Fixed prosthodontics is contraindicated because the distance between the maxillary and mandibular teeth is too great to be effectively corrected with crowns.

equally, creating a stable position for the cusp. With some techniques a cusp contacts an embrasure between two opposing marginal ridges, resulting in two reciprocating contacts (bipodization). The final result is often the development of 10 to 12 contacts per molar restoration (see Fig. 20-4, *A*). Academically, the technique is sound. However, practically it has many disadvantages. Often it is difficult to develop and maintain all the reciprocating contacts through the fabrication and delivery phase. If during fabrication the final crown is missing one or more contacts, reciprocation is lost and the stability of the tooth can be jeopardized. Tripodization is also difficult to accomplish when a restoration is being fabricated to occlude with the relatively flat amalgam restoration. In other words, this technique is best suited when the opportunity exists to develop opposing restorations. It is also difficult when the guidance is not immediately provided during eccentric movements or when there is an immediate lateral translation movement present. In both instances posterior teeth will move laterally before being disoccluded by the anterior teeth. Eliminating posterior contacts in the laterotrusive movement when the cusps are already contacting adjacent inclines in the ICP is difficult.

2. *Cusp tip–to–flat surface contact:* A second acceptable method of developing posterior tooth contacts is by using cusp tips to flat surfaces (see Fig. 20-4, *B*). Achieving this allows occlusal forces to be directed through the long axes of the teeth. Even if during the fabrication of a restoration a contact is lost, the remaining contacts will provide the necessary stability while directing forces through the long axes. Cusp tip–to–flat surface contacts can be satisfactorily accomplished against amalgams, and when an immediate lateral translation movement is present, the fossa can be easily widened to eliminate any potential eccentric contacts.

In summary, both techniques produce a stable occlusal contact relationship. Tripodization is better used when guidance is immediate and opposing surfaces can be controlled. In other words, it is indicated more in full reconstruction of the dental arches. However, it can be a difficult procedure to accomplish. Success is more readily achieved with a cusp tip–to–flat surface technique, which can be used regardless of the extent of restoration needs. Therefore it is a more practical and widely applicable procedure.

On occasion, a cusp-fossa relationship will lend itself to one or the other of these techniques. Using both in the same restoration when appropriate conditions exist is possible. The following section describes in detail the technique for developing cusp tip–to–flat surface contacts while providing good tooth form.

Waxing Technique. In this wax-added technique,[1] a pattern is created by developing and blending specific tooth components. It can be used for single restorations as well as complete posterior reconstructions.

To simplify the discussion, the development of a right maxillary molar wax pattern is demonstrated as follows:

1. Begin with accurate diagnostic casts mounted in CR on a semiadjustable articulator. Develop a removable die for the right maxillary first molar preparation and trim appropriately (Fig. 20-10).

2. Apply a separating medium to the die so that the final wax pattern can be easily removed. Using waxing instruments, a source of heat, and

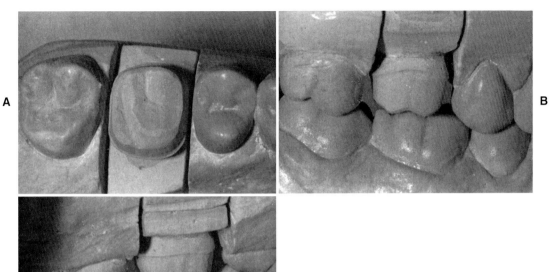

Fig. 20-10 **A,** Die for a full gold crown preparation (occlusal view). **B,** Buccal and **C,** lingual views.

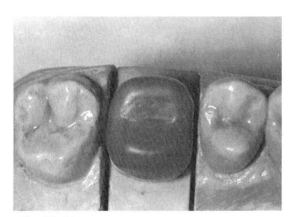

Fig. 20-11 Wax coping over the entire preparation.

inlay wax, form a wax coping that will cover the entire preparation (Fig. 20-11).

3. Examine the occlusal surface of the maxillary right posterior quadrant, noting the buccolingual, linguoocclusal, and central fossa lines.

Using the position of the adjacent cusp tips as a guide, scratch these three lines across the occlusal table that has been developed in the wax coping (Fig. 20-12).

Remember that the centric cusps (lingual) are located approximately one third of the distance into the occlusal surface of the tooth and the noncentric cusps (buccal) one sixth of the distance. The central fossa line is generally through the center of the tooth. These markings will offer guidelines in the appropriate placement of cusps.

4. Close the casts together and try to visualize the most appropriate mesiodistal locations of the centric cusps. Each cusp tip of the molar tooth should contact on a flat surface, either in a fossa or on a marginal ridge of the opposing tooth. The position of this tooth will permit the mesiolingual cusp to contact in the central fossa of the opposing molar, whereas the distolingual cusp contacts the distal marginal ridge of the opponent (Fig. 20-13).

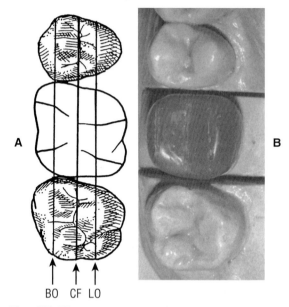

Fig. 20-12 A, The buccoocclusal *(BO)*, linguoocclusal *(LO)*, and central fossa *(CF)* lines are drawn. **B,** These lines are marked on the occlusal surface of the wax coping.

The contact location of each cusp tip is determined individually according to the position and relations of the teeth. In another patient these cusps might contact in different locations. Remember that each centric cusp tip must contact on a flat surface, which may be at the base of the central fossa or at the crest of a marginal ridge as dictated by tooth alignment and intercuspation.

Step 1: Centric Cusp (Lingual) Tips. Using appropriate waxing instruments and ivory wax, develop the centric cusp cones. Different-colored waxes are helpful in demonstrating this technique. Once the components of the tooth are learned, a single-colored wax is used to expedite the procedure. Place the centric cones at the appropriate mesiodistal position on the linguoocclusal lines. The height and direction of the cusps can be determined by closing the articulator and visualizing the occlusal relationships from the lingual. The diameter of the base of the cone will be approximately one third the mesiodistal diameter of the respective cusp.

Sufficient space must be allowed to wax the lingual cusp ridge and triangular ridges. Wax the mesiolingual cusp to contact a flat area located in the central fossa of the mandibular first molar. Wax the distolingual cusp to contact on the crest of the distal marginal ridge of the mandibular first molar. These contacts are developed only on the cusp tips and do not involve any inclines (Fig. 20-14). Once the cones are developed, move the mandibular cast through the various laterotrusive and protrusive excursions. The cones should not contact any opposing surface during these movements.

Step 2: Mesial and Distal Marginal Ridges. The next portion of the wax pattern to be developed is the marginal ridges. In visualizing the occluded casts from the lingual, it is determined

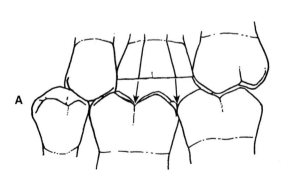
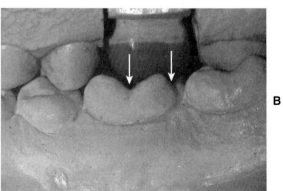

Fig. 20-13 A, The mesiolingual cusp of the maxillary molar will contact in the central fossa area of the mandibular molar, and the distolingual cusp of the maxillary molar will contact on the distal marginal ridge of the mandibular molar. **B,** Same cusp locations from the lingual of the wax coping.

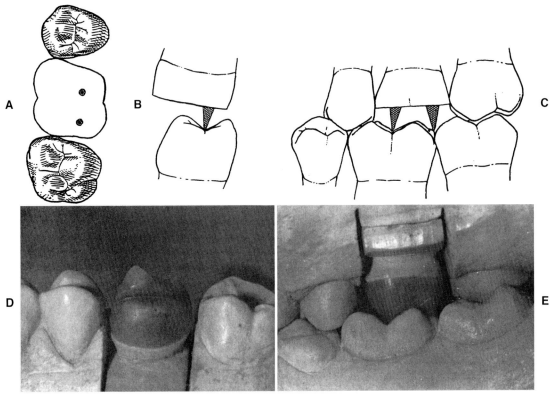

Fig. 20-14 DEVELOPMENT OF THE LINGUAL CENTRIC CUSP CONES. Occlusal **(A)**, proximal **(B)**, and lingual **(C)** views. **D,** Lingual centric cusp cones developed on the wax coping. **E,** Mesiolingual cusp contacting in the central fossa; distolingual cusp on the distal marginal ridge is demonstrated.

that the mesiobuccal cusp of the mandibular first molar will most appropriately contact the mesial marginal ridge of the maxillary first molar. It also appears that the distal marginal ridge will be unopposed because the mesiobuccal cusp of the mandibular second molar contacts the mesial marginal ridge of the maxillary second molar (see Fig. 20-14, *C*).

Using blue wax, develop the mesial and distal marginal ridges in a triangular shape with the apex of the triangle at the occlusal pit. The mesial marginal ridge should contact the opposing cusp on the central fossa line (Fig. 20-15). Make the distal marginal ridge in good form to the same height as the adjacent marginal ridges. From the occlusal

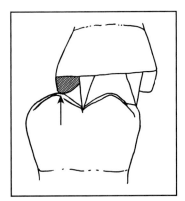

Fig. 20-15 The mesial marginal ridge is developed so that the mandibular centric cusp tip will contact on a flat surface (the crest of the marginal ridge).

view the marginal ridges of a tooth should converge toward the lingual, creating a greater lingual than buccal embrasure. The proximal contact areas should be located slightly buccal to the central fossa line. The contour from the crest of the marginal ridge to the apex of the triangle represents a portion of the fossa and is a convex surface sloping from the crest of the ridge to the apex of the triangle (Fig. 20-16).

Step 3: Central Fossa Contact Area. The next portion of the wax pattern to be developed is the central fossa contact area. This represents the final occlusal contact area for the tooth.

Again, examine the occluded casts from the lingual and visualize whether the distobuccal cusp of the mandibular first molar is in an appropriate position to contact the central fossa of the maxillary first molar (see Fig. 20-16, *C*). Develop a central fossa contact area in blue wax. It should have

a superior surface that is slightly convex, with the highest point at the center (the contact area). From the occlusal view this area is rhomboid shaped, with each of its apexes fitting into a developmental occlusal groove. The mesiodistal and buccolingual diameters of the area should be approximately 2 mm (Fig. 20-17).

After this step is completed, all the occluding surfaces of the wax pattern have been established. The remaining portions of the tooth need to be developed to good tooth form without any centric or eccentric contacts.

Step 4: Lingual Cusp Ridges. Develop the lingual cusp ridges in red wax. These should have a definite convexity between the lingual height of contour and the cusp tip. From the lingual view they should be triangular shaped with the apex at the cusp tip and base at the wax coping. The addition of these ridges should in no way modify the

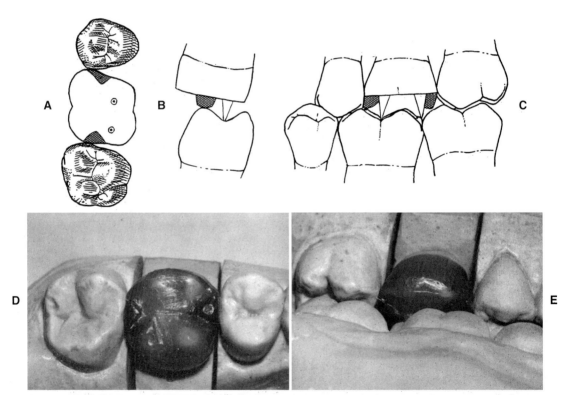

Fig. 20-16 DEVELOPMENT OF THE MARGINAL RIDGES. Occlusal **(A)**, proximal **(B)**, and lingual **(C)** views. **D,** Marginal ridge on the wax pattern. The contact on the mesial ridge is demonstrated. **E,** Marginal ridge in occlusion.

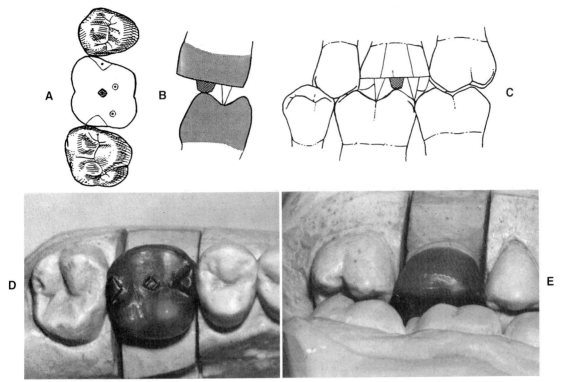

Fig. 20-17 DEVELOPMENT OF THE CENTRAL FOSSA CONTACT AREA. Occlusal **(A)**, proximal **(B)**, and lingual **(C)** views. **D** and **E,** Central fossa contact area on the wax pattern and in occlusion.

existing cusp tips (in ivory wax) because they do not contact the opposing teeth in any centric or eccentric position (Fig. 20-18).

Step 5: Mesial and Distal Lingual Cusp Ridges. Develop the mesial and distal cusp ridges in green wax. Each lingual cusp should have a mesial and a distal lingual cusp ridge that does not alter the cusp tip (ivory wax). The mesiolingual and distolingual cusp ridges should provide physiologic occlusal embrasures and proper transitional line angles (Fig. 20-19). They must not contact the opposing tooth in any centric or eccentric position. Development of mesiolingual and distolingual cusp ridges should leave sufficient space for the triangular and oblique ridges.

Step 6: Lingual Cusp Triangular Ridges. Develop a lingual cusp triangular ridge for each lingual cusp that extends from the cusp tip to the central fossa (Fig. 20-20). The triangular ridges should

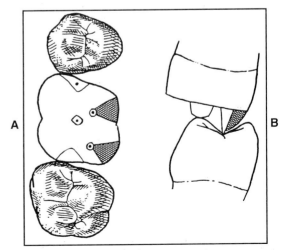

Fig. 20-18 DEVELOPMENT OF THE LINGUAL CUSP RIDGES. Occlusal **(A)** and proximal **(B)** views.

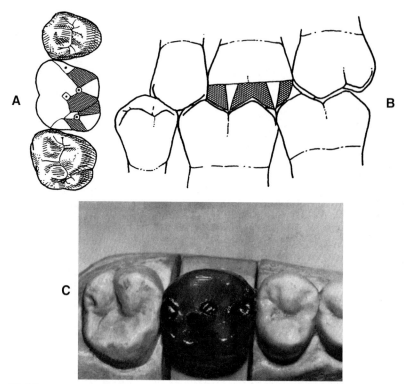

Fig. 20-19 DEVELOPMENT OF THE MESIOLINGUAL AND DISTOLINGUAL CUSP RIDGES. Occlusal **(A)** and proximal **(B)** views. **C,** Wax pattern with the mesial and distal cusp ridges added.

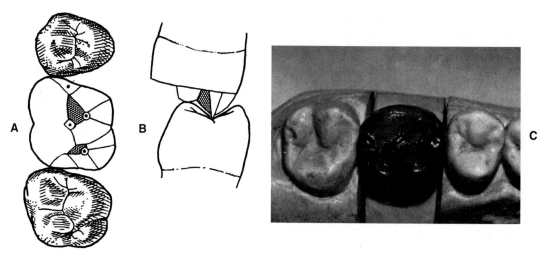

Fig. 20-20 DEVELOPMENT OF THE LINGUAL CUSP TRIANGULAR RIDGES. Occlusal **(A)** and proximal **(B)** views. **C,** Wax pattern with the lingual triangular ridge added.

be convex both from the cusp tip to the fossa line and from the mesial aspect to the distal aspect. Each lingual cusp triangular ridge should have a greater mesiodistal width at the central fossa than at the cusp tip and should slope down from the cusp tip to the fossa. The lingual cusp triangular ridge in no way modifies the existing cusp tip (ivory wax). Develop supplementary grooves to separate the mesial and distal aspects of the lingual cusp ridges from the respective inner aspects of the mesiolingual and distolingual cusp ridges. The triangular ridge of the mesiolingual cusp should angle slightly distally as it approaches the central developmental groove. The triangular ridge

of the distobuccal cusp should angle markedly mesially as it approaches the lingual developmental groove. As with the other cusp inclines, the lingual cusp triangular ridges must not contact the opposing teeth in any centric or eccentric position.

Step 7: Noncentric (Buccal) Cusp Tips. Develop the mesial and distal noncentric (buccal) cusp tips in ivory wax on the buccoocclusal line. The buccal cusp tip should vertically and horizontally overlap the opposing tooth in the occluded position (Fig. 20-21). During laterotrusive movement these cusps are developed to pass through the embrasures and grooves of the opposing tooth

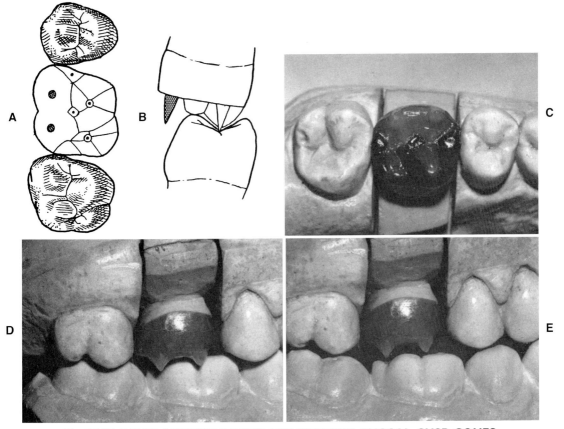

Fig. 20-21 DEVELOPMENT OF THE NONCENTRIC BUCCAL CUSP CONES. Occlusal **(A)** and proximal **(B)** views. **C,** Wax pattern with the buccal cusp cones added. **D,** Buccal cusp cones with the teeth in occlusion. **E,** The buccal cusp cones are disoccluded during a laterotrusive movement.

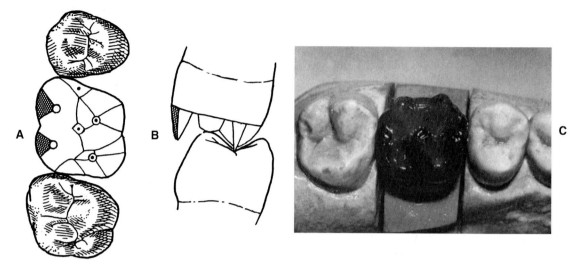

Fig. 20-22 DEVELOPMENT OF THE BUCCAL CUSP RIDGES. Occlusal **(A)** and proximal **(B)** views. **C,** Wax pattern with the buccal cusp ridges added.

without contact. Sufficient room must be allowed to wax the surrounding cuspal ridges.

Step 8: Buccal Cusp Ridges. With red wax, develop the buccal cusp ridges and blend them to the buccal cusp cones. They should be triangular with their apex at the cusp tip and the base on the wax coping (Fig. 20-22). Each buccal cusp ridge has a slight convexity between the crest of the contour and the cusp tip. It should not modify the existing cusp tip. There is no contact with any opposing tooth in any centric or eccentric position.

Step 9: Mesiobuccal and Distobuccal Cusp Ridges. Each buccal cusp has a mesial and a distal ridge that is developed with green wax. Each mesiobuccal and distobuccal cusp ridge has a slight convexity between the buccal crest of contour and the buccoocclusal line. The mesiobuccal and distobuccal cusp ridges do not modify the existing cusp tip or contact any opposing tooth surface in any centric or eccentric position.

The mesiobuccal and distobuccal transitional line angles should be continuous with the remaining wax pattern, providing physiologic buccal embrasures (Fig. 20-23). The inner aspect of the mesiobuccal ridge of the mesiobuccal cusp and the distobuccal cusp ridge of the distobuccal cusp are convex surfaces that slope down into the

marginal ridges and form the buccal portion of the mesioocclusal and distoocclusal fossae. The mesiobuccoocclusal and distobuccoocclusal point angles should align buccolingually with the point angle of the adjacent teeth, providing a physiologic occlusal embrasure.

Step 10: Buccal Cusp Triangular Ridges. Complete the wax pattern by developing the buccal cusp triangular ridges in red wax. Each buccal cusp triangular ridge should be convex in all dimensions, both from the cusp tip to the central fossa line and from the mesial aspect to the distal. The buccal cusp triangular ridge has greater mesiodistal width at the central fossa line than at the cusp tip and does not modify the existing cusp tip (Fig. 20-24). Supplemental grooves are developed to separate the mesial and distal aspects of the buccal cusp triangular ridges from the respective inner aspects of the mesiobuccal and distobuccal cusp ridges. The buccal cusp triangular ridges do not contact the opposing teeth in any centric or eccentric position.

After this step, the wax pattern is complete. Reevaluating the pattern for occlusal contacts and verifying that these contact areas occur between cusp tips and opposing flat surfaces are appropriate. The mandibular casts are moved through the

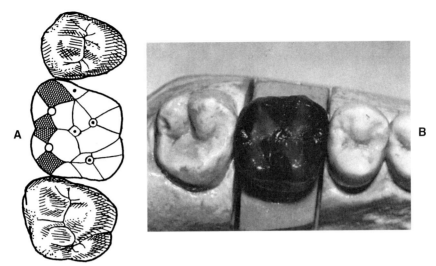

Fig. 20-23 DEVELOPMENT OF THE MESIAL AND DISTAL BUCCAL CUSP RIDGES. A, Occlusal view. **B,** Wax pattern.

various eccentric positions to verify the absence of any contacts on the wax pattern. Care is taken that all information received from the patient and stored in the articulator is transferred in the movements of the wax pattern. When the various colored waxes are used, the final wax pattern is developed as depicted in Fig. 20-25.

Once the occlusal portion of the wax pattern is correctly developed, the anatomic form of the entire pattern is evaluated. When sound tooth contours are refined and margins perfected, the pattern is removed, invested, cast, and prepared for the patient's mouth. Remember that the purpose of the restoration is not to fit the articulator but to fit the patient's mouth. The clinician must be prepared, therefore, to make any necessary adjustments in the mouth that will make up for the shortcomings of the articulator, as well as any other errors that have been introduced.

When the casting is placed in the mouth, proximal contacts and margins are evaluated first. Once these requirements are satisfied, the occlusal aspect of the restoration is evaluated. The patient closes in the desired contact position, and the adjacent teeth are observed for occlusal contacts. This helps identify the degree of adjustment required to bring the new restoration into harmony with the other teeth. If space is observed between adjacent occluding teeth, extensive grinding is likely to be indicated. Red marking paper is placed between the dried teeth, and any heavy red contact areas are identified and reduced. Care must be taken to maintain the desired form of the contact (either flat surface or cusp tip) during the adjustment. The adjustment of the restoration in the ICP is complete if shim stock (0.0005-inch cellophane tape) binds between the adjacent teeth when the patient closes. The patient can provide valuable information regarding contact of the restoration, especially when anesthesia is not necessary for the adjustment phase. Once the restoration is adequately adjusted in the desired closure position, eccentric movements are evaluated.

If the restoration has been developed in the maximum ICP, the mandible is positioned in CR and the CR-to-ICP slide is evaluated. The new restoration should not alter in any way the pre-existing slide. If CR contacts have been created on the restoration, they are eliminated. When the restoration has been fabricated in the CR position, these adjustments are already incorporated in the fabrication of the wax pattern and should need only slight intraoral refinements.

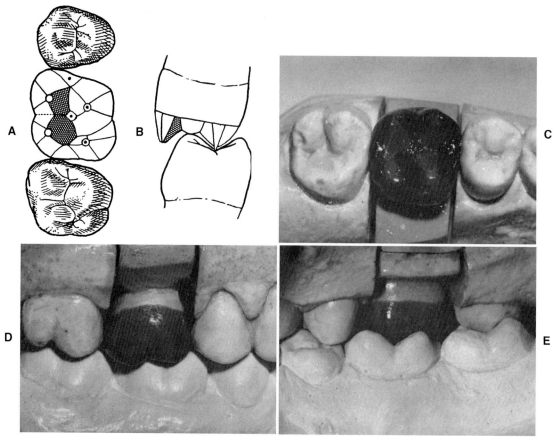

Fig. 20-24 Development of the buccal cusp triangular ridge, which completes the waxing procedure. Occlusal **(A)** and proximal **(B)** views. The wax pattern is completed by the addition of the buccal cusp triangular ridges. Occlusal **(C)**, buccal **(D)**, and lingual **(E)** views.

Laterotrusive and protrusive eccentric movements are evaluated next. As in the selective grinding procedure, two different-colored marking papers are helpful in the adjustment of eccentric movements. Blue articulating paper is placed between the dried teeth. The patient closes in the ICP and then moves the mandible through left and right laterotrusive, as well as straight, protrusive excursions. (It is helpful to assist the mandible with extraoral force on the mediotrusive side so that the protective reflex system does not avoid mesiotrusive contacts.) Red marking paper is then placed, and the patient again closes into ICP. When adequate anterior guidance is present, all blue marks are eliminated. If it is necessary to provide

laterotrusive guidance on certain posterior teeth, the desired guidance contacts are identified and the remaining blue marks eliminated.

It is worth reemphasizing that all TMDs cannot be resolved by restorative procedures. First, the occlusal condition must be determined to be a significant contributing factor or it must be established that occlusal alterations are necessary to restore function. Once the need for treatment has been established, it must be decided through appropriate treatment planning that restorative procedures can successfully accomplish the treatment goals. If doubt exists regarding the feasibility of restorative procedures, diagnostic cast analysis and waxing procedures are indicated to provide

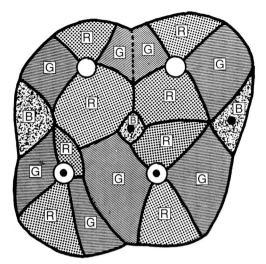

Fig. 20-25 FINAL WAX PATTERN WHEN COLORED WAXES ARE USED. The cusp tips are in ivory wax. The other areas are red (*R*), blue (*B*), and green (*G*).

insight regarding the success of treatment. When it is finally decided that the alignment of teeth is preventing successful restorative procedures, orthodontics or orthognathic surgery may need to be considered. Likewise, as the number of missing teeth increases, partial or complete removable dentures may need to be considered as options in achieving the treatment goals.

Reference

1. Kemper JT, Okeson JP: *Development of occlusal anatomy,* Lexington, 1982, University of Kentucky Press.

Appendix

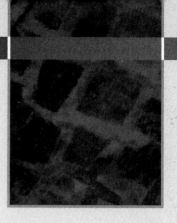

Diagnostic Algorithm for Masticatory Muscle Disorders
SUBCLASS: PROTECTIVE CO-CONTRACTION; LOCAL MUSCLE SORENESS

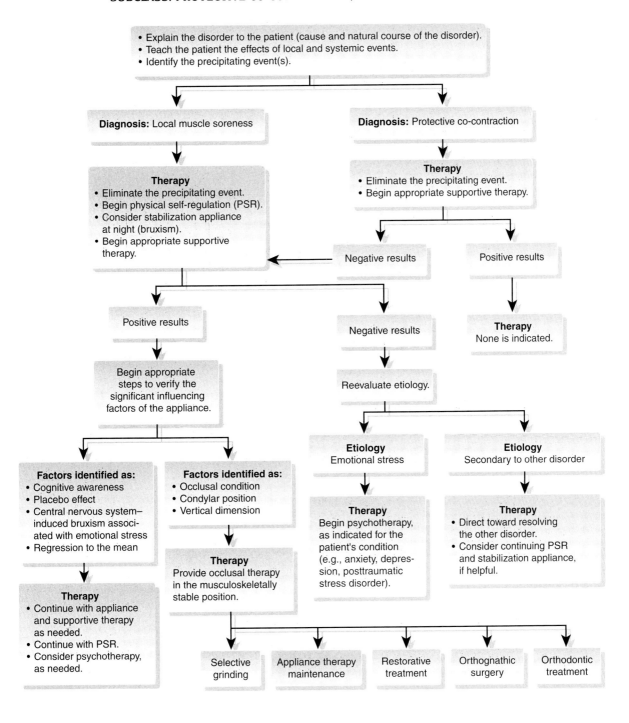

- Explain the disorder to the patient (cause and natural course of the disorder).
- Teach the patient the effects of local and systemic events.
- Identify the precipitating event(s).

Diagnosis: Local muscle soreness

Diagnosis: Protective co-contraction

Therapy
- Eliminate the precipitating event.
- Begin physical self-regulation (PSR).
- Consider stabilization appliance at night (bruxism).
- Begin appropriate supportive therapy.

Therapy
- Eliminate the precipitating event.
- Begin appropriate supportive therapy.

Negative results

Positive results

Positive results

Negative results

Therapy
None is indicated.

Begin appropriate steps to verify the significant influencing factors of the appliance.

Reevaluate etiology.

Factors identified as:
- Cognitive awareness
- Placebo effect
- Central nervous system–induced bruxism associated with emotional stress
- Regression to the mean

Factors identified as:
- Occlusal condition
- Condylar position
- Vertical dimension

Etiology
Emotional stress

Etiology
Secondary to other disorder

Therapy
- Continue with appliance and supportive therapy as needed.
- Continue with PSR.
- Consider psychotherapy, as needed.

Therapy
Provide occlusal therapy in the musculoskeletally stable position.

Therapy
Begin psychotherapy, as indicated for the patient's condition (e.g., anxiety, depression, posttraumatic stress disorder).

Therapy
- Direct toward resolving the other disorder.
- Consider continuing PSR and stabilization appliance, if helpful.

Selective grinding

Appliance therapy maintenance

Restorative treatment

Orthognathic surgery

Orthodontic treatment

Diagnostic Algorithm for Masticatory Muscle Disorders
SUBCLASS: MYOFASCIAL PAIN

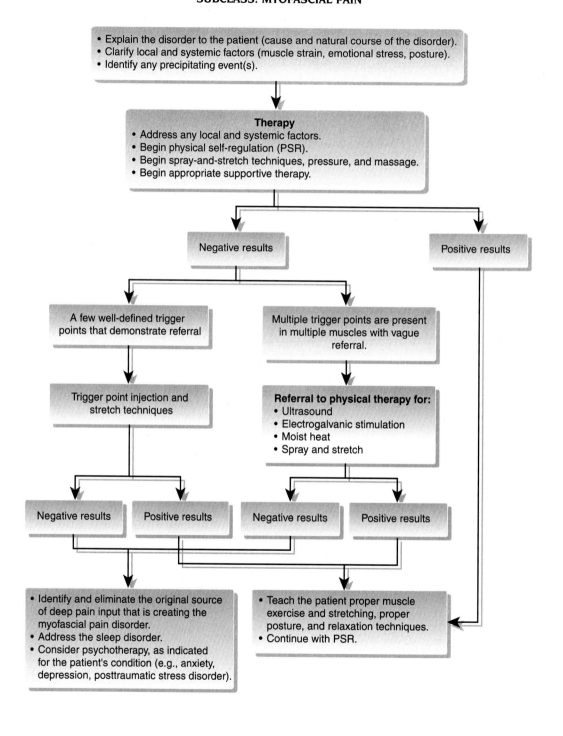

- Explain the disorder to the patient (cause and natural course of the disorder).
- Clarify local and systemic factors (muscle strain, emotional stress, posture).
- Identify any precipitating event(s).

Therapy
- Address any local and systemic factors.
- Begin physical self-regulation (PSR).
- Begin spray-and-stretch techniques, pressure, and massage.
- Begin appropriate supportive therapy.

Negative results

Positive results

A few well-defined trigger points that demonstrate referral

Multiple trigger points are present in multiple muscles with vague referral.

Trigger point injection and stretch techniques

Referral to physical therapy for:
- Ultrasound
- Electrogalvanic stimulation
- Moist heat
- Spray and stretch

Negative results

Positive results

Negative results

Positive results

- Identify and eliminate the original source of deep pain input that is creating the myofascial pain disorder.
- Address the sleep disorder.
- Consider psychotherapy, as indicated for the patient's condition (e.g., anxiety, depression, posttraumatic stress disorder).

- Teach the patient proper muscle exercise and stretching, proper posture, and relaxation techniques.
- Continue with PSR.

Diagnostic Algorithm for Masticatory Muscle Disorders
SUBCLASS: MYOSPASM

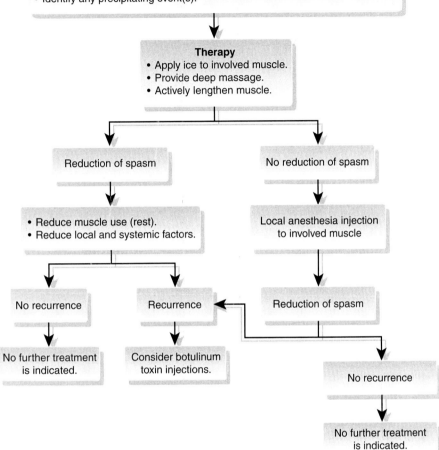

Diagnostic Algorithm for Masticatory Muscle Disorders
SUBCLASS: CHRONIC CENTRALLY MEDIATED MYALGIA

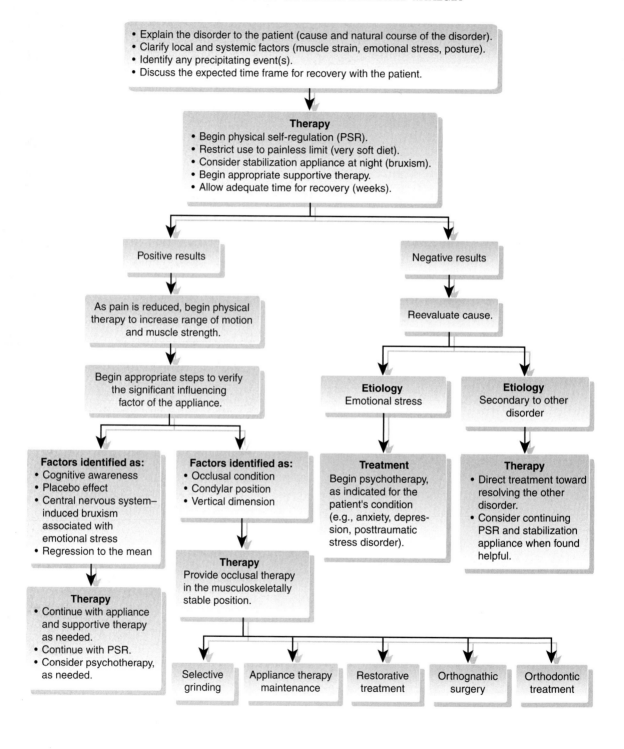

- Explain the disorder to the patient (cause and natural course of the disorder).
- Clarify local and systemic factors (muscle strain, emotional stress, posture).
- Identify any precipitating event(s).
- Discuss the expected time frame for recovery with the patient.

Therapy
- Begin physical self-regulation (PSR).
- Restrict use to painless limit (very soft diet).
- Consider stabilization appliance at night (bruxism).
- Begin appropriate supportive therapy.
- Allow adequate time for recovery (weeks).

Positive results

Negative results

As pain is reduced, begin physical therapy to increase range of motion and muscle strength.

Reevaluate cause.

Begin appropriate steps to verify the significant influencing factor of the appliance.

Etiology
Emotional stress

Etiology
Secondary to other disorder

Factors identified as:
- Cognitive awareness
- Placebo effect
- Central nervous system–induced bruxism associated with emotional stress
- Regression to the mean

Factors identified as:
- Occlusal condition
- Condylar position
- Vertical dimension

Treatment
Begin psychotherapy, as indicated for the patient's condition (e.g., anxiety, depression, posttraumatic stress disorder).

Therapy
- Direct treatment toward resolving the other disorder.
- Consider continuing PSR and stabilization appliance when found helpful.

Therapy
- Continue with appliance and supportive therapy as needed.
- Continue with PSR.
- Consider psychotherapy, as needed.

Therapy
Provide occlusal therapy in the musculoskeletally stable position.

Selective grinding

Appliance therapy maintenance

Restorative treatment

Orthognathic surgery

Orthodontic treatment

Diagnostic Algorithm for Temporomandibular Joint Disorders
SUBCLASS: DERANGEMENT OF THE CONDYLE-DISC COMPLEX (DISC DISPLACEMENT AND DISC DISLOCATION WITH REDUCTION)

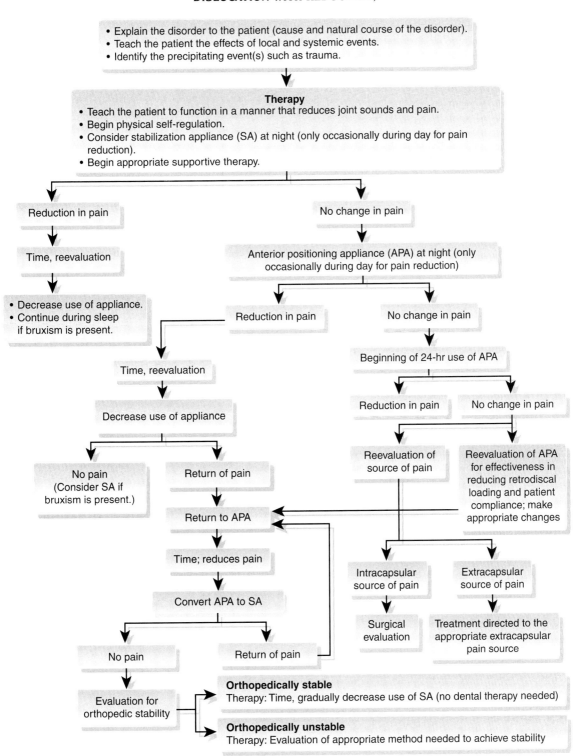

Diagnostic Algorithm for Temporomandibular Joint Disorders
SUBCLASS: DERANGEMENT OF THE CONDYLE-DISC COMPLEX (DISC DISLOCATION WITHOUT REDUCTION)

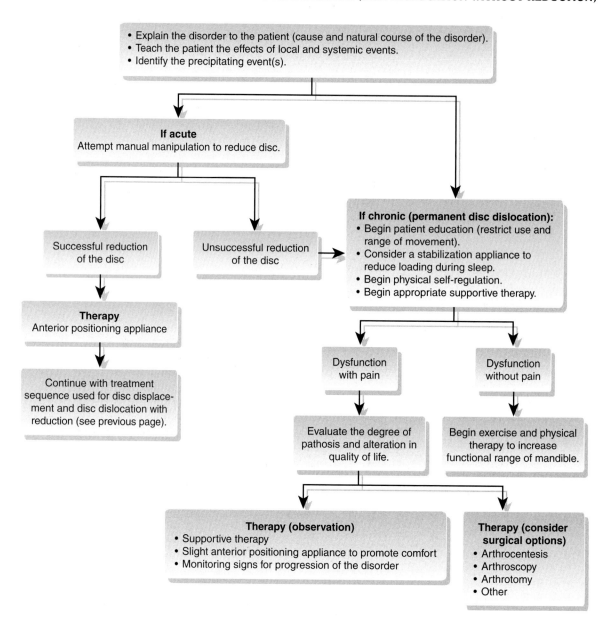

- Explain the disorder to the patient (cause and natural course of the disorder).
- Teach the patient the effects of local and systemic events.
- Identify the precipitating event(s).

If acute
Attempt manual manipulation to reduce disc.

Successful reduction of the disc

Unsuccessful reduction of the disc

If chronic (permanent disc dislocation):
- Begin patient education (restrict use and range of movement).
- Consider a stabilization appliance to reduce loading during sleep.
- Begin physical self-regulation.
- Begin appropriate supportive therapy.

Therapy
Anterior positioning appliance

Continue with treatment sequence used for disc displacement and disc dislocation with reduction (see previous page).

Dysfunction with pain

Dysfunction without pain

Evaluate the degree of pathosis and alteration in quality of life.

Begin exercise and physical therapy to increase functional range of mandible.

Therapy (observation)
- Supportive therapy
- Slight anterior positioning appliance to promote comfort
- Monitoring signs for progression of the disorder

Therapy (consider surgical options)
- Arthrocentesis
- Arthroscopy
- Arthrotomy
- Other

Diagnostic Algorithm for Temporomandibular Joint Disorders
SUBCLASS: STRUCTURAL INCOMPATIBILITY (DEVIATION IN FORM AND ADHESIONS)

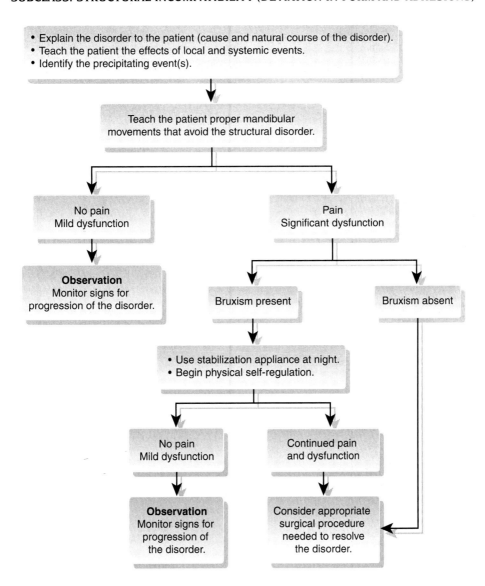

- Explain the disorder to the patient (cause and natural course of the disorder).
- Teach the patient the effects of local and systemic events.
- Identify the precipitating event(s).

Teach the patient proper mandibular movements that avoid the structural disorder.

No pain
Mild dysfunction

Observation
Monitor signs for progression of the disorder.

Pain
Significant dysfunction

Bruxism present

Bruxism absent

- Use stabilization appliance at night.
- Begin physical self-regulation.

No pain
Mild dysfunction

Continued pain and dysfunction

Observation
Monitor signs for progression of the disorder.

Consider appropriate surgical procedure needed to resolve the disorder.

Diagnostic Algorithm for Temporomandibular Joint Disorders
SUBCLASS: STRUCTURAL INCOMPATIBILITY (SUBLUXATION AND SPONTANEOUS DISLOCATION)

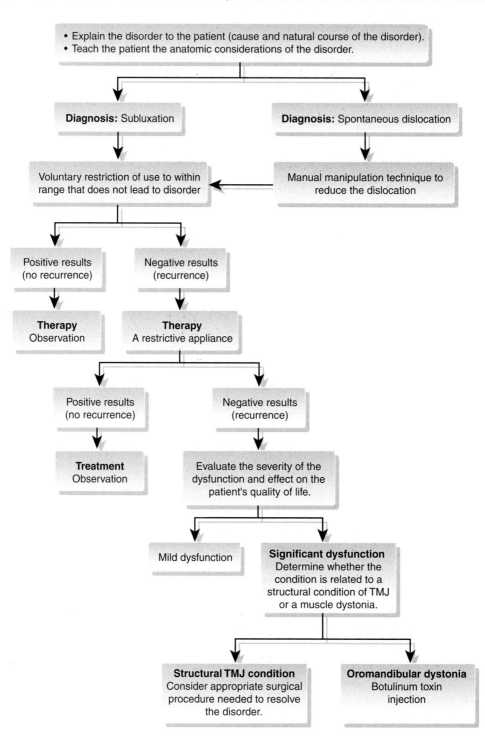

- Explain the disorder to the patient (cause and natural course of the disorder).
- Teach the patient the anatomic considerations of the disorder.

Diagnosis: Subluxation

Diagnosis: Spontaneous dislocation

Voluntary restriction of use to within range that does not lead to disorder

Manual manipulation technique to reduce the dislocation

Positive results (no recurrence)

Negative results (recurrence)

Therapy
Observation

Therapy
A restrictive appliance

Positive results (no recurrence)

Negative results (recurrence)

Treatment
Observation

Evaluate the severity of the dysfunction and effect on the patient's quality of life.

Mild dysfunction

Significant dysfunction
Determine whether the condition is related to a structural condition of TMJ or a muscle dystonia.

Structural TMJ condition
Consider appropriate surgical procedure needed to resolve the disorder.

Oromandibular dystonia
Botulinum toxin injection

Diagnostic Algorithm for Temporomandibular Joint Disorders

SUBCLASS: INFLAMMATORY DISORDERS OF THE TEMPOROMANDIBULAR JOINT (CAPSULITIS AND SYNOVITIS, RETRODISCITIS, AND TRAUMATIC ARTHRITIS)

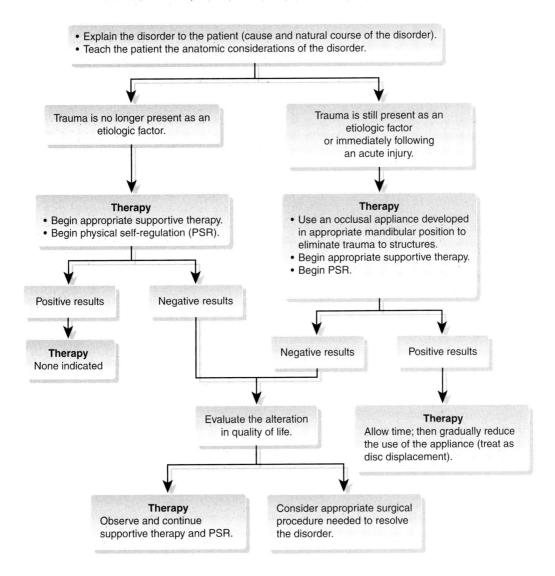

- Explain the disorder to the patient (cause and natural course of the disorder).
- Teach the patient the anatomic considerations of the disorder.

Trauma is no longer present as an etiologic factor.

Trauma is still present as an etiologic factor or immediately following an acute injury.

Therapy
- Begin appropriate supportive therapy.
- Begin physical self-regulation (PSR).

Therapy
- Use an occlusal appliance developed in appropriate mandibular position to eliminate trauma to structures.
- Begin appropriate supportive therapy.
- Begin PSR.

Positive results

Negative results

Therapy
None indicated

Negative results

Positive results

Evaluate the alteration in quality of life.

Therapy
Allow time; then gradually reduce the use of the appliance (treat as disc displacement).

Therapy
Observe and continue supportive therapy and PSR.

Consider appropriate surgical procedure needed to resolve the disorder.

Diagnostic Algorithm for Temporomandibular Joint Disorders
SUBCLASS: INFLAMMATORY DISORDERS OF THE TEMPOROMANDIBULAR JOINT (OSTEOARTHRITIS)

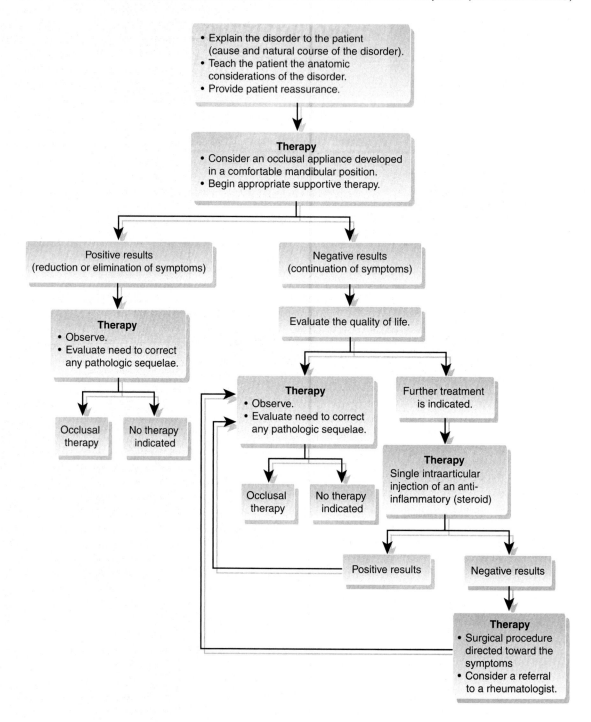

Diagnostic Algorithm for Temporomandibular Joint Disorders
**SUBCLASS: INFLAMMATORY DISORDERS OF THE TEMPOROMANDIBULAR JOINT
(INFECTIOUS ARTHRITIS)**

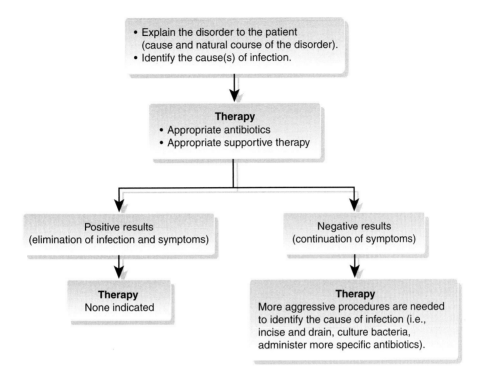

- Explain the disorder to the patient
  (cause and natural course of the disorder).
- Identify the cause(s) of infection.

Therapy
- Appropriate antibiotics
- Appropriate supportive therapy

Positive results
(elimination of infection and symptoms)

Negative results
(continuation of symptoms)

Therapy
None indicated

Therapy
More aggressive procedures are needed
to identify the cause of infection (i.e.,
incise and drain, culture bacteria,
administer more specific antibiotics).

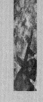

Page numbers followed by *f* indicate figures; *t*, tables; *b*, boxes.

596